D0919497

Neurogenetic Developmental Disorders

Issues in Clinical and Cognitive Neuropsychology
Jordan Grafman, series editor

Neurogenetic Developmental Disorders

Variation of Manifestation in Childhood

edited by Michèle M. M. Mazzocco and Judith L. Ross

The MIT Press
Cambridge, Massachusetts
London, England

© 2007 Massachusetts Institute of Technology

All rights reserved. No part of this book may be reproduced in any form by any electronic or mechanical means (including photocopying, recording, or information storage and retrieval) without permission in writing from the publisher.

For information about special quantity discounts, please email special_sales@mitpress.mit.edu

This book was set in Times New Roman on 3B2 by Asco Typesetters, Hong Kong.
Printed and bound in the United States of America.

Library of Congress Cataloging-in-Publication Data

Neurogenetic developmental disorders : variation of manifestation in childhood /
Michèle M. M. Mazzocco and Judith L. Ross, editors.
    p. ; cm. — (Issues in clinical and cognitive neuropsychology)
Includes bibliographical references and index.
ISBN 978-0-262-13480-4 (hc : alk. paper)
1. Developmental disabilities—Genetic aspects. 2. Chromosome abnormalities. 3. Neurogenetics.
4. Pediatric neuropsychology. I. Mazzocco, Michèle M. M. II. Ross, Judith L. III. Series.
[DNLM: 1. Genetic Diseases, Inborn—diagnosis. 2. Child. 3. Genetic Counseling—methods.
4. Heredodegenerative Disorders, Nervous System—diagnosis. 5. Sex Chromosome Disorders—
diagnosis. WS 200 N494 2007]

RJ506.D47N486   2007
619.92′8588—dc22   2006046910

10   9   8   7   6   5   4   3   2   1

The real voyage of discovery consists not in seeking new landscapes but in having new eyes.
—Marcel Proust

Contents

Note that although the chapter case reports represent real individuals, the names of the individuals described in all case reports have been assigned by the volume editor, alphabetically.

Foreword

Finally there are some answers. They cover not only the etiologies of a variety of neurodevelopmental disorders but they give us new insight as to how behavior and cognition are created from the genome. When I entered this field more than 25 years ago there were very few researchers interested in the children who had syndromes that were beginning to be characterized into behavioral phenotypes. Our clinics were relegated into the basement or temporary buildings of the hospital and they were always a financial loss for the institution. However, the children were fascinating because you could see the biology in their behavior. There were amazing consistencies from one child to the next with the same disorder even though there were many individual differences. The clinician felt empowered to predict and sometimes prevent some of the problems associated with the phenotype. The families were always wonderful; very grateful for your knowledge and supportive for whatever clinical studies and molecular research that could be done. Over time we also realized that there were consistencies in how children with a given disorder responded to medication, a psychopharmacological phenotype that could help to guide treatment for new families with the same problem. This is all part of the gift that children with neurodevelopmental disorders have given to neurosciences. They are a treasure chest of specific lesions to the genome that have a discrete influence on the developing brain eventually leading to the phenotypes that we know so well and are brilliantly described in this book.

We are so lucky to live in a time of breathtaking advances in genetics and neurobiology. Every month the genetics journals describe multiple new genes and even just bits of RNA and DNA that control the expression of genes. What was previously thought of as junk DNA has turned into complex regulatory elements whose pathways are so complex that I thank God I am a clinician. The explosion in neurosciences riding the coat tails of the human genome project and the new technologies in neuroimaging allow us to visualize how the brain works. The chapters in this book describe the latest findings in the neurobiology and the neuroimaging for each of the disorders.

If you appreciate the expertise from multiple fields including pediatrics, psychiatry, psychology, genetics, molecular biology, neurosciences, radiology, education, speech and language pathology, occupational therapy, physical therapy, computer sciences, and assistive technology, then this is the book for you. The information contained here is too hard to pull from multiple sources even if you subscribe to multiple journals every month. All of the fields are expanding so quickly that even full time reading would not be enough. For those of you who have tried out there even with just one area of expertise or one disorder, you know what I mean. Drs. Mazzocco and Ross and the authors of the individual chapters are to be congratulated for their excellence and expertise in writing this marvelous book.

Reading about multiple disorders all in one book gives you insight to the commonalities across disorders that are beginning to emerge. Each chapter touches on autism, ADHD, executive function deficits, visual spatial deficits and even math problems that so many disorders have in common. Elegant theories can then be studied in other disorders with similar phenotypic aspects regarding math and visual spatial deficits, such as fragile X syndrome, Turner syndrome, Williams syndrome, etc.

Neurodevelopmental disorders are now hot topics and significant resources from communities, families, and the NIH have been dedicated for their study. With the rise in autism, people realize that these disorders are not rare and new centers are dedicated to treatment. Some of these disorders are becoming model subtypes for better understanding the mechanisms leading to common psychopathology, such as psychosis (22q deletions), autism (fragile X syndrome), and dyslexia (Kleinfelter syndrome). The variations that are seen among individuals with the same disorder are leading to analyses of secondary genetic effects such as the Val^{158} Met allelic differences in the COMT gene that influences executive function deficits in VCFS. These changes may be informative for many other neurodevelopmental disorders in addition to the general population.

This book also delves into the Pandora's box of environmental toxins. They are not only a common cause of neurodevelopment disorders, but they further influence the individual differences that are seen in genetic disorders and in the general population. The detailed descriptions by Lidsky et al. regarding mechanisms of involvement from lead, mercury and manganese demonstrate further commonalities with genetic disorders regarding influences on synaptic plasticity and gene expression. The interplay between environmental toxicity and gene expression will only become more intense as our environment deteriorates in the future.

On a more positive side is treatment, and the last section of this book is devoted to how to help families after the diagnosis. The breadth of this section is appealing, covering genetic counseling, support to the family, and targeted education intervention. Perhaps the greatest benefit from the multidisciplinary study of neurodevelopmental disorders is just now emerging, and that is targeted medical treatment. The ability to reverse the neurochemical changes of a genetic disorder is exciting and is detailed in some of the chapters where this research is pushing forward. For instance, farnyseal transferases and statins are helping with tumor growth and cognitive impairments in neurofibromatosis. The metabotropic glutamate receptor 5 (mGluR5) antagonists have been helpful in reversing cognitive deficits and seizures in the fragile X animal models and are now being tried in patients with fragile X. These are exciting times and the treatment endeavors will further push early identification and even newborn screening so that treatment can be initiated immediately after birth. Now if we can just resolve the obstacles to research being supported so that these studies will be funded and also save our environment we will be in good shape, so start reading and get to work.

Randi J. Hagerman, MD

Preface

The idea for this book evolved from discussions with parents, teachers, researchers, and clinicians—discussions for which the common thread was the potential for misinterpretation of phenotype descriptions. While the specific topics of discussion were highly variable, the lesson reinforcing the notion that genetic disorders may have highly variable effects was, perhaps, not so obvious. Indeed, it is the within-group homogeneity observed in each of these populations that is of inherent interest, to both clinicians and researchers. This book was the result of our need to expand the discussion of the *differences* represented in populations with well-characterized phenotypes.

As this story was unfolding, the pervasive emphases on genetics and brain development in science continued and altered the phenotypic description of various developmental disorders. But this increase in knowledge does not automatically translate into increased awareness in practice, even for common disorders, such as fragile X syndrome. One obstacle to early identification of a disorder is the phenotypic variation that differs significantly from a "typical" case. For this reason, the emphasis in each chapter of this volume is on reporting the full breadth of phenotypes such that "subtle" or "atypical" variants are also described.

To address the needs of practitioners and researchers alike, we report on disorders that each have a wide-ranging cognitive phenotype, including relatively common disorders (fragile X, Turner, and Klinefelter syndromes) and other disorders for which a genetic etiology is fairly well understood (as seen in Section I), but we also report on the broader categories of congenital hypothyroidism and metabolic disorders. Together, this combination of disorders has implications for understanding influences on development that apply to all human beings. Indeed, the wide range of phenotypic characteristics within each disorder presented affords the opportunity to study such influences whether via gene mapping studies (such as for Turner syndrome) or gene dosage effects (such as for fragile X syndrome).

Part I includes chapters on the common disorders that have an established etiology. For each disorder, there is an explanation of the genotype leading to the syndrome, the medical implications, and the behavioral or psychological consequences directly related to the disorder. Within each chapter, there is an emphasis on how much variability is observed across individuals with the disorder as well as changes that occur during development.

Part II deals with broader categories of etiologies: congenital hypothyroidism, metabolic diseases, and environmental neurotoxins. What these distinct categories have in common is their widespread implications for brain and behavioral sequelae.

Part III deals with potential reactions to, and interactions with, diagnostic information, such as the role of genetic counseling after a diagnosis is made, the family's adaptation to a diagnosis that includes mental retardation or learning disability, and navigation of the early intervention options during the preschool or school-age years. Each of these chapters is intended to serve as a resource for the specialist whose expertise may not include these general issues beyond the identification and diagnosis of specific genetic disorder(s) in question.

We are grateful for the contributions made by the chapter authors, in our joint attempt to compile a useful, informative, interdisciplinary volume. We are also grateful to Barbara Murphy at MIT Press who guided this project.

Acknowledgments

My work on this book has been supported by my research grants from the National Institute of Child Health and Human Development (NICHD), specifically Grants R01-HD034061-01 to -09, and R03-HD044082. I am grateful for the support that the NICHD has provided me over the last decade. I am also grateful to the children and families who have participated in my research throughout these years, and who have been among my most important teachers.

I am grateful for the support and guidance of my colleagues and mentors at the Johns Hopkins University School of Medicine, specifically Drs. Paul McHugh, and Richard Kelley; to my outstanding former Project Coordinator, Gwen Friday Myers; and to my mentor, Susan Somerville, who nurtured my passion for precision in science and in all matters large and small. I am especially grateful to my husband, Michael, for his unwavering support of all my endeavors.

M.M.M.M.

My efforts in this book have been supported by research grants from National Institute for Neurological Disorders and Stroke (NINDS). I am grateful for the support of the National Institutes of Health for the past 20 years. These research efforts were enriched by interactions with wonderful children and their families. I appreciate the support of my husband, Richard, and my daughters, Carly, Anna, and Lizzie. I also acknowledge the inspiration provided by my mentor, Gordon Cutler, Jr., who taught me about asking the right questions.

J.L.R.

I COMMON GENETIC DISORDERS: WIDELY RANGING OUTCOMES FROM A SPECIFIC ETIOLOGY

1 Turner Syndrome in Childhood

Marsha L. Davenport, Stephen R. Hooper, and Martha Zeger

Turner syndrome, like other sex chromosome abnormalities, has high morbidity due to associated congenital abnormalities, neurodevelopmental disturbances, neurocognitive deficits, and social–behavioral problems. Many individuals with Turner syndrome are not diagnosed. Those who are identified may be subject to inadequate care, bias, and discrimination because of a poor understanding among families, health care providers, and educators of the condition, especially regarding developmental profiles and outcomes.

This chapter provides an up-to-date informational source on the broad spectrum of phenotypes associated with Turner syndrome. It provides information pertinent to the definition, karyotype abnormalities, and prevalence of this disorder. An in-depth discussion of the pathophysiology of Turner syndrome, along with associated physical/medical, neurocognitive, and psychosocial findings in childhood, are also presented. Although much of the early literature was limited to the classic phenotypic presentation of Turner syndrome, the contemporary literature describes an enlarging range of variability in all domains: medical/physical, neurocognitive, and psychosocial. This variability is accentuated by our increasing knowledge of the neurodevelopmental processes that permit the expression of selected functions and behaviors during specific developmental epochs. The chapter concludes with specific practice recommendations to enhance the early identification of Turner syndrome.

Definition

Turner syndrome describes phenotypic females who have clinical problems caused by loss of all of the X chromosome or loss of the tip of the short arm of the X chromosome that contains the pseudoautosomal region (PAR) (figure 1.1). Virtually all individuals with Turner syndrome have short stature and some degree of gonadal failure. Other common problems include left-sided cardiovascular abnormalities, renal anomalies, conductive and sensorineural hearing losses, and nonverbal learning

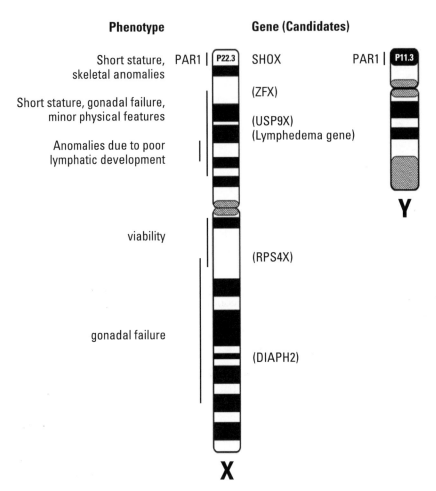

Figure 1.1
Cartoon illustrating the homologous pseudoautosomal regions (PAR1) on the X (p22.3) and Y (p11.3) chromosomes. For the X chromosome, regions that correlate with the phenotype of Turner syndrome are listed to the left with their candidate genes to the right. Modified with permission from Zinn, A. R. (1997). *Nature Genetics, 16*(3).

disabilities (Davenport & Calikoglu, 2004; Sybert & McCauley, 2004; Elsheikh et al., 2002; Lippe & Saenger, 2002).

Karyotype Abnormalities

In most Turner syndrome clinics and studies, 45%–60% of the population are monosomic for the X chromosome (45,X) (Sybert & McCauley, 2004; Soriano-Guillen et al., 2005; Savendahl & Davenport, 2000). Another 35%–50% are mosaic, that is, they contain a 45,X cell line and one or more additional cell lines. The second cell line most commonly contains one normal X chromosome and one structurally abnormal X or Y chromosome such as an isochromosome X (46,X,i(Xq)), ring X (46,X,r(X)), or isochromosome Y (46,X,i(Y)) (figure 1.2), but it may contain a normal 46,XX or 46,XY cell line. The other 5%–10% of individuals with Turner syndrome have one cell line containing a normal X and a structural abnormal X or Y, most often 46,X,i(X). A summary of the karyotypes of patients followed in the Turner syndrome clinic at the University of North Carolina is listed in table 1.1 (Savendahl & Davenport, 2000).

A cell line with a Y chromosome component is found in ∼5% of patients when using a routine karyotype alone, but is found in ∼10% when the analysis is supplemented by fluorescent in situ hybridization (FISH) studies for Y material (Gravholt et al., 2000; figure 1.3). These studies are essential if marker chromosome material is present. Ascertainment of Y material is important because it places the patient at an approximately 30% risk for the development of gonadoblastoma. This gonadal tumor, which occurs almost exclusively in dysgenetic gonads containing Y material, is composed of aggregates of germ cells and sex cord stromal derivatives that resemble immature granulosa and Sertoli cells. Malignant transformation, most often to a dysgerminoma, occurs in about 60% of the cases (Scully et al., 1998). The gonadoblastoma gene has not been definitely identified, but a candidate region (Vogt et al., 1997) and genes (Horn et al., 2005) on the Y chromosome have been proposed. Except under special circumstances, girls with all or some of a Y chromosome should undergo prophylactic gonadectomy.

The sex chromosomes are thought to be particularly susceptible to both structural and nondisjunctional errors during male gametogenesis because of the absence of pairing along the greater part of the XY bivalent during paternal meiosis I (Jacobs et al., 1997). This most likely explains why the X is maternal in origin in ∼75% of those with a 45,X karyotype (the paternal X was lost) and the majority of X deletions and rings are of paternal origin as well. Isochromosomes are equally likely to involve the paternal or maternal chromosome. There are no known relationships between Turner syndrome and maternal or paternal age.

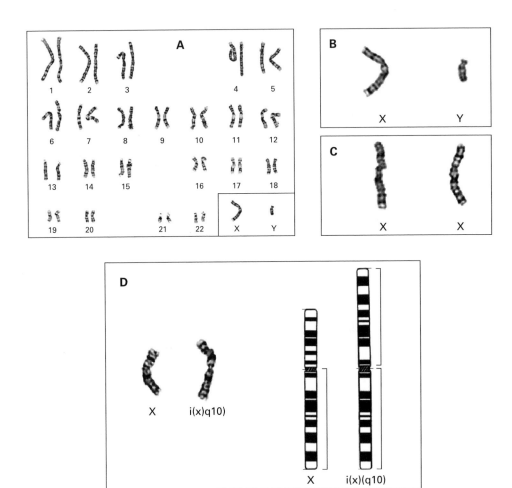

Figure 1.2
Normal male karyotype (A). X and Y chromosomes from the normal male karyotype enlarged (B); two X chromosomes from a normal female karyotype (C). Normal X and isochromosome X from a patient with 46,X,i(X) Turner syndrome with their ideotypes (D).

Table 1.1
Karyotypes in a Turner syndrome clinic population ($n = 81$)

Category	Percent	Karyotype	Number of participants
45,X	54		44
Mosaic	37	45,X/46,X,r(X)	7
		45,X/46,XX	6
		45,X/46,X,i(X)	3
		45,X/46,XY	3
		45,X/46,X,i(Y)	3
		45,X/del(Y)	1
		45,X/46,X,del(X)	1
		45,X/46,X,rea(X)	1
		45,X/47,XY,+8	1
		45,X/47,XYY	1
		45,X/46,X,del(X)/46,X,r(X)	1
		45,X,t(1;12)/46,XX,t(1;12)/46,X,i(X),t(1;12)(q23;13)	1
		45,X/46,X,i(Y)/46,X,r(Y)	1
Other	9	46,X,i(X)	6
		46,X,der(X)t(X;Y)(p22.31;q11.2)	1

Abbreviations: del, deletion; der, derivative; i, isochromosome; p, short arm; q, long arm; r, ring; rea, rearrangement; t, translocation.
Source: Based on the population reported on in Savendahl, L., & Davenport, M. L. (2000). *Journal of Pediatrics, 137*, 455–459.
Reprinted from Davenport, M. L. & Calikoglu, A. S. (2004) Turner syndrome. In O. H. Pescovitz & E. A. Eugster (Eds.), *Pediatric endocrinology: Mechanisms, manifestations, and management* (pp. 203–223). Philadelphia: Lippincott Williams & Wilkins.

Prevalence

Turner syndrome occurs in approximately 1:1,900 female live births. Prevalence rates have been calculated from studies in which karyotypes were performed on the blood of thousands of consecutively live born infants in Denmark (Nielsen & Wohlert, 1991) and the United Kingdom (Jacobs et al., 1974; Nielsen & Wohlert, 1991). Although only five metaphases were routinely analyzed, all but one of the 11 girls identified as having Turner syndrome had mosaicism. Therefore, the prevalence of 45,X individuals in the Turner syndrome population is estimated to be less than 10%, far fewer than the 50% found in a typical clinic or study population. The relatively small percentage of individuals in clinics with mosaicism, especially ones with a normal cell line, suggests that many, if not most, individuals with Turner syndrome remain undiagnosed because their phenotype is normal or mild. In a recent study Gunther et al. (2004) classified patients into two groups, one that had been diagnosed incidentally (on the basis of a prenatal karyotype performed for reasons unrelated to suspicion of Turner syndrome, usually advanced maternal age) or "traditionally"

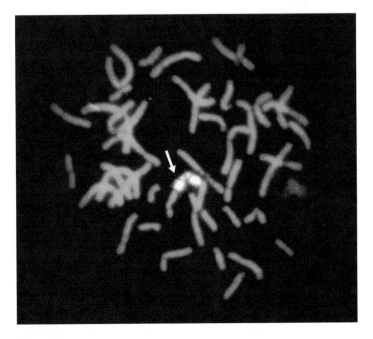

Figure 1.3
Karyotype of a girl with 45X/46X,dic(Y). Yellow fluorescence is positive for centromeric Y material.

diagnosed for clinical findings suggestive of Turner syndrome. The incidental group had fewer cardiac anomalies (19%) than the traditional group (74%), as well as fewer phenotypic features. When subgrouped by karyotype, 45,X subjects had the greatest number of phenotypic features, 45,X/46,XX had the fewest, and those with "other" karyotypes had an intermediate number. The study populations on which we base our knowledge of Turner syndrome are skewed toward the 45,X karyotype and a more severe phenotype. This is important to keep in mind when counseling parents about a prenatal diagnosis of Turner syndrome, especially one diagnosed "incidentally" by amniocentesis or chorionic villous sampling.

Pathophysiology

There are multiple mechanisms by which abnormalities of the sex chromosome contribute to the Turner syndrome phenotype.

Genes That Escape X Inactivation

The X chromosome carries over 1,000 genes, while the Y chromosome has but a few (Ross et al., 2005). To equalize gene dosage, the maternal or paternal X is randomly inactivated in somatic cells during the late blastocyst stage and all descendants of that cell have the same inactive X as hypothesized by Lyon (1961). If the second X chromosome were totally inactive, there would not be a Turner syndrome phenotype. However, the X-inactivation process is not complete. Although most genes on the inactive X are stably silenced, as many as 25% of X-linked genes are expressed from the "inactive X" in some females. Placental mammals have small regions of X–Y homology on the tips of both short and long arms that remain capable of meiotic re-combination. Genes inside these regions are shared between the sex chromosomes, and their behavior is therefore described as "pseudoautosomal." However, not all genes that escape inactivation in humans have Y homologues. That is, they are expressed by the single X in males and both Xs in females. It has been postulated that gene dosage differences may be inconsequential at certain of these loci or that differences in gene expression at the RNA level may not predict difference at the pro-tein level. Alternatively, these genes could confer female-specific functions and pro-vide a fundamental source of differences in the genetic output of males and females (Brown & Greally, 2003; Carrel & Willard, 1999; Chow et al., 2005). Many of these genes are localized to the pseudoautosomal region on the tip of the short arm. Al-though most of the clinical features of Turner syndrome are thought to be caused by the loss of genes that escape inactivation, only one such gene, the short stature homeobox-containing (SHOX) gene, has been identified to date.

Stature

The SHOX gene belongs to a family of transcriptional regulators, homeobox genes that are major controllers of developmental processes. SHOX mRNA and protein are found in all zones of fetal and childhood growth plates (Munns et al., 2004), an expected finding given its importance in growth. In addition, its expression during embryogenesis correlates with many of the phenotypic abnormalities found in Turner syndrome. SHOX gene expression is localized to the developing limbs (particularly at the elbow, knee, and wrist) and the first and second pharyngeal arches that form the maxillary shelves, mandible, ossicles, and the external auditory meatus (Clement-Jones et al., 2000; Blaschke & Rappold, 2000; Ellison et al., 1997).

Lymphatics

It is likely that another pseudoautosomal gene exists that is critical to lymphatic development. Most fetuses with a 45,X karyotype have absence or hypoplasia of pe-ripheral lymphatics and delayed timing in the connection of the lymphatic system to the jugular vein. A delay in the connection of the lymphatic system to the jugular vein causes large cystic hygromas (collections of lymph fluid in the posterior neck) to form. Severe lymphatic obstruction causes hydrops fetalis with thoracic, pericar-dial, and peritoneal effusions, and cardiac failure (Kajii et al., 1980). It is estimated that 99% of conceptuses with a 45,X karyotype are spontaneously aborted through such a mechanism. In fact, some have postulated that 45,X fetuses that do survive actually have "hidden" mosaicism. In those that survive, some of the dysmorphic features such as webbed neck, low upward sweeping hairline, and low-set prominent ears result from a resolving cystic hygroma. Lymphedema of the hands and feet as well as nail dysplasia may result from the more peripheral process (Kajii et al., 1980) of lymphatic hypoplasia. Structural abnormalities of the heart and vascular system are much more common in girls with coexistent cystic hygroma or lymphedema, suggesting that abnormal lymphatics might be involved in their development (Berdahl et al., 1995; Lacro et al., 1988; Loscalzo et al., 2005).

Ovarian Function

Gonadal dysgenesis occurs in the vast majority of individuals with Turner syndrome (Pasquino et al., 1997). Ovarian differentiation requires only one X chromosome so that germ cell formation proceeds normally. However, there is rapid atresia of germ cells, and the ovaries are replaced by fibrous streaks (Reynaud et al., 2004; Speed, 1986). Genes on both the short and long arms of X are important for maintenance of ovarian function and perhaps meiotic pairing (Zinn, 2001; Frank, 2003; Simpson & Rajkovic, 1999). Unlike somatic cells, both X chromosomes remain active in oocytes. Although the rapid rate of oocyte loss in X monosomy could be caused by nonspecific, generalized meiotic pairing errors (Ogata & Matsuo, 1995), haploinsufficiency of genes involved in ovarian function appears to be the principle mechanism for failure. Other mammals with 45X monosomy have relatively normal ovarian development (Simpson & Rajkovic, 1999). Besides the obvious psychosocial challenges that ovarian failure brings, it also makes the hormonal milieu in which development occurs one that is both estrogen- and androgen-deficient.

Neurocognition

The X chromosome carries a disproportionately high number of genes affecting cognition (Skuse, 2005). Indeed, males have a 30% higher incidence of mental disability than females (Zechner et al., 2001) in the general population. Ross et al. hypothesized that deletion of one or more pseudoautosomal genes causes the neurocognitive problems associated with Turner syndrome. In 2000, Ross and colleagues identified a small 10-Mb interval of the distal Xp (Xp22.33) that they described as sufficient for expression of the Turner syndrome neurocognitive phenotype (Ross et al., 2000c). More recently, Good et al. have identified a 4.96-Mb locus at Xp11.3 that contains at least one dosage-sensitive X-linked gene influencing amygdala structure and function (Good et al., 2003). The neurocognitive phenotype will be discussed in more detail in the Neurocognitive and Psychosocial Phenotypic Expression section.

Imprinting

For imprinted genes, one allele is silenced according to its parental origin. This means that imprinted traits are passed down the maternal or paternal line, in contrast to the more frequent Mendelian mode of inheritance that is indifferent to the parental origin of the allele. Until recently, imprinting was not thought to occur on the X chromosome with the notable exception of the Xist gene, which is central to X-chromosome inactivation. For example, physical phenotype and response to growth hormone (GH) in Turner syndrome do not differ in those with a paternal or maternal X (Tsezou et al., 1999). In 1997, however, Skuse et al. proposed that a paternally expressed allele was associated with enhanced social–cognitive abilities in normal females. This year, two separate research groups demonstrated locus-specific imprinting on the mouse X chromosome (Davies et al., 2005; Raefski & O'Neill, 2005). Both used microarray analyses to compare gene expression of the brain tissue from 39,X mice with an X of paternal origin versus that from 39,X mice with an X of maternal origin. Davies et al. (2005) identified Xlr3b and Raefski and O'Neill (2005) identified Xlr3b and two nearby Xlr4c genes as maternally expressed imprinted genes, respectively. In addition, Davies et al. used a maze-based, visual, nonspatial, serial reversal learning paradigm to study the effect of parental origin on mouse behavior. Parental origin of the X chromosome influenced the ability of mice to inhibit response to a previously correct but now incorrect cue and to form new associations with the previously incorrect but now correct cue. Thus, XLr3b is a candidate gene for the deficits in behavioral flexibility seen in many individuals with monosomy X.

Functional Disomy

Individuals with small ring X chromosomes often have a severe phenotype that is not typical of Turner syndrome and includes mental retardation (Migeon et al., 1993; Turner et al., 2000). In these cases, the loss of the XIST gene, which is involved in X inactivation, may allow for normally inactivated genes to be expressed, thereby causing functional disomy.

X-Linked Recessive Disorder

Girls with Turner syndrome are at increased risk for X-linked recessive disorders, such as color blindness, that are typically restricted to males. Because roughly one fourth of all diseases associated with mental retardation listed in the Online Mendelian Inheritance of Man (OMIM) have been mapped to the X chromosome, it is expected that girls with Turner syndrome would be at higher risk for disorders of cognition (Skuse, 2005).

Key Physical Findings

The key physical features of girls with Turner syndrome (figure 1.4) and the ability of health care personnel to recognize them vary widely, affecting if and when they will be diagnosed (Lippe, 1996; Massa & Vanderschueren Lodeweyckx, 1991; Savendahl & Davenport, 2000). The features of individuals with Turner syndrome differ depending upon the period in which they are diagnosed: (a) prenatal life, (b) infancy, (c) childhood, (d) adolescence, or (e) adulthood.

Most girls who are diagnosed with Turner syndrome in prenatal life are diagnosed "incidentally" when a karyotype is obtained by chorionic villous sampling or amniocentesis for advanced maternal age, a chromosomal abnormality in a previous pregnancy, or an abnormal maternal triple screen (case 1.1).

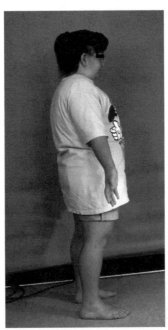

Short stature (99%)
Epicanthal folds (44%)
Ptosis (33%)
Strabismus (32%)
Prominent ears (63%)
High-arched palate (71%)
Retrognathia (55%)
Low hairline (57%)
Webbed neck (44%)
Pectus excavatum (24%)
Kyphosis (40%)
Scoliosis (19%)
Cubitus valgus (47%)
Madelung's deformity (1.8%)
Short 4th metacarpal (33%)
Nail dysplasia (44%)
Genu valgum
Multiple nevi (44%)
Lymphedema as newborn (51%)
Flat feet (33%)

Savendahl L, et. al J Pediatr. 2000
Elder DA, et al. Pediatrics. 2002 [figure]

Figure 1.4
Physical findings in Turner syndrome (TS). The percentage of girls in a TS clinic population with each of those findings is indicated in parentheses. From Savendahl, L. & Davenport, M. L. (2000). *Journal of Pediatrics, 137,* 455–459; except for kyphosis and scoliosis from Elder, D. A., et al. (2002). *Pediatrics, 109*(6), e93.

Case 1.1: Abigail   Abigail was diagnosed with Turner syndrome (45,X/46,X,del(X)(q21.2) prenatally when a routine amniocentesis was performed for advanced maternal age. At birth, she weighed 7 lbs., 8 oz. and her physical exam was notable only for epicanthal folds, retrognathia, and mild auricular abnormalities. On renal ultrasound, she had a small left kidney with mild ureteral reflux. Her echocardiogram was normal. Her history was unremarkable throughout early childhood. When she was 8 years old, Abigail received a comprehensive neuropsychological evaluation as part of a research study on Turner syndrome. Findings from this evaluation revealed above average abilities—even in the area of math, and relatively even cognitive abilities. Despite an earlier history of positive social–behavioral functions, however, Abigail was then showing emergent difficulties in processing affective information, which were beginning to be evident in social difficulties with her 8 year old peers. She developed mild scoliosis and fell to below the 5th percentile in height at age 10 years, at which time she was started on growth hormone.

Occasionally, girls with Turner syndrome are diagnosed in prenatal life because of fetal problems, including increased nuchal thickness, a cystic hygroma, generalized edema or a cardiac defect (figure 1.5). Girls with Turner syndrome who are

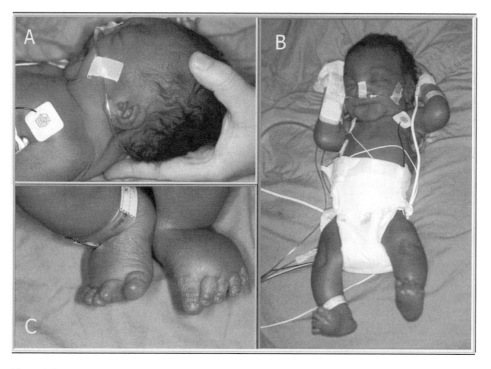

Figure 1.5
Premature 45,X infant diagnosed in utero for cystic hygroma. Photos taken at 2 days of life, before surgical repair of coarctation of the aorta. A. Lateral view of the head and neck. Note the low-set ears and redundant skin over the posterior neck. B. Full body photo. C. Peripheral lymphedema of the feet.

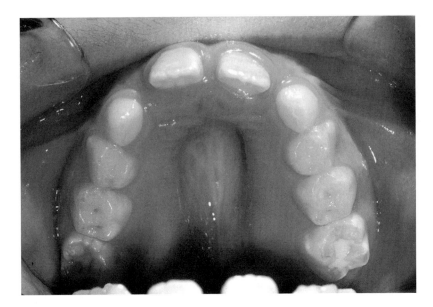

Figure 1.6
High, narrow palate.

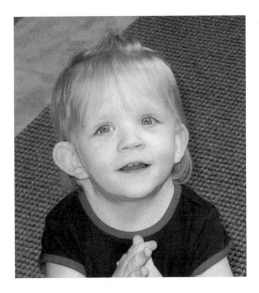

Figure 1.7
Twenty-five-month-old girl with Turner syndrome diagnosed at birth for lymphedema. Note the epicanthal folds, prominent and low-set ears, and webbed neck.

diagnosed at birth are likely to demonstrate many of the "classic features" including puffy hands and feet and/or a webbed neck (redundant skin on the back of her neck from a resolving hygroma). These girls often have dysmorphic features such as malformed, low set and prominent ears, epicanthal folds, short neck, high arched palate (figure 1.6), retrognathia, low and upsweeping hairline, a broad ("shield") chest, and peripheral lymphedema (figure 1.7) (case 1.2).

Case 1.2: Betty   Betty is a 7-year-old girl with 45,X Turner syndrome who was diagnosed at birth when a karyotype was obtained for lymphedema. Other stigmata of Turner syndrome included a left epicanthal fold, high arched palate, retrognathia, low-set and prominent ears, low hairline, shield chest, and nail dysplasia. A renal ultrasound was normal, and an echocardiogram revealed a bicuspid aortic valve and mild narrowing of the aortic isthmus. During early infancy, she had gastroesophageal reflux and failure to thrive. Later, despite adequate weight gain, linear growth failure persisted. She fell below the 5th percentile in length by 12 months of age, and she was started on growth hormone at age 4 years. She has had persistent lymphedema in her left foot, complicated by several episodes of cellulitis. She has required tympanostomy tube placement for recurrent otitis media and conductive hearing loss. At age 24 months she received a developmental assessment that revealed relatively intact functioning across both cognitive and social–behavioral domains. She did not have evidence of any emergent problems with visual reception; however, her fine-motor capabilities fell at the lower end of the normal range. As a toddler, she had abnormally high stranger anxiety, and in elementary school she has required special services in reading and math.

Girls lacking classic physical features of Turner syndrome are often not diagnosed until late childhood or adolescence when they are investigated for short stature and/or delayed puberty (case 1.3).

Case 1.3: Cathy   Cathy was diagnosed with Turner syndrome (45,X/46,XX) at age $12\frac{1}{2}$ years when she was evaluated for the absence of breast development. On careful physical exam, she was noted to have subtle features of Turner syndrome including a height between the fifth and tenth percentile, high palate, short neck, low hairline, auricular malformations, nail dysplasia, flat feet, and multiple nevi. She had chronic otitis media that required tympanostomy tubes and obstructive sleep apnea for which she underwent tonsillectomy and adenoidectomy. After her diagnosis of Turner syndrome, an echocardiogram showed a bicuspid aortic valve. A comprehensive neuropsychological assessment revealed average intellectual abilities, with significantly higher verbal than nonverbal abilities. Specifically, Cathy evidenced poorer short-term visual memory, mild problems with visual discrimination, and slippages in her visual selective attention. In addition, she showed visual working memory deficits and problems with visual organization. Social–behavioral ratings by her parents suggested the emergence of mild social difficulties with her peers. She already had been diagnosed with a learning disability in mathematics and was receiving specific services for these needs.

Table 1.2
Clinical features of Turner syndrome according to age at diagnosis

Clinical Features	Childhood $N = 24$		Adolescence $N = 15$		Infancy $N = 33$		Prenatal $N = 9$		All patients $N = 81$	
Early growth failure (<5th percentile by age 4)	19/23	83%	7/15	47%	26/33	79%	6/8	75%	58/79	73%
Recurrent otitis media	17/24	71%	11/15	73%	31/33	94%	5/7	71%	64/79	81%
High arched palate	16/23	70%	8/15	53%	27/32	84%	4/7	57%	55/77	71%
Delayed puberty	6/10	60%	10/15	66%	14/15	93%	0/0	0%	30/40	75%
Nail dysplasia	12/21	57%	12/15	80%	27/33	90%	4/9	57%	55/73	75%
Lowset ears	13/23	56%	7/12	58%	19/26	73%	3/6	40%	42/67	63%
Retrognathia	10/18	56%	4/11	36%	20/29	67%	2/6	33%	36/65	55%
Learning difficulties	11/20	55%	3/10	30%	14/27	52%	1/3	33%	29/60	48%
Cubitus valgus	9/17	53%	5/10	50%	13/25	52%	0/5	0%	27/57	47%
Feeding problems	6/14	43%	1/7	14%	9/16	56%	2/8	25%	18/45	40%
Strabismus	10/23	43%	3/13	23%	11/33	33%	0/6	0%	24/75	32%
Epicanthal folds	9/22	41%	4/13	31%	12/27	44%	5/6	83%	30/68	44%
Low posterior hairline	9/23	39%	9/12	75%	22/29	76%	1/8	13%	41/72	57%
Obstructive sleep apnea	7/20	35%	1/10	10%	6/18	33%	1/5	20%	15/53	28%
Multiple nevi (>40)	8/23	35%	10/13	77%	11/27	41%	1/6	17%	30/69	44%
Kidney malformation	6/21	29%	3/12	25%	6/30	20%	4/9	44%	20/72	28%
Flat feet	5/18	28%	4/12	33%	10/24	42%	0/3	0%	19/57	33%
Webbed neck	6/23	26%	4/14	28%	22/30	73%	1/8	13%	33/74	44%
Scoliosis	6/23	26%	0/11	0%	6/29	21%	1/5	20%	13/68	19%
Short 4th metacarpal	5/20	25%	7/14	50%	9/24	37%	0/5	0%	21/63	33%
Ptosis	4/20	20%	3/12	25%	14/27	52%	1/6	17%	22/65	33%
Lymphedema as newborn	4/22	18%	2/14	14%	32/33	97%	2/9	22%	40/78	51%
Bicuspid aortic valve	4/24	17%	1/11	9%	8/30	27%	0/7	0%	13/72	18%
Pectus excavatum	3/22	14%	3/13	23%	9/26	35%	1/5	20%	16/66	24%
Aortic coarctation	3/24	13%	0/11	0%	8/31	26%	1/8	13%	12/74	16%
Hypothyroidism	3/24	12%	2/14	14%	3/33	9%	0/9	0%	8/80	10%
Inverted nipples	2/22	9%	4/12	33%	7/26	27%	0/6	0%	13/66	20%

Source: Reprinted from Savendahl, L., & Davenport, M. L. (2000). *Journal of Pediatrics, 137,* 455–459.

Finally, some individuals with Turner syndrome are diagnosed in adulthood during a workup for premature ovarian failure or infertility. It is clear that the phenotype can be mild, and even the most sophisticated clinician can miss the diagnosis based on appearance alone. Therefore, it is important to evaluate any girl with unexplained short stature for Turner syndrome.

In addition to short stature, haploinsufficiency of the SHOX gene causes disproportionate growth and/or developmental abnormalities of specific bones, which can also be useful in diagnosis. In a Danish study of adult women with Turner syndrome whose average height was almost -4 *SD*, measurements of hands and feet were only -1.8 *SD*; weight, head, and shoulders were average; and pelvis was actually

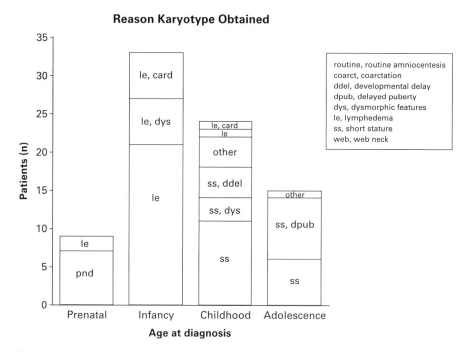

Figure 1.8
Reasons karyotype obtained by age at diagnosis. Reproduced from Savendahl, L. & Davenport, M. L. (2000). *Journal of Pediatrics, 137,* 455–459.

1.5 *SD* above the mean. Therefore, individuals with Turner syndrome generally appear stocky, with a wide body (shield chest) and relatively large hands and feet (Gravholt & Weis, 1997). SHOX may be involved in the development of the high arched palate. Developmental abnormalities of individual bones cause cubitus valgus (increased carrying angle at the elbows), which can be recognized by having the individual let her arms hang down with the palms facing forward, and genu valgum (knock-knees). A short fourth metacarpal can be recognized by the "knuckle sign" (a dimple rather than a knuckle is present when a fist is made).

Keys to Diagnosis in a Clinic Population

The clinical features of 81 children followed in the Turner syndrome Clinic at the University of North Carolina are shown in table 1.2 (Savendahl & Davenport, 2000). This population consisted of 9 girls diagnosed in prenatal life, 33 in infancy, 24 in childhood, and 15 in adolescence (figure 1.8), a distribution that appears to be comparable to that of other clinics.

Of the 9 girls diagnosed in prenatal life, 7 were diagnosed incidentally. Of the 7 that were diagnosed incidentally, the karyotype was 45,X/46,XX in 4, 45,X/46,X,del(X) in 1, 46,Xi(X) in 1, and 45X in 1. No one had an abnormal cardiac exam. All but 1 girl had growth failure, but 2 girls did not fall below the 5th percentile until 9–10 years of age (see case 1.1).

Of the 33 girls diagnosed in infancy, all but 1 was diagnosed for lymphedema with or without dysmorphic features or cardiac abnormalities.

Of the 24 girls diagnosed in childhood, the primary reason for obtaining a karyotype was short stature in 18 (75%) and lymphedema in 2 (8%). Of the remaining 4 (17%), 1 was karyotyped for developmental delay alone, 1 for developmental delay and dysmorphic features, 1 for developmental delay and a cardiac lesion, and 1 for a cardiac lesion alone. Developmental delay was the driving force for diagnosis in 5 of the 10 girls who were diagnosed between the ages of 1 and 4 years (case 1.4).

Case 1.4: Diane   Diane was diagnosed with 45,X Turner syndrome at age $3\frac{1}{2}$ years during a workup for developmental delay. She was a 7 lbs., 1 oz. term infant and first rolled over at age 4–5 months, sat alone and crawled at 11 months, and walked alone at 17 months. Her language skills were delayed one year and her behavior problems included spitting, biting, and pinching. She was diagnosed with an auditory processing disorder, autism, and attention deficit/hyperactivity disorder (ADHD). Her history was positive for severe food allergies, chronic suppurative otitis media requiring four sets of tympanostomy tubes and an adenoidectomy, and strabismus requiring surgery. Careful physical exam at diagnosis was notable for mild features of Turner syndrome including height at the 5th percentile, a high arched palate, mild scoliosis, an increased carrying angle, and clinodactyly. She also had low tone and vitiligo. Treatment with growth hormone was initiated. A developmental assessment during the preschool years revealed mild mental retardation. Social–behavioral functioning was disproportionately low when compared to her developmental level. She has received services in psychology, behavior/play therapy, physical therapy, and occupational therapy.

There were 15 girls diagnosed in adolescence. Short stature with or without delayed puberty was responsible for the diagnosis in all but 1 girl.

Key Medical Issues

Unfortunately, there are numerous medical issues in Turner syndrome that need to be addressed. Alone or in concert with others, many of these medical conditions negatively impact the cognitive, emotional, and social development of these girls.

Short Stature

Short stature is a hallmark of Turner syndrome. Growth failure, primarily the result of SHOX haploinsufficiency, begins in utero and continues at a rapid pace postnatally (Davenport et al., 2002a; Rongen-Westerlaken et al., 1997; Karlberg et al., 1991; Even et al., 2000). In one study, the average girl with Turner syndrome fell below the 5th percentile in length/height by 1.8 years of age (Savendahl & Davenport, 2000). Untreated individuals achieve an average adult stature 8 in. (20 cm) shorter than their target height, which is about 3 *SD*s below the mean (Sybert, 1984; Ranke et al., 1983). In the United States, the average height for an untreated adult with Turner syndrome is 4 ft, 8 in. (148 cm) (Even et al., 2000; Davenport et al., 1999; Karlberg et al., 1991). Because of estrogen deficiency, bone maturation is delayed and growth may proceed slowly into the early 20s without treatment.

Growth hormone therapy is considered the standard of care in Turner syndrome for those who would not otherwise obtain a normal height. It increases final adult stature in Turner syndrome (The Canadian Growth Hormone Advisory Committee, 2005), and the magnitude of effect is most dependent on age at initiation and length of therapy. Preliminary data from the Toddler Turner Study, in which 88 girls between the ages of 9 months and 4 years of age (mean age = 2.0 years) were randomized to GH or no-GH therapy, indicate that it is safe and effective when begun as early as 9 months of age (Davenport et al., 2005). Therefore, treatment with GH should begin as soon as growth failure is demonstrated. The psychosocial implications of being closer to peers in length/height throughout life are likely to be more important than achieving a near-normal height beginning in late childhood or adolescence. Most girls who are started on GH therapy in early childhood at a dose approved by the FDA (0.054 mg/kg sc daily) should be able to start estrogen therapy at a normal pubertal age and achieve a normal adult stature. Clinical observation has suggested, but not proven, that women treated with GH during childhood and achieving a height near or within the normal range face fewer obstacles, have higher self-esteem, and are more successful in social life and careers (Van Pareren et al., 2005). However, physicians must be careful that families and patients have realistic expectations of the height to be gained, as it is likely to still be below average.

Other medical consequences of abnormal bone include an increased risk for scoliosis and kyphosis, which may be severe enough to require orthopedic intervention, including surgery (Elder et al., 2002). Individuals with Turner syndrome are also at increased risk for osteoporosis.

Gonadal Dysgenesis

The majority of girls with Turner syndrome have gonadal dysgenesis and pubertal delay in addition to short stature. Girls with pubertal delay generally have pubic hair stimulated by androgens of adrenal origin, but no breast development. In a large retrospective Italian study of over 500 patients older than 12 years of age, only 14% of 45,X individuals and 32% of those with cells lines containing more than one X initiated puberty spontaneously (Pasquino et al., 1997). Sixteen percent

had spontaneous menarche, although many of those developed secondary amenor-
rhea. Unassisted pregnancies are very rare.

To maximize adult height, families and physicians may be compromising the
child's quality of life during adolescence by waiting until 15 years of age or later to
induce puberty. With early GH therapy, systemic estrogens may be initiated at a
relatively normal age, 12 years, allowing girls with Turner syndrome to develop sex-
ually with their peers.

Lymphedema

Lymphedema tends to be most severe at birth and improves over the first year or two
of life. In some individuals, however, chronic lymphatic stasis causes thickening and
tightening of the skin, decreased flexibility of the limb, ingrown toenails, and soft tissue infections. Therapeutic modalities include compressive stockings/garments, manual lymphatic drainage, salt restriction, and diuretics.

Cardiovascular Malformations and Hypertension

Although symptomatic congenital heart disease is the key to diagnosis in some girls
with Turner syndrome, many more have asymptomatic cardiac lesions. Structural
abnormalities of the cardiovascular system, predominantly left-sided defects, are
found in approximately 40% of individuals with Turner syndrome. In one study
(Sybert, 1998), aortic coarctation with or without a bicuspid valve was present in
14%, a bicuspid valve alone in 10%, aortic stenosis and/or regurgitation in 5%, and
other structural defects such as hypoplastic left heart, ASD, and VSD were present in
10%. In another study, partial anomalous pulmonary venous drainage was found in
2.9% of patients, giving it the highest relative risk compared to heart defects in the
general population (Mazzanti & Cacciari, 1998). Hypertension is common, and the
risk of aortic dissection (generally fatal) exists at any age. In the published literature,
about half of those with aortic dissection were children (Elsheikh et al., 2001a).
Therefore, all individuals with Turner syndrome should receive an echocardiogram
or magnetic resonance imaging (MRI) to screen for the presence of cardiac malformations at the time of diagnosis.

Renal Malformations

All girls with Turner syndrome should also have a screening renal ultrasound at the
time of diagnosis. Renal and renovascular abnormalities occur in over a third of individuals with Turner syndrome (Gravholt et al., 1998; Bilge et al., 2000; Lippe et al.,
1988; Chang et al., 2000). Of those with malformations, about half have abnormalities of the collecting system and half have positional abnormalities. Luckily, many
structural malformations do not cause functional problems.

Strabismus and Other Eye Problems

Strabismus (crossed eyes) occurs in about one third of individuals with Turner syndrome (Adhikary, 1981; Chrousos et al., 1984; Savendahl & Davenport, 2000). Strabismus is usually an accommodative esotropia for farsightedness. This can occur as early as 6 months but most commonly develops around age 2.5 years. If left uncorrected, amblyopia (loss of vision in the deviated eye) may occur.

Conductive and Sensorineural Hearing Losses

Hearing loss is a problem that plagues the Turner syndrome population through the life span and may have a serious impact on development and socialization. Havercamp et al. (2003) reported that hearing impairment was a predictor of neuromotor proficiency in children with Turner syndrome. Most children (60%–80%) suffer from conductive hearing loss secondary to chronic otitis media (Sculerati et al., 1990; Stenberg et al., 1998), and most adults suffer from sensorineural hearing loss. Chronic otitis media may be the result of a short, more horizontally oriented Eustachian tube. This results in poor drainage and ventilation of the middle ear space and may allow more nasopharyngeal microorganisms to reach the middle ear. In a study of 56 girls with Turner syndrome ages 4–15 years, 61% had had recurrent acute otitis media; 32% had been treated with ventilation tubes; and 57% had evidence of eardrum pathology, such as effusion, myringosclerosis, atrophic scars, retraction pockets, and perforations. In addition, a midfrequency sensorineural hearing loss was present in over half of the girls, and 2 of the 56 had hearing aids (Stenberg et al., 1998). Middle ear disease should be aggressively treated in Turner syndrome, and girls should be warned to avoid exposure to loud noises.

Gastrointestinal Disease

Feeding Difficulties   Many infants with Turner syndrome have early feeding difficulties. Gagging and regurgitation with refusal to eat solid food is quite common and has been attributed to oral-motor dysfunction. The causes may be multifactorial, including the high arched palate, low orofacial tone, and poor jaw strength, as well as velopharyngeal and lower gastroesophageal tract dysfunction (Mathisen et al., 1992).

Celiac Disease   Celiac disease, an immune-mediated disease of the small intestines triggered by the ingestion of gluten-containing grains (wheat, barley, and rye), occurs in about 6% of individuals with Turner syndrome, which is 10 times more prevalent than in the general population (Bonamico et al., 1998). Celiac disease can cause growth failure, bloating, abdominal pain, and malabsorption. It is treated by excluding all gluten-containing foods from the diet.

Inflammatory Bowel Disease   Inflammatory bowel disease occurs in about 3% of individuals with Turner syndrome (Williams et al., 1966; Weinrieb et al., 1976; Keating et al., 1978; Gravholt et al., 1998; Elsheikh et al., 2002), with Crohn's disease being at least as common as ulcerative colitis (Manzione et al., 1988; Hayward et al., 1996). In Turner syndrome, the median age of onset has been reported as 16 years. Diagnosis is often delayed. Growth retardation is often present, while classical symptoms such as bloody diarrhea, abdominal pain and weight loss may not be. Osteoporosis is a common complication, resulting from many factors including the inflammatory process itself, poor nutrition, corticosteroids, and calcium and vitamin D deficiencies (Lichtenstein, 2001).

GI Bleeding   Some girls with Turner syndrome have GI bleeding as the result of vascular lesions in the intestines, generally telangiectasias (localized dilations of capillaries and venules) on the serosal surface of the small bowel (Eroglu et al., 2002). GI bleeding is usually intermittent and self-limited; however, brisk, life-threatening bleeding may also occur. Bleeding generally begins in childhood and resolves with age, perhaps as the result of estrogen supplementation.

Liver Problems   Many individuals with Turner syndrome have elevated liver enzymes, even in childhood (Salerno et al., 1999). The causes appear to be multifactorial, and the disorder does not usually progress to cirrhosis (Hanson et al., 2002; Larizza et al., 2000; Ostberg et al., 2005; Roulot et al., 2004). Overall, gastrointestinal diseases are common in Turner syndrome and should be thought of not only when there is GI symptomatology but when growth is poorer than expected or when nonspecific problems such as malaise and depression are present.

Hypothyroidism and Other Thyroid Disease

Autoimmune thyroiditis is the most prevalent autoimmune disorder in patients with Turner syndrome. Thyroid dysfunction, usually hypothyroidism, is more common in those with karyotypes containing a structurally abnormal X chromosome (Elsheikh et al., 2001b; de Kerdanet et al., 1994; El-Mansoury et al., 2005; Medeiros et al., 2000; Radetti et al., 1995). Thyroid function should be monitored routinely because the consequences of its abnormality are often insidious (see also Rovet and Brown, this volume, chapter 8). Therefore, it is generally suggested that thyroid function be monitored yearly, beginning in early childhood, in girls with Turner syndrome.

Orthodontic Problems

Most patients with Turner syndrome have significant orthodontic problems associated with many abnormalities of the orofacial region. Although the high palate is well known (figure 1.6), other common abnormalities include hypoplasia of the mandible and cranial base, lateral crossbite, and anterior open bite (Simmons, 1999). Because most girls with Turner syndrome have orthodontic problems, consultation with an orthodontist is suggested by age 7 years. The timing of any orthodontic treatment should take into consideration growth-promoting therapies that may alter tooth and jaw alignment. In addition, because the dental roots are short, unnecessary tooth movement should be minimized to avoid root resorption and loss of teeth (Townsend et al., 1984).

Skin Disorders

Individuals with Turner syndrome are at increased risk for several skin disorders. These include hypertrophic scar (keloid) formation, increased numbers of nevi (Zvulunov et al., 1998; Becker et al., 1994), and hemangiomas. Other common skin problems include atopic dermatitis, seborrheic dermatitis, keratosis pilaris, and immune-related dermatological conditions such as psoriasis, alopecia, and vitiligo. Plastic surgery is an option for those with severe webbed neck, ptosis, prominent ears, and so forth. However, the increased possibility of keloid formation needs to be taken into account (Thomson et al., 1990).

Diabetes Mellitus and the Metabolic Syndrome

Both type 1 and type 2 diabetes mellitus are much more common in women with Turner syndrome compared with the general population (Gravholt et al., 1998). Recently, individuals of all ages with Turner syndrome were found to have decreased insulin secretory function (Bakalov et al., 2004); therefore, diabetes tends to develop at a younger age. Individuals with Turner syndrome are at increased risk for developing the metabolic syndrome (e.g., hypertension, dyslipidemia, type 2 diabetes obesity, insulin resistance, and hyperuricemia), as well as ischemic heart disease, and stroke. These factors contribute to the decreased life span of these individuals (Gravholt et al., 1998).

Neurocognitive and Psychosocial Phenotypic Expression

The word "phenotype" denotes a set of observable physical characteristics of an individual organism, although a single trait also can also be referred to as a phenotype. A phenotype is the result of many factors, including an individual's genotype, environment, and lifestyle, and the interactions among these factors (also see Mazzocco, this volume, chapter 13). As noted in table 1.2, individuals with Turner syndrome can manifest a variety of phenotypic features such as poor growth, gonadal failure, hearing loss, and cardiovascular abnormalities. The following sections will describe the neurocognitive and psychosocial phenotypic features that are associated with

Turner syndrome including deficits in visual perception (visual attention, visual–spatial, visual/nonverbal memory), selected executive functions (e.g., visual working memory), and social skills.

Neurological Underpinnings

Several neurostructural differences in individuals with Turner syndrome have been documented over the past decade. Structural studies have described reduced volumes of the parietal lobe bilaterally, particularly in the anterior and superior regions (Brown et al., 2004) and the right hippocampus (Kesler et al., 2004) when compared to controls. Larger volumes are described for the right superior temporal gyrus (Kesler et al., 2003) and left amygdala gray matter volumes (Kesler et al., 2004). Evidence also has begun to surface that links many of these neurostructural findings to specific neurocognitive deficits. For example, reduced parietal, parietal–occipital (Murphy et al., 1993; Reiss et al., 1995), and prefrontal volumes have been associated with higher order visuospatial processing difficulties. Furthermore, impaired performance on higher order cognitive tasks in individuals with Turner syndrome, such as arithmetic calculation, recently has been linked to selective structural pathology in the intraparietal sulcus (Molko et al., 2004).

Similarly, functional imaging studies using positron-emission tomography and functional MRI (fMRI) methods have reported reduced activation in parietal regions at rest (Clark et al., 1990) and abnormal engagement of parietal and prefrontal areas during more challenging tasks (Kesler et al., 2004; Tamm et al., 2003). For example, Haberecht et al. (2001) found that individuals with Turner syndrome showed decreased activation in the dorsolateral prefrontal cortex, caudate, and inferior parietal lobes during the high-load condition of a visuospatial working memory task, but not during the low-load condition (Haberecht et al., 2001). Using fMRI, our group (Hart et al., 2006) found impaired performance across both verbal and spatial domains in persons with Turner syndrome, with greater impairment on tasks with working memory demands. Frontoparietal regions in controls showed significantly sustained levels of activation during visuospatial working memory, but this was significantly reduced in the group with Turner syndrome. Activation of temporal regions, in contrast, did not differ between the two groups. Participants with Turner syndrome also showed differentially reduced prefrontal activation during the visuospatial task compared to controls. The results suggest impaired frontoparietal circuitry recruitment during visuospatial executive processing in persons with Turner syndrome, perhaps indicating a unique role for the X chromosome in the development of these pathways.

The consistent abnormalities across functional and structural neuroimaging studies suggest that deficient engagement of frontoparietal circuits is a key component of the Turner syndrome cognitive and psychosocial phenotype. Given these neurological underpinnings, this section reviews the empirical findings on the neurocognitive and psychosocial manifestations of Turner syndrome, with a particular focus on the heterogeneity of expression that can be seen during childhood.

Neurocognitive Manifestations

Findings in School-Age Children and Adolescents   Although the overall level of intellectual functioning in Turner syndrome is generally within the average range, individuals with Turner syndrome typically demonstrate an uneven profile of cognitive strengths and weaknesses suggestive of right-hemispheric dysfunction. Generally speaking, many individuals with Turner syndrome have greater difficulties in visuospatial processing but relative preservation of verbal abilities (McCauley et al., 1987). This pattern is evident in Cathy, case 1.3.

Over 40 years ago, Shaffer first reported that a population of adults with Turner syndrome had Verbal IQ (VIQ) scores on the Wechsler scales that averaged 18 points higher than those on the Performance IQ (PIQ). More recently, studies have demonstrated this VIQ > PIQ intellectual pattern in school-age and adolescent girls with Turner syndrome, with the typical difference in scores ranging from 12–15 points. On intellectual testing using one of the frequently employed Wechsler intelligence scales, individuals with Turner syndrome generally perform below normal controls on Arithmetic, Digit Span, Picture Completion, Coding, Object Assembly, and Block Design subtests (Rovet, 2004; Shaffer, 1962).

One of the primary assertions for the consistency of this VIQ > PIQ difference in the intellectual arena is that individuals with Turner syndrome manifest significant disruption of many of their visual processing abilities. Specific deficits have been reported in higher order visual–spatial functions (Downey et al., 1991; Money, 1993; Rovet, 1993; Temple & Carney, 1995), visual memory (Downey et al., 1991; Lewandowski, 1985), visuoconstructive abilities (Downey et al., 1991; McCauley et al., 1987; Temple & Carney, 1995), and visual attention (Ross et al., 2000a; Rovet, 1990). Visual-motor and fine-motor coordination difficulties also have been described (Nijhuis-Van der Sanden et al., 2004; Romans et al., 1998; Nijhuis-Van der Sanden et al., 2003; see case 1.1, Abigail) although the fine-motor speed deficits have been linked more to problems with motor initiation than to problems in motor planning (Nijhuis-Van der Sanden et al., 2004). Using the model of visual information processing first proposed by Ungerleider and Mishkin (Mishkin & Ungerleider, 1982; Ungerleider & Haxby, 1994), Hart et al. (2006) also noted that adolescents with Turner syndrome showed deficits in functions tapping the "where" pathway (i.e., visual–spatial abilities or where the object is), but not necessarily the "what" pathway (i.e., visual recognition abilities or what the object is). These pathways have been associated with specific neuroanatomical connections in the brain. The "what" pathway projects from the primary visual region of the occipital cortex to the inferior temporal cortex (ventral stream), while the "where" pathway projects from the primary visual region of the occipital cortex to the posterior region of the parietal cortex (dorsal stream). This latter model also has been used to demonstrate emergent evidence for impairment in both pathways, despite intact performance on some tasks within each pathway as well, thus implicating deficits that are pervasive with respect to both "what" and "where" pathways, but that are not representative of gross deficits in overall visual processing capabilities in girls with Turner syndrome (Mazzocco et al., 2006).

Furthermore, cognitive deficits in Turner syndrome, especially in visuospatial processing, appear to become most pronounced under high task demand conditions, such as those using working memory (see case 1.3; Hart et al., 2006), and seem to manifest most significantly in the development of early skills in mathematics (Murphy et al., 2006). Consequently, selected problems in executive functioning also have been suggested in girls with Turner syndrome (Kirk et al., 2005), with the classic visuospatial deficits and associated math problems both being secondary to the executive dysfunction (Mazzocco & McCloskey, 2005). These problems in visual processing have been reported in children as young as 4 years of age, in adolescents, and in adults. When these neurocognitive deficits are present early, they typically continue into adulthood (Downey et al., 1991; Ross et al., 2002; Rovet, 2004).

The neurobehavioral profile of Turner syndrome almost certainly involves changes in cerebral organization caused by insufficient expression of genes on the X chromosome and low levels of sex steroids. Because most girls with Turner syndrome have gonadal dysgenesis, physicians caring for them have a unique opportunity to control much of their sex steroid environment. Generally, estrogen replacement therapy is begun after age 12 to induce feminization and improve bone accrual. However, Ross et al. have demonstrated that estrogen therapy in early adolescence is also important in cognition. Deficits in short-term memory (Ross et al., 2000b), reaction time (Ross et al., 1998), and nonverbal processing speed (Ross et al., 1998), but not visuospatial task performance (Ross et al., 2002), can be partially reversed with estrogen therapy. At least in adulthood, there are marked differences in the cognitive function of estrogen-replaced women with premature ovarian failure (POF), those of estrogen-replaced women with Turner syndrome, and normal controls. In a study by Ross et al. (2004), the phenotypes of women with POF and normal controls were similar. The women with Turner syndrome, however, had deficits in spatial/perceptual skills, visual–motor integration, affect recognition, visual memory, attention, and executive function. The absence of estrogen effects in this study, however, does not preclude estrogen effects in Turner syndrome on these same parameters. Effects may depend upon the type of estrogen preparation, the route of administration, the length of therapy, and the age at which it is administered. Androgen replacement therapy is not routinely given in childhood or adolescence; however, oxandrolone, a nonaromatizable androgen, is sometimes given to enhance growth. Ross et al. (2003) reported a positive effect of oxandrolone on verbal working memory, but not on verbal abilities, spatial cognition, or executive function.

In contrast to many other chromosomal disorders, children with Turner syndrome generally do not have mental retardation. Recently, however, 11% of 500 patients with Turner syndrome reported in one university center's experience had mental retardation (Sybert & McCauley, 2004). As described in the pathophysiology section of this chapter, the X chromosome is enriched in genes affecting cognition (Skuse, 2005), and loss of gene expression on the X chromosome has been linked to mental retardation (Ross et al., 2000c; Good et al., 2003). Interestingly, though, persons with Turner syndrome who are at highest risk for mental retardation are those with structural abnormalities that cause genes that are normally silenced to continue to be expressed (functional disomy). This most frequently occurs in cases of ring X or X/autosome translocations (Leppig et al., 2004; Bouayed et al., 2004), in which X inactivation is disrupted or the abnormal X is preferentially expressed in cells. Kuntsi et al. (2000) examined the cognitive and educational functioning of 47 females with ring X chromosome and found that the possession of a ring X chromosome was associated with increased risks for learning problems, behavioral difficulties, and needs for special education assistance. They also reported a negative correlation between nonverbal IQ and the proportion of cells in peripheral blood containing an inactivated ring X chromosome; however, failure of X inactivation was not found to be associated with severe cognitive or social–behavioral deficits. Yorifuji et al. (1998) described uniparental disomy in persons with Turner syndrome with X-derived marker chromosomes and mental retardation.

Creswell and Skuse (2000) also noted the risk for autism to be rather high in Turner syndrome, with rates being at least 200 times more than is seen in the normal population. When Wassink et al. (2001) reviewed the records of subjects diagnosed with autism in their child and adolescent psychiatry clinic over an 18-year period, 278 of 898 had been referred for karyotype. Of those, 25 (9%) had a chromosomal abnormality, the most common being fragile X, other sex chromosome anomalies (including Turner syndrome), and chromosome 15 abnormalities. Given some of the neurocognitively based psychosocial manifestations of Turner syndrome, particularly the problems with eye gaze and face and emotion recognition deficits (Lawrence et al., 2003), the relationship to autism spectrum disorders, such as autism and Asperger syndrome, becomes clearer (Skuse, 2005). Indeed, case 1.4, Diane, would be consistent with these reports with this youngster having a co-occurrence of Turner syndrome and autism.

Although severe developmental disorders do not predominate Turner syndrome, the initial recognition of a significant developmental delay actually may create a pathway wherein children receive a karyotype, a subsequent diagnosis of Turner syndrome and, perhaps, earlier interventions. Our case 1.4 would fit this pathway of diagnosis.

Finally, given the neuropsychological difficulties manifested by many children with Turner syndrome, the alignment of these features with the nonverbal learning disabilities model has been proposed (Rovet & Schowalter, 1995). Although there are many differences within the population of individuals with Turner syndrome, the general pattern of cognitive, behavioral, and psychosocial functioning is quite similar to the one described by the nonverbal learning disabilities model (NLD; Rovet, 2004). In fact, in the Rourke et al. (2002) description of the NLD model, they classify 45,X Turner syndrome as "level 1," that is, as having virtually all of the NLD assets and deficits. Although making an NLD "diagnosis" probably is not warranted, nor even evidence-based, conceptualizing children with Turner syndrome within an NLD framework can help to provide a heuristic for better understanding the problems experienced by many individuals with Turner syndrome and it should help to frame this disorder for health care providers and educators. In fact, it was demonstrated over a decade ago that some persons with Turner syndrome may benefit from problem-solving strategy training in a manner similar to children with nonverbal learning disabilities (Williams et al., 1992). More complete features of NLD as defined by Rourke et al. (2002) are listed in table 1.3. Note that many other disorders are also associated with the NLD profile and that the limitation of this diagnostic category is discussed further in chapter 13 (Mazzocco, this volume, chapter 13).

In accordance with the NLD model (Rourke et al., 2002), many children with Turner syndrome manifest problems with mathematics. In addition to relatively poorer performance on the Arithmetic subtest of the Wechsler scales, Downey et al. (1991) and Rovet and Schowalter (1995) reported their samples of girls with Turner syndrome to be at least two grade levels below grade placement, with specific problems in the nonverbal reasoning and application of specific math facts. This finding subsequently has been echoed by other researchers (Kesler et al., 2005; Mazzocco, 1998, 2001; Siegel et al., 1998). Most recently, Murphy, Mazzocco, Gerner, and Henry (2006) demonstrated that young girls with Turner syndrome manifested a higher rate of math disabilities when compared to a grade-matched comparison group, although the persistence of the math disability through elementary school was not different. On a positive note, elementary-school-age girls did not differ from their grade-matched comparison group on many formal and informal math skills. Interestingly, reading disabilities can occur in children with Turner syndrome, but they may occur only in the presence of a math disability (Rovet, 1993). This profile was apparent in our case 1.3, Cathy, where a wide variety of visual–perceptual deficits were apparent, including problems in mathematics. However, it is certainly not the case that all—or even most—girls with Turner syndrome who have math disability also have dyslexia (Mazzocco, 2001).

Table 1.3
Diagnostic criteria for research in nonverbal learning disabilities

1. Bilateral deficits in tactile perception, usually more marked on the left side of the body. Simple tactile perception may reach normal levels as the child ages, but interpreting complex tactile stimulation remains impaired.

2. Bilateral deficits in psychomotor coordination, usually more marked on the left side of the body. Simple, repetitive motor skills may reach normal levels with age, but complex motor skills remain impaired or worsen relative to age norms.

3. Extremely impaired visual–spatial–organizational abilities. Simple visual discrimination can reach normal levels with age, particularly when stimuli are simple. Compared to age norms, complex visual–spatial–organizational abilities worsen with advancing years.

4. Substantial difficulty in dealing with novel or complex information or situations. A strong tendency to rely on rote, memorized reactions, approaches, and responses (often inappropriate for the situation), and failure to learn or adjust responses according to informational feedback. Also, especially frequent use of verbal responses in spite of the requirements of the novel situation. These tendencies remain or worsen with age.

5. Notable impairments in nonverbal problem solving, concept formation, and hypothesis testing.

6. Distorted sense of time. Estimating elapsed time over an interval and estimating time of day are both notably impaired.

7. Well-developed rote verbal abilities (e.g., single-word reading and spelling), frequently superior to age norms, in the context of notably poor reading comprehension abilities (particularly so in older children).

8. High verbosity that is rote and repetitive, with content disorders of language and deficits in functional/pragmatic aspects of language.

9. Substantial deficits in mechanical arithmetic and reading comprehension relative to strengths in single-word reading and spelling.

10. Extreme deficits in social perception, judgment, and interaction, often leading to eventual social isolation/withdrawal. Easily overwhelmed in novel situations, with a marked tendency toward extreme anxiety, even panic, in such situations. High likelihood of developing internalized forms of psycho-pathology (e.g., depression) in later childhood and adolescence.

Source: Reprinted from Drummond, C. R. (2005). *Archives of Clinical Neuropsychology, 20,* 171–182.

Findings in Early Childhood Relatively little is known about the neuropsychological profile of infants, toddlers, and preschoolers with Turner syndrome and factors that might contribute to their phenotypic presentation. In one of the few studies to examine these issues from birth, Bender et al. (1993) identified a small sample ($n = 9$) of newborns with Turner syndrome using neonatal screening. These investigators reported that 6 of their children evidenced a diffuse pattern of cognitive difficulties, with problems eventually arising in both verbal and nonverbal IQ, problem solving, and reading, while 3 fell within the average range. In addition to having a small sample size, this study did not provide information relative to the developmental trajectory of cognitive functions during the preschool years, nor did it provide key information related to factors that could predict the cognitive functions in this sample.

Our research group has been involved in a longitudinal study examining the cognitive phenotypic features of a sample of young girls with Turner syndrome. We recently presented preliminary baseline findings describing the cognitive/developmental functioning of our sample (Hooper et al., 2005). The prospective sample included 89 females with Turner syndrome ranging in age from 9 months to 48 months at baseline. The sample was mostly Caucasian and generally fell within the middle socioeconomic strata as determined by maternal education. Most of the participants had the classic 45X karyotype ($n = 56$), 14 had a 45X/46XX karyotype, and the remaining 19 had other karyotypes. At enrollment, participants were administered the Mullen scale of Early Learning. The Mullen scale provides age-based standard scores for Fine-Motor, Gross Motor, Receptive Language, Expressive Language, Visual Reception, and a Total Score.

Preliminary examination of the Mullen showed the group with Turner syndrome to be significantly below the normative means for all five subtests as well as the composite score, with approximately 20% of the sample being 2 *SD*s below the mean on the Mullen Total Score. The developmental trajectories of the cognitive abilities of these individuals will continue to be followed as they progress into the school-age years. Recognizing specific developmental lags at an earlier developmental period may lead to more aggressive neurodevelopmental surveillance and earlier deployment of intervention strategies—even for the typically developing children. This is particularly important where underlying neuropsychological deficits remain silent until they are challenged later in development. This was nicely illustrated in clinical case 1.2, Betty, who manifested no evidence of problems early in development but later experienced significant difficulties with learning-related activities.

Psychosocial Manifestations

Findings in School-Age Children and Adolescents   A common social–behavioral feature reported for children with Turner syndrome is the presence of attention deficits, with many of them showing symptoms of inattention, impulsivity, and hyperactivity (McCauley et al., 1986; Rovet & Schowalter, 1995; Rovet & Ireland, 1994). Swillen et al. (1993) noted that these symptoms tend to be more pronounced in early school-age children and later diminished to hypoactivity around the age of normal puberty. In contrast, McCauley et al. (2001) reported that even in adolescence, girls with Turner syndrome were more likely to be diagnosed with ADHD than their peers (see cases 1.3 and 1.4).

In addition, a variety of psychosocial problems have been described that tend to include internalizing types of problems (e.g., anxiety, depression, social withdrawal), with such problems being apparent even in sibling control research designs attempting to control for sociodemographic and other familial influences (Mazzocco et al., 1998). In addition, social adjustment problems clearly begin to surface during adolescence, perhaps secondary to growing differences with peers in terms of secondary sex characteristics, stature, long-standing neurocognitive and learning issues, and the presence of hearing impairments. Several investigators, including McCauley and colleagues (Downey et al., 1989; McCauley et al., 1986; McCauley et al., 1995; McCauley et al., 2001), reported problems with immaturity, a lack of connectedness with peers, poor social competence, and low self-esteem. Interestingly, some research also has suggested an increased risk of anorexia nervosa in adolescents (Muhs & Lieberz, 1993; Taipale et al., 1982), while another study found a negative correlation between self-esteem in children and increasing numbers of physical anomalies (el Abd et al., 1995). These problems are not solely due to short stature (McCauley et al., 1986). Although some positive psychosocial benefits appear to be derived from GH therapy, body attitude and self-perception issues have been reported to persist even after treatment for short stature (Van Pareren et al., 2005).

Social–behavioral problems may be potentiated by deficits in affective expression and reception. Girls with Turner syndrome may experience significant challenges in accurately and/or efficiently reading social cues, particularly in rapidly paced social interactions (McCauley et al., 1987; Waber, 1979; Lesniak-Karpiak et al., 2003). Lesniak-Karpiak and colleagues reported that their sample of females with Turner syndrome made fewer facial movements in their role-play interaction than did a typical group, or even a comparison group of individuals with fragile X syndrome. Lawrence et al. (2003) reported face and emotion recognition deficits in women with Turner syndrome when compared to typical peers, although normal configural face-processing abilities were present. Women with Turner syndrome also had deficits in their fear recognition accuracy. Three of our case examples had difficulties with affective processing (cases 1.1, 1.3, and 1.4, Abigail, Cathy, & Diane). Abigail and Diane showed no social–behavioral difficulties early in development but later demonstrated emergent concerns in their affective processing and social functioning. Cathy showed the pattern of nonverbal learning disabilities but did not evidence any major social–behavioral issues, at least into the latency years.

Taken together, there appears to be a wide range of social–behavioral issues that can be evidenced in girls with Turner syndrome. Available research suggests that these difficulties can increase through childhood and adolescence (Skuse, 2005). These can lead to social isolation and, later in life, to the appearance of mild depressive symptoms (Delooz et al., 1993) and a lower likelihood of positive adult relationships and marriage (Orten, 1990).

Findings in Early Childhood   Similar to the relative dearth of neurocognitive findings for young children with Turner syndrome, we are unaware of published studies that have examined the psychosocial manifestations in toddlers and preschool children with Turner syndrome. From the longitudinal study presented above (Hooper et al., 2005), Davenport, Quigley, Hooper, and the Toddler Turner Study Group

(Davenport et al., 2002b) presented initial baseline findings on the psychosocial functioning of a prospective sample of 89 preschool girls with Turner syndrome. At enrollment, the caregivers of the participants completed two measures of social–behavioral functioning: the Vineland Social–Emotional Early Scales and the Carey Temperament Scales. The Vineland Social–Emotional Early Scales provide age-based standard scores for Interpersonal Relationships, Play and Leisure, Communication, and an overall score, while the Carey Temperament Scales provide age-based standard scores for nine different temperament dimensions (e.g., Distractibility, Intensity, and Mood). Preliminary data on the Vineland Social–Emotional Early Scales showed the group with Turner syndrome to fall largely at the lower end of the average range of functioning, with the scores for Interpersonal Relationships, Play and Leisure, and the Composite being significantly below the normative means. In contrast, the Coping Skills Scale was slightly above average when compared to the normative mean. A greater number of children had scores that fell 2 SDs below the mean for the Interpersonal Relationships and Play and Leisure scales than expected, with approximately 8.5% of the sample falling 2 SDs below the mean on the Vineland Composite scale. A similar trend was noted on the Carey Temperament Scales, with three of the nine temperament scales being significantly below the normative mean: Persistence, Approach, and Adaptability. Specifically, girls with Turner syndrome were described as less persistent, more cautious in their approach to new situations, and slower to adapt to these situations.

Heterogeneity of Expression

Reports describing the phenotype of children with Turner syndrome are generally based on populations ascertained postnatally because of specific development and/or medical problems; therefore, the phenotypic descriptions in these reports are likely to be based on more severely involved individuals. Indeed, the relatively smaller numbers of patients that have been identified in utero have had a milder phenotypic expression than those diagnosed postnatally. This was evident in Diane, case 1.4. In a small retrospective study of 12 girls prenatally diagnosed with mosaic (45,X/46,XX) Turner syndrome, Koeberl et al. (1995) found that all but 3 had a completely normal appearance and none would have warranted chromosomal analysis for Turner syndrome. All of them had normal growth in early childhood (median age at last follow-up = 4 years; range = 7 months–10 years) and only 1 of 8 had evidence of gonadal failure. In contrast, in girls with Turner syndrome diagnosed postnatally, we would anticipate that essentially all of them would have growth failure and about three fourths would have delayed puberty. Failure of reports to include the milder end of the phenotypic spectrum perpetuates the inability of physicians to make the diagnosis of Turner syndrome in those with milder phenotypes.

Other challenges to understanding Turner syndrome stem from the heterogeneity of the syndrome in terms of karyotypes and gene expression. Even individuals with the same karyotypes may differ profoundly because of different degrees of mosaicism, differences in gene inactivation, different hormonal milieus, different modifier genes, and, perhaps, the effect of imprinting. While individuals with 45,X may evidence more neurocognitive and psychosocial involvement than individuals with mosaicism (Bender et al., 1994; Bender et al., 1984; Temple & Carney, 1993; Rovet & Ireland, 1994), the degree of phenotypic variability remains quite large due to dosage-sensitive X-linked gene involvement. This assertion was quite evident in our selection of case illustrations. Further, these factors do not even include the amount of variance that could be accounted for by social-demographic factors.

Summary

Although there are "classic" phenotypic features in Turner syndrome, care should be taken in assuming that all children with Turner syndrome will manifest these neurocognitive and psychosocial characteristics. A definite ascertainment bias toward a more severe phenotype is present in the current literature (Gunther et al., 2004), and a truer depiction of the phenotypic range will not be possible until all girls with Turner syndrome are diagnosed, for example, by neonatal screening (Meng et al., 2005). The literature is clear that if a phenotypic feature is present, then it likely will persist throughout the life span. These specific difficulties may create different challenges for individuals at different developmental epochs, and a developmental perspective is absolutely essential for working with these individuals. How the presence of visual–spatial deficits affects a youngster during the preschool years will be different than how it may affect specific issues in their life during the school-age and adolescent time periods. Further, as noted by Ross et al. (2000a), the interaction between the neurocognitive deficits—even if mild—with the psychosocial functions may serve to potentiate selected learning and social–behavioral concerns.

Finally, comprehensive assessment strategies, hopefully as part of an interdisciplinary team process, are critical to understanding the phenotypic manifestations of children with Turner syndrome. In addition to the requisite medical monitoring and necessary treatments (Frias & Davenport, 2003; Saenger et al., 2001), and the need for more aggressive diagnostic strategies at an earlier age (Savendahl & Davenport, 2000; Massa et al., 2005), neurodevelopmental surveillance of the cognitive and psychosocial functions of children with Turner syndrome should be part of the standard of care for these children. As argued by a number of investigators, the earlier the diagnosis is made, the earlier neurodevelopmental surveillance and subsequent interventions can be initiated. From our case illustrations, this certainly proved true for

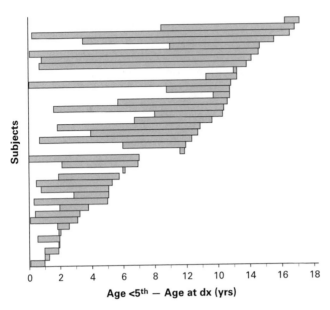

Figure 1.9
Delay in diagnosis for each patient diagnosed after infancy ($n = 40$) in the Turner syndrome (TS) population reported in Savendahl & Davenport (2000). *Journal of Pediatrics, 137,* 455–459. The time (in years) between the age at which each patient fell below the 5th percentile for height and the age at which the patient was diagnosed with TS is represented by a bar.

cases 1.1, 1.2, and 1.4, where early diagnosis facilitated neurodevelopmental surveillance as well as the pursuit of a variety of clinical and community-based services.

Recommendations to Enhance Early Identification

Early identification of girls with Turner syndrome is critical to their success and depends largely on educating and raising the index of suspicion for Turner syndrome in the many health care providers that they commonly encounter early in life—pediatricians, family practitioners, geneticists and genetic counselors, developmental specialists, physical and occupation therapists, audiologists, and so forth. Unfortunately, many girls with Turner syndrome are diagnosed late (figure 1.9). The most important guideline is that Turner syndrome should be considered in all girls with unexplained short stature or growth failure. The range of phenotypes is very broad (figure 1.10) and many girls with Turner syndrome will lack the obvious stigmata. The following guidelines by Savendahl and Davenport (2000) were adapted to include nonverbal learning disabilities in secondary criteria for obtaining a karyotype (Savendahl & Davenport, 2000).

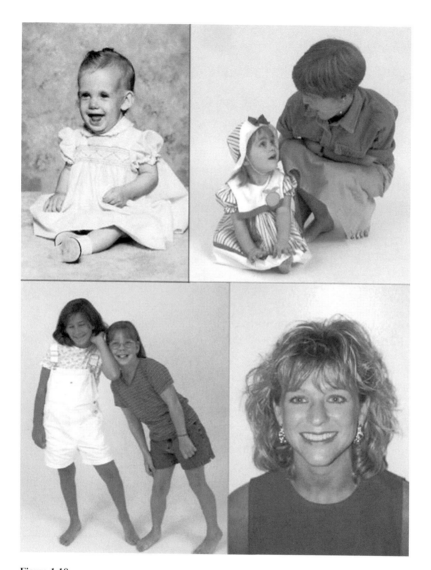

Figure 1.10
Five individuals with Turner syndrome (TS) demonstrating the variability in TS phenotype. Patients diagnosed as a newborn (top left) to adulthood (lower right).

A karyotype to evaluate a girl for Turner syndrome should be obtained in any girl with one or more of the following:

Unexplained short stature or growth failure

Webbed neck

Peripheral lymphedema

Delayed puberty

Coarctation of the aorta

Or any girl with two or more of the following:

Nail dysplasia

High arched palate

Short fourth metacarpal

Strabismus

Nonverbal learning disorder

Other suggestive features include epicanthal folds, ptosis, cubitus valgus, multiple nevi, renal malformations, bicuspid aortic valve, recurrent otitis media, and need for glasses.

Conclusions

The absence of some or all of a sex chromosome causes abnormalities in almost every organ system, including the brain. Although some girls with Turner syndrome have classic dysmorphic features, short stature and gonadal failure, the phenotype is less severe for most girls. Optimal health care requires a thorough knowledge of the unique health risks, psychoeducational needs, functional capabilities, and phenotypic variation associated with Turner syndrome. Early diagnosis is important because it allows patients and health care providers to place their problems into an understandable framework, to receive social support, and to receive screening and treatment for problems for which girls with Turner syndrome are at increased risk. Turner syndrome-specific health care should complement standard preventive health care recommendations. Health care checklists to help health care providers and families track these evaluations are available and should be routinely used. Internet resources and support groups such as the Turner Syndrome Society, Magic Foundation, and Human Growth Foundation are often tremendously helpful to affected individuals and their families.

Children with Turner syndrome should undergo a baseline developmental evaluation at the time of initial diagnosis or, at latest, during the preschool years. Academic tutoring, occupational therapy, and training in problem-solving strategies can help girls and women with Turner syndrome cope with their visual–spatial and cognitive challenges. Individual psychotherapy may be required to address the social and emotional difficulties commonly experienced by individuals with Turner syndrome (Boman et al., 1998). Because an understanding of these developmental issues as they specifically pertain to Turner syndrome may be limited in any given community, many families may benefit from using general books on learning disabilities (Thompson, 1997) and Web sites (e.g., www.nldontheweb.org). Physicians should keep in mind that virtually all of their associated medical problems impact on their social–emotional welfare and that some therapies, such as sex hormone replacement, may have a fundamental impact on cognition as well. Advancements such as sequencing of the X chromosome and dissection of neural pathways through fMRI have allowed quantum leaps in our understanding of Turner syndrome and its neurodevelopmental abnormalities over the past few years. The outlook for girls with Turner syndrome continues to improve as this understanding is translated into clinical practice.

References

Adhikary, H. P. (1981). Ocular manifestations of Turner's syndrome. *Transactions of the Ophthalmological Societies of the United Kingdom, 101,* 395–396.

Bakalov, V. K., Cooley, M. M., Quon, M. J., Luo, M. L., Yanovski, J. A., Nelson, L. M., et al. (2004). Impaired insulin secretion in the Turner metabolic syndrome. *Journal of Clinical Endocrinology and Metabolism, 89,* 3516–3520.

Becker, B., Jospe, N., & Goldsmith, L. A. (1994). Melanocytic nevi in Turner syndrome. *Pediatric Dermatology, 11,* 120–124.

Bender, B., Puck, M., Salbenblatt, J., & Robinson, A. (1984). Cognitive development of unselected girls with complete and partial X monosomy. *Pediatrics, 73,* 175–182.

Bender, B. G., Linden, M. G., & Robinson, A. (1993). Neuropsychological impairment in 42 adolescents with sex chromosome abnormalities. *American Journal of Medical Genetics, 48,* 169–173.

Bender, B. G., Linden, M. G., & Robinson, A. (1994). Neurocognitive and psychosocial phenotypes associated with Turner syndrome. In S. H. Broman & J. Grafman (Eds.), *Atypical cognitive deficits in developmental disorders: Implications for brain function,* chapter 10, pp. 197–216. Hillsdale, NJ: Lawrence Erlbaum Associates.

Berdahl, L. D., Wenstrom, K. D., & Hanson, J. W. (1995). Web neck anomaly and its association with congenital heart disease. *American Journal of Medical Genetics, 56,* 304–307.

Bilge, I., Kayserili, H., Emre, S., Nayir, A., Sirin, A., Tukel, T., et al. (2000). Frequency of renal malformations in Turner syndrome: Analysis of 82 Turkish children. *Pediatric Nephrology, 14,* 1111–1114.

Blaschke, R. J., & Rappold, G. A. (2000). SHOX: Growth, Leri-Weill and Turner syndromes. *Trends in Endocrinology and Metabolism, 11,* 227–230.

Boman, U. W., Moller, A., & Albertsson-Wikland, K. (1998). Psychological aspects of Turner syndrome. *Journal of Psychosomatic Obstetrics & Gynaecology, 19,* 1–18.

Bonamico, M., Bottaro, G., Pasquino, A. M., Caruso-Nicoletti, M., Mariani, P., Gemme, G., et al. (1998). Celiac disease and Turner syndrome. *Journal of Pediatric Gastroenterology & Nutrition, 26,* 496–499.

Bouayed, Abdelmoula N., Portnoi, M. F., Amouri, A., Arladan, A., Chakroun, M., Saad, A., et al. (2004). Turner syndrome female with a small ring X chromosome lacking the XIST, an unexpectedly mild phenotype and an atypical association with alopecia universalis. *Annales de Génétique, 47,* 305–313.

Brown, C. J., & Greally, J. M. (2003). A stain upon the silence: Genes escaping X inactivation. *Trends in Genetics, 19,* 432–438.

Brown, W. E., Kesler, S. R., Eliez, S., Warsofsky, I. S., Haberecht, M., & Reiss, A. L. (2004). A volumetric study of parietal lobe subregions in Turner syndrome. *Developmental Medicine & Child Neurology, 46,* 607–609.

Canadian Growth Hormone Advisory Committee. (2005). Impact of growth hormone supplementation on adult height in Turner syndrome: Results of the Canadian Randomized Controlled Trial. *Journal of Clinical Endocrinology Metabolism, 90,* 3360–3366.

Carrel, L., & Willard, H. F. (1999). Heterogeneous gene expression from the inactive X chromosome: An X-linked gene that escapes X inactivation in some human cell lines but is inactivated in others. *Proceedings of the National Academy of Sciences, U.S.A., 96,* 7364–7369.

Chang, P., Tsau, Y. K., Tsai, W. Y., Tsai, W. S., Hou, J. W., Hsiao, P. H., et al. (2000). Renal malformations in children with Turner's syndrome. *Journal of the Formosan Medical Association, 99,* 796–798.

Chow, J. C., Yen, Z., Ziesche, S. M., & Brown, C. J. (2005). Silencing of the mammalian X chromosome. *Annual Review of Genomics and Human Genetics, 6,* 69–92.

Chrousos, G. A., Ross, J. L., Chrousos, G. C., Chu, F. C., Kenigsberg, D., Cutler, G., et al. (1984). Ocular findings in Turner syndrome: A prospective study. *Ophthalmology, 91,* 926–928.

Clark, C., Klonoff, H., & Hayden, M. (1990). Regional cerebral glucose metabolism in Turner syndrome. *Canadian Journal of Neurological Sciences, 17,* 140–144.

Clement-Jones, M., Schiller, S., Rao, E., Blaschke, R. J., Zuniga, A., Zeller, R., et al. (2000). The short stature homeobox gene SHOX is involved in skeletal abnormalities in Turner syndrome. *Human Molecular Genetics, 9,* 695–702.

Creswell, C., & Skuse, D. (2000). Autism in association with Turner syndrome: Implications for male vulnerability. *Neurocase, 5,* 511–518.

Davenport, M. L., & Calikoglu, A. S. (2004). Turner syndrome. In O. H. Pescovitz & E. A. Eugster (Eds.), *Pediatric endocrinology: Mechanisms, manifestations, and management* (pp. 203–223). Philadelphia: Lippincott Williams & Wilkins.

Davenport, M. L., Punyasavatsut, N., Gunther, D., Savendahl, L., & Stewart, P. W. (1999). Turner syndrome: A pattern of early growth failure. *Acta Paediatrica Supplement, 88,* 118–121.

Davenport, M. L., Punyasavatsut, N., Stewart, P. W., Gunther, D. F., Savendahl, L., & Sybert, V. P. (2002a). Growth failure in early life: An important manifestation of Turner syndrome. *Hormone Research, 57,* 157–164.

Davenport, M. L., Quigley, C. A., Bryant, C. G., Rubin, K., Travers, S. H., Geffner, M. E., et al. (2005). *Effect of early growth hormone (GH) treatment in very young girls with Turner syndrome (TS).* Paper presented at the 7th Joint ESPE/LWPES meeting, Lyon, France.

Davenport, M. L., Quigley, C. A., Hooper, S. R., & the Toddler Turner Study Group. (2002b). Social behavior of infants and toddlers with Turner syndrome [Abstract]. *Pediatric Research, 51*(4), 115A.

Davies, W., Isles, A., Smith, R., Karunadasa, D., Burrmann, D., Humby, T., et al. (2005). Xlr3b is a new imprinted candidate for X-linked parent-of-origin effects on cognitive function in mice. *Nature Genetics, 37,* 625–629.

de Kerdanet, M., Lucas, J., Lemee, F., & Lecornu, M. (1994). Turner's syndrome with X-isochromosome and Hashimoto's thyroiditis. *Clinical Endocrinology (Oxford), 41,* 673–676.

Delooz, J., Van den Berghe, H., Swillen, A., Kleczkowska, A., & Fryns, J. P. (1993). Turner syndrome patients as adults: A study of their cognitive profile, psychosocial functioning and psychopathological findings. *Genetic Counseling, 4,* 169–179.

Downey, J., Ehrhardt, A. A., Gruen, R., Bell, J. J., & Morishima, A. (1989). Psychopathology and social functioning in women with Turner syndrome. *The Journal of Nervous and Mental Disease, 177,* 191–201.

Downey, J., Elkin, E. J., Ehrhardt, A. A., Meyer Bahlburg, H. F., Bell, J. J., & Morishima, A. (1991). Cognitive ability and everyday functioning in women with Turner syndrome. *Journal of Learning Disabilities, 24*, 32–39.

el Abd, A. S., Turk, J., & Hill, P. (1995). Psychological characteristics of Turner syndrome. *Journal of Child Psychology and Psychiatry, 36*, 1109–1125.

El-Mansoury, M., Bryman, I., Berntorp, K., Hanson, C., Wilhelmsen, L., & Landin-Wilhelmsen, K. (2005). Hypothyroidism is common in Turner syndrome: Results of a five-year follow-up. *Journal of Clinical Endocrinology and Metabolism, 90*, 2131–2135.

Elder, D. A., Roper, M. G., Henderson, R. C., & Davenport, M. L. (2002). Kyphosis in a Turner syndrome population. *Pediatrics, 109*, e93.

Ellison, J. W., Wardak, Z., Young, M. F., Gehron, R. P., Laig-Webster, M., & Chiong, W. (1997). PHOG, a candidate gene for involvement in the short stature of Turner syndrome. *Human Molecular Genetics, 6*, 1341–1347.

Elsheikh, M., Casadei, B., Conway, G. S., & Wass, J. A. (2001a). Hypertension is a major risk factor for aortic root dilatation in women with Turner's syndrome. *Clinical Endocrinology (Oxford), 54*, 69–73.

Elsheikh, M., Dunger, D. B., Conway, G. S., & Wass, J. A. (2002). Turner's syndrome in adulthood. *Endocrine Reviews, 23*, 120–140.

Elsheikh, M., Wass, J. A., & Conway, G. S. (2001b). Autoimmune thyroid syndrome in women with Turner's syndrome—The association with karyotype. *Clinical Endocrinology (Oxford), 55*, 223–226.

Eroglu, Y., Emerick, K. M., Chou, P. M., & Reynolds, M. (2002). Gastrointestinal bleeding in Turner's syndrome: A case report and literature review. *Journal of Pediatric Gastroenterology & Nutrition, 35*, 84–87.

Even, L., Cohen, A., Marbach, N., Brand, M., Kauli, R., Sippell, W., et al. (2000). Longitudinal analysis of growth over the first 3 years of life in Turner's syndrome. *Journal of Pediatrics, 137*, 460–464.

Frank, G. R. (2003). Role of estrogen and androgen in pubertal skeletal physiology. *Medical and Pediatric Oncology, 41*, 217–221.

Frias, J. L., & Davenport, M. L. (2003). Health supervision for children with Turner syndrome. *Pediatrics, 111*, 692–702.

Good, C. D., Lawrence, K., Thomas, N. S., Price, C. J., Ashburner, J., Friston, K. J., et al. (2003). Dosage-sensitive X-linked locus influences the development of amygdala and orbitofrontal cortex, and fear recognition in humans. *Brain, 126*, 2431–2446.

Gravholt, C. H., Fedder, J., Naeraa, R. W., & Muller, J. (2000). Occurrence of gonadoblastoma in females with Turner syndrome and Y chromosome material: A population study. *Journal of Clinical Endocrinology and Metabolism, 85*, 3199–3202.

Gravholt, C. H., Juul, S., Naeraa, R. W., & Hansen, J. (1998). Morbidity in Turner syndrome. *Journal of Clinical Epidemiology, 51*, 147–158.

Gravholt, C. H., & Weis, N. R. (1997). Reference values for body proportions and body composition in adult women with Ullrich–Turner syndrome. *American Journal of Medical Genetics, 72*, 403–408.

Gunther, D. F., Eugster, E., Zagar, A. J., Bryant, C. G., Davenport, M. L., & Quigley, C. A. (2004). Ascertainment bias in Turner syndrome: New insights from girls who were diagnosed incidentally in prenatal life. *Pediatrics, 114*, 640–644.

Haberecht, M. F., Menon, V., Warsofsky, I. S., White, C. D., Dyer-Friedman, J., Glover, G. H., et al. (2001). Functional neuroanatomy of visuo–spatial working memory in Turner syndrome. *Human Brain Mapping, 14*, 96–107.

Hanson, L., Bryman, I., Janson, P. O., Jakobsen, A. M., & Hanson, C. (2002). Fluorescence in situ hybridisation analysis and ovarian histology of women with Turner syndrome presenting with Y-chromosomal material: A correlation between oral epithelial cells, lymphocytes and ovarian tissue. *Hereditas, 137*, 1–6.

Hart, S. J., Davenport, M. L., Hooper, S. R., & Belger, A. (2006). Visuospatial executive function in Turner syndrome: Functional MRI and neurocognitive findings. *Brain, 129*, 1125–1136.

Haverkamp, F., Keuker, T., Woelfle, J., Kaiser, G., Zerres, K., Rietz, C., et al. (2003). Familial factors and hearing impairment modulate the neuromotor phenotype in Turner syndrome. *European Journal of Pediatrics, 162,* 30–35.

Hayward, P. A., Satsangi, J., & Jewell, D. P. (1996). Inflammatory bowel disease and the X chromosome. *Quarterly Journal of Medicine, 89,* 713–718.

Hooper, S. R., Davenport, M. L., & Ross, J. L. (2005). *Neurocognitive and psychosocial dysfunction in preschool children with Turner syndrome.* Paper presented at the 113th Annual Convention of the American Psychological Association, Washington, DC.

Horn, L. C., Limbach, A., Hoepffner, W., Trobs, R. B., Keller, E., Froster, U. G., et al. (2005). Histologic analysis of gonadal tissue in patients with Ullrich–Turner syndrome and derivative Y chromosomes. *Pediatric and Developmental Pathology, 8,* 197–203.

Jacobs, P., Dalton, P., James, R., Mosse, K., Power, M., Robinson, D., et al. (1997). Turner syndrome: A cytogenetic and molecular study. *Annals of Human Genetics, 61,* 471–483.

Jacobs, P. A., Melville, M., Ratcliffe, S., Keay, A. J., & Syme, J. (1974). A cytogenetic survey of 11,680 newborn infants. *Annals of Human Genetics, 37,* 359–376.

Kajii, T., Ferrier, A., Niikawa, N., et al. (1980). Anatomic and chromosomal anomalies in 639 spontaneous abortuses. *Human Genetics, 55,* 87–98.

Karlberg, J., Albertsson-Wikland, K., Nilsson, K. O., Ritzen, E. M., & Westphal, O. (1991). Growth in infancy and childhood in girls with Turner's syndrome. *Acta Paediatrica Scandinavica, 80,* 1158–1165.

Keating, J. P., Ternberg, J. L., & Packman, R. (1978). Association of Crohn disease and Turner syndrome. *Journal of Pediatrics, 92,* 160–161.

Kesler, S. R., Blasey, C. M., Brown, W. E., Yankowitz, J., Zeng, S. M., Bender, B. G., et al. (2003). Effects of X-monosomy and X-linked imprinting on superior temporal gyrus morphology in Turner syndrome. *Biological Psychiatry, 54,* 636–646.

Kesler, S. R., Garrett, A., Bender, B., Yankowitz, J., Zeng, S. M., & Reiss, A. L. (2004). Amygdala and hippocampal volumes in Turner syndrome: A high-resolution MRI study of X-monosomy 17. *Neuropsychologia, 42,* 1971–1978.

Kesler, S. R., Menon, V., & Reiss, A. L. (2005). Neurofunctional differences associated with arithmetic processing in Turner syndrome. *Cerebral Cortex, 16,* 849–856.

Kirk, J. W., Mazzocco, M. l. M. M., & Kover, S. T. (2005). Assessing executive dysfunction in girls with fragile X or Turner syndrome using the Contingency Naming Test (CNT). *Developmental Neuropsychology, 28,* 755–777.

Koeberl, D. D., McGillivray, B., & Sybert, V. P. (1995). Prenatal diagnosis of 45,X/46,XX mosaicism and 45,X: Implications for postnatal outcome. *American Journal of Human Genetics, 57,* 661–666.

Kuntsi, J., Skuse, D., Elgar, K., Morris, E., & Turner, C. (2000). Ring-X chromosomes: Their cognitive and behavioural phenotype. *Annals of Human Genetics, 64,* 295–305.

Lacro, R. V., Jones, K. L., & Benirschke, K. (1988). Coarctation of the aorta in Turner syndrome: A pathologic study of fetuses with nuchal cystic hygromas, hydrops fetalis, and female genitalia. *Pediatrics, 81,* 445–451.

Larizza, D., Locatelli, M., Vitali, L., Vigano, C., Calcaterra, V., Tinelli, C., et al. (2000). Serum liver enzymes in Turner syndrome. *European Journal of Pediatrics, 159,* 143–148.

Lawrence, K., Kuntsi, J., Coleman, M., Campbell, R., & Skuse, D. (2003). Face and emotion recognition deficits in Turner syndrome: A possible role for X-linked genes in amygdala development. *Neuropsychology, 17,* 39–49.

Leppig, K. A., Sybert, V. P., Ross, J. L., Cunniff, C., Trejo, T., Raskind, W. H., et al. (2004). Phenotype and X inactivation in 45,X/46,X,r(X) cases. *American Journal of Medical Genetics, A, 128,* 276–284.

Lesniak-Karpiak, K., Mazzocco, M. M., & Ross, J. L. (2003). Behavioral assessment of social anxiety in females with Turner or fragile X syndrome. *Journal of Autism and Developmental Disorders, 33,* 55–67.

Lewandowski, L. J. (1985). Clinical syndromes among the learning disabled. *Journal of Learning Disabilities, 18,* 177–178.

Lichtenstein, G. R. (2001). Management of bone loss in inflammatory bowel disease. *Seminars in Gastrointestinal Disease, 12,* 275–283.

Lippe, B., Geffner, M. E., Dietrich, R. J., Boechat, M. I., & Kangarloo, H. (1988). Renal malformations in patients with Turner syndrome: Imaging in 141 patients. *Pediatrics, 82,* 852–856.

Lippe, B. M. (1996). Turner syndrome. In M. A. Sperling (Ed.), *Pediatric endocrinology* (1st ed., pp. 387–421). Philadelphia: Saunders.

Lippe, B. M., & Saenger, P. H. (2002). Turner syndrome. In M. A. Sperling (Ed.), *Pediatric endocrinology* (2nd ed., pp. 519–564). Philadelphia: Saunders.

Loscalzo, M. L., Van, P. L., Ho, V. B., Bakalov, V. K., Rosing, D. R., Malone, C. A., et al. (2005). Association between fetal lymphedema and congenital cardiovascular defects in Turner syndrome. *Pediatrics, 115,* 732–735.

Lyon, M. F. (1961). Gene action in the X-chromosome of the mouse (*Mus musculus L.*). *Nature, 190,* 372–373.

Manzione, N. C., Kram, M., Kram, E., & Das, K. M. (1988). Turner's syndrome and inflammatory bowel disease: A case report with immunologic studies. *American Journal of Gastroenterology, 83,* 1294–1297.

Massa, G., Verlinde, F., De, S. J., Thomas, M., Bourguignon, J. P., Craen, M., et al. (2005). Trends in age at diagnosis of Turner syndrome. *Archives in Disease in Childhood, 90,* 267–268.

Massa, G. G., & Vanderschueren-Lodeweyckx, M. (1991). Age and height at diagnosis in Turner syndrome: Influence of parental height. *Pediatrics, 88,* 1148–1152.

Mathisen, B., Reilly, S., & Skuse, D. (1992). Oral-motor dysfunction and feeding disorders of infants with Turner syndrome. *Developmental Medicine and Child Neurology, 34,* 141–149.

Mazzanti, L., & Cacciari, E. (1998). Congenital heart disease in patients with Turner's syndrome. Italian Study Group for Turner Syndrome (ISGTS). *Journal of Pediatrics, 133,* 688–692.

Mazzocco, M. M. M. (1998). A process approach to describing mathematics difficulties in girls with Turner syndrome. *Pediatrics, 102,* 492–496.

Mazzocco, M. M. M. (2001). Math learning disability and math LD subtypes: Evidence from studies of Turner syndrome, fragile X syndrome, and neurofibromatosis type 1. *Journal of Learning Disabilities, 34,* 520–533.

Mazzocco, M. M. M., Baumgardner, T., Freund, L. S., & Reiss, A. L. (1998). Social functioning among girls with fragile X or Turner syndrome and their sisters. *Journal of Autism & Developmental Disorders, 28,* 509–517.

Mazzocco, M. M. M., Bhatia, N. S., & Lesniak-Karpiak, K. (2006). Visuospatial skills and their association with math performance in girls with fragile X or Turner syndrome. *Child Neuropsychology, 12,* 87–110.

Mazzocco, M. M. M., & McCloskey, M. (2005). Mathematics problem solving in girls with fragile X or Turner syndrome. In J. Campbell (Ed.), *Handbook of mathematical cognition* (pp. 269–297). Hove, England: Psychology Press.

McCauley, E., Feuillan, P., Kushner, H., & Ross, J. L. (2001). Psychosocial development in adolescents with Turner syndrome. *Journal of Developmental and Behavioral Pediatrics, 22,* 360–365.

McCauley, E., Ito, J., & Kay, T. (1986). Psychosocial functioning in girls with Turner's syndrome and short stature: Social skills, behavior problems, and self-concept. *Journal of the American Academy of Child Psychiatry, 25,* 105–112.

McCauley, E., Kay, T., Ito, J., & Treder, R. (1987). The Turner syndrome: Cognitive deficits, affective discrimination, and behavior problems. *Child Development, 58,* 464–473.

McCauley, E., Ross, J. L., Kushner, H., & Cutler, G., Jr. (1995). Self-esteem and behavior in girls with Turner syndrome. *Journal of Developmental and Behavioral Pediatrics, 16,* 82–88.

Medeiros, C. C., Marini, S. H., Baptista, M. T., Guerra, G., Jr., & Maciel-Guerra, A. T. (2000). Turner's syndrome and thyroid disease: A transverse study of pediatric patients in Brazil. *Journal of Pediatric Endocrinology and Metabolism, 13,* 357–362.

Meng, H., Hager, K., Rivkees, S. A., & Gruen, J. R. (2005). Detection of Turner syndrome using high-throughput quantitative genotyping. *Journal of Clinical Endocrinology and Metabolism, 90,* 3419–3422.

Migeon, B. R., Luo, S., Stasiowski, B. A., Jani, M., Axelman, J., Van Dyke, D. L., et al. (1993). Deficient transcription of XIST from tiny ring X chromosomes in females with severe phenotypes. *Proceedings of the National Academy of Sciences, U.S.A., 90,* 12025–12029.

Mishkin, M., & Ungerleider, L. G. (1982). Contribution of striate inputs to the visuospatial functions of parieto-preoccipital cortex in monkeys. *Behavioural Brain Research, 6,* 57–77.

Molko, N., Cachia, A., Riviere, D., Mangin, J. F., Bruandet, M., LeBihan, D., et al. (2004). Brain anatomy in Turner syndrome: Evidence for impaired social and spatial-numerical networks. *Cerebral Cortex, 14,* 840–850.

Money, J. (1993). Specific neuro-cognitive impairments associated with Turner (45,X) and Klinefelter (47,XXY) syndromes: A review. *Social Biology, 40,* 147–151.

Muhs, A., & Lieberz, K. (1993). Anorexia nervosa and Turner's syndrome. *Psychopathology, 26,* 29–40.

Munns, C. J., Haase, H. R., Crowther, L. M., Hayes, M. T., Blaschke, R., Rappold, G., et al. (2004). Expression of SHOX in human fetal and childhood growth plate. *Journal of Clinical Endocrinology and Metabolism, 89,* 4130–4135.

Murphy, D. G., DeCarli, C., Daly, E., Haxby, J. V., Allen, G., White, B. J., et al. (1993). X-chromosome effects on female brain: A magnetic resonance imaging study of Turner's syndrome [see comments]. *Lancet, 342,* 1197–1200.

Murphy, M. M., Mazzocco, M. M. M., Gerner, G., & Henry, A. E. (2006). Mathematics learning disability in girls with Turner syndrome or fragile X syndrome. *Brain and Cognition, 61,* 195–210.

Nielsen, J., & Wohlert, M. (1991). Chromosome abnormalities found among 34,910 newborn children: Results from a 13-year incidence study in Arhus, Denmark. *Human Genetics, 87,* 81–83.

Nijhuis-Van der Sanden, M. W., Eling, P. A., & Otten, B. J. (2003). A review of neuropsychological and motor studies in Turner syndrome. *Neuroscience and Biobehavioral Reviews, 27,* 329–338.

Nijhuis-Van der Sanden, M. W., Eling, P. A., Van Asseldonk, E. H., & Van Galen, G. P. (2004). Decreased movement speed in girls with Turner syndrome: A problem in motor planning or muscle initiation? *Journal of Clinical and Experimental Neuropsychology, 26,* 795–816.

Ogata, T., & Matsuo, N. (1995). Turner syndrome and female sex chromosome aberrations: Deduction of the principal factors involved in the development of clinical features. *Human Genetics, 95,* 607–629.

Orten, J. L. (1990). Coming up short: The physical, cognitive, and social effects of Turner's syndrome. *Health and Social Work, 15,* 100–106.

Ostberg, J. E., Thomas, E. L., Hamilton, G., Attar, M. J., Bell, J. D., & Conway, G. S. (2005). Excess visceral and hepatic adipose tissue in Turner syndrome determined by magnetic resonance imaging: Estrogen deficiency associated with hepatic adipose content. *Journal of Clinical Endocrinology and Metabolism, 90,* 2631–2635.

Pasquino, A. M., Passeri, F., Pucarelli, I., Segni, M., & Municchi, G. (1997). Spontaneous pubertal development in Turner's syndrome. Italian Study Group for Turner's Syndrome. *Journal of Clinical Endocrinology and Metabolism, 82,* 1810–1813.

Radetti, G., Mazzanti, L., Paganini, C., Bernasconi, S., Russo, G., Rigon, F., et al. (1995). Frequency, clinical and laboratory features of thyroiditis in girls with Turner's syndrome. The Italian Study Group for Turner's syndrome. *Acta Paediatrica, 84,* 909–912.

Raefski, A. S., & O'Neill, M. J. (2005). Identification of a cluster of X-linked imprinted genes in mice. *Nature Genetics, 37,* 620–624.

Ranke, M. B., Pfluger, H., Rosendahl, W., Stubbe, P., Enders, H., Bierich, J. R., et al. (1983). Turner syndrome: Spontaneous growth in 150 cases and review of the literature. *European Journal of Pediatrics, 141,* 81–88.

Reiss, A. L., Mazzocco, M. M. M., Greenlaw, R., Freund, L. S., & Ross, J. L. (1995). Neurodevelopmental effects of X monosomy: A volumetric imaging study. *Annals of Neurology, 38,* 731–738.

Reynaud, K., Cortvrindt, R., Verlinde, F., De, S. J., Bourgain, C., & Smitz, J. (2004). Number of ovarian follicles in human fetuses with the 45,X karyotype. *Fertility and Sterility, 81,* 1112–1119.

Romans, S. M., Stefanatos, G., Roeltgen, D. P., Kushner, H., & Ross, J. L. (1998). Transition to young adulthood in Ullrich–Turner syndrome: Neurodevelopmental changes. *American Journal of Medical Genetics, 79,* 140–147.

Rongen-Westerlaken, C., Corel, L., van, D., Broeck, J., Massa, G., Karlberg, J., et al. (1997). Reference values for height, height velocity and weight in Turner's syndrome. Swedish Study Group for GH treatment. *Acta Paediatrica, 86,* 937–942.

Ross, J., Zinn, A., & McCauley, E. (2000a). Neurodevelopmental and psychosocial aspects of Turner syndrome. *Mental Retardation and Developmental Disabilities Research Reviews, 6,* 135–141.

Ross, J. L., Roeltgen, D., Feuillan, P., Kushner, H., & Cutler, G. B., Jr. (1998). Effects of estrogen on nonverbal processing speed and motor function in girls with Turner's syndrome. *Journal of Clinical Endocrinology and Metabolism, 83,* 3198–3204.

Ross, J. L., Roeltgen, D., Feuillan, P., Kushner, H., & Cutler, G. B., Jr. (2000b). Use of estrogen in young girls with Turner syndrome: Effects on memory. *Neurology, 54,* 164–170.

Ross, J. L., Roeltgen, D., Kushner, H., Wei, F., & Zinn, A. R. (2000c). The Turner syndrome-associated neurocognitive phenotype maps to distal Xp. *American Journal of Human Genetics, 67,* 672–681.

Ross, J. L., Roeltgen, D., Stefanatos, G. A., Feuillan, P., Kushner, H., Bondy, C., et al. (2003). Androgen-responsive aspects of cognition in girls with Turner syndrome. *Journal of Clinical Endocrinology and Metabolism, 88,* 292–296.

Ross, J. L., Stefanatos, G. A., Kushner, H., Bondy, C., Nelson, L., Zinn, A., et al. (2004). The effect of genetic differences and ovarian failure: Intact cognitive function in adult women with premature ovarian failure versus Turner syndrome. *Journal of Clinical Endocrinology and Metabolism, 89,* 1817–1822.

Ross, J. L., Stefanatos, G. A., Kushner, H., Zinn, A., Bondy, C., & Roeltgen, D. (2002). Persistent cognitive deficits in adult women with Turner syndrome. *Neurology, 58,* 218–225.

Ross, M. T., Grafham, D. V., Coffey, A. J., Scherer, S., McLay, K., Muzny, D., et al. (2005). The DNA sequence of the human X chromosome. *Nature, 434,* 325–337.

Roulot, D., Degott, C., Chazouilleres, O., Oberti, F., Cales, P., Carbonell, N., et al. (2004). Vascular involvement of the liver in Turner's syndrome. *Hepatology, 39,* 239–247.

Rourke, B. P., Ahmad, S. A., Collins, D. W., Hayman-Abello, B. A., Hayman-Abello, S. E., & Warriner, E. M. (2002). Child clinical/pediatric neuropsychology: Some recent advances. *Annual Review of Psychology, 53,* 309–339.

Rovet, J. (2004). Turner syndrome: A review of genetic and hormonal influences on neuropsychological functioning. *Child Neuropsychology: A Journal on Normal and Abnormal Development in Childhood and Adolescence, 10,* 262–279.

Rovet, J., & Ireland, L. (1994). Behavioral phenotype in children with Turner syndrome. *Journal of Pediatric Psychology, 19,* 779–790.

Rovet, J. F. (1990). The cognitive and neuropsychological characteristics of females with Turner syndrome. In D. B. Berch & B. G. Berger (Eds.), *Sex chromosome abnormalities and human behavior* (pp. 38–77). Boulder, CO: Western Press.

Rovet, J. F. (1993). The psychoeducational characteristics of children with Turner syndrome. *Journal of Learning Disabilities, 26,* 333–341.

Rovet, J. F., & Schowalter, J. E. (1995). The psychoeducational characteristics of children with Turner syndrome. *Yearbook of Psychiatry & Applied Mental Health, 2,* 25–26.

Saenger, P., Wikland, K. A., Conway, G. S., Davenport, M., Gravholt, C. H., Hintz, R., et al. (2001). Recommendations for the diagnosis and management of Turner syndrome. *Journal of Clinical Endocrinology and Metabolism, 86,* 3061–3069.

Salerno, M., Di Maio, S., Gasparini, N., Rizzo, M., Ferri, P., & Vajro, P. (1999). Liver abnormalities in Turner syndrome. *European Journal of Pediatrics, 158,* 618–623.

Savendahl, L., & Davenport, M. L. (2000). Delayed diagnoses of Turner's syndrome: Proposed guidelines for change. *Journal of Pediatrics, 137,* 455–459.

Sculerati, N., Ledesma Medina, J., Finegold, D. N., & Stool, S. E. (1990). Otitis media and hearing loss in Turner syndrome. *Archives of Otolaryngology—Head & Neck Surgery, 116,* 704–707.

Scully, R. E., Young, R. H., & Clemente, C. D. (1998). Mixed germ cell-sex cord-stromal tumors. In R. E. Scully, R. H. Young, & C. D. Clemente (Eds.), *Tumors of the ovary, maldeveloped gonads, fallopian tube and broad ligament* (pp. 307–400). Washington, DC: Armed Forces Institute of Pathology.

Shaffer, J. W. (1962). A specific cognitive deficit observed in gonadal aplasia (Turner's syndrome). *Journal of Clinical Psychology, 18,* 403–406.

Siegel, P. T., Clopper, R., & Stabler, B. (1998). The psychological consequences of Turner syndrome and review of the National Cooperative Growth Study psychological substudy. *Pediatrics, 102*(2 Pt 3), 488–491.

Simmons, K. E. (1999). Growth hormone and craniofacial changes: Preliminary data from studies in Turner's syndrome. *Pediatrics, 104,* 1021–1024.

Simpson, J. L., & Rajkovic, A. (1999). Ovarian differentiation and gonadal failure. *American Journal of Medical Genetics, 89,* 186–200.

Skuse, D. H. (2005). X-linked genes and mental functioning. *Human Molecular Genetics, 14,* R27–R32.

Skuse, D. H., James, R. S., Bishop, D. V., Coppin, B., Dalton, P., Aamodt-Leeper, G., et al. (1997). Evidence from Turner's syndrome of an imprinted X-linked locus affecting cognitive function. *Nature, 387,* 705–708.

Soriano-Guillen, L., Coste, J., Ecosse, E., Leger, J., Tauber, M., Cabrol, S., et al. (2005). Adult height and pubertal growth in Turner syndrome after treatment with recombinant growth hormone. *Journal of Clinical Endocrinology and Metabolism, 90,* 5197–5204.

Speed, R. M. (1986). Ooctye develoment in XO foetuses of man and mouse: The possible role of heterologous X-chromosome pairing in germ cell survival. *Chromosoma, 94,* 115–124.

Stenberg, A. E., Nylen, O., Windh, M., & Hultcrantz, M. (1998). Otological problems in children with Turner's syndrome. *Hearing Research, 124,* 85–90.

Swillen, A., Fryns, J. P., Kleczkowska, A., Massa, G., Vanderschueren Lodeweyckx, M., & Van den Berghe, H. (1993). Intelligence, behaviour and psychosocial development in Turner syndrome. A cross-sectional study of 50 pre-adolescent and adolescent girls (4–20 years). *Genetic Counseling, 4,* 7–18.

Sybert, V. P. (1984). Adult height in Turner syndrome with and without androgen therapy. *Journal of Pediatrics, 104,* 365–369.

Sybert, V. P. (1998). Cardiovascular malformations and complications in Turner Syndrome. *Pediatrics, 101,* e11.

Sybert, V. P., & McCauley, E. (2004). Turner's syndrome. *New England Journal of Medicine, 351,* 1227–1238.

Taipale, V., Niittymaki, M., & Nevalainen, I. (1982). Turner's syndrome and anorexia nervosa symptoms. *Acta Paedopsychiatrica, 48,* 231–238.

Tamm, L., Menon, V., & Reiss, A. L. (2003). Abnormal prefrontal cortex function during response inhibition in Turner syndrome: Functional magnetic resonance imaging evidence. *Biological Psychiatry, 53,* 107–111.

Temple, C. M., & Carney, R. A. (1993). Intellectual functioning of children with Turner syndrome: A comparison of behavioural phenotypes. *Developmental Medicine and Child Neurology, 35,* 691–698.

Temple, C. M., & Carney, R. A. (1995). Patterns of spatial functioning in Turner's syndrome. *Cortex, 31,* 109–118.

Thompson, S. (1997). *The source for nonverbal learning disorders.* East Moline, IL: LinguiSystems.

Thomson, S. J., Tanner, N. S., & Mercer, D. M. (1990). Web neck deformity: Anatomical considerations and options in surgical management. *British Journal of Plastic Surgery, 43,* 94–100.

Townsend, G., Jensen, B. L., & Alvesalo, L. (1984). Reduced tooth size in 45,X (Turner syndrome) females. *American Journal of Physical Anthropology, 65,* 367–371.

Tsezou, A., Hadjiathanasiou, C., Gourgiotis, D., Galla, A., Kavazarakis, E., Pasparaki, A., et al. (1999). Molecular genetics of Turner syndrome: Correlation with clinical phenotype and response to growth hormone therapy. *Clinical Genetics, 56,* 441–446.

Turner, C., Dennis, N. R., Skuse, D. H., & Jacobs, P. A. (2000). Seven ring (X) chromosomes lacking the XIST locus, six with an unexpectedly mild phenotype. *Human Genetics, 106,* 93–100.

Ungerleider, L. G., & Haxby, J. V. (1994). 'What' and 'where' in the human brain. *Current Opinions in Neurobiology, 4,* 157–165.

Van Pareren, Y. K., Duivenvoorden, H. J., Slijper, F. M., Koot, H. M., Drop, S. L., & de Muinck Keizer-Schrama, S. M. (2005). Psychosocial functioning after discontinuation of long-term growth hormone treatment in girls with Turner syndrome. *Hormone Research, 63,* 238–244.

Vogt, P. H., Affara, N., Davey, P., Hammer, M., Jobling, M. A., Lau, Y. F., et al. (1997). Report of the Third International Workshop on Y Chromosome Mapping 1997. Heidelberg, Germany, April 13–16, 1997. *Cytogenetics and Cell Genetics, 79,* 1–20.

Waber, D. P. (1979). Neuropsychological aspects of Turner's syndrome. *Developmental Medicine and Child Neurology, 21,* 58–70.

Wassink, T. H., Piven, J., & Patil, S. R. (2001). Chromosomal abnormalities in a clinic sample of individuals with autistic disorder. *Psychiatric Genetics, 11,* 57–63.

Weinrieb, I. J., Fineman, R. M., & Spiro, H. M. (1976). Turner syndrome and inflammatory bowel disease. *New England Journal of Medicine, 294,* 1221–1222.

Williams, E. D., Engel, E., Taft, P. D., & Forbes, A. P. (1966). Gonadal dysgenesis and ulcerative colitis: A case report with clinical, cytogenetic, and post-mortem studies. *Journal of Medical Genetics, 3,* 51–55.

Williams, J. K., Richman, L. C., & Yarbrough, D. B. (1992). Comparison of visual–spatial performance strategy training in children with Turner syndrome and learning disabilities. *Journal of Learning Disabilities, 25,* 658–664.

Yorifuji, T., Muroi, J., Kawai, M., Uematsu, A., Sasaki, H., Momoi, T., et al. (1998). Uniparental and functional X disomy in Turner syndrome patients with unexplained mental retardation and X derived marker chromosomes. *Journal of Medical Genetics, 35,* 539–544.

Zechner, U., Wilda, M., Kehrer-Sawatzki, H., Vogel, W., Fundele, R., & Hameister, H. (2001). A high density of X-linked genes for general cognitive ability: A run-away process shaping human evolution? *Trends in Genetics, 17,* 697–701.

Zinn, A. R. (2001). The X chromosome and the ovary. *Journal of the Society of Gynecologic Investigation, 8,* S34–S36.

Zvulunov, A., Wyatt, D. T., Laud, P. W., & Esterly, N. B. (1998). Influence of genetic and environmental factors on melanocytic naevi: A lesson from Turner's syndrome. *British Journal of Dermatology, 138,* 993–997.

2 Klinefelter Syndrome

Judith L. Ross, Gerry A. Stefanatos, and David Roeltgen

Definition

Klinefelter syndrome was first described by Klinefelter et al. (1942) on the basis of males demonstrating testicular failure, breast enlargement, and an inability to produce sperm. The genetic basis of Klinefelter syndrome was characterized 14 years later by observation of an abnormal chromosome karyotype 47,XXY (see figure 2.1; Bradbury et al., 1956). About 80% of individuals with Klinefelter syndrome demonstrate the karyotype 47,XXY, while the remaining 20% have 47,XXY/46,XY mosaicism, higher grade aneuploidy, or structural abnormalities of the X chromosomes. The Klinefelter syndrome phenotype includes childhood onset testicular failure, tall stature, and characteristic cognitive and behavioral features. In this chapter, we will review the current literature on the development of individuals with Klinefelter syndrome and attempt to integrate current knowledge regarding genetic and endocrine aspects of Klinefelter syndrome and their potential influence on the emergence of the behavioral phenotype.

Diagnosis and Identification

The primary clinical physical characteristics of Klinefelter syndrome emerge during puberty as a constellation of symptoms that include underdeveloped secondary sexual characteristics, small testes, and aspermatogenesis (Klinefelter et al., 1942). Other commonly observed clinical features include symptoms of androgen deficiency, tall stature, gynecomastia, and castrate (elevated) levels of gonadotropins. Although individuals with Klinefelter syndrome may show a tendency toward long limbs and tall stature during childhood, symptoms are typically difficult to discern prior to mid-puberty (Salbenblatt et al., 1985). Identification often does not occur until late puberty or early adulthood when signs and symptoms of hypogonadism prompt endocrine testing. Even in adulthood, the defining clinical characteristics show substantial

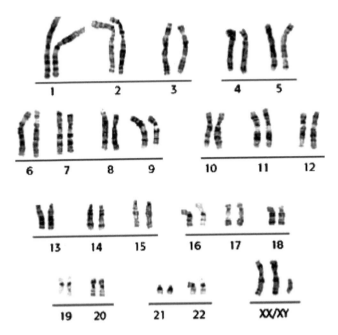

Figure 2.1
47,XXY Klinefelter syndrome chromosome karyotype.

variation (Smyth & Bremner, 1998), and up to 64% of males with Klinefelter syndrome may go unrecognized throughout the life span.

The clinical spectrum for the testicular failure phenotype ranges from nearly complete, fetal onset androgen deficiency and gonadal failure, manifested by small testes and penis early in infancy or childhood (Laron & Hochman, 1971; Ross et al., in press; Salbenblatt et al., 1985; Stewart et al., 1990; Stewart et al., 1982a; Stewart et al., 1982b) to mild androgen deficiency with azoospermia in adulthood (Kamischke et al., 2003). Testes tend to be small at all ages in boys with Klinefelter syndrome (Muller et al., 1995; Ratcliffe et al., 1982b; Wikstrom et al., 2004), because both testicular germ cells and interstitial cells fail to develop normally. Despite the presence of small testes, only one fourth of males with Klinefelter syndrome are diagnosed in childhood (Bojesen et al., 2003; Kamischke et al., 2003). About 10% are diagnosed prenatally (Abramsky & Chapple, 1997). In a Danish national registry study, the reason for referral was generally hypogonadism or infertility. Most were not suspected of having Klinefelter syndrome by primary and secondary referral sources (Bojesen et al., 2003).

While the prominent features of the physical phenotype are testicular failure and tall stature, other physical anomalies such as smaller head circumference (Stewart et al., 1982a) and mild alterations in craniofacial structure have also been noted. Additional Klinefelter syndrome–associated phenotypic findings include increased risk for osteoporosis, breast cancer, autoimmune thyroid disorders, and type 2 diabetes mellitus (Price et al., 1985). Chromosome analysis performed in lymphocytes (Jacobs, 1979) is the genetic standard for the diagnosis. Increasing numbers are now detected through routine antenatal or newborn chromosome screening. Still, many individuals with Klinefelter syndrome are diagnosed later in life or remain undetected.

The underdiagnosis of Klinefelter syndrome may be due, at least in part, to the focus on endocrine and reproductive abnormalities. Earlier diagnosis of Klinefelter syndrome would permit earlier intervention for the behavioral and neurocognitive developmental issues that are described below (Jones, 1997). Specifically, Klinefelter syndrome is characteristically associated with impaired language development including early problems with expressive speech, word retrieval, and phonemic processing (Bender et al., 1983; Graham et al., 1988; Netley & Rovet, 1984; Nielsen et al., 1980; Walzer, 1985). In addition, the disorder is linked with a characteristic personality style that includes immaturity, insecurity, and shyness (Mandoki et al., 1991; Ratcliffe et al., 1982a). These developmental neurobehavioral symptoms have long-term implications for social and academic development and often persist into adulthood.

The precise nature and extent of anomalies in brain development associated with Klinefelter syndrome are not completely understood. Brain development may be altered by androgen deficiency early in life, X-chromosome gene excess dosage effects, or both. Neuropsychological studies as well as structural and functional neuroimaging results suggest that the neurocognitive problems observed in Klinefelter syndrome are not secondary to diffuse brain dysfunction but instead probably reflect dysfunction of specific neural systems.

Case 2.1: Edgar   Edgar was first diagnosed with Klinefelter syndrome at 9 years of age, on the basis of tall stature. His developmental history was notable for his being slower to walk and talk, particularly relative to his three older brothers. He had received educational support for reading in first grade but was otherwise performing at grade level. Edgar was described as having a more sensitive personality, such as crying more easily than his brothers. He was quite shy and had to be encouraged to interact with other boys his age. He did not participate in athletic pursuits unless he was actively encouraged by his father. The case of Edgar exemplifies the difficulty in diagnosing Klinefelter syndrome in childhood. Although he had many features consistent with Klinefelter syndrome, there was no single diagnostic feature that would have permitted earlier diagnosis. This case also illustrates some of the key learning and personality issues that have been reported in boys with Klinefelter syndrome. Earlier anticipatory guidance, as well as school-based interventions, would have perhaps eased the course of development for this child.

Case 2.2: Frank The case of Frank exemplifies an even later diagnosis of Klinefelter syndrome. He was diagnosed with Klinefelter syndrome in adolescence when he presented with small testicular size. He has since been treated with testosterone replacement therapy and has done well. He is currently a junior in high school and shows relative strength in the area of carpentry and machine shop. Frank has participated in sports activities and reports having friends his own age. This young man does not appear to have any particular social issues. Although he has not achieved academically at the level comparable to that of his siblings, Frank will graduate from high school and plans to attend college.

Epidemiology and Prevalence

Klinefelter syndrome is currently recognized as the most common sex-linked genetic disorder, occurring in 0.1%–0.2% of the general population and in 1 per 426 to 1,000 males (Bojesen et al., 2003; Jacobs, 1979; MacLean et al., 1961; Nielsen & Wohlert, 1990; Visootsak et al., 2001). It accounts for 3.1% of infertile males and is the most prevalent cause of male hypogonadism and chromosomal aneuploidy in humans. Although Klinefelter syndrome is equally distributed in socioeconomic levels and racial groups, ascertainment is lower in minority populations (Bojesen et al., 2003; Jacobs, 1979; MacLean et al., 1961; Nielsen & Wohlert, 1990).

Karyotypes and Genetic Mechanisms

Klinefelter syndrome is associated with an extra X chromosome, resulting in a 47,XXY karyotype (figure 2.1). The extra X chromosome in Klinefelter syndrome is usually acquired though nondisjunction during maternal or paternal gametogenesis (MacDonald et al., 1994) or, less commonly, from errors in division during mitosis of the zygote (Jacobs et al., 1988). The primary genetic basis for the phenotypic abnormalities of Klinefelter syndrome is the expression of genes on the extra X chromosome. Another genetic factor that could account for variation in the Klinefelter syndrome phenotype is the pattern of X inactivation (defined in chapter 1 of this volume). In one study (Iitsuka et al., 2001), 31% of individuals with Klinefelter syndrome had skewed X inactivation (>80%), which could be a factor in the subset of individuals with Klinefelter syndrome that is most severely affected. Last, parent-of-origin or imprinting effects have been postulated to affect the Klinefelter syndrome phenotype (Jacobs et al., 1988; Skuse, 2000). However, studies on imprinting effects are inconsistent: In one study, no correlation was found between the severity of the Klinefelter syndrome phenotype and the parental origin of the X chromosome (Ratcliffe et al., 1990).

Klinefelter syndrome variants with additional chromosomal abnormalities such as 48,XXYY and 48,XXXY account for one per 50,000 male births. The most severe variant, 49,XXXXY, is thought to occur in 1 per 85,000 to 100,000 male births. These variants are associated with some genetic and endocrine features of Klinefelter syndrome and manifest generally more severe cognitive deficits.

Endocrinology

Growth of the penis in utero and during childhood represents a bioassay for the levels of endogenous testosterone. A burst of testosterone synthesis by the normal fetal male testis in the last trimester of pregnancy, which stimulates penile growth, is deficient in males with Klinefelter syndrome and may result in their small penile size at birth (Forest et al., 1974; Main et al., 2000; Ross et al., 2005). Boys with Klinefelter syndrome also lack the normal infant male postnatal surge in testosterone that peaks at 2 to 4 months of age (Forest et al., 1973a, 1973b; Lahlou et al., 2004).

Poor penile growth in early childhood implies early testosterone deficiency. For example, in a unique set of monozygotic male twins cytogenetically discordant for Klinefelter syndrome (Ratcliffe, 1982), the testes and penis of only the Klinefelter syndrome–affected twin were small at birth and throughout adolescence, consistent with what is reported in other Klinefelter syndrome boys (Caldwell & Smith, 1972; Laron & Hochman, 1971; Ratcliffe, 1982; Ratcliffe et al., 1982a; Salbenblatt et al., 1981; Stewart et al., 1990; Stewart et al., 1982a; Stewart et al., 1982b). There is a reported decrease in testosterone levels in blood measured prenatally and in infancy, based on studies with small samples of males with Klinefelter syndrome (Ratcliffe, 1982; Ross et al., 2005; Topper et al., 1982). Testosterone levels are low normal (Sorensen et al., 1981) and remain low in childhood and adulthood (Ross et al., 2005; Schiavi et al., 1978; Sorensen et al., 1981; Topper et al., 1982). Testicular biopsy specimens of infants with Klinefelter syndrome demonstrate decreased or absent germ cells (Ferguson-Smith, 1959; Kamischke et al., 2003; Mikamo et al., 1968; Muller et al., 1995) and abnormal seminiferous tubules in infancy; this is also observed in boys with Klinefelter syndrome ages 10 to 14 years (Ferguson-Smith, 1959; Kamischke et al., 2003; Mikamo et al., 1968; Muller et al., 1995; Wikstrom et al., 2004).

Testosterone measurements in childhood are difficult to interpret because the levels are typically low, there is a wide range of normative values, and there is variability of individual assays. Moreover, the presence of reduced levels of testosterone in prepubertal and pubertal boys seems to have functional significance. Diurnal rhythms of testosterone with higher levels in the early morning hours were observed in boys with normal testicular function as young as 4 to 5 years of age (Mitamura et al.,

1999; Sorensen et al., 1981). In addition, testosterone levels are higher in 4- to 5-year-old boys than same-age girls (Mitamura et al., 1999, 2000; Sorensen et al., 1981). Thus, testosterone is likely to act physiologically at low levels in childhood, before the onset of puberty.

Characteristics of Individuals with Klinefelter Syndrome

Physical Phenotype

Boys with Klinefelter syndrome tend to be tall (average adult height of 186 cm, or approximately 6 ft, 2 in., Ratcliffe, 1999; Visootsak et al., 2001), with disproportionately long legs (Caldwell & Smith, 1972; Ratcliffe, 1982; Ratcliffe et al., 1994a, 1986). The childhood-onset tall stature is likely related to the presence of three copies of the X-chromosome height-determining gene, SHOX (see also chapter 1 of this volume), as well as delayed epiphyseal fusion on the basis of decreased sex hormone levels (Rao et al., 1997). Other sex chromosome trisomies, 47,XYY males and 47,XXX females, also tend be tall and have three copies of the SHOX gene (Linden, 2002). Signs of testicular failure and testosterone deficiency in adolescents with Klinefelter syndrome include gynecomastia; eunuchoidal body proportion with relatively longer legs and increased arm span; decreased facial, pubic, and body hair; and decreased muscle mass (figure 2.2). Other physical features include clinodactyly (curved) fifth finger and hypertelorism (widely spaced eyes; table 2.1, figure 2.3). Skeletal anomalies associated with Klinefelter syndrome include osteoporosis, scoliosis, and pectus excavatum. Males with Klinefelter syndrome also have an increased risk for obesity (Ratcliffe, 1999).

Motor Function   Motor dysfunction is a cardinal feature in Klinefelter syndrome, reflected in performance on measures of strength, fine motor coordination, speed, and dexterity. Boys and adults with Klinefelter syndrome have decreased strength and reduced muscle mass compared to males without Klinefelter syndrome (Robinson et al., 1986; Salbenblatt et al., 1987). Specifically, they commonly have impairments in gross and fine motor skills, upper limb coordination, and speed and dexterity (Robinson et al., 1986; Salbenblatt et al., 1987) evident on a variety of measures including reduced hip flexor, shoulder abductor, and shoulder adductor muscle strength (Robinson et al., 1990). Additionally, we have recently observed decreased motor tone in infants with Klinefelter syndrome (Ross et al., 2005; Zinn et al., 2005).

In addition to decreased strength, infants and boys with Klinefelter syndrome are also more likely to have decreased muscle tone and mass, impaired motor praxis, decreased motor activity, atypical movement patterns, and delayed motor milestones

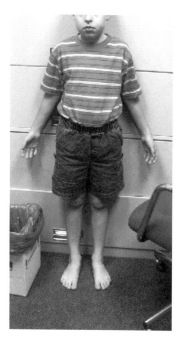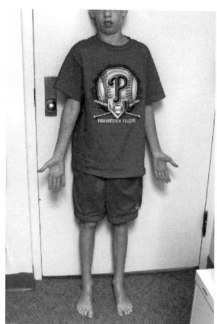

Figure 2.2
Decreased muscle mass in boys with Klinefelter syndrome.

Table 2.1
Features of Klinefelter syndrome (KS) in a population of 87 males (ages infant–adults) seen at Thomas Jefferson University, 36 with cognitive evaluations

	Clinical features	Frequency (%)	Unique to KS
Testicular failure	Testes smaller than average for age	80	Usually
	Phallus smaller than average for age	93	No
Facial features	High arched palate	33	No
	Hypertelorism	66	No
Extremities	Fifth finger clinodactyly	70	No
	Long arms and legs	50	Usually
Skeleton	Pectus	10	No
	Tall stature $> 1\ SD$	50	No
Other	Breast tissue	15	No
Development	Speech and motor delays	70	No
Personality	Shyness/social anxiety—Conners shyness < 85 SS	60	No
Academic	Reading difficulty—WRAT3 < 85 SS	22	No
	Attention disorders—Conners inattention < 85 SS	66	No

WRAT3, Wide Range Achievement Test; SD, standard deviation; SS, standard score.

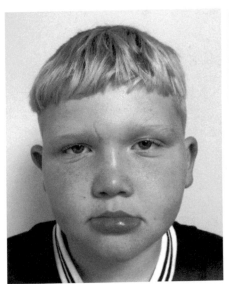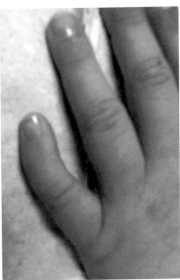

Figure 2.3
Physical Klinefelter syndrome (KS) features in boys with KS: Hypertelorism (left) and fifth finger clinodactyly (right).

(figures 2.2 and 2.4; Salbenblatt et al., 1987; Simpson et al., 2003). Impaired coordination, as demonstrated by problems in balance, jumping, and hopping, remain evident throughout childhood, as reflected in performance on measures of strength, fine
motor coordination, speed, and dexterity (Robinson et al., 1986; Salbenblatt et al.,
1987; Samango-Sprouse, 2001). Finger joint hypermobility and poor grasp specifically hinder early writing ability (Salbenblatt et al., 1987) in boys with Klinefelter
syndrome. The combination of motor slowing and poor coordination, along with
diminished muscle mass and elongated legs and arms, commonly results in poor athletic skills, particularly evident in comparison to peers during adolescence (figure
2.2).

Aspects of motor function, including motor speed and coordination, have been
shown to improve with androgen replacement in adolescents and adults with Klinefelter syndrome. Other androgen-deficient populations also respond to this treatment
(Alexander et al., 1998; Brill et al., 2002; Hines et al., 2003; Nielson, 1988; O'Connor
et al., 2001). Early androgen effects on developing musculature may explain the superior motor performance, relative to female controls, observed in females with congenital adrenal hyperplasia who have elevated testosterone levels in utero and early
in life (Hines et al., 2003). Therefore, testosterone replacement before puberty may
be beneficial, although this remains to be demonstrated empirically in Klinefelter
syndrome.

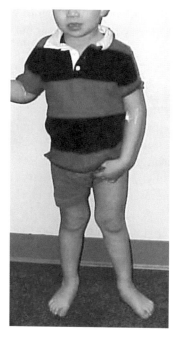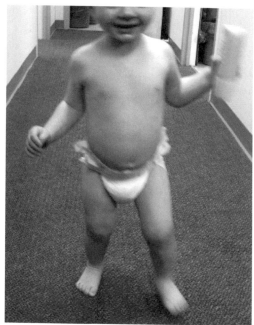

Figure 2.4
Decreased lower extremity muscle tone in boys with Klinefelter syndrome.

In addition, Netley and Rovet (1984) suggest that individuals with X-chromosome aneuploidy have atypical lateral dominance, specifically an excess of non-right-handedness. They observed that 8 out of 47 boys with Klinefelter syndrome (24%) followed in a Toronto study were not right-handed, compared with 10% of children in a comparison group. These researchers interpreted their finding as consistent with evidence that individuals with Klinefelter syndrome demonstrate atypical patterns of cerebral dominance. However, Ratcliffe et al. (1982b) found no difference in patterns of lateral dominance in a follow-up of 33 individuals with Klinefelter syndrome who had been identified as newborns.

Cognitive Phenotype

Klinefelter syndrome has been reported to be a common cause of developmental delay of unknown etiology among prepubertal boys (Khalifa & Struthers, 2002). In contrast to conditions such as fragile X syndrome (see chapter 3, this volume), which can result in mild to moderate mental retardation, Klinefelter syndrome results in rather selective cognitive impairment described below (Ratcliffe, 1999; Robinson et al., 1986; Rovet et al., 1995; Walzer et al., 1990). Exceptions to this general trend can occur when the disorder is accompanied by additional conditions with cognitive implications (e.g., a seizure disorder) or when there is increased numerical chromosome loading (e.g., 48,XXXY).

Intelligence   The natural history of cognitive development in Klinefelter syndrome has been derived from several prospective, population-based longitudinal studies (Ratcliffe, 1999; Robinson et al., 1986; Rovet et al., 1995). General intelligence as measured by a Full Scale IQ (FSIQ) score varies greatly but is typically within normal limits. While FSIQ estimates in children and adolescents with Klinefelter syndrome tend to be lower than siblings or other comparison groups (Ratcliffe, 1999; Robinson et al., 1986; Rovet et al., 1995; Walzer et al., 1990), this disparity is not as apparent in adults with Klinefelter syndrome (Geschwind et al., 1998; Porter et al., 1988).

Despite having average FSIQ scores, Verbal IQ (VIQ) is often depressed relative to Performance IQ (PIQ). This discrepancy has been observed in both children and adults with Klinefelter syndrome (Graham et al., 1988; Porter et al., 1988; Ratcliffe et al., 1986; Robinson et al., 1986; Rovet et al., 1996; Walzer et al., 1990), although this profile may vary across the life span. For example, in one study of 35 males with Klinefelter syndrome who were 16 to 61 years old, the younger men had decreased VIQ versus PIQ, motor impairment, and language dysfunction, consistent with the VIQ/PIQ difference, whereas the older men had decreased PIQ versus VIQ, intact language function, and impairment of visual–spatial and executive function skills (Boone et al., 2001). This change in the VIQ relative to PIQ pattern may reflect improved language processing possibly related to androgen treatment in the older males with Klinefelter syndrome (Stewart et al., 1982b).

Academic Abilities   A survey of early studies suggested that learning disabilities associated with Klinefelter syndrome are primarily verbal in nature and are evident early in the school-age years. By 7 years, boys with Klinefelter syndrome have moderate to severe problems with reading, spelling, and writing, but not with arithmetic (Nielsen et al., 1981; Stewart et al., 1979; Walzer, 1985). As children progress through elementary and middle school, problems in other areas of achievement become more evident. By age 10, many boys with Klinefelter syndrome show delays in arithmetic of comparable severity to their problems in reading and spelling (Leonard & Sparrow, 1986; Stewart et al., 1982b). With the emergence of math difficulties and the reported limitations in acquiring general knowledge in other academic content areas in later grades, very few older boys with Klinefelter syndrome have pure reading or arithmetic problems. Instead, these boys may demonstrate a generalized learning disability, performing several grades below expected grade levels in basic areas of achievement (Rovet et al., 1996). Approximately 50%–75% of boys with Klinefelter syndrome demonstrate a specific reading disability at some point in their development (Bender et al., 1993; Graham et al., 1988), and 60%–86% require some special education (Robinson et al., 1986; Walzer, 1985). Although most succeed in graduating from high school, many repeat at least one grade and relatively few complete higher levels of education (Leonard & Sparrow, 1986).

Language Abilities   Longitudinal studies have consistently revealed that 70%–80% of males with Klinefelter syndrome demonstrate difficulties with language development and language-based learning. These anomalies are often initially observed as delays in early expressive language and speech milestones (Walzer et al., 1982; Bender et al., 1983; Nielsen & Sorensen, 1984; Graham et al., 1988). In a follow-up of 40,000 births at a public hospital in Denver, Robinson et al. (1979) noted that children with Klinefelter syndrome demonstrated delayed speech at 24 months of age, while others have reported that delays in language and speech development may be apparent by age 2 to 3 years (Bender et al., 1993; Ratcliffe, 1999; Robinson et al., 1979).

Among most boys with Klinefelter syndrome, problems in expressive language remain evident, in some form, at all ages. Speech sound production is not consistently impaired (Graham et al., 1988; Walzer et al., 1990). Rather, as children develop, significant impairments are frequently observed in higher order aspects of expressive language, particularly in deficits with word retrieval, expressive grammar, and narrative formulation (Graham et al., 1988; Robinson et al., 1986; Walzer et al., 1990). These problems reflect difficulties accessing, retrieving, and applying linguistic information. Difficulties in some aspect of language output frequently persist into adulthood (Boone et al., 2001; Geschwind et al., 2000; Nielsen & Pelsen, 1987; Porter et al., 1988).

Aspects of receptive processing of language are also commonly impaired in males with Klinefelter syndrome. Several studies have noted relative deficiencies in phonemic discrimination (Bender et al., 1993; Graham et al., 1988; Nielsen et al., 1980; Walzer, 1985), slower verbal processing speed, and difficulties in understanding the grammatical and morphological aspects of language (Walzer et al., 1990). It has been suggested that problems with receptive language are most evident on tasks requiring the perception and short-term memory of sequential auditory information. Some researchers propose that this pattern of difficulties stems from primary processing deficits in auditory temporal processing and working memory (Rovet et al., 1996), while others propose that these language-based problems cannot be explained in terms of these cognitive impairments (Geschwind et al., 2000).

Neuropsychological studies have further suggested that the cognitive phenotype of Klinefelter syndrome may be related to anomalous development of functional hemispheric asymmetries in cerebral development. Although most typically developing right-handed children demonstrate left-hemisphere dominance in processing language from an early age, the results of dichotic listening tests (Alexander et al., 1998; Netley & Rovet, 1984; Netley et al., 1995) suggest that individuals with Klinefelter syndrome have greater than usual right-hemisphere (vs. left-hemisphere) involvement in processing language. This alteration in hemispheric organization may be related to altered fetal brain growth rates and the failure of the left hemisphere to gain dominance in language processing (Netley & Rovet, 1984). D. H. Geschwind and colleagues (1998) suggest that anomalous cerebral dominance in Klinefelter syndrome may be related to alterations in gene dosage in the pseudoautosomal region of the X chromosome.

Anomalous cortical processing of speech is also reflected in the increased latency of late components of event-related responses to phonemic probes (Netley & Rovet, 1984). In addition, a volumetric study of brain structure by Patwardhan and colleagues (2000, 2002) revealed that, relative to typically developing children, individuals with Klinefelter syndrome demonstrate significant reductions in left temporal lobe gray matter volume and in the amygdala (but not in the hippocampus). These researchers speculate that their findings may provide a structural basis for the observed neuropsychological deficits in Klinefelter syndrome, as evident in reduced performance on measures of word retrieval, reading skill, auditory short-term memory, and verbal IQ. Interestingly, a subgroup of males with Klinefelter syndrome who were treated with testosterone showed relative preservation of temporal lobe gray matter bilaterally and demonstrated relative sparing of verbal skills in comparison to the untreated subgroup of males with Klinefelter syndrome.

These testosterone treatment effects on structural neuroimaging must be interpreted with considerable caution, because they are based on a small number of boys (5 treated, 5 untreated). Yet multiple studies have examined the relationship between certain verbal abilities and the response to testosterone in androgen-deficient, hypogonadal adolescents and adults. In general, testosterone replacement for intervals ranging from 2 to 12 months or more has been associated with improved verbal fluency (Alexander et al., 1998; Cherrier et al., 2004; O'Connor et al., 2001; Patwardhan et al., 2000), VIQ (Netley, 1992), and verbal memory (Cherrier et al., 2001; Cherrier et al., 2003; Moffat et al., 2002).

Attention and Executive Function   Attentional deficits are frequently detected on neuropsychological assessment of males with Klinefelter syndrome. Behavioral or anecdotal observations have included reports of increased distractibility and problems with concentration that some researchers interpret as a reflection of a language-based learning disability rather than comorbid attentional problems (Rovet et al., 1996; Theilgaard, 1984). The Klinefelter syndrome cognitive phenotype also includes impaired working memory (Bender et al., 1993; Boone et al., 2001; Fales et al., 2003) and executive function (Bender et al., 1993; Boone et al., 2001; Temple & Sanfilippo,

2003) that is not limited to logical, conceptual, and relational reasoning (Fales et al., 2003).

There are few studies of executive function in children with Klinefelter syndrome, but several reports in adults have suggested that deficiencies in this area are as marked as are the language-based difficulties (Boone et al., 2001; D. H. Geschwind et al., 2000). Temple and Sanfilippo (2003) examined the performance of three 10-year-old boys with Klinefelter syndrome on measures of (a) problem solving and conceptual shifting, (b) speeded responding and (c) planning. They also examined inhibitory processes, measures of problem solving and conceptual shifting as assessed with the Wisconsin Card Sort Test, and the Trail-Making Test. Compared to boys without Klinefelter syndrome, all three boys with Klinefelter syndrome demonstrated difficulty on at least two of the four measures used to assess inhibitory function.

In addition, on speeded tasks such as word fluency and figural fluency, the boys with Klinefelter syndrome made more errors (including perseverative errors) than did boys without Klinefelter syndrome, despite generating an adequate number of responses. No measurable impairment was observed among the boys with Klinefelter syndrome on other measures of executive function such as the Tower of London task, self-ordered pointing, and the Rey-Osterreith Complex Figure Test. Although these results are based on a very small number of participants (including one boy with a co-diagnosis of Asperger syndrome), the findings suggest that deficits in executive function are evident in school-age boys with Klinefelter syndrome and that these difficulties are limited to faulty inhibitory processes, in both inhibiting responses to distraction and in an exaggerated degree of rigid inhibition. These results differ in some important respects from the findings in adults with Klinefelter syndrome, in whom a more pervasive involvement of executive dysfunction has been reported (Boone et al., 2001; D. H. Geschwind et al., 2000). The dissimilarity across age groups may relate to methodological differences or simply to variability inherent in this population.

Behavioral Phenotype

Social Development   Klinefelter syndrome is associated with a fairly characteristic behavioral profile that includes quiet, shy, and unassertive personalities; diminished self-esteem (Ratcliffe et al., 1982a; Stewart et al., 1986); increased anxiety; and increased social isolation (table 2.1; Mandoki et al., 1991; Nielsen & Pelsen, 1987; Ratcliffe, 1999). The role of androgen deficiency in the emergence of these characteristics has not been established, but indirect evidence suggests a possible contribution. For example, testosterone replacement in boys with delayed puberty has been associated with improved self-perceived competence (Schwab et al., 2001), energy level, and mood (Wang et al., 1996, 2000). Interestingly, testosterone replacement therapy does not make androgen-deficient males aggressive. High doses (three times the replacement dose) of testosterone administered to men without Klinefelter does not lead to increased aggression or mood disturbances. In contrast, hypogonadal men who received testosterone replacement have reduced negative mood (tension, anger, fatigue) and increased vigor (O'Connor et al., 2002).

Salbenblatt et al. (1981) noted that boys with Klinefelter syndrome demonstrate problems with emotional adjustment, evident in poor relationships with peers and increased anger and depression. While emotional problems may be more evident in boys with Klinefelter syndrome during times of stress, this may reflect chronic behavioral and emotional adjustment problems. Manifestations of the behavioral disturbances in more chronically maladjusted individuals may include encopresis, suicidal thoughts, and acting out against persons and property. These behavior problems are less common in children diagnosed at birth perhaps because awareness of the diagnosis results in greater attention and support for the associated problems that can emerge with learning and language development.

The Toronto study of males with Klinefelter syndrome revealed decreased sexual interest, perhaps related to reduced serum levels of testosterone. Males with Klinefelter syndrome lack self-confidence and are easily misled, are more reserved and aloof, and are more likely to disregard rules than participants in the comparison group (Stewart et al., 1990). As adolescents, males with Klinefelter syndrome appear to have greater difficulty in both impulse control and conforming to societal guidelines. While early maladjustment does not necessarily predict later maladjustment, school performance in early adolescence is a predictor of later personal and social concerns. The ability to perform successfully in school is regarded as a major determinant of long-term adjustment.

A compelling and insightful personal account of the interaction of physical, neuropsychological, and personality characteristics was recently provided by Grace (2004), who noted that high school was both an academic and social struggle. By sixth grade (at 12 years of age), his extremely tall stature (180 m) and skinny frame made him an easy mark for the teasing and taunts of his peers. The stigma of his image as a social outcast was further exacerbated by slow academic progress, the need for special education, and his teachers' opinion that he was lazy. His Klinefelter syndrome–associated problems extended into adulthood. Lack of upper-body strength for manual work left him short of stamina. Social interaction with work colleagues continued to be difficult.

Brain Development: Neurophysiological Correlates

Event-Related Potentials

Netley et al. (1995) described the results of a longitudinal event-related potential study carried out with a sample of 18 males with Klinefelter syndrome. They used a stimulus oddball procedure to measure response inhibition during orthographic and phonemic discrimination tasks. Both N2 and P3 response latencies and amplitude measures were obtained as independent variables. From other studies, it is evident that these N2 and P3 waveforms are the key indicators of active inhibitory processing (e.g., Roche et al., 2005) and that the frontal N2 measures may correspond to response suppression while P3 may measure intent to respond. Netley and colleagues reported that P3 response latencies were highly correlated with VIQ but not PIQ scores among males with Klinefelter syndrome. Moreover, the discrepancy between VIQ and PIQ scores was strongly associated with P3 latency, but only for latencies obtained during the phonemic discrimination task and not during the more visual, orthographic task. These associations emerged at all three ages during which they were examined, including before, during, and after puberty. Netley and colleagues argue that these associations contrast with the lack of any such associations observed between P3 latencies and IQ scores in the general population. The P3 component is thought to reflect stimulus classification or updating of information in working memory. Increased P3 latencies seemed to reflect prolonged processing times and indicated problems with working memory that impact on verbal skill development in males with Klinefelter syndrome.

Structural Neuroimaging

There appear to be early genetic effects of the additional X chromosome on brain growth and development, resulting in relative microcephaly at birth in males with Klinefelter syndrome that persists and correlates with IQ. Support for relative microcephaly being related to genetic rather than hormonal mechanisms comes from the genetic model of females with the karyotype 47,XXX (Ratcliffe et al., 1986; Ratcliffe et al., 1994b) who are not androgen-deficient but who tend to have relatively small heads. In addition, both males with Klinefelter syndrome and females with 47,XXX have increased speech and language problems, decreased coordination, and increased academic difficulties (Linden, 2002).

Persistent microcephaly has not been demonstrated in all studies (Ross et al., 2005). Radcliffe et al. (1994a) suggest that head circumference is significantly lower at birth (-0.7 SD) in males with Klinefelter syndrome, but is not evident by 9 years of age. The velocity of head growth in the first 6 months is slightly below that of controls but increases at ages 2 to 3 years.

Although head circumference may normalize with age, structural neuroimaging studies suggest persistent anomalies of brain development. Shen et al. (2004) performed an automated voxel-based morphometric parcellization and volumetric analysis of 34 males with Klinefelter syndrome ranging in age from 5 to 19 years. Compared to 62 males without Klinefelter syndrome, males with Klinefelter syndrome demonstrated relative reductions in brain volume in the insula temporal gyri, amygdala, hippocampus, cingulate gyrus, and occipital gyri. These local reductions in volume resulted in overall enlargement of lateral ventricles and diminished overall white and gray matter volumes. Similar findings were also reported by Warwick et al. (1999, 2003).

Functional Neuroimaging

Itti et al. (2003) obtained single photon emission computed tomography (SPECT) scans from 9 men with Klinefelter syndrome, ages 18 to 37 years. SPECT images obtained at rest showed significant leftward blood flow asymmetry in right-handed individuals without Klinefelter syndrome. Specifically, these asymmetries were evident in perirolandic gyri (precentral, middle, and postcentral), perisylvian areas (insula, superior, middle, and transverse temporal), the cuneus, superior and inferior parietal gyri, and cerebellum. By contrast, the adults with Klinefelter syndrome demonstrated symmetric activation in most volumes of interest with the exception of the central gyrus, transverse temporal gyrus, and cerebellum. Overall, the males with Klinefelter syndrome appeared to lack the leftward cerebral perfusion asymmetry evident in normally developing right-handed individuals.

Hormonal Factors Influencing Development

Testosterone influences brain development and function, beginning in utero. It continues to exert apparent organizational effects in childhood and adulthood. Both animal and human studies have shown clear-cut structural effects of androgen on subcortical nuclear regions such as the hypothalamic/preoptic area and the forebrain regions (Juraska, 1991; Matsumoto, 1991; Rasika et al., 1994). Therefore, decreased testosterone levels in males with Klinefelter syndrome may influence functional outcome. Androgen alterations during the perinatal period and puberty influence cognitive function and behavior in animal and human models. Gonadal steroids during human fetal development lead to select gender differences in cognition (D. H. Geschwind et al., 1998; N. Geschwind & Galaburda, 1985). For instance, in the general population, males tend to outperform females (on average) in performance during very specific spatial tasks involving mental rotation, spatial perception, targeting (e.g., throwing darts or catching a ball), or spatial visualization (D. H. Geschwind et al., 1998; N. Geschwind & Galaburda, 1985).

   Table 2.1 is a summary of the aspects of the Klinefelter syndrome motor function and cognitive phenotypes that may be due to androgen deficiency and to respond to androgen treatment. Muscle weakness, motor dysfunction, working memory impairment, and attentional deficits represent major problem areas in the development of boys with Klinefelter syndrome, and these are the most likely aspects of the phenotype to be androgen responsive.

The most commonly reported positive effects of androgen replacement therapy in androgen-deficient males have been in the area of muscle function and body composition. Most adolescents and adults with Klinefelter syndrome who have been treated with testosterone report improved endurance and strength (Robinson et al., 1986; Salbenblatt et al., 1987). Testosterone replacement in hypogonadal men is associated with increased lean body mass, increased muscle mass and strength, and faster speed of walking 30 m and climbing stairs (Brill et al., 2002; Herbst & Bhasin, 2004), without change in lipids, liver, or kidney function (Bhasin et al., 1997; Brodsky et al., 1996; Ly et al., 2001; Wang et al., 2000). In normal healthy young men, testosterone treatment for 20 weeks increases both muscle strength and leg power (Storer et al., 2003), and testosterone treatment in adult males who received systemic glucocorticoids also improves muscle mass and strength (Crawford et al., 2003). Additionally, androgen oxandrolone has been used in boys (mean age = 7 years) with muscular dystrophy, who demonstrate improved arm muscle strength after 6 months (Fenichel et al., 2001). Oxandrolone treatment (12 weeks) of males with inclusion body myositis is associated with improved upper extremity strength and stair climbing (Rutkove et al., 2002). Oxandrolone has been demonstrated to safely induce improvement in lean body mass, muscle area, and strength in elderly men (Schroeder et al., 2003).

Androgen effects on muscle are initiated by testosterone, the androgen present in males in the highest concentration, binding to the androgen receptor (AR) and leading to transcription of specific genes affecting myogenesis. Motor neurons and skeletal muscle fibers both have ARs and are potential sites of androgen action. Initially, testosterone increases motor neuron size, and later in life it maintains the relative size of the motor neurons and muscle fibers (Kadi & Thornell, 2000; Sinha-Hikim et al., 2002). On the basis of in vivo laboratory tests and extensive clinical information, oxandrolone, a synthetic androgen, also acts at the level of the AR, is an AR agonist in vivo, and affects androgen-responsive target tissues (Kemppainen et al., 1999). Different androgens have distinct promoter activation profiles and vary in their biological actions on androgen-responsive target tissues. Oxandrolone is much less virilizing, less hepatotoxic, and less active at a cellular level compared to testosterone (Hart et al., 2001). Short-term testosterone and oxandrolone administration both increase skeletal muscle protein synthesis (Barrow et al., 2003; Bhasin et al., 1996; Sheffield-Moore et al., 1999). The critical interaction of androgen and motor neurons in males is demonstrated by Kennedy's disease, in which an abnormality in the AR is associated with degeneration of motor neurons (Sperfeld et al., 2002).

Androgens may also influence brain structural development and function. Multiple studies have examined the relationship between aspects of attention and working memory and response to testosterone in androgen-deficient, hypogonadal adolescents and adults. In general, testosterone replacement for intervals ranging from 2 to 12 months or more has been associated with improved attention (Cherrier et al., 2002;

Kenny et al., 2002) and working memory (Janowsky et al., 2000). Androgen replacement in the androgen-deficient population of girls with Turner syndrome has also been associated with improved working memory after 2 years of treatment (Ross et al., 2003).

Brain development in males with Klinefelter syndrome may be altered by androgen deficiency early in life, X-chromosome gene excess dosage effects, or both. N. Geschwind and Galaburda (1985) proposed that cerebral dominance for language is related to prenatal testosterone levels. They hypothesized that higher levels of testosterone in utero create greater hemispheric asymmetry that in turn leads to better language ability. Since males with Klinefelter syndrome have decreased testosterone during fetal development, brain differentiation would theoretically be affected. Functional neuroimaging studies of males with Klinefelter syndrome have shown altered left hemisphere metabolism (Itti et al., 2003) consistent with the verbal and language deficits and reduced left temporal and amygdala volumes on structural brain scans (Warwick et al., 1999). These findings appear to be associated with alterations in lateral asymmetries in brain development (Patwardhan et al., 2002; Patwardhan et al., 2000). Language ability is asymmetrically organized in the brain, with nearly all right-handers and two thirds of left-handers demonstrating left-hemisphere language dominance (Galaburda et al., 1978). By contrast, there is evidence to suggest reduced involvement of the left hemisphere in language-processing tasks in males with Klinefelter syndrome. To some extent, these differences may be amenable to alteration with hormone replacement therapy (N. Geschwind & Galaburda, 1985). Androgen replacement in males with Klinefelter syndrome (and others with androgen deficiency) has been associated with relatively increased left temporal cortical volumes (Patwardhan et al., 2000) and altered brain perfusion or morphology (Alexander et al., 1998; Itti et al., 2003; Netley & Rovet, 1984; Netley et al., 1995). However, there have been very few studies of the relationship between cognition, brain function, and testosterone replacement in males with Klinefelter syndrome.

Early Androgen Replacement in Males with Klinefelter Syndrome

In 1942, Klinefelter et al. suggested that testosterone therapy (available since the 1930s) be used for the hypoandrogenism, noting that this intervention did not improve fertility or gynecomastia. Subsequently, considerable interest has been devoted to the possibility that androgen replacement may influence aspects of motor and cognitive function in boys with Klinefelter syndrome. Earlier testosterone replacement may possibly contribute to improved motor and cognitive skills with potential educational impact such as reduced need for special education. In addition, alterations in structural or functional cerebral organization may be more likely to occur in younger than older brains.

Adrenarche in Klinefelter Syndrome

A question could be raised about the contribution of adrenal androgens to the testosterone deficiency phenotype in boys with Klinefelter syndrome. Adrenarche, a developmental change in the adrenal glands (that occurs at about age 7–9 years in boys) is characterized by an increase in adrenal 17-ketosteroid production (de Peretti & Forest, 1978; Korth-Schutz et al., 1976). It is synchronized with the onset of sexual hair growth (pubarche) and is separate and distinct from pubertal development of gonadal function (gonadarche; Counts et al., 1987). The biomarker of this process is a rise in serum dehydroepiandrosterone (DHEA) and its sulfate (DHEAS). DHEA is a precursor to both testosterone and estradiol and is considered to be a weak androgen because neither DHEA nor DHEAS acts directly via the AR but must first be converted to testosterone. The circulating concentration of testosterone rises minimally during adrenarche (40–50 ng/dl in prepubertal boys), compared with levels attained in normal male puberty (200–1,000 ng/dl; Auchus & Rainey, 2004). Adrenarche occurs independent of puberty/gonadarche such that even children with gonadal failure undergo adrenarche (Martin et al., 2004; Sklar et al., 1980). Adrenarche or pubarche has been reported as normal in boys with Klinefelter syndrome at ages 5–10 years (Sperling, 2002; Topper et al., 1982), despite their low testosterone levels. Therefore, it is unlikely that the adrenal androgens have a significant effect on the phenotype in boys with Klinefelter syndrome.

Summary

Klinefelter syndrome has been studied for more than 50 years. The phenotype includes muscle weakness and motor and cognitive dysfunction that is probably due to both genetic and hormonal abnormalities. The disorder can be identified early in life and is associated with early androgen deficiency. Multiple lines of evidence support the contention that androgen replacement may influence brain development and have an impact on motor and cognitive function. There is a strong rationale for identifying boys with this disorder early in childhood.

The distinctive behavioral and cognitive features have suggested the existence of perturbations in the normative unfolding of multiple developmental competencies and reflect perturbations in brain development. There is growing evidence from both the neuropsychological profiles as well as structural and functional neuroimaging studies that the problems observed in Klinefelter syndrome are not related to widespread or diffuse aberrations in neurodevelopment but instead may reflect maldevelopment or dysfunction of neural systems distributed in the left cerebral hemisphere. The goal of this chapter has been to characterize this rather common disorder. Early identification and intervention will help children with Klinefelter syndrome achieve normal adult milestones.

Acknowledgment

This work was supported in part by National Institutes of Health Grant NS050597.

References

Abramsky, L., & Chapple, J. (1997). 47,XXY (Klinefelter syndrome) and 47,XYY: Estimated rates of and indication for postnatal diagnosis with implications for prenatal counselling. *Prenatal Diagnosis, 17,* 363–368.

Alexander, G. M., Swerdloff, R. S., Wang, C., Davidson, T., McDonald, V., Steiner, B., et al. (1998). Androgen–behavior correlations in hypogonadal men and eugonadal men: II. Cognitive abilities. *Hormones and Behavior, 33*(2), 85–94.

Auchus, R. J., & Rainey, W. E. (2004). Adrenarche—Physiology, biochemistry and human disease. *Clinical Endocrinology (Oxf), 60,* 288–296.

Barrow, R. E., Dasu, M. R., Ferrando, A. A., Spies, M., Thomas, S. J., Perez-Polo, J. R., et al. (2003). Gene expression patterns in skeletal muscle of thermally injured children treated with oxandrolone. *Annals of Surgery, 237,* 422–428.

Bender, B., Fry, E., Pennington, B., Puck, M., Salbenblatt, J., & Robinson, A. (1983). Speech and language development in 41 children with sex chromosome anomalies. *Pediatrics, 71,* 262–267.

Bender, B. G., Linden, M. G., & Robinson, A. (1993). Neuropsychological impairment in 42 adolescents with sex chromosome abnormalities. *American Journal of Medical Genetics, 48,* 169–173.

Bhasin, S., Storer, T. W., Berman, N., Callegari, C., Clevenger, B., Phillips, J., et al. (1996). The effects of supraphysiologic doses of testosterone on muscle size and strength in normal men. *New England Journal of Medicine, 335*(1), 1–7.

Bhasin, S., Storer, T. W., Berman, N., Yarasheski, K. E., Clevenger, B., Phillips, J., et al. (1997). Testosterone replacement increases fat-free mass and muscle size in hypogonadal men. *Journal of Clinical Endocrinology and Metabolism, 82*(2), 407–413.

Bojesen, A., Juul, S., & Gravholt, C. H. (2003). Prenatal and postnatal prevalence of Klinefelter syndrome: A national registry study. *Journal of Clinical Endocrinology and Metabolism, 88,* 622–626.

Boone, K. B., Swerdloff, R. S., Miller, B. L., Geschwind, D. H., Razani, J., Lee, A., et al. (2001). Neuropsychological profiles of adults with Klinefelter syndrome. *Journal of the International Neuropsychological Society, 7,* 446–456.

Bradbury, J., Bunge, R. G., & Boccabella, R. A. (1956). Chromatin test in Klinefelter's syndrome. *Journal of Clinical Endocrinology and Metabolism, 16,* 689.

Brill, K. T., Weltman, A. L., Gentili, A., Patrie, J. T., Fryburg, D. A., Hanks, J. B., et al. (2002). Single and combined effects of growth hormone and testosterone administration on measures of body composition, physical performance, mood, sexual function, bone turnover, and muscle gene expression in healthy older men. *Journal of Clinical Endocrinology and Metabolism, 87,* 5649–5657.

Brodsky, I. G., Balagopal, P., & Nair, K. S. (1996). Effects of testosterone replacement on muscle mass and muscle protein synthesis in hypogonadal men—A clinical research center study. *Journal of Clinical Endocrinology and Metabolism, 81,* 3469–3475.

Caldwell, P. D., & Smith, D. W. (1972). The XXY (Klinefelter's) syndrome in childhood: Detection and treatment. *Journal of Pediatrics, 80,* 250–258.

Cherrier, M. M., Anawalt, B. D., Herbst, K. L., Amory, J. K., Craft, S., Matsumoto, A. M., et al. (2002). Cognitive effects of short-term manipulation of serum sex steroids in healthy young men. *Journal of Clinical Endocrinology and Metabolism, 87,* 3090–3096.

Cherrier, M. M., Asthana, S., Plymate, S., Baker, L., Matsumoto, A. M., Peskind, E., et al. (2001). Testosterone supplementation improves spatial and verbal memory in healthy older men. *Neurology, 57,* 80–88.

Cherrier, M. M., Craft, S., & Matsumoto, A. H. (2003). Cognitive changes associated with supplementation of testosterone or dihydrotestosterone in mildly hypogonadal men: A preliminary report. *Journal of Andrology, 24,* 568–576.

Cherrier, M. M., Plymate, S., Mohan, S., Asthana, S., Matsumoto, A. M., Bremner, W., et al. (2004). Relationship between testosterone supplementation and insulin-like growth factor: I. levels and cognition in healthy older men. *Psychoneuroendocrinology, 29*(1), 65–82.

Counts, D. R., Pescovitz, O. H., Barnes, K. M., Hench, K. D., Chrousos, G. P., Sherins, R. J., et al. (1987). Dissociation of adrenarche and gonadarche in precocious puberty and in isolated hypogonadotropic hypogonadism. *Journal of Clinical Endocrinology and Metabolism, 64,* 1174–1178.

Crawford, B. A., Liu, P. Y., Kean, M. T., Bleasel, J. F., & Handelsman, D. J. (2003). Randomized placebo-controlled trial of androgen effects on muscle and bone in men requiring long-term systemic glucocorticoid treatment. *Journal of Clinical Endocrinology and Metabolism, 88,* 3167–3176.

de Peretti, E., & Forest, M. G. (1978). Pattern of plasma dehydroepiandrosterone sulfate levels in humans from birth to adulthood: Evidence for testicular production. *Journal of Clinical Endocrinology and Metabolism, 47,* 572–577.

Fales, C. L., Knowlton, B. J., Holyoak, K. J., Geschwind, D. H., Swerdloff, R. S., & Gonzalo, I. G. (2003). Working memory and relational reasoning in Klinefelter syndrome. *Journal of the International Neuropsychological Society, 9,* 839–846.

Fenichel, G. M., Griggs, R. C., Kissel, J., Kramer, T. I., Mendell, J. R., Moxley, R. T., et al. (2001). A randomized efficacy and safety trial of oxandrolone in the treatment of Duchenne dystrophy. *Neurology, 56,* 1075–1079.

Ferguson-Smith, M. (1959). The prepubertal testicular lesion in chromatin positive Klinefelter's Syndrome (primary micro-orchidism) as seen in mentally handicapped children. *Lancet, 1,* 219–222.

Forest, M. G., Cathiard, A. M., & Bertrand, J. A. (1973a). Evidence of testicular activity in early infancy. *Journal of Clinical Endocrinology and Metabolism, 37*(1), 148–151.

Forest, M. G., Cathiard, A. M., & Bertrand, J. A. (1973b). Total and unbound testosterone levels in the newborn and in normal and hypogonadal children: Use of a sensitive radioimmunoassay for testosterone. *Journal of Clinical Endocrinology and Metabolism, 36,* 1132–1142.

Forest, M. G., Sizonenko, P. C., Cathiard, A. M., & Bertrand, J. (1974). Hypophyso-gonadal function in humans during the first year of life: I. Evidence for testicular activity in early infancy. *Journal of Clinical Investigation, 53,* 819–828.

Galaburda, A. M., LeMay, M., Kemper, T. L., & Geschwind, N. (1978). Right–left asymmetrics in the brain. *Science, 199,* 852–856.

Geschwind, D. H., Boone, K. B., Miller, B. L., & Swerdloff, R. S. (2000). Neurobehavioral phenotype of Klinefelter syndrome. *Mental Retardation and Developmental Disabilities Research Reviews, 6*(2), 107–116.

Geschwind, D. H., Gregg, J., Boone, K., Karrim, J., Pawlikowska-Haddal, A., Rao, E., et al. (1998). Klinefelter's syndrome as a model of anomalous cerebral laterality: Testing gene dosage in the X chromosome pseudoautosomal region using a DNA microarray. *Developmental Genetics, 23*(3), 215–229.

Geschwind, N., & Galaburda, A. M. (1985). Cerebral lateralization. Biological mechanisms, associations, and pathology: II. A hypothesis and a program for research. *Archives of Neurology, 42,* 521–552.

Grace, R. J. (2004). Klinefelter's syndrome: A late diagnosis. *Lancet, 364*(9430), 284.

Graham, J. M., Jr., Bashir, A. S., Stark, R. E., Silbert, A., & Walzer, S. (1988). Oral and written language abilities of XXY boys: Implications for anticipatory guidance. *Pediatrics, 81,* 795–806.

Hart, D. W., Wolf, S. E., Ramzy, P. I., Chinkes, D. L., Beauford, R. B., Ferrando, A. A., et al. (2001). Anabolic effects of oxandrolone after severe burn. *Annals of Surgery, 233,* 556–564.

Herbst, K. L., & Bhasin, S. (2004). Testosterone action on skeletal muscle. *Current Opinion in Clinical Nutrition and Metabolic Care, 7*(3), 271–277.

Hines, M., Fane, B. A., Pasterski, V. L., Mathews, G. A., Conway, G. S., & Brook, C. (2003). Spatial abilities following prenatal androgen abnormality: Targeting and mental rotations performance in individuals with congenital adrenal hyperplasia. *Psychoneuroendocrinology, 28,* 1010–1026.

Iitsuka, Y., Bock, A., Nguyen, D. D., Samango-Sprouse, C. A., Simpson, J. L., & Bischoff, F. Z. (2001). Evidence of skewed X-chromosome inactivation in 47,XXY and 48,XXYY Klinefelter patients. *American Journal of Medical Genetics, 98*(1), 25–31.

Itti, E., Gaw Gonzalo, I. T., Boone, K. B., Geschwind, D. H., Berman, N., Pawlikowska-Haddal, A., et al. (2003). Functional neuroimaging provides evidence of anomalous cerebral laterality in adults with Klinefelter's syndrome. *Annals of Neurology, 54,* 669–673.

Jacobs, P. A. (1979). The incidence and etiology of sex chromosme abnormalities in man. *Birth Defects Original Article Series, 15,* 3–14.

Jacobs, P. A., Hassold, T. J., Whittington, E., Butler, G., Collyer, S., Keston, M., et al. (1988). Klinefelter's syndrome: An analysis of the origin of the additional sex chromosome using molecular probes. *Annals of Human Genetics, 52*(Pt 2), 93–109.

Janowsky, J. S., Chavez, B., & Orwoll, E. (2000). Sex steroids modify working memory. *Journal of Cognitive Neuroscience, 12,* 407–414.

Jones, D. L. (1997). *Smith's recognizable patterns of human malformation* (5th ed.). Philadelphia: Saunders.

Juraska, J. M. (1991). Sex differences in "cognitive" regions of the rat brain. *Psychoneuroendocrinology, 16*(1–3), 105–109.

Kadi, F., & Thornell, L. E. (2000). Concomitant increases in myonuclear and satellite cell content in female trapezius muscle following strength training. *Histochemistry and Cell Biology, 113*(2), 99–103.

Kamischke, A., Baumgardt, A., Horst, J., & Nieschlag, E. (2003). Clinical and diagnostic features of patients with suspected Klinefelter syndrome. *Journal of Andrology, 24,* 41–48.

Kemppainen, J. A., Langley, E., Wong, C. I., Bobseine, K., Kelce, W. R., & Wilson, E. M. (1999). Distinguishing androgen receptor agonists and antagonists: Distinct mechanisms of activation by medroxyprogesterone acetate and dihydrotestosterone. *Molecular Endocrinology, 13,* 440–454.

Kenny, A. M., Bellantonio, S., Gruman, C. A., Acosta, R. D., & Prestwood, K. M. (2002). Effects of transdermal testosterone on cognitive function and health perception in older men with low bioavailable testosterone levels. *The Journals of Gerontology. Series A, Biological Sciences and Medical Sciences, 57,* M321–325.

Khalifa, M. M., & Struthers, J. L. (2002). Klinefelter syndrome is a common cause for mental retardation of unknown etiology among prepubertal males. *Clinical Genetics, 61,* 49–53.

Klinefelter, H., Reifenstein, E. C., & Albright, F. (1942). Syndrome characterized by gynecomastia, aspermatogenesis, without a-Leydigism and increased excretion of follicle stimulating hormone. *Journal of Clinical Endocrinology and Metabolism, 2,* 615–627.

Korth-Schutz, S., Levine, L. S., & New, M. I. (1976). Serum androgens in normal prepubertal and pubertal children and in children with precocious adrenarche. *Journal of Clinical Endocrinology and Metabolism, 42,* 117–124.

Lahlou, N., Fennoy, I., Carel, J. C., & Roger, M. (2004). Inhibin b and anti-Mullerian hormone, but not testosterone levels, are normal in infants with nonmosaic Klinefelter syndrome. *Journal of Clinical Endocrinology and Metabolism, 89,* 1864–1868.

Laron, Z., & Hochman, I. H. (1971). Small testes in prepubetal boys with Klinefelter's syndrome. *Journal of Clinical Endocrinology and Metabolism, 32,* 671–672.

Leonard, M. F., & Sparrow, S. (1986). Prospective study of development of children with sex chromosome anomalies: New Haven study: IV. Adolescence. *Birth Defects Original Article Series, 22*(3), 221–249.

Linden, M., and Bender, B. G. (2002). Fifty-one prenatally diagnosed children and adolescents with sex chromosome abnormalities. *American Journal of Medical Genetics, 110,* 11–18.

Ly, L. P., Jimenez, M., Zhuang, T. N., Celermajer, D. S., Conway, A. J., & Handelsman, D. J. (2001). A double-blind, placebo-controlled, randomized clinical trial of transdermal dihydrotestosterone gel on muscular strength, mobility, and quality of life in older men with partial androgen deficiency. *Journal of Clinical Endocrinology and Metabolism, 86,* 4078–4088.

MacDonald, M., Hassold, T., Harvey, J., Wang, L. H., Morton, N. E., & Jacobs, P. (1994). The origin of 47,XXY and 47,XXX aneuploidy: Heterogeneous mechanisms and role of aberrant recombination. *Human Molecular Genetics, 3,* 1365–1371.

MacLean, J., Harnden, D. G., and CourtBrown, W. M. (1961). Abnormalities of sex chromosome constitution in newborn babies. *Lancet, 2,* 7199.

Main, K. M., Schmidt, I. M., & Skakkebaek, N. E. (2000). A possible role for reproductive hormones in newborn boys: Progressive hypogonadism without the postnatal testosterone peak. *Journal of Clinical Endocrinology and Metabolism, 85,* 4905–4907.

Mandoki, M. W., Sumner, G. S., Hoffman, R. P., & Riconda, D. L. (1991). A review of Klinefelter's syndrome in children and adolescents. *Journal of the American Academy of Child and Adolescent Psychiatry, 30*(2), 167–172.

Martin, D. D., Schweizer, R., Schwarze, C. P., Elmlinger, M. W., Ranke, M. B., & Binder, G. (2004). The early dehydroepiandrosterone sulfate rise of adrenarche and the delay of pubarche indicate primary ovarian failure in turner syndrome. *Journal of Clinical Endocrinology and Metabolism, 89,* 1164–1168.

Matsumoto, A. (1991). Synaptogenic action of sex steroids in developing and adult neuroendocrine brain. *Psychoneuroendocrinology, 16,* 25–40.

Mikamo, K., Aguercif, M., Hazeghi, P., & Martin-Du Pan, R. (1968). Chromatin-positive Klinefelter's syndrome: A quantitative analysis of spermatogonial deficiency at 3, 4, and 12 months of age. *Fertility and Sterility, 19,* 731–739.

Mitamura, R., Yano, K., Suzuki, N., Ito, Y., Makita, Y., & Okuno, A. (1999). Diurnal rhythms of luteinizing hormone, follicle-stimulating hormone, and testosterone secretion before the onset of male puberty. *Journal of Clinical Endocrinology and Metabolism, 84,* 29–37.

Mitamura, R., Yano, K., Suzuki, N., Ito, Y., Makita, Y., & Okuno, A. (2000). Diurnal rhythms of luteinizing hormone, follicle-stimulating hormone, testosterone, and estradiol secretion before the onset of female puberty in short children. *Journal of Clinical Endocrinology and Metabolism, 85,* 1074–1080.

Moffat, S. D., Zonderman, A. B., Metter, E. J., Blackman, M. R., Harman, S. M., & Resnick, S. M. (2002). Longitudinal assessment of serum free testosterone concentration predicts memory performance and cognitive status in elderly men. *Journal of Clinical Endocrinology and Metabolism, 87,* 5001–5007.

Muller, J., Skakkebaek, N. E., & Ratcliffe, S. G. (1995). Quantified testicular histology in boys with sex chromosome abnormalities. *International Journal of Andrology, 18*(2), 57–62.

Netley, C. (1992). Time of pubertal onset, testosterone levels and intelligence in 47,XXY males. *Clinical Genetics, 42,* 31–34.

Netley, C., & Rovet, J. (1984). Hemispheric lateralization in 47,XXY Klinefelter's syndrome boys. *Brain and Cognition, 3*(1), 10–18.

Netley, C., Taylor, M. J., & Molan, M. (1995). Event-related potentials (ERPs) and intelligence in neonatally identified 47,XXY males. *Clinical Genetics, 47,* 150–154.

Nielsen, J., Johnsen, S. G., & Sorensen, K. (1980). Follow-up 10 years later of 34 Klinefelter males with karyotype 47,XXY and 16 hypogonadal males with karyotype 46,XY. *Psychological Medicine, 10,* 345–352.

Nielsen, J., & Pelsen, B. (1987). Follow-up 20 years later of 34 Klinefelter males with karyotype 47,XXY and 16 hypogonadal males with karyotype 46,XY. *Human Genetics, 77,* 188–192.

Nielsen, J., Sorensen, A. M., & Sorensen, K. (1981). Mental development of unselected children with sex chromosome abnormalities. *Human Genetics, 59,* 324–332.

Nielsen, J., & Wohlert, M. (1990). Sex chromosome abnormalities found among 34,910 newborn children: Results from a 13-year incidence study in Arhus, Denmark. *Birth Defects Original Article Series, 26*(4), 209–223.

Nielson, J., and Sorensen, K. (1988). Follow-up of 30 Klinefelter males treated with testosterone. *Clinical Genetics, 33,* 362–369.

O'Connor, D. B., Archer, J., Hair, W. M., & Wu, F. C. (2001). Activational effects of testosterone on cognitive function in men. *Neuropsychologia, 39,* 1385–1394.

O'Connor, D. B., Archer, J., Hair, W. M., & Wu, F. C. (2002). Exogenous testosterone, aggression, and mood in eugonadal and hypogonadal men. *Physiology and Behavior, 75,* 557–566.

Patwardhan, A. J., Brown, W. E., Bender, B. G., Linden, M. G., Eliez, S., & Reiss, A. L. (2002). Reduced size of the amygdala in individuals with 47,XXY and 47,XXX karyotypes. *American Journal of Medical Genetics, 114,* 93–98.

Patwardhan, A. J., Eliez, S., Bender, B., Linden, M. G., & Reiss, A. L. (2000). Brain morphology in Klinefelter syndrome: Extra X chromosome and testosterone supplementation. *Neurology, 54,* 2218–2223.

Porter, M. E., Gardner, H. A., DeFeudis, P., & Endler, N. S. (1988). Verbal deficits in Klinefelter (XXY) adults living in the community. *Clinical Genetics, 33,* 246–253.

Price, W. H., Clayton, J. F., Wilson, J., Collyer, S., & De Mey, R. (1985). Causes of death in X chromatin positive males (Klinefelter's syndrome). *Journal of Epidemiology and Community Health, 39,* 330–336.

Rao, E., Weiss, B., Fukami, M., Rump, A., Niesler, B., Mertz, A., et al. (1997). Pseudoautosomal deletions encompassing a novel homeobox gene cause growth failure in idiopathic short stature and Turner syndrome. *Nature Genetics, 16*(1), 54–63.

Rasika, S., Nottebohm, F., & Alvarez-Buylla, A. (1994). Testosterone increases the recruitment and/or survival of new high vocal center neurons in adult female canaries. *Proceedings of the National Academy of Sciences, U.S.A., 91,* 7854–7858.

Ratcliffe, S. (1999). Long-term outcome in children of sex chromosome abnormalities. *Archives of Diseases in Childhood, 80,* 192–195.

Ratcliffe, S. G. (1982). The sexual development of boys with the chromosome constitution 47,XXY (Klinefelter's syndrome). *Journal of Clinical Endocrinology and Metabolism, 11,* 703–716.

Ratcliffe, S. G., Bancroft, J., Axworthy, D., & McLaren, W. (1982a). Klinefelter's syndrome in adolescence. *Archives of Diseases in Childhood, 57,* 6–12.

Ratcliffe, S. G., Butler, G. E., & Jones, M. (1990). Edinburgh study of growth and development of children with sex chromosome abnormalities: IV. *Birth Defects Original Article Series, 26*(4), 1–44.

Ratcliffe, S. G., Masera, N., Pan, H., & McKie, M. (1994a). Head circumference and IQ of children with sex chromosome abnormalities. *Developmental Medicine and Child Neurology, 36,* 533–544.

Ratcliffe, S. G., Murray, L., & Teague, P. (1986). Edinburgh study of growth and development of children with sex chromosome abnormalities: III. *Birth Defects Original Article Series, 22*(3), 73–118.

Ratcliffe, S. G., Read, G., Pan, H., Fear, C., Lindenbaum, R., & Crossley, J. (1994b). Prenatal testosterone levels in XXY and XYY males. *Hormone Research, 42*(3), 106–109.

Ratcliffe, S. G., Tierney, I., Nshaho, J., Smith, L., Springbett, A., & Callan, S. (1982b). The Edinburgh study of growth and development of children with sex chromosome abnormalities. *Birth Defects Original Article Series, 18*(4), 41–60.

Robinson, A., Bender, B. G., Borelli, J. B., Puck, M. H., Salbenblatt, J. A., & Winter, J. S. (1986). Sex chromosomal aneuploidy: Prospective and longitudinal studies. *Birth Defects Original Article Series, 22*(3), 23–71.

Robinson, A., Bender, B. G., & Linden, M. G. (1990). Summary of clinical findings in children and young adults with sex chromosome anomalies. *Birth Defects Original Article Series, 26*(4), 225–228.

Robinson, A., Puck, M., Pennington, B., Borelli, J., & Hudson, M. (1979). Abnormalities of the sex chromosomes: A prospective study on randomly identified newborns. *Birth Defects Original Article Series, 15*(1), 203–241.

Roche, R. A. P., Garavan, H., Foxe, J. J., & O'Mara, S. M. (2005). Individual differences discriminate event-related potentials but not performance during response inhibition. *Experimental Brain Research, 160,* 60–70.

Ross, J. L., Roeltgen, D., Stefanatos, G. A., Feuillan, P., Kushner, H., Bondy, C., et al. (2003). Androgen-responsive aspects of cognition in girls with Turner syndrome. *Journal of Clinical Endocrinology and Metabolism, 88,* 292–296.

Ross, J. L., Samango-Sprouse, C., Lahlou, N., Kowal, K., Elder, F. F., & Zinn, A. (2005). Early androgen deficiency in infants and young boys with 47,XXY Klinefelter syndrome. *Hormone Research, 64*(1), 39–45.

Ross, J. L., Samango-Sprouse, C., Lahlou, N., Kowal, K., Elder, F., & Zinn, A. R. (2005). The phenotype of early androgen deficiency in young boys with 47,XXY Klinefelter syndrome. *Hormone Research, 64,* 39–45.

Rovet, J., Netley, C., Bailey, J., Keenan, M., & Stewart, D. (1995). Intelligence and achievement in children with extra X aneuploidy: A longitudinal perspective. *American Journal of Medical Genetics, 60,* 356–363.

Rovet, J., Netley, C., Keenan, M., Bailey, J., & Stewart, D. (1996). The psychoeducational profile of boys with Klinefelter syndrome. *Journal of Learning Disabilities, 29*(2), 180–196.

Rutkove, S. B., Parker, R. A., Nardin, R. A., Connolly, C. E., Felice, K. J., & Raynor, E. M. (2002). A pilot randomized trial of oxandrolone in inclusion body myositis. *Neurology, 58*, 1081–1087.

Salbenblatt, J. A., Bender, B. G., Puck, M. H., Robinson, A., Faiman, C., & Winter, J. S. (1985). Pituitary-gonadal function in Klinefelter syndrome before and during puberty. *Pediatric Research, 19*(1), 82–86.

Salbenblatt, J. A., Bender, B. G., Puck, M. H., Robinson, A., & Webber, M. L. (1981). Development of eight pubertal males with 47,XXY karyotype. *Clinical Genetics, 20*, 141–146.

Salbenblatt, J. A., Meyers, D. C., Bender, B. G., Linden, M. G., & Robinson, A. (1987). Gross and fine motor development in 47,XXY and 47,XYY males. *Pediatrics, 80*, 240–244.

Samango-Sprouse, C. (2001). Mental development in polysomy X Klinefelter syndrome (47,XXY; 48,XXXY): Effects of incomplete X inactivation. *Seminars in Reproductive Medicine, 19*(2), 193–202.

Schiavi, R. C., Owen, D., Fogel, M., White, D., & Szechter, R. (1978). Pituitary-gonadal function in XYY and XXY men identified in a population survey. *Clinical Endocrinology (Oxf), 9*(3), 233–239.

Schroeder, E. T., Zheng, L., Yarasheski, K. E., Qian, D., Stewart, Y., Flores, C., et al. (2004). Treatment with oxandrolone and the durability of effects in older men. *Journal of Applied Physiology, 96*, 1056–1062.

Schwab, J., Kulin, H. E., Susman, E. J., Finkelstein, J. W., Chinchilli, V. M., Kunselman, S. J., et al. (2001). The role of sex hormone replacement therapy on self-perceived competence in adolescents with delayed puberty. *Child Development, 72*, 1439–1450.

Sheffield-Moore, M., Urban, R. J., Wolf, S. E., Jiang, J., Catlin, D. H., Herndon, D. N., et al. (1999). Short-term oxandrolone administration stimulates net muscle protein synthesis in young men. *Journal of Clinical Endocrinology and Metabolism, 84*, 2705–2711.

Shen, D., Liu, D., Liu, H., Clasen, L., Giedd, J., & Davatzikos, C. (2004). Automated morphometric study of brain variation in XXY males. *Neuroimage, 23*, 648–653.

Simpson, J. L., De La Cruz, F., Swerdloff, R. S., Samango-Sprouse, C., Skakkebaek, N. E., Graham, J. M., Jr., et al. (2003). Klinefelter syndrome: Expanding the phenotype and identifying new research directions. *Genetics and Medicine, 5*, 460–468.

Sinha-Hikim, I., Artaza, J., Woodhouse, L., Gonzalez-Cadavid, N., Singh, A. B., Lee, M. I., et al. (2002). Testosterone-induced increase in muscle size in healthy young men is associated with muscle fiber hypertrophy. *American Journal of Physiology: Endocrinology and Metabolism, 283*(1), E154–164.

Sklar, C. A., Kaplan, S. L., & Grumbach, M. M. (1980). Evidence for dissociation between adrenarche and gonadarche: Studies in patients with idiopathic precocious puberty, gonadal dysgenesis, isolated gonadotropin deficiency, and constitutionally delayed growth and adolescence. *Journal of Clinical Endocrinology and Metabolism, 51*, 548–556.

Skuse, D. H. (2000). Imprinting, the X-chromosome, and the male brain: Explaining sex differences in the liability to autism. *Pediatric Research, 47*(1), 9–16.

Smyth, C. M., & Bremner, W. J. (1998). Klinefelter syndrome. *Archives of Internal Medicine, 158*, 1309–1314.

Sorensen, K., Nielsen, J., Wohlert, M., Bennett, P., & Johnsen, S. G. (1981). Serum testosterone of boys with karyotype 47,XXY (Klinefelter's syndrome) at birth. *Lancet, 2*, 1112–1113.

Sperfeld, A. D., Karitzky, J., Brummer, D., Schreiber, H., Haussler, J., Ludolph, A. C., et al. (2002). X-linked bulbospinal neuronopathy: Kennedy disease. *Archives of Neurology, 59*, 1921–1926.

Sperling, M. A. (2002). *Pediatric endocrinology* (2nd ed.). Philadelphia: Saunders.

Stewart, D. A., Bailey, J. D., Netley, C. T., & Park, E. (1990). Growth, development, and behavioral outcome from mid-adolescence to adulthood in subjects with chromosome aneuploidy: The Toronto study. *Birth Defects Original Article Series, 26*(4), 131–188.

Stewart, D. A., Bailey, J. D., Netley, C. T., Rovet, J., & Park, E. (1986). Growth and development from early to midadolescence of children with X and Y chromosome aneuploidy: The Toronto study. *Birth Defects Original Article Series, 22*(3), 119–182.

Stewart, D. A., Bailey, J. D., Netley, C. T., Rovet, J., Park, E., Cripps, M., et al. (1982a). Growth and development of children with X and Y chromosome aneuploidy from infancy to pubertal age: The Toronto study. *Birth Defects Original Article Series, 18*(4), 99–154.

Stewart, D. A., Netley, C. T., Bailey, J. D., Haka-Ikse, K., Platt, J., Holland, W., et al. (1979). Growth and development of children with X and Y chromosome aneuploidy: A prospective study. *Birth Defects Original Article Series, 15*(1), 75–114.

Stewart, D. A., Netley, C. T., & Park, E. (1982b). Summary of clinical findings of children with 47,XXY, 47,XYY, and 47,XXX karyotypes. *Birth Defects Original Article Series, 18*(4), 1–5.

Storer, T. W., Magliano, L., Woodhouse, L., Lee, M. L., Dzekov, C., Dzekov, J., et al. (2003). Testosterone dose-dependently increases maximal voluntary strength and leg power, but does not affect fatigability or specific tension. *Journal of Clinical Endocrinology and Metabolism, 88*, 1478–1485.

Temple, C. M., & Sanfilippo, P. M. (2003). Executive skills in Klinefelter's syndrome. *Neuropsychologia, 41*, 1547–1559.

Theilgaard, A. (1984). A psychological study of the personalities of XYY- and XXY-men. *Acta Psychiatrica Scandinavica Supplementum, 315*, 1–133.

Topper, E., Dickerman, Z., Prager-Lewin, R., Kaufman, H., Maimon, Z., & Laron, Z. (1982). Puberty in 24 patients with Klinefelter syndrome. *European Journal of Pediatrics, 139*(1), 8–12.

Visootsak, J., Aylstock, M., & Graham, J. M., Jr. (2001). Klinefelter syndrome and its variants: An update and review for the primary pediatrician. *Clinical Pediatrics (Phila), 40*, 639–651.

Walzer, S. (1985). X chromosome abnormalities and cognitive development: Implications for understanding normal human development. *Journal of Child Psychology and Psychiatry, 26*(2), 177–184.

Walzer, S., Bashir, A. S., & Silbert, A. R. (1990). Cognitive and behavioral factors in the learning disabilities of 47,XXY and 47,XYY boys. *Birth Defects Original Article Series, 26*(4), 45–58.

Wang, C., Alexander, G., Berman, N., Salehian, B., Davidson, T., McDonald, V., et al. (1996). Testosterone replacement therapy improves mood in hypogonadal men—A clinical research center study. *Journal of Clinical Endocrinology and Metabolism, 81*, 3578–3583.

Wang, C., Swedloff, R. S., Iranmanesh, A., Dobs, A., Snyder, P. J., Cunningham, G., et al. (2000). Transdermal testosterone gel improves sexual function, mood, muscle strength, and body composition parameters in hypogonadal men. Testosterone gel study group. *Journal of Clinical Endocrinology and Metabolism, 85*, 2839–2853.

Warwick, M. M., Doody, G. A., Lawrie, S. M., Kestelman, J. N., Best, J. J., & Johnstone, E. C. (1999). Volumetric magnetic resonance imaging study of the brain in subjects with sex chromosome aneuploidies. *Journal of Neurology, Neurosurgery, and Psychiatry, 66*, 628–632.

Warwick, M. M., Lawrie, S. M., Beveridge, A., & Johnstone, E. C. (2003). Abnormal cerebral asymmetry and schizophrenia in a subject with Klinefelter's syndrome (XXY). *Biological Psychiatry, 53*, 627–629.

Wikstrom, A. M., Raivio, T., Hadziselimovic, F., Wikstrom, S., Tuuri, T., & Dunkel, L. (2004). Klinefelter syndrome in adolescence: Onset of puberty is associated with accelerated germ cell depletion. *Journal of Clinical Endocrinology and Metabolism, 89*, 2263–2270.

Zinn, A. R., Ramos, P., Elder, F. F., Kowal, K., Samango-Sprouse, C., & Ross, J. L. (2005). Androgen receptor CAGn repeat length influences phenotype of 47,XXY Klinefelter syndrome. *Journal of Clinical Endocrinology and Metabolism, 90*, 5041–5046.

3 Fragile X Syndrome: The Journey from Genes to Behavior

Kimberly M. Cornish, Andrew Levitas, and Vicki Sudhalter

Case 3.1: Harold   Harold is a 6-year-old boy recently evaluated by his pediatrician for developmental delay and autistic-like features. Harold's mother reported early problems with speech production, hyperactivity, and aggressive outbursts. More recently the behavioral problems have intensified, and Harold has begun to hand bite. On physical examination, the pediatrician notes that Harold has a slightly longer face, larger ears, and more prominent jaw than would be expected for a boy his age but nothing too unusual. A family history reveals that Harold's sister and maternal cousin, both females, have mild learning difficulties including attention problems, chronic shyness, and social anxiety. Molecular analysis revealed fragile X syndrome.

Fragile X syndrome is the most prevalent known inherited cause of developmental delay in humans, affecting 1 in 4,000 males and 1 in 8,000 females (de Vries, Halley, Oostra, & Niermeijer, 1998; Kooy, Willesden, & Oostra, 2000; Turner, Webb, Wake, & Robinson, 1996). Elongated face, large prominent ears and forehead, and macroorchidism (postpuberty) can characterize some children with the condition (Lachiewicz, Dawson, & Spiridigliozzi, 2000), alongside more subtle features that include narrow intereye distance, a highly arched palate of the mouth, and hyperextensible metacarpophalangeal joints. However, the wide variability in expression, in both males and females, makes diagnosis on physical features alone almost impossible. See figure 3.1, which illustrates the facial features of two siblings, both with the full mutation, ranging in age from 4–9 years. The most defining feature of fragile X syndrome, especially in boys with the condition, is mental retardation and the resulting behavioral phenotype. It is precisely because of their quite normal appearance that many affected children are not recognized until relatively later in development as having fragile X, which is why a close examination of the phenotypic signature and its developmental timeline is crucial in helping clinicians toward an early diagnosis. See table 3.1 for a summary of the clinical and medical problems associated with fragile X syndrome.

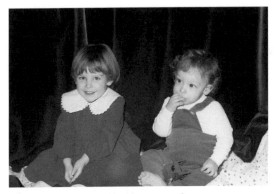

sister and brother (L–R) aged 4 & 2 years

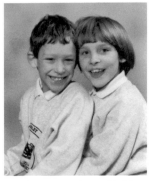

brother and sister (L–R)
aged 7 and 9 years

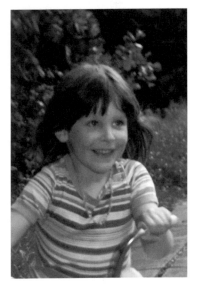

sister – 4 years

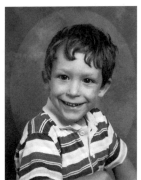

brother – 6 years

Figure 3.1
Siblings with fragile X syndrome. Abbreviations: L, left; R, right.

Table 3.1
Prevalence of characteristic physical, cognitive, and behavioral symptoms in children with fragile X syndrome and prevalence of fragile X syndrome among persons with clinical presentation of these symptoms

Characteristic/Symptom	% of Cases in All Individuals with Fragile X Syndrome	% of Fragile X Cases Among Persons with Symptom	
		Males	Females
Epilepsy	13–20[8] 23[14] 0[13]	No studies found	
Cardiac abnormalities	1[8]	No studies found	
Macroorchidism	68[5]	39[12]	
Mental retardation	70[8] 50–70 (full mutation females)[6] 100[7]	0.9–8.9[1] 2–3[11]	0.3–1[1]
Elongated face	50[7]	No studies found	
Large ears	100[7]	No studies found	
Language delay	75[8]	0.56[9]	
Speech problems	70[8]	No studies found	
Attention and concentration difficulties	100[8]	No studies found	
Autism	24–33[2] 15–33[3]	2–16[2]	
Autistic-like features	90[8] 58[7]	7.5[10]	
Attention deficit/hyperactivity disorder	80[4] 67[7]	1[4]	
Social anxiety and hyperarousal	100[8]	No studies found	

	% of Cases in All Individuals with Fragile X Syndrome	% of Non-Fragile X Syndrome Cases with Fragile X Symptom
Mental retardation and:		
Elongated face	51[5]	7[5]
Large ears	27[5]	11[5]
Hyperextensible finger joints	41[5]	23[5]
Soft/smooth skin	22[5]	4[5]
Macroorchidism	68[5]	16[5] 27[11]
Characteristic personality	63[5]	4[5]

1. Pooled data, numerous worldwide studies 1983–2005.
2. Pooled data, reviewed in the following: Demark, J. L., Feldman, M. A., & Holden, J. J. A. (2003). Behavioral relationship between autism and fragile X syndrome. *American Journal on Mental Retardation, 108,* 314–326.
3. Pooled data, reviewed in this chapter.
4. Bastain, T. M., Lewczyk, C. M., Sharp, W. S., James, R. S., Long, R. T., Eagen, P. B., et al. (2002). Cytogenetic abnormalities in attention-deficit/hyperactivity disorder. *Journal of the American Academy of Child and Adolescent Psychiatry, 41,* 806–810.
5. de Vries, B. B. A., Mohkamsing, S., van den Ouweland, A. M. W., Mol, E., Gelsema, K., van Rijn, M., et al. (1999). Screening for the fragile X syndrome among the mentally retarded: A clinical study. *Journal of Medical Genetics, 36,* 467–470.

Table 3.1
(continued)

6. de Vries, B. B. A., Wiegers, A. M., Smits, A. P. T., Mohkamsing, A., Duivenvoorden, H. J., Fryns, J.-P., et al. (1996). Mental status of females with an FMR1 gene full mutation. *American Journal of Human Genetics, 58,* 1025–1032.

7. Giangreco, C. A., Steele, M. W., Aston, C. E., Cummins, J. H., & Wenger, S. L. (1996). A simplified six-item checklist for screening for fragile X syndrome in the pediatric population. *Journal of Pediatrics, 129,* 611–614.

8. Hagerman, R. J., & Cronister, A. (Eds.). (1996). *Fragile X syndrome: Diagnosis, treatment and research* (2nd ed.). Baltimore: Johns Hopkins University Press.

9. Mazzocco, M. M., Myers, G. F., Hamner, J. L., Panoscha, R., Shapiro, B. K., & Reiss, A. L. (1998). The prevalence of the FMR1 and FMR2 mutations among preschool children with language delay. *Journal of Pediatrics, 132,* 795–801.

10. Sherman, S. (1996). Epidemiology. In R. J. Hagerman & A. Cronister (Eds.), *Fragile X syndrome: Diagnosis, treatment and research* (2nd ed., pp. 165–192). Baltimore: Johns Hopkins University Press.

11. Slaney, S. F., Wilkie, A. O. M., Hirst, M. C., Charlton, R., McKinley, M., Pointon, J., et al. (1995). DNA testing for fragile X syndrome in schools for learning difficulties. *Archives of Disease in Childhood, 72,* 33–37.

12. Vatta, S., Cigui, I., Demori, E., Morgutti, M., Pecile, V., Benussi, D. G., et al. (1998). Fragile X syndrome, mental retardation and macroorchidism [Letter to the Editor]. *Clinical Genetics, 54,* 366–367.

13. Vieregge, P., & Froster-Iskenius, U. (1989). Clinico–neurological investigations in the fra(X) form of mental retardation. *Journal of Neurology, 236,* 85–92.

14. Wisniewski, K. E., Segan, S. M., Miezejeski, C. M., Sersen, E. A., & Rudelli, R. D. (1991). The Fra(X) syndrome: Neurological, electrophysiological, and neuropathological abnormalities. *American Journal of Medical Genetics, 38,* 476–480.

Fragile X syndrome's single-gene etiology affords us the unique opportunity to begin to understand the relationships among genes, brain, and behavior. To that end, we provide a description of the recent advances that define the syndrome at the genetic and brain level, a description of the defining clinical features, and profile of cognitive strengths and weaknesses. We conclude with some ideas for medical and educational interventions.

Fragile X Syndrome—Genetic and Brain-Level Considerations

By virtue of its single-gene etiology, fragile X syndrome represents an important model for understanding the impact of the fragile X mental retardation gene—1 (FMR1) expression on the development and normal functioning of the central nervous system. While it is becoming commonplace to investigate the phenotypic effects resulting from the loss of a single gene product in animal models, few naturally occurring genetic anomalies exist in humans that allow us to examine the specific contribution of a single gene to behavior, although that contribution might be by way of modification of the action of many other genes. The syndrome is caused by the silencing of a single gene on the X chromosome, FMR1 (Verkerk et al., 1991). The FMR1 gene carries a CGG trinucleotide repeat in the 5′ untranslated region. The American College of Medical Genetics guidelines define unaffected individuals as having between 7 and 55 repeats, with 30 repeats the most common allele and a "gray zone" of ~45–54 CGG repeats with lesser size instability on transmission (Hagerman & Hagerman, 2004). In fully clinically affected individuals the CGG region expands to over 200 repeats, resulting in the silencing of the gene and loss of the encoded protein, fragile X mental retardation protein (FMRP). Due to X linkage, almost all affected males present with mental retardation compared to approximately one half of affected females. In nearly all cases, the disorder is caused by an expansion of the CGG repeat at the beginning of the FMR1 gene on the X chromosome, leading to methylation of the promoter sequence and loss of the FMRP in individuals with 200 or more repeats (Turner et al., 1996; Verkerk et al., 1991).

Alleles with between 55~200 repeats are called "premutations" and typically are associated with normal or slightly reduced levels of protein production, generating some protein. However, these premutations can be unstable through successive generations, giving rise to the fragile X syndrome phenotype upon full expansion (Kooy, 2003; O'Donnell & Warren, 2002). When 200 or more CGG repeats are present, usually (unless there is a failure of methylation) there is hypermethylation and a subsequent silencing of the FMR1 gene. This is commonly referred to as the FMR1 *full mutation*. Although both males and females can be carriers of fragile X syndrome, inheritance of the full mutation can only be from a female who carries either a full mutation or a premutation that is *unstable* on female transmission. In contrast, male carriers can only transmit their premutation to their daughters. Figure 3.2 illustrates the pattern of inheritance and its expansion over generations.

The abnormal CGG repeat sequences can be detected and quantified using restriction endonuclease digestion and Southern blot technology. Cleavage of the FMR1 gene by EcoR1 yields a 5.2-kb fragment; this is further cleaved by Eag1 into 2.4- and 2.8-kb fragments if unmethylated. Abnormal-sized DNA fragments caused by increases in numbers of CGG repeats in the 5' untranslated region are detected and quantified by migration on Southern blot (see figures 3.3, 3.4, and 3.5).

It is now established that the FMR1 gene is the major contributor to the pathogenesis of fragile X syndrome and that the key issues relate to a lack of messenger RNA (mRNA) and a lack or absence of the protein product of the FMR1 gene—FMRP—resulting in the fM. (See figure 3.6.) In contrast, premutation males and females possess unmethylated versions of the FMR1 gene and therefore have normal or near-normal levels of FMRP and the expanded (premutation) CGG repeat element results in both elevated FMR1 mRNA levels and slight to moderate reductions in FMRP.

The extent to which these discoveries explain some of the phenotypic outcomes of fragile X syndrome are beginning to be unraveled with converging evidence indicating a possible role in early neuronal development. First, FMRP is especially critical in the early embryonic stages of development including the neonatal stage (Bakker et al., 2000). And second, FMRP is an important regulator of synaptic activity and

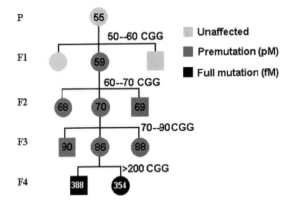

Figure 3.2
Hypothetical genogram of 5 generations of a family with fragile X syndrome. P: carrier female (premutation; pM) with 55 CGG repeats; unaffected. F1: A male and female inherit mother's normal X chromosome; a female pM with 59 CGG repeats. F2: a childless female pM with 68 CGG repeats, mild neuropsychological deficits, and hyperactivity; a childless male pM with 69 CGG repeats and attention deficit/hyperactivity disorder; a female pM with 70 CGG repeats, moderate neuropsychological deficits. F3: childless male pM with 90 CGG repeats, hyperactivity, borderline intellectual functioning; childless female pM with 88 CGG repeats, borderline intellectual functioning, and schizotypal disorder; a female pM with 86 CGG repeats, moderate neuropsychological deficits, generalized anxiety disorder, major depressive disorder. F4: male fM (full mutation) and female fM both with more than 200 CGG repeats, mental retardation and autistic disorder.

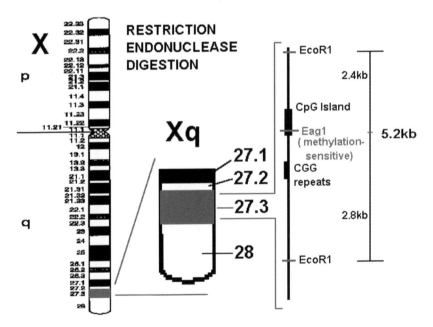

Figure 3.3
Endonuclease digestion of FMR1 yields a 2.8-kb DNA fragment if unmethylated.

FXS DNA DIAGNOSIS PROCEDURE

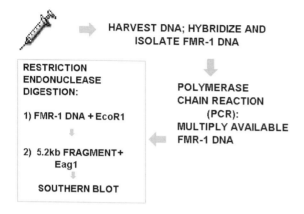

HARVEST DNA; HYBRIDIZE AND
ISOLATE FMR-1 DNA

**RESTRICTION
ENDONUCLEASE
DIGESTION:**

1) FMR-1 DNA + EcoR1

2) 5.2kb FRAGMENT+
   Eag1

   SOUTHERN BLOT

**POLYMERASE
CHAIN REACTION
(PCR):
MULTIPLY AVAILABLE
FMR-1 DNA**

Figure 3.4
Procedure for fragile X syndrome (FXS) DNA laboratory analysis.

FXS DNA DIAGNOSIS PROCEDURE
SOUTHERN BLOT

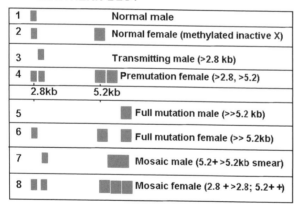

1	Normal male
2	Normal female (methylated inactive X)
3	Transmitting male (>2.8 kb)
4	Premutation female (>2.8, >5.2)
	2.8kb 5.2kb
5	Full mutation male (>>5.2 kb)
6	Full mutation female (>> 5.2kb)
7	Mosaic male (5.2+ >5.2kb smear)
8	Mosaic female (2.8 + >2.8; 5.2+ +)

Figure 3.5
DNA fragments in eight possible Southern Blot outcomes. Note the single FMR1 fragment seen in males (one X chromosome), the two in females (two X chromosomes, one normal X chromosome; the normal or the fragile X chromosome may be inactivated by methylation). Abbreviation: FXS, fragile X syndrome.

FXS MOLECULAR PATHOLOGY

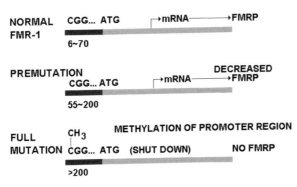

Figure 3.6
Fragile X syndrome (FXS) molecular pathology.

organization because of its role in the transportation of selective mRNAs molecules to dendrites in response to neural stimulation (Bardoni, Mandel, & Fisch, 2000; Irwin et al., 2001; see figure 3.7). Indeed, systematic studies of FMR1 knock-out mice and autopsied human brains of individuals with fragile X have indicated that the absence of the FMRP affects postsynaptic changes in dendrite spine morphology that include an abundance of long, thin, and tortuous spines; more spines with an immature-appearing structure; and a greater density of spines overall (e.g., Galvez & Green-ough, 2005; Irwin et al., 2002). One current theory, the mGluR theory, proposed by Bear, Huber, and Warren (2004), suggests that an early disruption to the molecular pathways involved in synaptic development and regulation may have a differential impact on early brain development to produce the phenotypic outcomes we associate with the syndrome. However, *development itself* will also play a critical role in defin-ing the fragile X syndrome phenotype (Cornish, Scerif, & Karmiloff-Smith, in press; Karmiloff-Smith, 1998).

At the brain level, studies have revealed decreased size of the posterior vermis of the cerebellum in males and females (Mostofsky et al., 1998; Reiss, Alyward, Freund, Joshi, & Bryan, 1991). Other structures affected by FMR1 status include the caudate nucleus (Eliez, Blasey, Freund, Hastie, & Reiss, 2001) and the hippo-campus (Kates, Abrams, Kaufmann, Breiter, & Reiss, 1997; Reiss, Lee, & Freund, 1994). In addition, several studies reported a correlation between neuroanatomical abnormalities and the degree of functional impairment in the full mutation. For example, posterior vermis volumes are positively correlated with performance on specific measures of intelligence, visual–spatial ability, and executive function, sug-gesting a putative functional role for this structure (Mostofsky et al., 1998). Taken

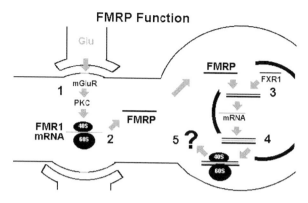

Figure 3.7
Normal fragile X mental retardation protein (FMRP) function. Activated metabotropic mGlu receptor (1) activates protein kinase C, which stimulates translation of prepositioned FMR1 messenger RNA (mRNA) ribonucleoprotein complexes at the synapse, producing FMRP (2). FMRP is imported into the nucleus, where, with FXR1 or FXR2 (3), it links to mRNA of other genes (4), transporting it to ribosomes where the mRNA is translated into as yet unknown proteins (5).

together, the purely structural and combined structural/functional studies implicate the cerebellum, caudate nucleus, and hippocampus as potential sites for phenotypic effects from abnormal FMR1 gene expression. However, it is important to stress that abnormal structures form part of widely distributed networks and that deficits may be observed across a broad range of activities.

In the following section we briefly describe the recent advances that have helped to define the fragile X syndrome phenotype at the behavioral and cognitive levels. We especially focus on the variations within the condition itself, most notably between affected males and females.

Fragile X Syndrome—Cognitive and Behavioral Considerations

Mental retardation is seen as the most defining clinical feature of boys with fragile X syndrome with almost all affected males presenting with IQs within the moderate–severe range of impairment with profiles emerging as young as 3 years of age (Skinner et al., 2005). In females, the phenotypic variation is such that some girls only show subclinical learning disabilities (Bennetto & Pennington, 2002), while approximately 50% display more moderate–severe mental retardation similar in profile to boys with fragile X syndrome. The X-inactivation status of females with fragile X is seen as the major contributor to the heterogeneity of intellectual disability and neuropsychological deficits. In some males, the presence of mosaicism may produce a higher level of cognitive functioning, but these cases are relatively rare, although well documented (Hagerman, Hull et al., 1994; Merenstein et al., 1996).

Behavioral Concerns

Severity of behavioral difficulties in boys and girls with fragile X syndrome will vary across and within gender. In addition, there is the added complication of comorbidities that have implications for early diagnosis and treatment. Here we target three areas of behavioral difficulties that have been frequently documented in boys and girls with fragile X.

Social Anxiety and Hyperarousal   Hypersensitivity and hyperarousal are recognized as early prominent behavioral features of children with fragile X syndrome, with and without autism (Belser & Sudhalter, 1995; Hagerman, 1996; Miller et al., 1999). Keysor, Mazzocco, McLeod, and Hoehn-Saric (2002) demonstrated higher arousal levels at baseline for girls with fragile X relative to girls with Turner syndrome or typical developing children, with a small rise on anxiety-provoking cognitive tasks compared to that seen in girls with Turner syndrome, resulting in eventual comparable anxiety in both groups on these tasks. Despite an evident desire for social contact (Simon & Finucane, 1996; Turk & Cornish, 1998), children with fragile X syndrome (with and without autism) show social anxiety, with delay in initiating interaction, gaze avoidance, and failure to understand gaze direction (Garrett, Menon, MacKenzie, & Reiss, 2004; Kau, Reider, Payne, Meyer, & Freund, 2000; Turk, 1998; Wolff, Gardner, Paccia, & Lappen, 1989) associated with their greater difficulty (Lachiewicz, 1992; Lachiewicz & Dawson, 1994).

Lesniak-Karpiak, Mazzocco, and Ross (2003) demonstrated different manifestations of social anxiety/social deficit in girls with fragile X versus girls with Turner syndrome. In a pilot study using psychophysiological and behavioral measures, Belser and Sudhalter (1995) demonstrated that males with fragile X syndrome were more aroused by eye contact than their matched cohorts with either mental retardation or attention deficit/hyperactivity disorder (ADHD). It was additionally demonstrated that the arousal disrupted the language of the males with fragile X syndrome.

Miller et al. (1999) investigated the relationship between hyperarousal as measured by electrodermal responses and reaction to sensory stimuli in individuals with fragile X syndrome. The research demonstrated that reactions in one modality predicted reactions in another; there was a negative relationship between FMRP expression and electrodermal responses, and the pattern of electrodermal responses did differentiate males with fragile X from normal controls. Taken together, these data suggested that males with fragile X syndrome may have a multimodal sensory defensiveness that may underlie or at least influence hyperarousal. The authors also suggest that the sympathetic nervous system may be affected in individual with fragile X based on the pattern of results from the research.

Roberts, Boccia, Bailey, Hatton, and Skinner (2001) present research comparing heart rate variability in boys with fragile X syndrome and typically developing boys matched for chronological age. They predicted that boys with fragile X would display higher levels of heart activity and different patterns of modulation, as measured by shorter interbeat intervals (IBIs) than chronologically matched controls. In addition, they hypothesized that the heart activity of boys with fragile X would reflect lower vagal tone estimates and different patterns of modulation than chronologically matched controls. The participants completed a 30-min procedure consisting of alternating passive (i.e., watching a video) and active (i.e., completing cognitive tasks) phases. Heart rate activity was collected while the participants were engaged in these activities. Post hoc tests confirmed hypotheses. Boys with fragile X displayed shorter IBIs and higher sympathetic tone estimates during the passive tasks than the control group and displayed lower vagal tone estimates across all phases of the task and showed no modulation of vagal tone, while the typically developing boys showed higher level of vagal tone and suppression during phrases of increased demand. Finally, the typically developing boys displayed coordinated responses between the vagal and sympathetic systems, while the boys with fragile X did not. The authors suggest that these results demonstrate that boys with fragile X do not discriminate between phases of a task and modulate their heart rate activity through increased sympathetic tone rather than suppression of vagal tone, which is the demonstrated pattern of typically developing boys. This pattern of increased sympathetic input is in accordance with the findings of other studies (Belser & Sudhalter, 1995; Miller et al., 1999). The authors also suggest that the inefficient self-regulation mechanisms demonstrated by individuals with fragile X syndrome may help explain the behavioral arousal problems evidenced in the population.

The bases for hyperarousal, anxiety, and social anxiety/deficit may differ markedly among genetic syndromes, but hypersensitivity in all sensory modalities, low threshold for anxious or catastrophic reaction, and social anxiety may make separation from parents, experiences in crowds or noisy, echoing spaces, new clothing, all but a few foods (in some children), and some odors, especially when unexpected, very problematic to the point of severe "tantrum" behavior. Children with fragile X syndrome may be overwhelmed by the demands created by social involvement, novel or unexpected situations, and changes, even by the common transitions of daily life. Generalized anxiety and/or panic disorder may occur (Hagerman, Hull et al., 1994). Recently, Turk, Robbins, and Woodhead (2005) described two cases of posttraumatic stress disorder (PTSD) in persons with fragile X syndrome, one a 13-year-old boy.

Autism   There are currently very few single-gene studies for which there is a certainty of the involvement of autism; fragile X is one of those disorders. Although still controversial, a plethora of recent studies using a variety of standardized measures (e.g., Autism Diagnostic Observation Schedule-Generic [ADOS-G], Autism Diagnostic Interview-revised [ADI], Childhood Autism Rating Scale [CARS]) indicate a range of between 15%~33% of individuals with fragile X syndrome will fulfill a clinical diagnosis of autism (Bailey et al., 1998; Bailey, Hatton, Mesibov, Ament, & Skinner, 2000; Bailey, Hatton, Skinner, & Mesibov, 2001; Baumgardner, Reiss, Freund, & Abrams, 1995; Reiss & Freund, 1992; Rogers, Hepburn, Stackhouse, & Wehner, 2003). One argument is that the prevalence of autism in fragile X syndrome may simply be an artifact of general cognitive delay that is inherent in many disorders of mental retardation. However, closer examination of studies that have compared performance of children with fragile X syndrome and autism (fragile X syndrome + autism), children with fragile X without autism (fragile X alone), and children with autism without fragile X (autism alone) indicate quite different developmental profiles. For example, Hatton et al. (2003) observed lower adaptive scores as measured by the Vineland Adaptive Behavior Scales (Sparrow, Balla, & Cicchetti, 1984) in children with fragile X syndrome + autism compared to children with fragile X alone. In terms of social functioning, Kau et al. (2004) found children with fragile X syndrome + autism to display a distinct social profile that differentiated them from children with idiopathic autism and fragile X without autism. However, commonalities between fragile X syndrome + autism and idiopathic autism were striking on other domains, notably problem/aberrant behavior and adaptive behaviors. These domains were not as impaired in children with fragile X syndrome without autism. In the domain of language, Philofsky, Hepburn, Hayes, Hagerman, and Rogers (2004) report a relative strength in receptive language compared to expressive language for children with fragile X without autism. This pattern was not replicated in children with fragile X syndrome + autism, whose performance was much lower than children with fragile X alone but similar to that of children with idiopathic autism. They speculate that low receptive language may be a marker for autism symptoms in young children with fragile X syndrome.

Autistic-like Features   Although not all children with fragile X syndrome present with a clinical diagnosis of autism, almost all will display a range of "autistic-like" features, which include language delay, echolalia, and perseverative speech (see Cornish, Sudhalter, & Turk, 2004, for a review) alongside poor eye contact and stereotypic movements. However, the cause of these autistic-like behaviours in individuals with fragile X (without autistic disorder) may differ from the cause in individuals with autistic disorder who also have fragile X syndrome. It is well recognized that individuals with autistic disorder have a deficit in understanding social relationships, semantics, and pragmatics and in establishing interpersonal attachments. These deficits in turn interfere with the acquisition of social behaviors such as language, play, and empathy. On the other hand, males and females with fragile X syndrome are frequently described as friendly, loving, and extremely empathetic; however, they experience hyperarousal and social anxiety (as described above), which interferes with the expression of these emotions (Hagerman, 1996; Cohen, 1995; Cohen et al., 1991). Hyperarousal and social anxiety will cause the individuals to avert their eyes (so as to minimize social interactions or to avoid the sensory stimulation of eye contact), avoid parties and interactions, and produce atypical language (see below). Thus, males and females with fragile X syndrome will exhibit autistic-like behaviors, which are symptomatic of their hyperarousal and social anxiety rather than an inherent lack of understanding of the social situation.

Attention Deficit and Hyperactivity Disorder   Among the most distinctive and pervasive behavioral features of young boys with fragile X syndrome are attentional and hyperactivity problems (e.g., Baumgardner et al., 1995; Cornish, Munir, & Wilding, 2001; Hatton et al., 2002; Turk, 1998), the severity of which often leads to a clinical diagnosis of ADHD. Using the Child Behavior Checklist (CBCL; Achenbach, 1991), Hatton et al. (2002) report that approximately 57% of young boys with fragile X syndrome (4–12 years old) scored in the borderline or clinical range on the attention subscale of the CBCL. In a comparison study of 25 older boys with fragile X syndrome (ages 8–15 years) and 25 boys with Down syndrome (ages 7–15 years), Cornish, Munir, and Cross (2001) found greater attention problems (as measured by the CBCL attention subscale) and hyperactivity (as measured by the ADHD Comprehensive Teacher Rating [ACTeRs] scale; Ullman, Sleator, & Sprague, 1984) in boys with fragile X syndrome compared to boys with Down syndrome. In one of the most comprehensive studies to date, Turk (1998) compared the ADHD profiles of 49 boys with fragile X (ages 4–16 years) to that of 45 boys with Down syndrome (ages 4–16 years), and 42 boys with mental retardation of an unknown cause (ages 4–16 years). Although both groups of boys showed similar levels of motor activity, the boys with fragile X syndrome showed significantly more inattentiveness, restlessness, fidgetiness, distractibility, and impulsive tendencies as measured by the CBCL and the Parental Account of Childhood Symptoms questionnaire (Taylor, Schachar, & Hepstinall, 1993) than the group with unknown etiology. Furthermore, these features did not appear to improve spontaneously over time and are present early in development. Together, these findings highlight a distinctive ADHD profile in boys with fragile X that is not simply the artifact of mental retardation. In girls with fragile X, the profile is less well documented with more variability. Unlike affected boys, only about one third of girls appear to meet the *Diagnostic and Statistical Manual of Mental Disorders* (4th ed.) diagnostic criteria for ADHD (Freund, Reiss, & Abrams, 1993), although many will present with some ADHD symptomology, notably inattentiveness rather than hyperactivity (Hagerman et al., 1992; Mazzocco, Baumgardner, Freund, & Reiss, 1998). Other studies, however, using parental rating scales have reported significant problems with hyperactivity ranging from 38%–47% of affected girls.

Cognitive Profile

Although early reports indicated a slight verbal versus nonverbal discrepancy with better Verbal IQ scores than Performance IQ scores in males and females with fragile X syndrome (Theobald, Hay, & Judge, 1987; Veenema, Veenema, & Geraedts, 1987), it is now not regarded as a hallmark of the syndrome. Instead, and as will be described in detail below, the fragile X syndrome profile is characterized by uneven abilities within and across cognitive domains (Cornish et al., 2004). In essence, the cognitive dysfunction can be described as more "skill specific" rather than "global" in nature.

Cognitive Strengths and Difficulties

It is now well established that boys and girls with fragile X syndrome present with distinct cognitive profiles that differentiate them from children with other developmental disorders. Although mental retardation is a core clinical feature of fragile X, especially in boys, recent evidence clearly points to an uneven profile of cognitive strengths and difficulties that represents a developmental pathway that is atypical rather than simply delayed. Here we highlight recent findings from five cognitive domains known to be impaired in children with fragile X syndrome: speech and language, memory, motor, number, and attention. See table 3.2 for a summary of the fragile X syndrome cognitive phenotype. Note that strengths as well as deficits characterize this syndrome.

Speech and Language   It is well established that children with fragile X syndrome have delayed language acquisition (Fisch et al., 1999; Roberts, Mirrett, & Burchinal, 2001). There are at least four consequences of having fragile X syndrome that contribute to this delay. Individuals with fragile X syndrome are prone to recurrent ear infections (Hagerman, Altshul-Stark, & McBogg, 1987), low tone or hypotonia (Hagerman, Smith, & Mariner, 1983; Wisniewski, Segan, Miezejeski, Sersen, & Rudelli, 1991) sensory integration problems, and mental retardation. These consequences contribute to the late onset of language abilities. Once the individual with

Table 3.2
The fragile X syndrome cognitive phenotype

Strengths	Difficulties
Vocabulary acquisition	Speech (perseverative)
Memory for meaningful information	Memory for abstract information
Visuoperceptual processing	Visuomotor processing
Selective attention	Attentional control/inhibition
	Number processing

fragile X syndrome begins to speak, language is characterized by both delayed and atypical language/speech forms. An example of delayed language is the relatively spared semantic, morphological, and syntactic knowledge (Abbeduto et al., 2003; Sudhalter, Scarborough, & Cohen, 1991) of males with fragile X syndrome. Examples of the atypical language produced by males with fragile X are found within their social or conversational interactions. These interactions contain tangential language (Sudhalter & Belser, 2001), perseverative language (Ferrier, Bashir, Meryash, Johnston, & Wolff, 1991; Sudhalter, Cohen, Silverman, & Wolf-Schein, 1990), and repetitive speech (Hanson, Jackson, & Hagerman, 1986; Belser & Sudhalter, 2001). Each of these atypical language types is described below.

Tangential and Perseverative Language   Tangential language refers to off-topic questions, responses, or comments that do not logically follow the preceding conversational thread. Perseverative language refers to the reintroduction of favorite topics over and over, even in the presence of conflicting conversational demands. Studies comparing males with fragile X syndrome to verbal and chronologically matched individuals with mental retardation and individuals with autistic disorder demonstrated that males with fragile X syndrome produced significantly more tangential (Sudhalter & Belser, 2001) and perseverative language (Sudhalter et al., 1990; Ferrier et al., 1991) than either of the other cohorts. This suggests that these forms of atypical language production are not the consequence of being delayed or of undiagnosed autistic disorder.

Repetitive Speech   Repetitive speech refers to the repetition of sounds, words, or phrases within an utterance or conversational turn. In addition to the atypical types of language described above, another common linguistic characteristic of males with fragile X syndrome is repetitive speech (Belser & Sudhalter, 2001; Borghgraef, Frons, Dielkens, Pyck, & Van Den Berghe, 1987; Hanson et al., 1986). In studies comparing males with fragile X syndrome to chronologically and cognitively matched cohorts with either mental retardation or autistic disorder, it was demonstrated that males with fragile X produced significantly more repetitive speech than either of their matched cohorts.

We have suggested that one of the causes for these atypical language forms is the hyperarousal that social interactions cause in the males with fragile X. In a very small pilot study (described above) Belser and Sudhalter (1995) demonstrated that the language of males with fragile X syndrome was disturbed during periods of eye contact. When the males were not asked to maintain eye contact, their language contained significantly fewer examples of atypical language/speech. In subsequent papers, the authors suggested that the effects of hyperarousal induced the production of repetitive speech by causing the male to speak more quickly, thus interfering with productive abilities (Belser & Sudhalter, 2001), and additionally that hyperarousal interferes with the normal workings of the mental lexicon (a neural network of word meanings) thus promoting tangential language (Sudhalter & Belser, 2001).

The language of females with fragile X has not been described in the detail that the language of males has been. Lesniak-Karpiak et al. (2003) demonstrated that females with fragile X syndrome required significantly more time to initiate interactions than females with Turner syndrome, suggesting that females as well as males with fragile X are affected by social anxiety and that this anxiety may interfere with verbal production within social situations.

Memory   Not all components of memory are equally affected by fragile X syndrome. In boys, evidence clearly points to *relative* strengths in long-term and short-term recall for meaningful information including memory for faces (Turk & Cornish, 1998) and story recall (Munir, Cornish, & Wilding, 2000) with performance at a level equivalent to typical children matched on *developmental* level (but not chronological age level). No equivalent published studies have been conducted in girls with fragile X syndrome. In terms of *working memory* (the ability to retain and manipulate information "online" over short periods, which is crucial in guiding attention and behavior during the course of an activity), accumulating evidence points to a relative weakness in visuospatial working memory compared to verbal working memory (Cornish, Munir, & Cross, 1999; Munir et al., 2000). For example, Munir et al. (2000) examined working memory performance in 25 boys with fragile X syndrome, ages 8–15 years, 25 boys with Down syndrome (trisomy 21) ages 7–15 years, and two groups (25 in each) of typically developing children matched to the syndrome groups on developmental level (mental age) and on chronological age. At first glance the findings indicated general weaknesses across both verbal and visual memory skills that were not syndrome specific but suggestive of developmental delay. However, closer inspection revealed that the impairment of the group with fragile X syndrome relative to that of the Down syndrome group was significantly larger on tasks that tapped visuospatial memory skills than for tasks that tapped verbal memory skills. In comparison to boys with fragile, few studies have addressed working memory in affected girls and those that have focused almost exclusively on adult women. However, two recent studies by Mazzocco and colleagues highlight difficulties in working memory thresholds that also include a specific deficit in visual memory (Mazzocco, Bhatia, & Lesniak-Karpiak, 2006; Kirk, Mazzocco, & Kover, 2005). Less than 53% of affected girls (compared to 96% of typically developing females) were able to recreate the gestalt of a design by memory even though they could correctly identify the object. This finding lends some support to a tentative hypothesis that visuospatial impairment may be a defining feature of the phenotype in both boys and girls irrespective of degree of intellectual impairment. However, one must show some caution here in giving the impression that visual memory is a global person with weakness in fragile X syndrome. Variability, especially in the female phenotype, is inevitable, and studies of adult women have reported visual memory skills that are within the normal range (Mazzocco, Pennington, & Hagerman, 1993).

Visual–Motor Coordination   Another striking aspect of fragile X syndrome is the observed visuomotor deficits. In affected boys, there have been several reports of sensorimotor integration difficulties and visual–motor impairments (Busca Safont Tria, 2001; Cornish et al., 1999; Freund & Reiss, 1991). At a finer level of analysis, a number of recent neuropsychological studies have revealed lacunae in performance for tasks requiring the integration of visual information for effective motor control. For example, Cornish et al. (1999) recently demonstrated impairments in boys with fragile X syndrome (ages between 7 and 12 years) as compared to typical developing boys matched on developmental level for abstract visuoconstructive tasks, such as the Block Design subtest of the Wechsler Intelligence Scale for Children—Revised, and on a task of drawing (Draw-a-Person task). In contrast, these same boys did not show impairments in their performance on neuropsychological tasks that measure visuoperceptual abilities. A similar pattern of performance has been reported in girls with fragile X (Cornish et al., 1998). In contrast, relative strengths have been reported on visuoperceptual tasks and face recognition tasks (Hodapp et al., 1992; Cornish et al., 1999; Turk & Cornish, 1998). One possible explanation for this dissociation has come from a series of recent neurobiological studies by Kogan and colleagues (e.g., Kogan, Boutet et al., 2004; Kogan, Bertone et al., 2004) that speculate that fragile X syndrome is associated with selective deficits in magnocellular/dorsal stream visual functioning that result in an underlying impairment in regions of the brain devoted to processing visual information for the purpose of control of action. In contrast, the parvocellular/ventral stream is a transformer of visual input necessary for the conscious perception of visual information (e.g., color and recognition). Because fragile X syndrome is caused by a single gene, Kogan, Boutet et al. (2004) proposed that the protein normally expressed by the FMR1 gene and lacking in protein (FMRP) might be more important to normal magnocellular (M) neuron function or structure than parvocellular (P) function. Indeed, postmortem analyses did reveal FMRP to be expressed in greater abundance in the M pathway of monkey and human brains, suggesting that this pathway is more reliant on the protein for normal functioning. In contrast, postmortem analyses of an adult with fragile X syndrome revealed abnormal neuromorphology of LGN neurons such that they appear more like P neurons than M neurons. Kogan et al. concluded that abnormal visual–motor behavior in fragile X syndrome can be partially attributed to an M pathway deficiency in FMRP. These findings highlight the need for medical and pedagogical treatment to focus on improving early visual–motor coordination.

Number Processing Both boys and girls with fragile X syndrome experience considerable difficulty in acquiring math skills irrespective of academic attainment. Early work by Dykens and colleagues (e.g., Dykens, Hodapp, & Leckman, 1987; Hodapp, Dykens, Ort, Zelinsky, & Leckman, 1991) using the Kaufman Assessment Battery for Children (Kaufman & Kaufman, 1983) identified a specific deficit in arithmetic in boys with fragile X syndrome compared to the performance of boys with Down syndrome and typically developing children. Similar findings were also reported by Kemper, Hagerman, and Altshul-Stark (1988). Together, these findings suggest that poor arithmetic skills in boys with fragile X syndrome may not solely be attributed to general developmental delay but may be syndrome specific. More recent work has begun to define the math profile at a finer grained level. Roberts et al. (2005), for example, did not find a relative deficit in math skills in boys ages 3–14 years when the math problem was put into a meaningful context rather than requiring an abstract calculation. This finding is the first to suggest that context may place a crucial role in math development in boys with fragile. In girls with fragile X syndrome, math achievement is also an area of considerable difficulty, and problems have been reported as early as 5 years of age (Mazzocco, 2001). When present, the math difficulties are almost always persistent and thus do not diminish over time (Murphy, Mazzocco, Gerner, & Henry, 2006). Recent studies, however, highlight the variability in math performance among girls with fragile X by suggesting that not all math skills are comparably impaired. In the most recent study to date, Mazzocco et al. (2006) examined math performance in 15 girls with fragile X syndrome, 15 girls with Turner syndrome (a disorder that is caused by the partial or total loss of an X chromosome), and 15 IQ-matched comparison children (7–9 years of age). Although they found that girls with fragile X syndrome had a specific weakness on measures that tapped both formal, learned math (such as the procedures used in addition algorithms) and informal, intuitive math (recognizing which of two sets of items has more items), the impairment of the group with fragile X relative to that of the comparison group for tasks that required basic counting or calculating skills did not reach significance. When Mazzocco and colleagues (Murphy et al., 2006) examined counting skills more closely, they found that girls with fragile X had difficulty understanding counting rules and applications of counting knowledge, whereas rote counting skills were comparable to skills observed in an age- and grade-matched comparison group. Thus, while mathematics difficulties in girls with fragile X may not pertain to all aspects of mathematics, the persistence and nature of these difficulties suggest that mathematics achievement is likely to pose lifelong challenges and should thus be monitored periodically to determine appropriate educational support.

Attention Impairments in attentional focus alongside excessive distractibility and poor inhibitory control are well documented characteristics of both boys and girls with fragile X (see Cornish et al., 2004, for a review). Although the majority of research has focused on late childhood, recent evidence suggests that attention difficulties emerge early in development: Hooper, Hatton, Baranek, Roberts, and Bailey (2000) showed that children with fragile X from 4 years of age display striking difficulties in attention and memory subscales of the Leiter International Performance Scale Revised (Leiter-R; Roid & Miller, 1997), a nonverbal assessment tool. In a series of recent studies, Sceriff, Cornish, and Karmiloff-Smith have demonstrated even earlier difficulties in the control of attention in children with fragile X as young as 12 months of age (Scerif, Cornish, Wilding, Driver, & Karmiloff-Smith, 2004; Scerif et al., 2005; Cornish et al., in press). These studies aimed at tracing developmental trajectories of attentional control in children with fragile and in typically developing groups. While typically developing toddlers displayed gradual improvements in the accuracy with which they searched their visual environment, toddlers with fragile X tended to perseverate and were unable to shift attention away from previously correct responses, regardless of their overall developmental level. These findings replicate the pattern of difficulties seen in older boys (ages 7–12 years; Wilding, Cornish, & Munir, 2002) and in young adult men (ages 18–30 years; Cornish, Munir, & Cross, 2001). Similar difficulties in attention switching in girls with fragile X (ages 8–16 years) have also been reported (Kovar, 1993). Thus, difficulties in perseveration and in shifting attentional focus are core deficits in fragile X syndrome and appear to remain constant with age. In contrast, the ability to select relevant from irrelevant information (selective attention) is a relative strength at least in males with fragile X and this continues to develop linearly with increasing chronological age (Cornish et al., in press). Comparable developmental studies in females are needed to understand the range of attention dysfunction and its relation with age and IQ. To date, however, the current findings underscore the importance of recognizing and treating early attention deficits that left untreated will impact significantly across development and learning.

The Importance of Recognizing Comorbidities in Fragile X Syndrome and Their Impact on Early Identification

The child with fragile X syndrome and ADHD, alone or as part of an autism spectrum disorder, may display motor overactivity (sometimes seen as aimless activity or exploration), inability to concentrate or focus, distractibility, and inability to inhibit impulses (see section above). To some extent, these behaviors overlap with those seen in children with anxiety disorders, making it difficult to distinguish between them. The child with an anxiety disorder may have any or all of these symptoms, plus difficulty sleeping, obvious fright in some situations, signs of autonomic arousal not seen in ADHD (flushing, pallor, tachypnea [rapid breathing], tachycardia [rapid pulse], diaphoresis [sweating]), or frank panic episodes (sudden panicky running, aggression, or self-injury accompanied by signs of autonomic arousal). Both ADHD and anxiety disorders are part of the behavioral phenotype of fragile X syndrome, and it is possible for a child to have both ADHD and an anxiety disorder, evolving separately or together, making complete treatment a matter of a combined approach. Likewise, autistic-like features or a diagnosis of an autism spectrum disorder may precede an initial diagnosis of fragile X syndrome. DNA testing for fragile X is therefore an important part of the evaluation of any child with an autism spectrum disorder, and any child with ADHD, panic disorder, generalized anxiety disorder, and a maternal family history of developmental, learning, or anxiety disorders.

Interventions

Nonmedical Interventions

As with any disability, whether physical or cognitive, the sooner the child enters into early intervention the better. Some of the early symptoms of fragile X syndrome such as hypotonia, physical delays, oral motor difficulties, and speech delay can be addressed through speech and language therapy, oral motor therapy and occupational therapy. For instance, through oral motor therapy, boys or girls will learn how to eat more efficiently and produce language sounds. If the child has difficulty attaining motor milestones, physical and occupational therapy may assist in the acquisition of important daily living skills. Speech therapy will help the child to learn social interactive skills and to acquire vocabulary and syntax while the speech apparatus matures to the point that language sounds can be produced. It has been the experience of the fragile X community that combining therapies often produces beneficial results—that is, having the speech and language therapist use sensory motor techniques to calm the child while teaching language; similarly, the occupational therapist should encourage as much verbalization and communication as possible while teaching sensory techniques.

Many young boys and girls children with fragile X syndrome have difficulty with transitions, sensory stimulation, and hyperarousal (see above). These difficulties can manifest as behavior problems such as noncompliance, aggression, or tantrumming. Very often, a careful analysis of the environment within which the child is interacting can give clues as to both the reasons for the child's actions and appropriate remedies for the child's behavior. For instance if confronted with a visually and auditorily stimulating environment, the child may become uncomfortable. The easiest solution is to reduce the stimulation and place the child in a less stimulating place. Of course, preschools and elementary schools can be loud and youngsters cannot be asked to be quiet all the time. At those times when the environment does become loud, it will be important that the child have a quiet place to go or something he can do (e.g., put on earmuffs or sun glasses if tolerated) to help reduce the sensory stimulation. As the child gets older, when the teachers or parents know that the environment is going to become too overwhelming, the child should be allowed to go someplace safe and quiet (i.e., bedroom or library) to avoid the environment that may cause difficulties. Additionally, it will be important to give the child an awareness of what will and will not cause discomfort and support teaching the child effective strategies to cope with the environment. In this regard sensory integration techniques may be beneficial throughout the child's tenure in school. Transitions can be especially troublesome individuals with fragile X syndrome. Visual aids, sensory motor integrative techniques, and preparation for the transition can all be helpful tools to assist the child as he transitions through the day.

Individuals with fragile X syndrome are often misunderstood. The influence of the environment on their behavior is often overlooked. In addition, anticipatory anxiety, which is the awareness that some activity is looming, often influences behavior in individuals with fragile X (by causing either perseverative language or noncompliance) and is usually not appreciated. Often, all it takes to understand what is bothering the individual is to listen to the individual, who may tell you through perseverative language what is anticipated. Often times behavioral techniques can be very beneficial. However, it will be important that the behaviorist who is evaluating the child and interpreting behavior of a child with fragile X syndrome is familiar with the syndrome and understands the hyperarousal and anxiety associated with social situations for children affected by fragile X.

Psychopharmacological Interventions

Fragile X syndrome presents several potentially medication-responsive symptoms and comorbid psychiatric disorders. There are no drugs uniquely effective or uniquely ineffective for children with fragile X, nor are there drugs to treat the core symptoms of the syndrome itself. The targets of our available agents are common secondary disorders such as ADHD, or comorbid disorders such as anxiety disorders, or problems such as mood instability that may or may not be characteristic of fragile X but are exacerbated by it. Surveys of drug use at fragile X clinics (Amaria, Billeisen, & Hagerman, 2001; Tsiouris & Brown, 2004) show use of the wide variety of agents typical of any child psychiatric clinic or clinic for children with intellectual disabilities.

From the standpoint of the clinician, studies of these drugs, taken together, demonstrate only their safety and efficacy. A few studies have established the effectiveness of some classes of drugs in persons with fragile X syndrome (Hagerman, Murphy, & Wittenberger, 1988; Hagerman, Fulton et al., 1994; Hagerman et al., 1995). There are no studies of comparative efficacy (with a single exception: Riley,

Ikle, & Hagerman, 2000), and studies comparing one drug approach to another for a particular symptom or disorder are rare and almost never include persons with intellectual disabilities. The clinician is left to choose treatment from a catalog of agents, based upon psychiatric diagnosis and individual patient variables. Within classes of drugs (mood stabilizers, SSRIs) there is little to help the clinician choose among available agents. Even in the rare instances of comparative efficacy studies, only one has included patients with fragile X syndrome (Riley et al., 2000). The best guide to effective treatment is accurate diagnosis of the psychiatric symptom or comorbid disorder. Drug responsive components of the behavioral phenotype of fragile X syndrome—ADHD, obsessive–compulsive features of autism spectrum disorders, generalized anxiety disorder, panic disorder, PTSD, major depressive disorder, and bipolar disorder—can all be recognized from their effects on behavior, autonomic arousal, level of activity, and sleep and appetite (Levitas, Hurley, & Pary, 2001; Levitas & Silka, 2001). Family history of psychiatric disorder can be a guide to diagnosis, even within the behavioral phenotype of fragile X syndrome.

As important as diagnosing psychiatric disorder is ruling it out; isolated problem behaviors might proceed from environmental variables (inappropriate school setting or other demand, overstimulation or particular noxious events for a person with hyperarousal problems—e.g., fire drills—unfortunate family events, abuse, and other trauma) or may simply be based on hyperarousal. Many endocrine and neurological disorders have behavioral manifestations, and these must be ruled out as well. Such isolated behaviors are very unlikely to respond to medication or to medication alone. Family history of drug response may be a guide to choice of pharmacologic agent, but two family members might have completely different responses to the same drug. In the end, these may be guides to no more than a first choice of medication for trial, with many trials being necessary to establish the optimal treatment, or, more usually, a treatment that is "good enough" to allow the child and family to proceed with development.

Case 3.2: Ian   Ian is a 9-year-old boy with fragile X syndrome, referred for evaluation for possible ADHD. Until fourth grade he had been in a special class setting; he was now in a self-contained classroom with mainstreaming for some subjects, but was severely language impaired. Ian required repeated redirection to focus on classroom work, even with minimal demand and distraction. Motor overactivity was not severe. He showed some perseverative speech, was easily distracted, and demonstrated extreme social anxiety when meeting new people and in novel situations. Ian's maternal family history of fragile X was well-documented. His birth weight was 8 lbs. 2 oz. As an infant, Ian cuddled and breast-fed poorly, and he showed gaze-avoidance from a very early age. Speech and language were also delayed. He continued receiving speech and occupational therapies, and in second and third grade Ian attended a school for children with communication-based learning problems. Poor attention span and distractibility were noted. He could self-calm, and he denied anxieties. At interview Ian displayed mild gaze avoidance but was personable and outgoing. He acknowledged difficulty concentrating and ignoring distractions and was willing to consider a trial of medication for this. Diagnosis was ADHD.

Intervention   As stated above, ADHD is frequently documented in children with fragile X and can impact across many domains of learning and behavior both at home and school. In Ian's case, this child had already acquired some very important skills, such as self calming—which is very important in children with fragile X. It would be important to make Ian aware of those environmental and social variables that cause him to be uncomfortable. If, for instance, Ian has a school peer who makes a lot of noise (causing him to lose focus), he should learn how to ask for quiet. To that end, role play would be a very useful tool. Ian could practice routines that he would need in his everyday life. Once these verbal routines were practiced, he would then be able to access them when needed.

Role play may also help Ian with his language difficulties, as it would supply him with practiced routines which he could use when needed. The task of having to create language when anxious or upset usually results in repetitive or dysfluent language in individuals with fragile X. Ian would also benefit greatly from social skills training. To that end, Carol Gray stories are a very helpful component in that social skills training, as they are designed to build social awareness and help children learn social routines. Carol Gray first defined social stories in 1991. In her way of thinking, social stories address the needs of individuals with difficulties in understanding the social milieu within which they find themselves. There are four types of sentences found within social stories, each designed to help the reader understand the story, how the protagonist may feel, and how to act when confronted with a similar situation. For example, the social story is written with descriptive sentences that are truthful, opinion- and assumption-free statements of fact; perspective sentences refer to or describe a person's internal states; directive sentences help the reader find ways of responding or acting; and affirmative sentences enhance the meaning of the story by expressing the value structure of a given culture (Gray, 2000). These stories can not only be enjoyable but also help the child with social skills deficits begin to understand how to act in socially acceptable ways.

Ian may also benefit from continued occupational therapy until he has attained age-appropriate daily living skills and handwriting ability. Also the sensory motor techniques that he learns may be used when Ian begins to feel overwhelmed and overloaded in his classroom.

Ian's teachers should provide him with visual aids whenever possible. These visuals aids will assist with concentration and take some of the burden of school tasks off his auditory memory. A visual chart can also be created for the child so he can know what is expected of him at any given time. Once a task is completed, Ian can have the pleasure of taking the visual symbol of that task and placing it in a completed pile. He would also know what to go on to next. Visual aids can also be used to prompt the child through tasks. Children with ADHD have difficulty organizing their time; thus, these visual aids will be the external organizer the child needs in order to complete his work.

From a *medical perspective*, a stimulant should be tried; methylphenidate/Ritalin first; Dexedrine mixed salts/Adderall or Dexedrine could be tried if Ritalin proves ineffective, or an a-adrenergic if stimulants are poorly tolerated. Standard preparations should be tried first, in divided doses; these can be converted to long-acting preparations (Concerta, Adderall-XR) if desired.

Case 3.3: Jeremy   Jeremy was a 5-year-old boy referred for evaluation of aggressive episodes. He was described as "always going a hundred miles an hour," with distractibility and impulsivity. Episodes were precipitated by unwanted limits or interactions with siblings, transitions, or even pleasurable excitement, and consisted of screaming, crying, and various forms of self-injury or assault, usually on brother. Jeremy slept poorly, waking at least twice every night, and at 5 a.m. for the day. DNA testing revealed CGG > 200 at 36 months. Jeremy's mother's pregnancy was medically unremarkable, with labor induced at 40 weeks' gestation. His birth weight was 6 lbs., 15 oz., with Apgars 8/9. He was gaze avoidant and did not cuddle. Jeremy walked at 14 months, with toe walking, hand flapping, and other stereotypy. He ignored toys except to line them up or throw them, ignored peers, and exhibited hyperacusis. He began speech therapy at 19 months, finally speaking at 36 months; speech was a mix of communication and echolalia. Short attention span was noted in school and home. Jeremy's speech therapist noted that he greeted her with a mix of approach and anxious withdrawal, displaying "cluttering" in his speech. He rapidly explored her office, playing briefly and indiscriminately with both toys and office equipment. The diagnosis was autistic disorder, with comorbid ADHD.

Intervention   Many children with fragile X syndrome exhibit autistic-like behaviors similar to those described above. Many of the techniques that work with children with autism without fragile X will also be successful with Jeremy. These techniques include speech and language therapy, Applied Behavioral Analytic therapy and occupational therapy. However, it will be important for those individuals who work with this child to appreciate the differences between a child with autistic disorder and fragile X and a child with autistic disorder without fragile X. For instance, the child with only autistic disorder will not have the same response to the stimulation in his environment as the child with fragile X. The sensory stimulation may cause the child with autism but without fragile X to be distracted or not pay attention, whereas the sensory stimulation may cause the child with a dual diagnosis of autism and fragile X syndrome to become hyperaroused and therefore engage in maladaptive behaviors. It is likely that using only behavioral techniques to stop these maladaptive behaviors without "fixing" the environmental problems would not be effective in changing Jeremy's behavior.

Additionally, it is traditional to teach children with autism to maintain eye contact so that the child can focus and learn language. One would not want to encourage a child with fragile X syndrome to maintain eye contact. The maintenance of eye contact is aversive for the child as has been described above. The forcing of eye contact could also induce maladaptive behavior in the child with fragile X.

From a *medical perspective*, treatment must begin with consideration of which set of symptoms appears most in need of remediation and which medications type is most likely to be tolerated by the patient. Stimulants and a-adrenergics used for ADHD are better tolerated by younger children than are the SSRIs used to treat anxiety disorders; a-adrenergics may decrease anxiety by decreasing hyperarousal. Often a good strategy when both problems are present is to start by treating hyperactivity and adding an SSRI if necessary, bearing in mind the necessity to monitor cardiac side effects when a-adrenergics and SSRIs are used together.

Conclusion

Infants and children with fragile X syndrome represent a unique constellation of strengths and difficulties that impact across developmental time, affecting both cognitive and behavioral functioning. The last decade has seen tremendous advances in our understanding of this syndrome and its variability across many different levels— the genetic level, the brain level, and the cognitive and behavioral levels. Most recently, the role of environmental influences in helping define the "fragile X syndrome signature" has been explored (Hessl et al., 2001; Kuo, Reiss, Freund, & Huffman, 2002). Together, these advances highlight the importance of recognizing the distinct phenotypic outcomes that characterize a child with fragile X syndrome. They provide a multidisciplinary approach to investigating the developmental, cognitive, and behavioral symptoms of fragile X and to a recognition that the syndrome may co-occur with more common disorders such as ADHD and autism. Early diagnosis is crucial if educational and clinical interventions are to have maximum impact in enabling children with fragile X syndrome to develop to their maximum potential.

Acknowledgments

The authors gratefully acknowledge the help of Joshua Levitas with the illustrations. Cornish was supported by grants from the Canada Institute of Health Research, Social Sciences and Humanities Research Council, Canada, and the Mental Health Foundation, UK.

References

Abbeduto, L., Murphy, M. M., Cawthorn, S. W., Richmond, E. K., Weissman, M. D., Karadottir, S., et al. (2003). Receptive language skills of adolescents and young adults with Down or fragile X syndrome. *American Journal on Mental Retardation, 108,* 149–160.

Achenbach, T. M. (1991). *Manual for the Child Behaviour Checklist/4-18.* Burlington: University of Vermont, Department of Psychiatry.

Amaria, R. N., Billeisen, L. L., & Hagerman, R. J. (2001). Medication use in fragile X syndrome. *Mental Health Aspects of Developmental Disabilities, 4,* 143–147.

Bailey, D. B., Jr., Hatton, D. D., Mesibov, G., Ament, N., & Skinner, M. (2000). Early development, temperament, and functional impairment in autism and fragile X syndrome. *Journal of Autism and Developmental Disorders, 30,* 49–59.

Bailey, D. B., Jr., Hatton, D. D., Skinner, M., & Mesibov, G. B. (2001). Autistic behavior, FMR1 protein, and developmental trajectories in young males with fragile X syndrome. *Journal of Autism and Developmental Disorders, 31,* 65–174.

Bailey, D. B., Jr., Mesibov, G. B., Hatton, D. D., Clark, R. D., Roberts, J. E., & Mayhew, L. (1998). Autistic behavior in young boys with fragile X syndrome. *Journal of Autism and Developmental Disorders, 28,* 499–508.

Bakker, C. E., Otero, Y. D., Bonteko, C., Raghoe, P., Luteijn, T., Hoogeveen, A. T., et al. (2000). Immunocytochemical and biochemical characterization of FMRP, FXR1P, and FXR2P in the mouse. *Experimental Cell Research, 258,* 162–170.

Bardoni, B., Mandel, J. L., & Fisch, G. S. (2000). FMR1 gene and fragile X syndrome. *American Journal of Medical Genetics, 97,* 153–163.

Baumgardner, T. L., Reiss, A. L., Freund, L. S., & Abrams, M. T. (1995). Specification of the neurobehavioral phenotype in males with fragile X syndrome. *Pediatrics, 95,* 744–752.

Bear, M. F., Huber, K. M., & Warren, S. T. (2004). The mGluR theory of fragile X mental retardation. *Trends in Neuroscience, 27,* 370–377.

Belser, R. C., & Sudhalter, V. (1995). Arousal difficulties in males with fragile X syndrome: A preliminary report. *Developmental Brain Dysfunction, 8,* 252–269.

Belser, R. C., & Sudhalter, V. (2001). Conversational Characteristics of Children with Fragile X Syndrome: Repetitive Speech. *American Journal on Mental Retardation, 106,* 28–38.

Bennetto, L., & Pennington, B. F. (2002). Neuropsychology. In R. J. Hagerman, & P. J. Hagerman (Eds.), *Fragile X syndrome: Diagnosis, treatment, and research* (pp. 206–248). Baltimore: Johns Hopkins University Press.

Borghgraef, M., Frons, J. P., Dielkens, A., Pyck, K., & Van Den Berghe, H. (1987). Fragile X syndrome: A study of the psychological profile in 23 prepubertal patients. *Clinical Genetics, 32,* 179–186.

Busca Safont-Tria, N. (2002). Psychomotricity and fragile X syndrome. *Revista de Neurologia, 33* (Suppl. 1), S77–S81.

Cohen, I. L. (1995). Behavioral profiles of autistic and nonautistic fragile X males. *Developmental Brain Dysfunction, 8,* 252–269.

Cohen, I. L., Sudhalter, V., Pfadt, A., Jenkins, E. C., Brown, W. T., & Vietze, P. M. (1991). Why are autism and the fragile X syndrome associated? Conceptual and methodological issues. *American Journal of Human Genetics, 48,* 195–202.

Cornish, K. M., Munir, F., & Cross, G. (1998). The nature of the spatial deficit in young females with fragile-X syndrome: A neuropsychological and molecular perspective. *Neuropsychologia, 11,* 1239–1246.

Cornish, K. M., Munir, F., & Cross, G. (1999). Spatial cognition in males with fragile X syndrome: Evidence for a neuropsychological phenotype. *Cortex, 35,* 263–271.

Cornish, K. M., Munir, F., & Cross, G. (2001). Differential impact of the FMR-1 full mutation on memory and attention functioning: A neuropsychological perspective. *Journal of Cognitive Neuroscience, 13,* 1–7.

Cornish, K., Munir, F., & Wilding, J. (2001). A neuropsychological and behavioural profile of attention deficits in fragile X syndrome. *Revista de Neurologia, 33* (Suppl. 1), S24–S9.

Cornish, K., Scerif, G., & Karmiloff-Smith, A. (2007). Tracing syndrome-specific trajectories of attention across the lifespan. *Cortex.*

Cornish, K., Sudhalter, V., & Turk, J. (2004). Attention and language in fragile X. *Mental Retardation and Developmental Disabilities Research Reviews, 10,* 11–16.

de Vries, B. B., Halley, D. J., Oostra, B. A., & Niermeijer, M. F. (1998). Fragile X syndrome. *Journal of Medical Genetics, 7,* 579–589.

Dykens, E. M., Hodapp, R. M., & Leckman, J. F. (1987). Strengths and weaknesses in the intellectual functioning of males with fragile X syndrome. *American Journal of Mental Deficiency, 92,* 234–236.

Eliez, S., Blasey, C. M., Freund, L. S., Hastie, T., & Reiss, A. L. (2001). Brain anatomy, gender and IQ in children and adolescents with fragile X syndrome. *Brain, 24,* 1610–1618.

Ferrier, L. J., Bashir, A. S., Meryash, D. L., Johnston, J., & Wolff, P. (1991). Conversational skills of individuals with fragile-X syndrome: A comparison with autism and Down syndrome. *Developmental Medicine and Child Neurology, 33,* 776–788.

Fisch, G. S., Holden, J. J., Carpenter, N. J., Howard-Peebles, P. N., Maddalena, A., Pandya, A., et al. (1999). Age-related language characteristics of children and adolescents with fragile X syndrome. *American Journal of Medical Genetic, 83,* 253–256.

Freund, L. S., & Reiss, A. L. (1991). Cognitive profiles associated with the fra(X) syndrome in males and females. *American Journal of Medical Genetics, 38,* 542–547.

Freund, L. S., Reiss, A. L., & Abrams, M. T. (1993). Psychiatric disorders associated with fragile X in the young female. *Pediatrics, 91,* 321–329.

Galvez, R., & Greenough, W. T. (2005). Sequence of abnormal dendritic spine development in primary somatosensory cortex of a mouse model of the fragile X mental retardation syndrome. *American Journal of Medical Genetics, 135,* 155–160.

Garrett, A. S., Menon, V., MacKenzie, K., & Reiss, A. L. (2004). Here's looking at you, kid: Neural systems underlying face and gaze processing in fragile X syndrome. *Archives of General Psychiatry, 61,* 281–288.

Gray, C. (2000). *The new social story book.* Arlington, VA: Future Horizon.

Hagerman, R. J. (1996). Physical and behavioral phenotype. In R. J. Hagerman & A. C. Cronister (Eds.), *Fragile X syndrome: Diagnosis, treatment and research* (pp. 3–87). Baltimore: Johns Hopkins University Press.

Hagerman, R. J., Altshul-Stark, D., & McBogg, P. (1987). Recurrent otitis media in boys with fragile X syndrome. *American Journal of Disease of Children, 141,* 184–187.

Hagerman, R. J., Fulton, M. J., Leaman, A., Riddle, J., Hagerman, K., & Sobesky, W. (1994a). A survey of fluoxetine therapy in fragile X syndrome. *Developmental Brain Dysfunction, 7,* 155–164.

Hagerman, P. J., & Hagerman, R. J. (2004). The fragile X premutation: A maturing perspective. *American Journal of Human Genetics, 74,* 805–816.

Hagerman, R. J., Hull, C. E., Safanda, J. F., Carpenter, I., Staley, L. W., O'Connor, R. A., et al. (1994b). High functioning fragile X males: Demonstration of an unmethylated fully expanded FMR-1 mutation associated with protein expression. *American Journal of Medical Genetics, 51,* 298–308.

Hagerman, R. J., Jackson, C., Amiri, K., Silverman, A. C., O'Connor, R., & Sobesky, W. (1992). Girls with fragile X syndrome: Physical and neurocognitive status and outcome. *Pediatrics, 89,* 395–400.

Hagerman, R. J., Murphy, M. A., & Wittenberger, M. D. (1988). A controlled trial of stimulant medication in children with the fragile X syndrome. *American Journal of Medical Genetics, 30,* 377–392.

Hagerman, R. J., Riddle, J. E., Roberts, L. S., Brease, K., & Fulton, M. (1995). A survey of the efficacy of clonidine in fragile X syndrome. *Developmental Brain Dysfunction, 8,* 336–344.

Hagerman, R. J., Smith, A., & Mariner, R. (1983). Clinical features of the fragile X syndrome. In R. J. Hagerman, & P. McBogg (Eds.), *The fragile X syndrome: Diagnosis, biochemistry and intervention* (pp. 17–53). Dillon, CO: Spectra Publishing.

Hanson, D. M., Jackson, A. W., & Hagerman, R. J. (1986). Speech disturbances (cluttering) in mildly impaired males with Martin–Bell/fragile X syndrome. *American Journal of Medical Genetics, 23,* 195–206.

Hatton, D. D., Hooper, S. R., Bailey, D. B., Skinner, M. L., Sullivan, K. M., & Wheeler, A. (2002). Problem behavior in boys with fragile X syndrome. *American Journal of Medical Genetics, 108,* 105–116.

Hatton, D. D., Wheeler, A. C., Skinner, M. L., Bailey, D. B., Sullivan, K. M., Roberts, J. E., et al. (2003). Adaptive behavior in children with fragile X syndrome. *American Journal on Mental Retardation, 108,* 373–390.

Hessl, D., Dyer-Friedman, J., Glaser, B., Wisbeck, J., Barajas, R. G., Taylor, A., et al. (2001). The influence of environmental and genetic factors on behavior problems and autistic symptoms in boys and girls with fragile X syndrome. *Pediatrics, 108,* 88.

Hodapp, R. M., Dykens, E. M., Ort, S. I., Zelinsky, D. G., & Leckman, J. F. (1991). Changing patterns of intellectual strengths and weaknesses in males with fragile X syndrome. *Journal of Autism and Developmental Disorders, 21,* 503–516.

Hodapp, R. M., Leckman, J. F., Dykens, E. M., Sparrow, S. S., Zelinsky, D. G., & Ort, S. I. (1992). K-ABC profiles in children with fragile X syndrome, Down syndrome, and nonspecific mental retardation. *American Journal on Mental Retardation, 97,* 39–46.

Hooper, S. R., Hatton, D. D., Baranek, G. T., Roberts, J., & Bailey, D. B. (2000). Nonverbal assessment of cognitive abilities in children with fragile X syndrome: The utility of the Leiter International Performance Scale—Revised. *Journal of Psychoeducational Assessment, 18,* 255–267.

Irwin, S. A., Idupulapati, M., Gilbert, M. E., Harris, J. B., Chakravarti, A. B., Rogers, E. J., et al. (2002). Dendritic spine and dendritic field characteristics of layer V pyramidal neurons in the visual cortex of fragile-X knockout mice. *American Journal of Medical Genetics, 111,* 140–146.

Irwin, S. A., Patel, B., Idupulapati, M., Harris, J. B., Crisostomo, R. A., Larsen, B. P., et al. (2001). Abnormal dendritic spine characteristics in the temporal and visual cortices of patients with fragile-X syndrome: A quantitative examination. *American Journal of Medical Genetics, 98,* 161–167.

Karmiloff-Smith, A. (1998). Development itself is the key to understanding developmental disorders. *Trends in Cognitive Sciences, 2,* 389–399.

Kates, W. R., Abrams, M. T., Kaufmann, W. E., Breiter, S. N., & Reiss, A. L. (1997). Reliability and validity of MRI measurement of the amygdala and hippocampus in children with fragile X syndrome. *Psychiatry Research, 75,* 31–48.

Kau, A. S. M., Reider, E. E., Payne, L., Meyer, W. A., & Freund, L. (2000). Early behavior signs of psychiatric phenotypes in fragile X syndrome. *American Journal on Mental Retardation, 105,* 286–299.

Kau, A. S. M., Tierney, E., Bukelis, I., Stump, M., Kates, W. R., Trescher, W. H., et al. (2004). Social behavior profile in young males with fragile X syndrome: Characteristics and specificity. *American Journal of Medial Genetics, 126,* 9–17.

Kaufman, A. S., & Kaufman, N. L. (1983). *Kaufman Assessment Battery for Children (K-ABC).* Circle Pines, MN: American Guidance Service.

Kemper, M. B., Hagerman, R. J., & Altshul-Stark, D. (1988). Cognitive profiles of boys with the fragile X syndrome. *American Journal of Medical Genetics, 30,* 191–200.

Keysor, C. S., Mazzocco, M. M. M., McLeod, D. R., & Hoehn-Saric, R. (2002). Physiological arousal in females with fragile X or Turner syndrome. *Developmental Psychobiology, 41,* 133–146.

Kirk, J. W., Mazzocco, M. M. M., & Kover, S. T. (2005). Assessing executive dysfunction in girls with fragile X or Turner syndrome using the Contingency Naming Test (CNT). *Developmental Neuropsychology, 28,* 755–777.

Kogan, C. S., Bertone, A., Cornish, K., Boutet, I., Der Kaloustian, V. M., Andermann, E., et al. (2004). Integrative cortical dysfunction and pervasive motion perception deficit in fragile X syndrome. *Neurology, 63,* 1634–1639.

Kogan, C. S., Boutet, I., Cornish, K., Zangenehpour, S., Mullen, K. T., Holden, J. J., et al. (2004). Differential impact of the FMR1 gene on visual processing in fragile X syndrome. *Brain, 127,* 591–601.

Kooy, R. F. (2003). Of mice and the fragile X syndrome. *Trends in Genetics, 19,* 148–154.

Kooy, R. F., Willesden, R., & Oostra, B. A. (2000). Fragile X syndrome at the turn of the century. *Molecular Medicine Today, 6,* 193–198.

Kovar, C. (1993). *The neurocognitive phenotype of fragile X girls.* Unpublished master's thesis, University of Denver, Denver, CO.

Kuo, A. Y., Reiss, A. L., Freund, L. S., & Huffman, L. C. (2002). Family environment and cognitive abilities in girls with fragile-X syndrome. *Journal of Intellectual Disability Research, 46,* 328–339.

Lachiewicz, A. M. (1992). Abnormal behavior in young girls with fragile X syndrome. *American Journal of Medical Genetics, 43,* 72–77.

Lachiewicz, A. M., & Dawson, D. V. (1994). Behavior problems of young girls with fragile X: Scores on the Conners' Parents' Questionnaire. *American Journal of Medical Genetics, 51,* 364–369.

Lachiewicz, A. M., Dawson, D. V., & Spiridigliozzi, G. A. (2000). Physical characteristics of young boys with fragile X syndrome: Reasons for difficulties in making a diagnosis in young males. *American Journal of Medical Genetics, 5,* 229–236.

Lesniak-Karpiak, K., Mazzocco, M. M. M., & Ross, J. L. (2003). Behavioral assessment of social anxiety in females with Turner or fragile X syndrome. *Journal of Autism and Developmental Disorders, 33,* 55–67.

Levitas, A., Hurley, A., & Pary, R. (2001). The mental status examination in patients with mental retardation and developmental disabilities. *Mental Health Aspects of Developmental Disabilities, 4,* 2–16.

Levitas, A., & Silka, V. R. (2001). Mental health clinical assessment of persons with mental retardation and developmental disabilities. *Mental Health Aspects of Developmental Disabilities, 4,* 31–42.

Mazzocco, M. M. M. (2001). Math learning disability and math LD subtypes: Evidence from studies of Turner syndrome, fragile X syndrome, and neurofibromatosis type 1. *Journal of Learning Disabilities, 34,* 520–533.

Mazzocco, M. M. M., Baumgardner, T., Freund, L. S., & Reiss, A. L. (1998). Social functioning among girls with fragile X or Turner syndrome and their sisters. *Journal of Autism and Developmental Disorders, 28,* 509–517.

Mazzocco, M. M. M., Bhatia, N. S., & Lesniak-Karpiak, K. (2006). Visuo-spatial deficits in fragile X or Turner's syndrome. *Child Neuropsychology, 12,* 87–110.

Mazzocco, M. M. M., Pennington, B. F., & Hagerman, R. J. (1993). The neurocognitive phenotype of female carriers of fragile X: Additional evidence for specificity. *Journal of Developmental and Behavioral Pediatrics, 14,* 328–335.

Merenstein, S. A., Sobesky, W. E., Taylor, A. K., Riddle, J. E., Tran, H. X., & Hagerman, R. J. (1996). Molecular–clinical correlations in males with an expanded FMR1 mutation. *American Journal of Medical Genetics, 64,* 388–394.

Miller, L. J., McIntosh, D. N., McGrath, J., Shyu, V., Lampe, M., Taylor, A. K., et al. (1999). Electrodermal responses to sensory stimuli in individuals with fragile X syndrome: A preliminary report. *American Journal of Medical Genetics, 83,* 268–279.

Mostofsky, S. H., Mazzocco, M. M. M., Aakalu, G., Warsofsky, I. S., Denckla, M. B., & Reiss, A. L. (1998). Decreased cerebellar posterior vermis size in fragile X syndrome: Correlation with neurocognitive performance. *Neurology, 50,* 121–130.

Munir, F., Cornish, K. M., & Wilding, J. (2000). Nature of the working memory deficit in fragile-X syndrome. *Brain and Cognition, 44,* 387–401.

Murphy, M. M., Mazzocco, M. M. M., Gerner, G., & Henry, A. E. (2006). Mathematics learning disability in girls with Turner syndrome or fragile X syndrome. *Brain and Cognition, 61,* 195–210.

O'Donnell, W. T., & Warren, S. T. (2002). A decade of molecular studies of fragile X syndrome. *Annual Review of Neuroscience, 25,* 315–338.

Philofsky, A., Hepburn, S. L., Hayes, A., Hagerman, R., & Rogers, S. J. (2004). Linguistic and cognitive functioning and autism symptoms in young children with fragile X syndrome. *American Journal on Mental Retardation, 109,* 208–218.

Reiss, A., Alyward, E., Freund, L., Joshi, P. K., & Bryan, R. N. (1991). Neuroanatomy of fragile X syndrome: The posterior fossa. *Annals of Neurology, 29,* 26–32.

Reiss, A. L., & Freund, L. (1992). Behavioral phenotype of fragile X syndrome: *DSM–III–R* autistic behavior in male children. *American Journal of Medical Genetics, 43,* 35–46.

Reiss, A. L., Lee, J., & Freund, L. (1994). Neuroanatomy of fragile X syndrome: The temporal lobe. *Neurology, 44,* 1317–1324.

Riley, K., Ikle, L. O., & Hagerman, R. J. (2000). *A randomized, double-blind comparative trial of Adderall in the treatment of attention deficit disorder in children with fragile X.* Paper presented at the Seventh International Fragile X Conference, Los Angeles, CA.

Roberts, J. E., Boccia, M. L., Bailey, D. B., Jr., Hatton, D. D., & Skinner, M. (2001). Cardiovascular indices of physiological arousal in boys with fragile X syndrome. *Developmental Psychobiology, 39,* 107–123.

Roberts, J. E., Mirrett, P., & Burchinal, M. (2001). Receptive and expressive communication development of young males with fragile X syndrome. *American Journal on Mental Retardation, 106,* 216–240.

Roberts, J. E., Schaaf, J. M., Skinner, M., Wheeler, A., Hooper, S., Hatton, D. D., et al. (2005). Academic skills of boys with fragile X syndrome: Profiles and predictors. *American Journal Mental on Retardation, 110,* 107–120.

Rogers, S. J., Hepburn, S. L., Stackhouse, T., & Wehner, E. (2003). Imitation performance in toddlers with autism and those with other developmental disorders. *Journal of Child Psychology and Psychiatry, 44,* 763–781.

Roid, G. H., & Miller, L. J. (1997). *Leiter International Performance Scale—Revised.* Wood Dale, IL: Stoelting.

Scerif, G., Cornish, K., Wilding, J., Driver, J., & Karmiloff-Smith, A. (2004). Visual search in typically developing toddlers and toddlers with fragile X or Williams syndrome. *Developmental Science, 7,* 116–130.

Scerif, G., Karmiloff-Smith, A., Campos, R., Elsabbagh, M., Driver, J., & Cornish, K. (2005). To look or not to look? Typical and atypical development of oculomotor control. *Journal of Cognitive Neuroscience, 17,* 591–604.

Simon, E. W., & Finucane, B. M. (1996). Facial emotion identification in males with fragile X syndrome. *American Journal of Medical Genetics, 67,* 77–80.

Skinner, M., Hooper, S., Hatton, D. D., Robert, J., Mirrett, P., Schaaf, J., et al. (2005). Mapping nonverbal IQ in young boys with fragile X syndrome. *American Journal of Medical Genetics, 132A,* 25–32.

Sparrow, S., Balla, D., & Cicchetti, D. (1984). *Vineland Adaptive Behavior Scales.* Circle Pines, MN: American Guidance Service.

Sudhalter, V., & Belser, R. (2001). Conversational characteristics of children with fragile X syndrome: Tangential language. *American Journal on Mental Retardation, 106,* 389–400.

Sudhalter, V., Cohen, I. L., Silverman, W., & Wolf-Schein, E. G. (1990). Conversational analyses of males with fragile X, Down syndrome and autism: A comparison of the emergence of deviant language. *American Journal on Mental Retardation, 94,* 431–442.

Sudhalter, V., Scarborough, H., & Cohen, I. L. (1991). The syntactic delay and pragmatic deviance of the language of fragile X males. *American Journal of Medical Genetics, 38,* 493–497.

Taylor, E., Schachar, R., & Hepstinall, E. (1993). *Manual for Parental Account of Childhood Symptoms Interview.* London: Maudsley Hospital.

Theobald, T. M., Hay, D. A., & Judge, C. (1987). Individual variation and specific cognitive deficits in the fragile X syndrome. *American Journal of Medical Genetics, 28,* 1–11.

Tsiouris, J. A., & Brown, T. (2004). Neueropsychiatric symptoms of fragile X syndrome: Pathophysiology and pharmacotherapy. *CNS Drugs, 18,* 687–703.

Turk, J. (1998). Fragile X syndrome and attentional deficits. *Journal of Applied Research in Intellectual Disabilities, 11,* 175–191.

Turk, J., & Cornish, K. (1998). Face recognition and emotional perception in boys with fragile X syndrome. *Journal of Intellectual Disability Research, 42,* 490–499.

Turk, J., Robbins, I., & Woodhead, M. (2005). Post-traumatic stress disorder in young people with intellectual disability. *Journal of Intellectual Disability Research, 49,* 872–875.

Turner, G., Webb, T., Wake, S., & Robinson, H. (1996). Prevalence of fragile X syndrome. *American Journal of Medical Genetics, 64,* 196–197.

Ullman, R. K., Sleator, E. K., & Sprague, R. L. (1984). A new rating scale for diagnosis and monitoring of ADD children. *Psychopharmacology Bulletin, 20,* 160–164.

Veenema, H., Veenema, T., & Geraedts, J. P. M. (1987). The fragile X syndrome in a large family: Two psychological investigations. *Journal of Medical Genetics, 24,* 32–38.

Verkerk, A., Pieretti, M., Sutcliffe, J. S., Fu, Y. H., Kuhl, D. P., Pizzuti, A., et al. (1991). Identification of a gene (FMR-1) containing a CGG repeat coincident with a break-point cluster region exhibiting length variation in fragile X syndrome. *Cell, 65,* 905–914.

Wilding, J., Cornish, K., & Munir, F. (2002). Further delineation of the executive deficit in males with fragile X syndrome. *Neuropsychologia, 40,* 1343–1349.

Wisniewski, K. E., Segan, S. M., Miezejeski, C. M., Sersen, E. A., & Rudelli, R. D. (1991). The fra(X) syndrome: Neurological, electrophysiological and neuropathological abnormalities. *American Journal of Medical Genetics, 38,* 476–480.

Wolff, P. H., Gardner, J., Paccia, J., & Lappen, J. (1989). The greeting behavior in fragile X males. *American Journal on Mental Retardation, 93,* 406–411.

4 Duchenne Muscular Dystrophy

Veronica J. Hinton and Edward M. Goldstein

Duchenne muscular dystrophy is a devastating neurogenetic developmental disorder that occurs in about 1 in 3,500 male births (Emery, 1991). Duchenne is known primarily as a disease of muscle with an unforgivingly predictable course that is both progressive and fatal. Yet it affects far more than just muscles. Cognitive and behavioral characteristics are also associated with the disease, although their presentation is more variable than that of the physical characteristics. Children with Duchenne appear normal at birth and become weaker with age, and most die before their third decade. The weakness progresses at different rates in different individuals, but its course is constant—proximal muscles weaken before distal, legs weaken before arms, extensors weaken before flexors (McDonald et al., 1995). Duchenne also causes cognitive difficulties including mental retardation, yet the majority of affected boys are of normal intellectual level (Cotton et al., 2001). Further, Duchenne is associated with some behavioral characteristics, including limited social skills and depression (Hinton, Nereo, et al., 2006). Some behaviors are likely due to the underlying etiology, while others may be reactive responses to the condition. Duchenne impacts on more than just the affected individual; the diagnosis causes changes in families and family members' roles. Duchenne brings with it physical, emotional, and financial burdens. A child diagnosed with Duchenne will require multiple interventions on multiple levels, and the needs of the child will change with time.

The combination of symptoms, along with the progressive nature of the disease, makes characterizing the phenotype particularly problematic. In this chapter we will review what is known of Duchenne in the school-age child; we will review basic mechanisms, describe physical presentation and medical management of Duchenne, and give a particular emphasis to the cognitive and behavioral presentation. Four cases illustrating the combined impact of Duchenne on physical, cognitive, behavioral, and family status will be described, and potential interventions will be discussed at the chapter's end.

Duchenne and Becker Muscular Dystrophy

Duchenne is the most common neuromuscular disease of childhood, with prevalence rates ranging from 19 to 95 per million and an estimated overall prevalence of 63 per million, and affects all ethnic groups (Emery, 1991, 1992). It is X linked, and boys are primarily affected. Although there are cases of affected girls, they are very rare (Emery, 1992). Duchenne runs in families where women are carriers and have affected sons; yet about one third of all cases are spontaneous, new mutations. Duchenne is due to a mutated gene that inhibits the production of the protein dystrophin that normally is found in muscle and brain. Becker muscular dystrophy, a milder form of the disease with later onset and slower progression, has a lower incidence than Duchenne. In Becker muscular dystrophy, an abnormal dystrophin molecule is made that does not function in muscle as efficiently as the normal protein. Prevalence rates for Becker muscular dystrophy range from 12 to 27 per million (Emery, 1991).

Positive diagnosis for Duchenne is based on the following criteria: (a) male; (b) onset of weakness before age 5; (c) initial proximal muscle weakness; (d) muscle hypertrophy, most prominent in the calves; (e) elevated creatine kinase activity of at least 10 times above the upper limit of normal; and either (f) positive histopathological confirmation by muscle biopsy or (g) molecular characterization of a mutation within the gene for dystrophin.

History

In 1868, the French neurologist Guillaume-Benjamin-Amand Duchenne published detailed observations in 13 children with a progressive neuromuscular disorder (Duchenne, 1868). He referred to it as pseudohypertrophic dystrophy, due to the overdevelopment of calf muscles in boys with the disease. Duchenne was not the first to describe the illness, but his detailed report examining the signs and symptoms of the disease caused it to become known as Duchenne's muscular dystrophy. Duchenne noted that the disease ran in families and affected boys, and he deduced that it was inherited. Further, he noted that the boys with the disease were "mentally dull." The specific cause of the disease, however, was unknown, and the cognitive limitations were often thought to be associated with disability, but not disease specific.

Gene

In 1986, the gene for Duchenne muscular dystrophy was discovered on the short arm of the X chromosome at position Xp21 (Monaco et al., 1986). It was the first gene to be discovered using positional cloning techniques. The gene is the largest in the human genome, at greater than 2.5 Mb in length, and has a high proclivity for mutation (Beggs & Kunkel, 1990; Calvert et al., 1996; Drenckhahn et al., 1996; Hyser et al., 1987; Koenig et al., 1987; Wilton et al., 1998). One third of boys with Duchenne are the result of spontaneous mutations in the dystrophin gene, with the patient's mother maintaining a normal X chromosomal constitution. Deletion of genetic material in the dystrophin gene is detected by conventional polymerase chain reaction/gel electrophoresis technologies in about two thirds of boys with Duchenne. These deletions may occur at any point along the dystrophin gene, though there are two "hot spots" within the gene where the bulk of these mutations occur. In the remaining one third of affected males this testing is negative, due to the presence of point mutations or small deletions/insertions of genetic material (Mendell et al., 2001). The development of techniques to rapidly sequence the dystrophin gene now permits the detection of mutations in these patients for diagnostic purposes (Flanigan et al., 2003). Duchenne is associated with mutations that disrupt essential functional domains of the dystrophin molecule, or mutations that shift the reading frame of DNA transcription, resulting in a truncated, unstable, and nonfunctional dystrophin (Muntoni et al., 2003).

Dystrophin

A year after the discovery of the gene, its protein product, dystrophin, was identified (Hoffman et al., 1987). Dystrophin is a 427 kDa protein that is absent in the muscles of boys with Duchenne (Hoffman et al., 1987; Hoffman & Wang, 1993; Koenig et al., 1988). The gene also codes for other protein products that localize to other tissue types, including the brain (Boyce et al., 1991; Gorecki et al., 1992; Lederfein et al., 1992; Uchino et al., 1994a). Different internal promoters in the gene and posttranscriptional splicing regulate expression of the products. Three products are full-length 427 kDa molecules, and four are shorter with molecular weights of 260 kDa, 140 kDa, 116 kDa, and 71–78 kDa, respectively. Dp427, Dp140, Dp116, and Dp71 have been localized to brain tissue, and their absence in boys with Duchenne has been invoked as the reason for cognitive dysfunction in the context of their muscle disease (Felisari et al., 2000).

In muscles, dystrophin is localized to the sarcolemma in a glycoprotein complex. It serves to stabilize the plasma membrane during muscle contractions. In boys with Duchenne, dystrophin is missing, while in Becker muscular dystrophy an abnormal dystrophin molecule is made. With muscle use, tears develop in the cellular membrane and calcium ions enter into the cells, disrupting the intracellular homeostasis and causing the cells to break down. As a result, skeletal muscle fibers continually deteriorate and regenerate until they can no longer repair themselves and the muscle

Table 4.1
Duchenne muscular dystrophy affects multiple systems in the body that result in a range of disabilities requiring treatment

System/Organ	Impairment	Disability	Treatment
Skeletal muscle	Strength and endurance	Motor performance Mobility Fatigue	Corticosteroids Physical therapy
Bone and joint	Joint contractures Spine deformity	Function Pain and deformity	Physical therapy—stretching, Orthotics, surgery
Lungs	Pulmonary function	Restrictive lung disease Fatigue	Positive airway pressure, Cough assist, Nocturnal ventilation
Heart	Cardiomyopathy Conduction defects	Cardiopulmonary adaptations Fatigue	Pharmacologic intervention
Brain	Intellectual capacity Behavioral issues	Cognitive deficits Psychosocial adjustment Stress	Educational support, individual counseling, family therapy, Social support

fibers undergo irreversible degradation with replacement by fat and connective tissue. For the child with Duchenne, this presents as progressive weakness that is fatal. For the child with Becker muscular dystrophy, onset is later and disease progression is slower.

Physical Presentation

Natural history studies have been conducted to characterize the course of the disease. The Clinical Investigation of Duchenne Dystrophy group followed more than 200 individuals affected with Duchenne for more than 10 years (Brooke et al., 1983; Hyser et al., 1987; Mendell et al., 1987). The group measured numerous physical characteristics with standardized measures and developed a scoring system to allow for accurate assessment of severity, so that effects of interventions could be effectively tested. The results confirmed that the disease impacts multiple systems and organs as described in table 4.1. Moreover, although the rate of progression varies among boys, the course is markedly similar and all children progress through the same stages of the illness.

Initially, a boy with Duchenne will appear to be developing normally (figure 4.1). At age 2 to 3, he may have slight motor impairments and be perceived as being somewhat clumsy. His calf muscles will likely be overdeveloped or hypertrophic. He will have difficulty keeping up with his peers on the playground. He will be unable to jump from a standing position, will have difficulty climbing stairs, and will begin to have frequent falls. As the boy's muscles continue to weaken, he will have greater dif-

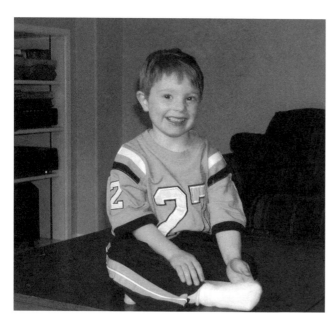

Figure 4.1
Youngsters with Duchenne muscular dystrophy are visually indistinguishable from other children. There are no dismorphic facial characteristics associated with the disorder. This boy walks but cannot jump or ride a bike like his peers.

ficulty walking. Specifically, as his quadriceps weaken, he will compensate by shifting his weight onto the balls of his feet and push his abdomen forward and shoulders back to steady himself. If he is asked to raise himself from a sitting position on the floor, he will generally do so by a typical sequence of movements. This involves him first raising his rear in the air and then, using his arms as supports, "walking" his hands up his legs to get into a standing position, a movement known as the Gower's maneuver. By age 12, he will tire easily and be dependant on a wheelchair for extended mobility (figures 4.2, 4.3). Over the next few years, he will lose significant skeletal muscle strength and will need assistance in all activities that require his legs, trunk, and arms. Additionally, he will develop multifocal joint contractures and scoliosis that may be painful. He will still be able to move his fingers, so he can operate his motorized wheelchair and use a computer, as long as his arms are properly supported. As he continues to age into his late teens, he may develop heart problems due to weakness in the myocardium. Additionally, as the muscles around his lungs weaken, he will lose the ability to cough independently and clear his lungs, putting him at increased risk for developing pneumonia. Without ventilator support, his death will occur before he reaches 30, usually due to respiratory or cardiac failure

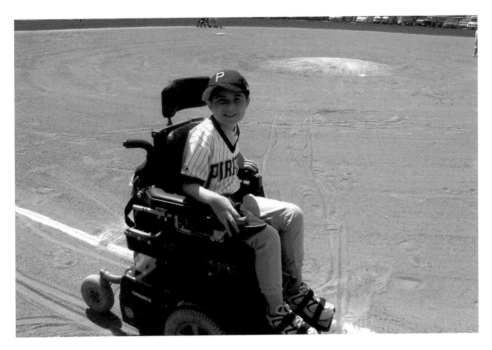

Figure 4.2
Most children with Duchenne muscular dystrophy share the interests and activities of their peers. Although
dependent on a wheelchair to get around, this boy lives a full and varied life. He is an avid baseball fan
and enjoys sharing his enthusiasm for his team with his friends.

resulting from extreme muscle weakness. Duchenne is the most common inherited
fatal childhood disorder.

Research supported by the National Institute on Disability and Rehabilitation further characterized the percentage of individuals with specific disease-related features
(McDonald et al., 1995). Table 4.2 is adapted from their findings and shows changes
in percentages of children affected with different symptoms over time.

Medical Management

There is currently no known cure for Duchenne, and treatment focuses on slowing
the disease progression and improving the quality of life of those affected. Medical
management involves multiple interventions to help ameliorate symptoms associated
with different systems involved (table 4.1). Protracted corticosteroid therapy in order
to slow the progression of muscle weakness is the primary treatment for Duchenne.
In 2005, the Quality Standards Subcommittee of the American Academy of Neurology and the Practice Committee of the Child Neurology Society published a review

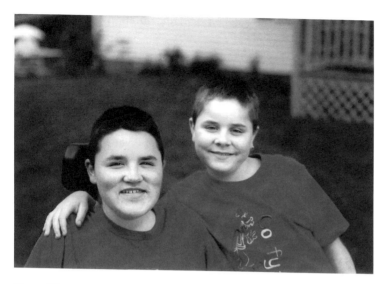

Figure 4.3
These brothers both have Duchenne muscular dystrophy. The older brother can no longer get around without the aid of a wheelchair, while his younger brother still walks independently. Both boys have the Cushingoid facial characteristics associated with long-term steroid use.

Table 4.2
The percentage of individuals affected with different physical symptoms of Duchenne muscular dystrophy varies according age

Impairment	Age (years)			
	<9	9–13	14–16	>16
Joint contractures (%)	18	68	97	100
Scoliosis (%)	15	50	70	90
Respiratory complications (%)	7	17	—	48
Cardiovascular complications (%)	—	9	24	67

Note: The above data show that as age increases, a greater percentage of affected boys will develop the listed impairments (McDonald et al., 1995).

of the relevant literature that confirmed that daily corticosteroid treatment with prednisone (0.75 or 1.5 mg/kg/day) increased muscle strength, performance, and pulmonary function and significantly decreased the progression of weakness (Moxley et al., 2005). In many boys with Duchenne, treatment with corticosteroids may also result in weight gain and development of Cushingoid facial appearance.

To maintain range of motion and optimize muscle strength and endurance, physical therapy consisting of a daily exercise program is also prescribed. Physical and occupational therapists assist with the mobilization of adaptive equipment to optimize function for children and their caregivers and to minimize complications such as skin breakdown and musculoskeletal pain. As weakness progresses, affected boys develop contractures in both the arms and legs. Range of motion exercises are performed to minimize their development, along with the application of braces where appropriate. Most commonly, night splints are employed to stretch the Achilles tendon and reduce forefoot gait.

If a functionally disabling contracture develops despite these interventions, consideration may be given to orthopedic surgery to improve joint range of motion. Regrettably, with wheelchair dependence, multifocal contractures develop in all boys with Duchenne. Additionally, scoliosis develops in the majority of boys who are wheelchair dependent. Left untreated, scoliosis produces pain and difficulty with positioning and may compromise respiratory status. As such, most boys with Duchenne will undergo spine fusion surgery in their early teen to midteen years.

Additional measures to maximize respiratory function include immunizations to reduce the frequency and severity of infections, chest physical therapy, aerosol treatments, cough assist machines, and the use of positive pressure ventilation.

Like the respiratory muscles, the heart may also be weakened by Duchenne and cardiac function must be carefully monitored. Regular electrocardiograms and echocardiograms are performed looking for evidence of cardiomyopathy. If heart muscle fails, pharmacologic therapies are invoked to improve heart contractility and reduce the heart's workload.

Finally, dietary management is critical to maintaining good health in boys with Duchenne. In addition to treating frequent problems like constipation, dietary intake must be carefully monitored to avoid obesity. Dietary management is particularly important in the setting of steroid therapy. Calcium and vitamin D supplements are prescribed to maintain bone density, while caloric restriction is frequently necessary to prevent weight gain.

Dystrophin and the Brain

The discovery that the mutated gene in Duchenne codes for multiple protein products that localize to separate tissue types, including the brain, offers a potential explanation for the cognitive manifestation of the Duchenne phenotype (Anderson et al., 2002; Mehler, 2000). In the brain, dystrophin isoforms normally localize to circumscribed cerebral and cerebellar cortical regions (Boyce et al., 1991; Gorecki et al., 1992; Kimura et al., 1997; Lederfein et al., 1992; Gorecki et al., 1998; Lidov et al., 1990; Tian et al., 1996; Uchino et al., 1994a; Uchino et al., 1994b) and are absent in autopsied brains of individuals affected with Duchenne. Brain dystrophins have been localized to specific cell types in both neurons and glia. In neurons, dystrophins have been clearly identified in pyramidal, stellate, and Purkinje cells (Tian et al., 1996; Uchino et al., 1994) and appear to be concentrated primarily in the postsynaptic region (Jancsik & Hajos, 1998; Lidov, Byers, Watkins, & Kunkel, 1990). Although the contribution of the dystrophin brain products to function is unknown, they have been hypothesized to play a structural role that aids in synaptic transmission (e.g., Jancsik & Hajos, 1998) and may modulate neuronal function (Gorecki et al., 1998; Kimura et al., 1997).

Brain dystrophins are also involved in developmental processes of the central nervous system. Transcripts have been found transiently during embryonic and fetal stages (Gorecki et al., 1998; Jones et al., 1998; Rodius et al., 1997; Ueda et al., 1995; Tian et al., 1996). Neuroradiologic studies reveal no obvious structural anomalies, although older patients may exhibit some cerebral atrophy (Echenne et al., 1998). Functional studies are limited but suggest central nervous system dysfunction secondary to dystrophin deficiency. Abnormal EEG findings have been demonstrated in about half of all patients with Duchenne (Uchino et al., 1994b). Flourodeoxyglucose positron emission tomography studies demonstrated cerebellar hypometabolism and variable involvement of the associative cortical areas (Lee et al., 2002). Metabolic abnormalities have also been demonstrated in the brains of patients with Duchenne; phosphorous-31 magnetic resonance spectroscopy of brain indicated a significantly increased ratio of inorganic phosphate to ATP (Koenig et al., 1988; Tracey et al., 1995). For the child with Duchenne, this is associated with lowered intellectual function preferentially affecting verbal skills and an increased incidence of mental retardation (Cotton et al., 2001).

IQ Scores

In general, the distribution of IQ scores among affected boys appears to be shifted down about 1 *SD* from the population mean. No epidemiological studies have been done to document the presentation of language or intellectual deficits among children diagnosed with Duchenne, so estimates of ranges of impairment are based on samples of children who are available and willing to participate in studies and may well overrepresent those with cognitive deficits. Table 4.3 presents information on the percentage of children affected with specific cognitive and behavioral characteristics derived from potentially biased convenience samples, rather than population based studies.

A meta-analysis of 32 published papers examining IQ among a total of 1,146 individuals with Duchenne found the mean full scale IQ value was 80.2 with a standard deviation of 19.3 (Cotton et al., 2001). Scores were shifted down from the normative population, but the frequency distribution did not differ significantly. Thus, as a

Table 4.3
The percentage of individuals with Duchenne muscular dystrophy who have significant cognitive and/or behavioral difficulties

Source	Diagnosis	% Found	% Expected in General Population
Emery, 1992	Mental retardation	19	2
Cotton, Voudouris, & Greenwood, 2001		35	2
Wu, Kuban, Allred, Shapiro, & Darras, 2005	Autism	3.8	0.2
Hinton, Batchelder, Cyrulnik, Fee, & Kiefel, 2006		13	0.2

Note: Data are from convenience samples, rather than a population survey, so numbers presented may be biased.

result of this downward shift, 35% of the children with Duchenne had IQ scores in the "mentally retarded" range (or scores less than 70). Most children, however, had normal intellectual level.

As a group, boys with Duchenne have significantly lower Verbal IQ scores than Performance IQ scores. When available data were collapsed across studies in a sample of 878 individuals affected with Duchenne, the mean group difference between the two scales was five points, which was statistically significant (Cotton et al., 2001). Given the motor and speed demands on many Performance (but not Verbal) subtests, the finding of higher Performance scores among a motor-impaired group is suggestive of even greater Verbal–Performance discrepancies than are reported.

Specific Cognitive Skills

The methods used to examine cognitive skills associated with Duchenne have differed across studies, and many have small samples with inadequate or no comparison groups. Given the variability in the disease presentation, multiple confounds may hamper the research in cognition. Physical disability, overall level of intellectual function, environmental background, and age variables may all influence results. Nonetheless, some findings appear to be consistent across studies. Overall, most studies have found that individuals with Duchenne have compromised verbal and reading skills and limited immediate verbal memory.

To control for the potentially confounding effects of physical impairment, a number of studies have compared test performance of children with Duchenne to those with spinal muscular atrophy (SMA), a different neuromuscular disorder. Results have demonstrated that the children with Duchenne have poorer verbal, immediate memory, and reading skills than their SMA peers (Billard et al., 1992; Billard et al., 1998; Ogasawara, 1989; Whelan, 1987). Specific findings included lowered scores on

Digit Span, Arithmetic, Similarities, Word Repetition, Supraspan, and Reading tests. Other areas, including many measures of basic language skill and nonverbal abilities, were not different between the two groups, highlighting the selective nature of the cognitive profile (Billard et al., 1992; Whelan, 1987).

To control for environmental background, we have compared performance of children with Duchenne to that of their unaffected siblings. These results also showed poorer verbal, immediate memory, and academic skills (Hinton et al., 2001; Hinton et al., 2004; Hinton et al., in press). Specifically, children with Duchenne did poorly on Digit Span, Comprehension, Story Memory, and Token Test when compared to their sibling controls, in addition to having lower reading and arithmetic skills. The main finding, however, was that most cognitive areas remained strong. Performance on tests of basic receptive vocabulary, naming, category fluency, and factual knowledge did not differ between the groups, clearly demonstrating that many basic language skills are not compromised. Likewise, problem solving, abstraction, categorization, and set shifting were also good; children with Duchenne performed similarly to their siblings on a range of "higher order" tests of "executive function." Similarly, there was no evidence of visual–spatial impairment among the boys with Duchenne, based on performance on a selection of puzzle completion tests that did not require manual dexterity but did require mental manipulations and/or familiarity with spatial features. There was also no evidence of impaired visual memory for details or learning and recall of spatial location.

Since the range of intellectual level among children with Duchenne is great, with as many as 35% manifesting pronounced cognitive deficits (Cotton et al., 2001), performance on measures of selective cognitive skills may be biased somewhat by those who are able to comply with testing. Even among those children who do not have mental retardation, IQ may have significant influence. To control for this, researchers have compared children with Duchenne to IQ-matched and age-matched children without Duchenne. On neuropsychological test batteries, the group with Duchenne generally performed more poorly than the comparison group on measures of memory (Cotton et al., 1998; Wicksell et al., 2004). The most striking finding of these comparisons, however, was the number of measures the two groups performed equivalently on, including measures of vocabulary, nonverbal reasoning, and a variety of visualspatial measures.

To determine whether individual strengths and weaknesses were similar across intellectual level, we examined boys with Duchenne by individually rank ordering their performance on standardized subtests and compared the relative rankings across individuals. The results demonstrated that boys with Duchenne have a selective cognitive profile such that subtests that tap verbal immediate recall (e.g., Digit Span and Story Memory) are consistently lowest, regardless of general intellectual function

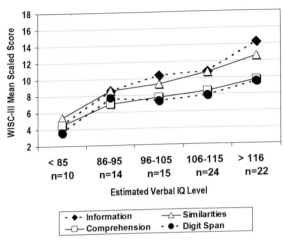

Figure 4.4
Children with Duchenne muscular dystrophy show relative weakness on Digit Span and Comprehension subtests, regardless of overall intellectual level. Participants (ages 6 to 16 years) are grouped according to their estimated Verbal IQ (as determined by performance on the Peabody Picture Vocabulary Test), and mean scaled scores on four subtests of the Wechsler Intelligence Scale for Children—III (WISC–III) are plotted. Note that scores on Digit Span and Comprehension are lowest across the IQ groups.

(Hinton et al., 2000). Plotting the data across IQ levels also shows that some scores are preferentially lower over the range of IQ (figures 4.4 and 4.5). Additionally, when data are examined covarying for the effects of IQ, the findings of poor performance on Digit Span and Story Memory were confirmed (Hinton et al., 2001). We hypothesized that for all children with Duchenne some skills are selectively compromised, but these reduced abilities may be detrimental only to those children of overall lower cognitive function.

The influence of age on selective cognitive skills in Duchenne is of interest. Although age is definitively associated with physical progression of the disease, there is no evidence of intellectual decline over time. Limited longitudinal data have shown no significant loss of skills over time (McDonald et al., 1995; Prosser et al., 1969). Moreover, there has been no evidence to indicate that more severely disabled individuals have more pronounced intellectual deficits (Glaub & Mechler, 1987; Leibowitz & Dubowitz, 1981; Zellweger & Hanson, 1967).

Interestingly, although there is no evidence of progressive decline of intellectual ability over time, there are data to support the idea that some cognitive skills selectively increase with age. Most studies have grouped children with Duchenne over wide age spans out of necessity due to a limited number of participants. Yet comparison of children at different developmental stages may be misleading. When

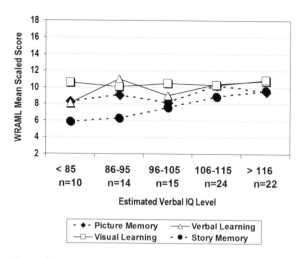

Figure 4.5
Children with Duchenne muscular dystrophy show relative weakness on Story Memory, irrespective of general intellectual level. Participants (ages 6 to 16 years) are grouped according to their estimated Verbal IQ (as determined by performance on the Peabody Picture Vocabulary Test), and mean scaled scores on four subtests of the Wide Range Assessment of Memory and Learning (WRAML) are plotted. Note that scores on Story Memory are lowest across the IQ groups.

younger children have been systematically compared to older children, the results have suggested that over time language skills may improve. Analysis of cross-sectional data across age groups from 32 published studies indicated increases in Verbal, but not Performance, IQ scores with age among boys with Duchenne (Cotton et al., 2005). Comparison of younger versus older affected children on a battery of tests showed the younger group to have more generalized impairments (Hinton et al., in submission; Sollee et al., 1985). Further, there is evidence to suggest that early language delays may be commonplace and may, at times, be even more pronounced than motor difficulties in the young child (Cyrulnik et al., in press; Kaplan et al., 1986; Smith et al., 1990). Reports of children who have been referred for language delays and later found to have Duchenne have been published (Kaplan et al., 1986), and we know of numerous anecdotal accounts of children with early language and behavioral concerns that predated any clear evidence of motor loss (Hinton, Batchelder, et al., 2006).

Thus, across studies, even when controlling for effects of physical involvement, environmental background, IQ, and age, the cognitive profile in Duchenne is defined by multiple strengths and deficits in language and immediate verbal memory skills. Moreover, contrary to the physical presentation that declines with age, the cognitive profile may show selective improvements in verbal skills over time.

Case 4.1: Kane   Kane, age 5, first came to medical attention when he said only single words at age 3. At that time, his pediatrician told his parents that Kane had unspecified developmental delay and recommended speech therapy. Kane's vocabulary has expanded dramatically since then. He names pictures of common items and speaks in sentences of about three words. For example, Kane says, "I want juice" and "ride in car." Kane has dark curls and large eyes. His parents have taken him to numerous developmental specialists who have concentrated on Kane's poor language and suggested different programs to augment his language development.

Kane looks physically fit and has large calf muscles that look like those of an athlete. Yet Kane tires easily when walking, and he has difficulty climbing stairs. At a recent visit to a pediatric neurologist, the physician noted Kane's enlarged calves and had blood taken to screen for creatine phosphokinase levels. The results showed levels of more than 10 times normal. Standard genetic testing was equivocal; no mutations were identified.

Kane attends nursery school. He does not "join in" the group activities and spends his free time playing with the train set. Kane takes all the engines and parks them next to each other. He becomes upset if the arrangement is disturbed or a classmate takes an engine. At home, Kane plays with his own trains similarly. He has special places on his shelves for each engine to go, and he enjoys arranging them.

Kane is an only child who lives with his parents. When he is introduced, Kane says, "ride in car." On standardized tests, Kane is generally not compliant. For single-word comprehension, he scores in the "impaired" range. On drawing tests, he scribbles but does not copy the items asked of him. When asked to solve a puzzle, Kane moves the pieces but shows no attempt to put them together, then gets up and says "ride in car!" When asked simple questions such as "How old are you?" or "What do you like to do?" Kane either does not respond or says, "ride in car."

Academic Skills

Children with Duchenne face considerable obstacles in maintaining a "normal" school life, including all the hardships associated with physical disability and "fitting in." Research suggests that they are at increased risk for poor academic achievement. Determining whether this is due to underlying cognitive deficits or adjustment issues is complex.

An early study by Worden and Vignos (1962) found that among boys with Duchenne, scores on academic achievement tests in reading and mathematics were about 1 *SD* lower than the general population. They reported that although the evaluation of 38 boys with Duchenne indicated decreased performance, it was commensurate with their IQ. The authors concluded that the boys with Duchenne were achieving as expected given their intellectual ability, and there was no evidence to indicate they had selective learning disabilities (Worden & Vignos, 1962).

Other researchers have focused solely on reading skills and have suggested that about half the children with Duchenne present with a form of developmental dyslexia. Liebowitz and Dubowitz (1981) tested 42 boys on reading tests and found the group had a mean standard score that was almost identical to their Verbal IQ mean score. Yet they note that the reading scores were very skewed, such that half of their sample did very poorly on the reading test. Dorman et al. (1988) tested 15 boys with Duchenne on reading tests and also demonstrated limited reading skills in about half of the children. Similarly, Billard et al. (1992) demonstrated that among a group of 24 older boys with Duchenne, about half of the children with Duchenne had severe reading disabilities, while none of the comparison group of children affected with a different neuromuscular disorder, spinal muscular atrophy, did. Further, the mean standard score on the Reading Index of the Duchenne group was about 1 *SD* lower than that of children with spinal muscular atrophy. Thus, across studies, children with Duchenne present with reading difficulties, yet group mean scores on reading tests are not substantially different from mean IQ scores.

In more detailed examinations of the components of reading, both Dorman and Billard report that phonological processing is particularly impaired in children with Duchenne. In Dorman's sample, the children with Duchenne had significantly reduced phonetic word attack skills (Dorman et al., 1988). Billard demonstrated the overall error rate was highest for the Duchenne group when reading nonwords, also implicating poor phonological processing skills (Billard et al., 1998). Billard's analyses compared boys with Duchenne to either children with spinal muscular atrophy or normal controls who were matched on age and socioeconomic level. They found the children with Duchenne had a reading age of about 2 years behind the comparison children, and they discussed possible contributions to the poor reading skills among the children with Duchenne. They noted that poor attention, difficulty with graphophonological conversion, reduction in short-term memory, a deficit on the level of speech production, or psychoaffective and cultural processes might each limit reading ability in the Duchenne group, and after careful consideration of each they concluded, "A deficit in graphophonological process seems to be the principal explanation of the reading disability" (Billard et al., 1998).

We have demonstrated that across academic areas, boys with Duchenne had lower scores than their siblings on achievement tests. Similarly to the other published studies, the children in our sample performed within normal limits, yet their mean scores were about 1 *SD* lower than that of their siblings. Examination of what contributed to the lower academic achievement test scores showed that age, physical disability, and behavior ratings did not significantly influence the outcome, while performance on tests of intellectual ability and Digit Span did. We hypothesized that a "core" deficit of limited verbal span (as evidenced by decreased digit recall on Digit Span) was the reason behind the lower academic skills (Hinton et al., 2004).

Case 4.2: Louis   Louis, age 7, is a sandy-haired little boy who was diagnosed with Duchenne when he was 4 years old, after his mother told the pediatrician he was having difficulty climbing stairs. The doctor examined Louis and had him sit on the floor and rise, and he observed Louis's Gower's maneuver, alerting him to the possible diagnosis of Duchenne. The pediatrician took blood samples from Louis and his two brothers and had them analyzed for possible mutations consistent with Duchenne. Both Louis and his infant brother were found to have large deletions spanning exons 49 through 63 in the dystrophin gene. Subsequent analysis of their mother showed that she too had the deletion and was therefore a carrier.

When Louis walks, his unusual posture is apparent; he has a broad gait and arched back, and he sticks his abdomen forward. When introduced, he shakes hands and briefly smiles. When queried about school and what he likes to do, Louis says, "School is okay," and he likes "to play fetch with my dog, Benji."

Louis repeated kindergarten and is now in the first grade. Currently, his teacher complains that he has attention problems. Louis has learned his alphabet but struggles with learning to sound out basic words. He has one friend who he seeks out during activity time. Louis sits near the other boy and they each play, yet there is little interaction between them.

Louis lives with his mother and two brothers. His parents separated 2 years before; his mother states that it was due, in part, to her husband's unwillingness to accept that anything was wrong with Louis and the baby. His mother describes Louis as "a good kid, but maddening at times" because he ignores her and does what he pleases. She oversees his daily stretching exercises and tries to get Louis to wear lower leg splints that keep his feet flexed and Achilles tendons stretched, but she says he is resistant to wearing them and she does not battle him over it. She reports that Louis does not "mind" her, and she often gets frustrated with him. She notes that his 9-year-old brother was always respectful and did as he was asked. She'd like Louis to behave more like him.

Louis's full scale IQ is in the "low average" range. Louis does well—at his appropriate age level—on tests of receptive vocabulary and naming. On more complex tests of language comprehension and expression, however, his limitations are evident. When asked a complex question, Louis repeats back the last few words instead of answering. When asked to make up a sentence about a picture, he names the picture and looks at the examiner. Similarly, when asked to point to a picture that best describes a sentence he has heard, he points to each choice and names something in the picture. He scores in the "borderline" range on tests of language. On nonverbal measures, his scores generally fall in the "low average" range.

Behavior

Research examining behavior in children with Duchenne has indicated two general areas that are susceptible to pathology: internalizing/depressive disorders and social problems. Similar to the other phenotypic characteristics of Duchenne, there is a range in presentation, and the behaviors observed in Duchenne are associated with numerous factors including age, disease progression, intellectual level, and environmental background.

Data collected using parent questionnaires has documented children with Duchenne have depressive signs that increased with age and less well-characterized antisocial tendencies (Fitzpatrick et al., 1986; Leibowitz & Dubowitz, 1981; Thompson et al., 1992). These studies showed that as children matured and became more physically disabled, parental ratings of depression and anxiety among the youths increased.

Harper (1983) directly investigated personality profiles of adolescents with Duchenne and compared them to those of children with other physical impairments. Both groups showed tendencies for increased social inhibitions and depressive symptoms. Physical disability and adjustment status were not linearly associated, but more rapid declines in the Duchenne group were associated with behaviors suggestive of increased stress. A later study replicated the finding that adolescents with Duchenne have significant adjustment difficulties (Reid & Renwick, 2001). Specifically, they found adolescents with Duchenne had poorer psychosocial adjustment than their healthy peers and that their adjustment was significantly associated with the level of stress reported by the family.

We examined parent ratings of behavior in a sample of 181 boys with Duchenne who were between 6 and 17 years old at the time of assessment and compared them to parental ratings from both unaffected siblings and children with cerebral palsy (Hinton, Nereo, et al., 2006). Parent ratings on the Child Behavior Checklist demonstrated that children with Duchenne were more likely to fall in the "clinically significant" range (as defined by being more common than 96% of the normative population) on the Social Problems scale than either comparison group. About a third of the boys were reported to have significant Social Problems (e.g., being immature, having poor peer relationships), and about a quarter reportedly had significant problems with being withdrawn and having poor attention. Of note is that the younger children were more likely to have increased Social Problems and the older children were more likely to have increased depression and anxiety (Hinton et al., manuscript in submission). We hypothesize that the social difficulties may be related to underlying etiology and associated with compromised verbal skills, while the depressive behaviors are likely a reactive response to the disease progression.

A few case studies describing children with Duchenne and autism have been published (Komoto et al., 1984; Zwaigenbaum & Tarnopolsky, 2003). Further, a recent screen by Wu and colleagues (2005) found that autism spectrum disorders in a Massachusetts muscular dystrophy clinic were considerably more common than expected among the general population. They reported a prevalence of 6/158 in their clinic compared to 1.6 in 1,000 in the general population. We too have observed multiple cases of children with Duchenne and autism spectrum disorders, with rates as high as 13% of the children participating in our studies meeting criteria (Hinton, Batchelder, et al., 2006). Although most children with Duchenne clearly are not autistic, the tendencies of being withdrawn and having poor peer relations may be mild behaviors on the spectrum.

Case 4.3: Muhhamad   Muhhamad, age 11, lives with his mother, father, and younger brother. Muhhamad was diagnosed with Duchenne at age 6 years, after his mother grew increasingly concerned about how often Muhhamad fell and was unable to keep up with his peers. Muhhamad was found to have elevated creatine kinase levels but a negative DNA test, so a muscle biopsy was performed. The results indicated that there was no positive staining for dystrophin in the muscle tissue examined, confirming the diagnosis of Duchenne. Muhhamad's parents have stated they do not agree with the diagnosis and refuse to accept that Muhhamad's motor difficulties will be fatal. They have no known family history of Duchenne but report on a number of relatives who had significant illnesses of various types who improved or "beat" the illness with time and proper diet. Muhhamad's parents have chosen to pursue physical therapy and orthopedic interventions for Muhhamad but have declined to give Muhhamad steroid medications because they are concerned that the side effects are too unpleasant and the benefits too uncertain. They also believe that a diet high in protein and low in fat will help Muhhamad and are careful about monitoring his food intake.

Muhhamad attends the sixth grade in a small school where he receives physical therapy two times a week. His school performance is average, and his teachers describe him a quiet and proud boy who keeps to himself. At home and at school Muhhamad uses long-leg braces and walks, but it is increasingly difficult for him and he gets fatigued. He has limited flexibility in his ankles, and they are painfully tight. Whenever he needs to go any distance, Muhhamad uses a wheelchair, but he does so reluctantly. At home, he sleeps in a room on the second floor, and Muhhamad relies on a family member to carry him up the stairs each night.

Muhhamad's family speaks Arabic at home. Muhhamad's manner is somewhat withdrawn, and he answers that he "is fine" and has "no problems" when asked. When asked how he likes to spend his time, he answers, "Draw." His younger brother asks "when will Muhhamad get well?" and states that their parents have said that Muhhamad will soon improve. During his evaluation, Muhhamad applies himself but rarely looks at the examiner. He does not initiate conversation but always answers any questions asked of him.

Muhhamad scores in the "average" range on IQ tests, yet there is scatter among his subtest scores and Digit Span and Arithmetic are notably low, while his Block Design and Picture Completion are impressively high. On most memory tests he also scores in the "average" range and demonstrates good long-term recall for both verbal and visual information. The exception to this is when he is read a story and asked to retell it. Muhhamad responds by stating some of the details in the story, but he does not give a cohesive narration. Further, on tests of reading comprehension and mathematics he struggles, but he tries everything asked of him and never states that he does not know an answer. His scores on academic achievement tests fall in the "borderline" range. His reading scores are particularly low; when asked to read words he was unfamiliar with, Muhhamad states words that begin with the same letter, but he shows no skill at decoding the word phonetically. On tests of reading comprehension, Muhhamad shows little understanding of more complex passages.

Stress

Duchenne, which is both chronic and terminal, may be characterized as a "complex chronic condition" in that it involves specialized and time-consuming care, even when the terminal phase lies years in the future (Gravelle, 1997). As such, it may be expected to have effects on the family similar to those of both chronic and terminal illnesses. Duchenne poses stressors in terms of daily care requirements, such as negotiating wheelchair transportation and meeting recommended physical therapy requirements. In addition, as with other complex chronic illnesses, many psychological adjustments become necessary, such as facing separation and loss; experiencing and expressing emotions (including anger, guilt, sadness, loss of control, resentment of increased demands); and changing values, expectations, roles, and responsibilities (Copeland, 1988).

In a study comparing ratings of parents of boys with Duchenne to ratings of parents of children with other "complex chronic conditions," parents of boys with Duchenne reported higher levels of stress than parents of children with cystic fibrosis or renal disease. All groups of children with a chronic disease reported more stress than parents of healthy children, and in patterns consistent with the care requirements of their child's disease (Holroyd & Guthrie, 1986).

In a study examining stress in 36 families with adolescents and Duchenne, familial stress was found to be associated with both psychosocial adjustment and intellectual function of the teen boys with Duchenne and not associated with sociodemographic variables (Reid & Renwick, 2001). The authors concluded that the effects of Duchenne extend well beyond the affected individual, and they recommended a holistic approach offering support for the whole family.

We also have examined parenting stress in 112 families with a son affected with Duchenne (Nereo et al., 2003) and compared it to stress reported in mothers of children with cerebral palsy and normative data. The results indicated that the mothers of boys with Duchenne report increased levels of stress relative to the normative sample, but the degree of the increase is comparable to that reported in mothers of children with cerebral palsy. Among the Duchenne group, there were high ratings of stress related to the difficult parent–child interaction, and these were associated with increased report of behavioral concerns in the children more than with physical disability.

Thus, with Duchenne, the family's adjustment to the disorder is also an important feature of the impact of the illness. How families adjust to and cope with illness and developmental disability in general has been repeatedly documented to be associated with improved psychological well-being (Copeland, 1988 see also chapter 12, this volume). In Duchenne, where the phenotype impacts on physical, intellectual, and behavioral attributes and involves substantial personal and financial burden associated with care giving, family's stress levels and adjustment are particularly salient.

Case 4.4: Ned   Ned, age 16 years, is a heavy teenager who states that he is self-conscious about his "chipmunk cheeks." Ned has taken prednisone since he was 7 years old, and his face has the typical Cushingoid characteristics. Ned used to be slim, but since he became wheelchair dependent at age 11, he has gained a significant amount of weight. Ned is friendly and polite and answers all questions asked of him. When asked to describe his interests, he readily discusses movies he has seen and describes favorites articulately and animatedly.

Ned originally received the diagnosis of Duchenne when he was 4 years old, and he tired easily and struggled on stairs or when running. His mother had had a brother who died of Duchenne, and she was the one to report her suspicions to Ned's physician. Ned was found to have elevated creatine kinase levels. Even with his mother's positive family history and strong suspicions, Ned's parents hoped the diagnosis was incorrect, so they chose to have Ned have muscle biopsy to be certain of the diagnosis. The results confirmed that Ned had no dystrophin in the muscle sample, and he was definitively diagnosed with Duchenne.

Ned's school performance is good. Ned has a small group of male friends who share his interests for movies and computer games. He attends a public school and is in the 11th grade. He feels shy and awkward around girls. He plans to go to college and hopes to study law to become a civil rights lawyer. Ned's school has ensured that he has handicap accessible facilities. Ned has a bulky motorized wheelchair, which he operates with proficiency, and he is able to move from classroom to classroom with his peers. Ned uses an adaptive keyboard for taking notes. He eats lunch with his 15-year-old sister, who helps him as needed. Ned has adaptive utensils and can feed himself, but it can be quite messy and he can no longer raise a glass to his lips. Ned relies on an aide to help with toileting. He is uncomfortable asking for such help and often holds his urine until he gets home at the end of the school day.

Ned lives at home with his parents and sister. At home, his mother helps him with many of his self-care needs, including dressing, washing, toileting, and turning him at night. She also monitors his nighttime ventilation, ensuring that he gets adequate pulmonary assistance during his sleep. The house has been adapted for his wheelchair; there is a ramp out front and the family had renovations to make all the doorways on the ground floor wider. The ground floor family room has been converted to a bedroom for Ned and the bathroom has a Hoyer lift to help with transferring him to the toilet or bath.

On an IQ test, Ned scores in the "high average" range. He is particularly adept at solving puzzles and reasoning tasks, and his knowledge of factual information is impressive. His academic achievement skills are a little lower than expected given his IQ, yet still well within normal limits. On tests of reading fluency he is slower than expected, and he has mild difficulty decoding nonsense words.

Quality of Life in Older Individuals with Duchenne

As individuals with Duchenne age, they become less independent physically. With treatment designed to prolong life, many become adults who are dependent on mechanical ventilation. Two studies examining these individuals have found the majority have positive affect and most self-report good quality of life (Rahbek et al., 2005; Bach et al., 1991). Moreover, the affected individuals rate their own life satisfaction and affect as considerably higher than health care professionals judge them to be. Among 82 ventilator-assisted young men with Duchenne in the United States, only 12.5% expressed dissatisfaction with their lives (compared to a rate of 7% in the general population), despite being unable to engage in activities that others their age do (Bach et al., 1991). Similarly, when 65 Danish young adults with Duchenne were surveyed, the majority responded that their quality of life was excellent, even while reporting lack of educational opportunity and a love life (Rahbek et al., 2005). These studies confirm the need to provide the older individuals with Duchenne with as many opportunities as possible to lead an involved and satisfying life, as well as highlight the difficulty families and professionals may have in judging another's quality of life.

Behavioral and Cognitive Interventions

One published study examined intervention to decrease social isolation among individuals affected with Duchenne (Soutter et al., 2004). The researchers provided 74 families with a son with Duchenne with a personal computer and e-mail and Internet connectivity, as part of the Golden Freeway project initiated in northern England to ameliorate the isolation experienced by families with a child with a life-limiting illness. The use of the computer and parental perceptions were recorded. Results indicated that social isolation was felt to have decreased and that boys with Duchenne enjoyed using the computers and did so both for helping with their schoolwork and for entertainment.

There are no published studies investigating systematic interventions for the cognitive aspects of Duchenne. As such, recommendations for treatment must be based on individual assessment, and application of interventions found to be beneficial for others with comparable difficulties are recommended. The published research delineates the areas of cognition and behavior that are at increased risk for being compromised in children with Duchenne. The cases presented earlier illustrate the spectrum of involvement. Potential interventions and hypothetical outcomes follow.

Case 4.1: Kane Kane's family is told of his probable diagnosis of Duchenne. At first, Kane's parents deny this possibility, as his primary problems appear to delayed language development. Moreover, the initial DNA test shows no evidence of mutation. A subsequent DNA test, screening the entire gene's length for possible mutations, is positive. Subsequent analysis of his mother does not show evidence of a similar mutation.

To help with adjustment to the overwhelming news of their son's diagnosis of Duchenne, Kane's parents are urged to attend supportive therapy. They do so and also read up on all aspects of the disease. After initially refusing to accept that the diagnosis was even possible in a son who looked so physically fit, Kane's parents start him on early treatment with corticosteroids and daily physical therapy. They meet individual families with children who are also diagnosed with Duchenne and became actively involved in parent advocacy and educational organizations.

Kane's parents learn that his behaviors are not commonplace among children with Duchenne, and they have him evaluated further. After interviews with his parents and observation of Kane in both his natural and a controlled setting, Kane receives a diagnosis of autism spectrum disorder in addition to Duchenne. Kane's poor reciprocal social interactions, limited communication, and a restricted range of interests all contribute to the diagnosis. Behavioral interventions, including applied behavior analysis and inclusion in a specialized preschool program, are initiated to help ameliorate the behaviors that are associated with autism spectrum disorder and that are of the greatest immediate concern for his family.

Case 4.2: Louis Louis and his younger brother had previously been diagnosed with Duchenne. Their mother was actively involved in the physical care of the boys but had been unaware that any cognitive or behavioral problems might co-occur with the disease. After a thorough neuropsychological evaluation, Louis is diagnosed with specific language impairment. Speech therapy and extra resource room help at school aimed at increasing Louis's familiarity with and discrimination of basic phonemes are initiated to help him improve his language skills. Louis's mother and teachers are advised of his limited auditory processing abilities, and they modify their interactions with him by speaking in shorter, more concise statements and repeating their verbal commands when he appears not to understand. At-home early reading and rhyming games (including computer games) are encouraged. Supportive family therapy is recommended to try to shift the focus away from Louis as "the problem" who caused the family to break apart and, instead, help everyone to adjust and cope with the diagnosis and the changing family dynamics. Additionally, increased focus on Louis's limited language comprehension helps remove the negative emphasis on Louis's behavior as willful disrespect. Instead, Louis's "maddening" behavior becomes more understandable as a disability that he struggles with, and he is understood to merit support with his struggles. In turn, relationships within the family improve considerably. With the reduction of stressful interaction, Louis becomes more compliant with physical therapy and wearing his night splints.

Case 4.3: Muhhamad A social worker with fluent knowledge of Arabic is recruited to help with Muhhamad's care. She speaks with his parents to describe Muhhamad's condition, relates medical information and advice from Muhhamad's treating physicians, and helps the family make adjustments to help Muhhamad cope. The family has known of Muhhamad's diagnosis of Duchenne for more than 5 years but have repeatedly stated, "Muhhamad is strong. He will get better." The social worker helps them face what he is going through. She recommends that Muhhamad's parents meet other parents of children with Duchenne and educates them as to the adaptive changes they must make to their home to help Muhhamad as he transitions to a wheelchair. She emphasizes the need for his increased physical therapy and compliance with treatment. She attempts to encourage them to speak with others in their community about Muhhamad and his illness to remove any stigma that they (and Muhhamad) might be feeling.

After a diagnostic interview with a clinical psychologist, Muhhamad is diagnosed with adjustment disorder and depression. Antidepressant medication and individual supportive therapy are initiated with positive results. Muhhamad becomes more animated, outgoing, and able to discuss his fears related to his physical decline and increasing need for assistance. Increasing Muhhamad's involvement in social activities outside of his home is also recommended. Muhhamad enrolls in a formal drawing class and finds that he enjoys it and is able to express himself more readily through drawing than speech. After a thorough neuropsychological evaluation, Muhhamad is also diagnosed with developmental dyslexia. Reading interventions to help Muhhamad increase his overall fluency and proficiency are offered at his school.

Case 4.4: Ned Open discussions about Ned's future and how best to facilitate his autonomy at a time while he is growing steadily less independent physically are encouraged. Ned begins individual counseling, and he and his family attend family therapy sessions. In individual counseling, Ned discusses feelings of being unattractive, desires for sexual experiences, and a need to be treated like a young man capable of making his own decisions—all issues considered perfectly normal for any 16-year-old youth. In the family sessions, focus is given to each individual's needs, as well as the whole family. Ned's mother is encouraged to devote more time to her interests by increasing the involvement of at-home health care workers. Ned's parents are recommended to take some time for themselves to focus on their relationship as partners and lovers rather than solely caregivers and parents. Ned's sister is supported to develop her own identity, separate and distinct from that of solely Ned's healthy sister. Additionally, carrier screening is recommended for his sister, so she can be aware of her status to help her with future family planning. Ned's plans for attending college and pursuing a career of his interest are reinforced. Together, they work out logistics of how to maintain a good quality of life for each family member.

Summary

A diagnosis of Duchenne brings with it an array of complications and adjustments that require input from multiple integrated specialties. Medical, neuropsychological, behavioral, and educational interventions are all necessary to ensure the best possible quality of life for those living with Duchenne. The genetic etiology of Duchenne and its resultant phenotype of progressive muscle weakness are well characterized, but a cure has yet to be found. In contrast to the severe physical manifestations of Duchenne, the cognitive and behavioral phenotypes seem relatively mild and, as such, have not been adequately studied. Families struggling with their child's educational difficulties feel the daily impact of these issues. Research characterizing the cognitive and behavioral phenotypes of Duchenne offers insight as to what specific domains may be involved. However, no intervention studies have been conducted to determine whether—and how—the neuropsychological aspects of the disease can be ameliorated. The disease provides a model for better known behavioral diagnoses such as developmental dyslexia and autism spectrum disorders, yet although Duchenne is associated with these disorders, most individuals with Duchenne do not have them. Continued characterization of the neuropsychological profile and investigation of ways to help children deal with their limitations are necessary to improve the quality of life for all individuals affected by Duchenne. Through its association with behavioral diagnoses such as developmental dyslexia and autism spectrum disorders, Duchenne provides a model for the study of the relationship between the molecular biology of dystrophin and cognitive development.

Acknowledgments

This work was supported in part by a National Institute of Neurological Disorders and Stroke grant to Veronica J. Hinton. We are most grateful to all the families we have worked with.

References

Anderson, J. L., Head, S. I., Rae, C., & Morley, J. W. (2002). Brain function in Duchenne muscular dystrophy. *Brain, 125,* 4–13.

Bach, J. R., Campagnolo, D. I., & Hoeman, S. (1991). Life satisfaction of individuals with Duchenne muscular dystrophy using long-term mechanical ventilatory support. *American Journal of Physical Medicine and Rehabilitation, 70*(3), 129–135.

Beggs, A. H., & Kunkel, L. M. (1990). Improved diagnosis of Duchenne/Becker muscular dystrophy. *Journal of Clinical Investigation, 85,* 613–619.

Billard, C., Gillet, P., Barthez, M., Hommet, C., & Bertrand, P. (1998). Reading ability and processing in Duchenne muscular dystrophy and spinal muscular atrophy. *Developmental Medicine and Child Neurology, 40,* 12–20.

Billard, C., Gillet, P., Signoret, J. L., Uicaut, E., Bertrand, P., Fardeau, M., et al. (1992). Cognitive functions in Duchenne muscular dystrophy: A reappraisal and comparison with spinal muscular atrophy. *Neuromuscular Disorders, 2,* 371–378.

Boyce, F. M., Beggs, A. H., Feener, C., & Kunkel, L. M. (1991). Dystrophin is transcribed in brain from a distant upstream promoter. *Proceedings of the National Academy of Sciences, U.S.A., 88,* 1276–1280.

Brooke, M. H., Fenichel, G. M., Griggs, R. C., Mendell, J. R., Moxley, R., Mller, J. P., & Province, M. (1983). Clinical investigation in Duchenne dystrophy: II. Determination of the "power" of therapeutic trials based on the natural history. *Muscle Nerve, 6,* 91–103.

Calvert, R., Kahana, E., & Gratzer, W. B. (1996). Stability of the dystrophin rod domain fold: Evidence for nested repeating units. *Biophysical Journal, 71,* 1605–1610.

Copeland, D. R. (1988). Stress and the patient's family. In M. L. Russell (Ed.), *Stress management for chronic diseases* (pp. 30–48). Pergamon: New York.

Cotton, S., Crowe, S. F., & Voudouris, N. (1998). Neuropsychological profile of Duchenne muscular dystrophy. *Child Neuropsychology, 4*(2), 110–117.

Cotton, S., Voudouris, N., & Greenwood, K. M. (2001). Intelligence and Duchenne muscular dystrophy: Full-scale, Verbal, and Performance intelligence quotients. *Developmental Medicine and Child Neurology, 43,* 497–501.

Cotton, S., Voudouris, N., & Greenwood, K. M. (2005). Association between intellectual functioning and age in children with Duchenne muscular dystrophy: Further results from a meta-analysis. *Developmental Medicine and Child Neurology, 73,* 257–265.

Cyrulnik, S., Fee, R., Goldstein, E., De Vivo, D. C., & Hinton, V. J. (in press). Delayed language developmental milestones reported by parents of children with Duchenne muscular dystrophy. *Journal of Pediatrics.*

Dorman, C., Hurley, A. D., & D'Avignon, J. (1988). Language and learning disorders of older boys with Duchenne muscular dystrophy. *Developmental Medicine and Child Neurology, 30,* 316–327.

Drenckhahn, D., Holbach, M., Ness, W., Schmitz, F., & Anderson, L. V. (1996). Dystrophin and the dystrophin-associated glycoprotein, beta-dystroglycan, co-localize in photoreceptor synaptic complexes of the human retina. *Neuroscience, 73,* 605–612.

Duchenne, G. B. A. (1968). Recherches sur la paralysie musculaire pseudohypertrophique, ou paralysie myo-sclerosique. [Studies on pseudohypertrophic muscular paralysis or myosclerotic paralysis] *Archives of Neurology, 19,* 629–636.

Echenne, B., Rivier, F., Tardieu, M., Brive, M., Robert, A., Pages, A. M., et al. (1998). Congenital muscular dystrophy and cerebellar atrophy. *Neurology, 50,* 1477–1480.

Emery, A. E. H. (1991). Population frequencies of inherited neuromuscular diseases—A world survey. *Neuromuscular Disorders, 1,* 19–29.

Emery, A. E. H. (1992). *Duchenne muscular dystrophy.* Oxford, England: Oxford Medical Publications.

Felisari, G., Martinelli Boneschi, F., Bardoni, A., Sironi, M., Comi, G. P., Robotti, M., et al. (2000). Loss of Dp140 dystrophin isoform and intellectual impairment in Duchenne dystrophy. *Neurology, 55,* 559–564.

Fitzpatrick, C., Barry, C., & Garvey, C. (1986). Psychiatric disorder among boys with Duchenne muscular dystrophy. *Developmental Medicine and Child Neurology, 28,* 589–595.

Flanigan, K. M., von Niederhausern, A., Dunn, D. M., Alder, J., Mendell, J. R., & Weiss, R. B. (2003). Rapid direct sequence analysis of the dystrophin gene. *American Journal of Human Genetics, 72,* 931–939.

Glaub, T., & Mechler, F. (1987). Intellectual function in muscular dystrophies. *European Archives of Psychiatry and Neurological Sciences, 236*(6), 379–382.

Gorecki, D. C., Lukasiuk, K., Szklarczyk, A., & Kaczmarek, L. (1998). Kainate-evoked changes in dystrophin messenger RNA levels in the rat hippocampus. *Neuroscience, 84,* 467–477.

Gorecki, D. C., Monaco, A. P., Derry, J. M., Walker, A. P., Barnard, E. A., & Barnard, P. J. (1992). Expression of four alternative dystrophin transcripts in brain regions regulated by different promoters. *Human Molecular Genetics, 1,* 505–510.

Gravelle, A. M. (1997). Caring for a child with a progressive illness during the complex chronic phase: Parents' experience of facing adversity. *Journal of Advanced Nursing, 25,* 738–745.

Harper, D. C. (1983). Personality correlates and degree of impairment in male adolescents with progressive and non-progressive physical disorders. *Journal of Clinical Psychology, 39,* 859–867.

Hinton, V. J., Batchelder, A., Cyrulnik, S., Fee, R., & Kiefel, J. (2006). Autism and Duchenne muscular dystrophy. *34th International Neuropsychological Society Annual Meeting Abstracts,* 66.

Hinton, V. J., Fee, R., DeVivo, D. C., Goldstein, E., & Stern, Y. (2004). Investigation of poor academic achievement in children with Duchenne muscular dystrophy. *Learning Disabilities Research & Practice, 19*(3), 146–154.

Hinton, V. J., Fee, R., DeVivo, D. C., & Goldstein, E. (in press). Verbal and memory skills in Duchenne muscular dystrophy. *Developmental Medicine and Child Neurology.*

Hinton, V. J., Kim, H., Fee, R., & Goldstein, E. Age-related changes in cognitive and behavioral characteristics associated with Duchenne muscular dystrophy. (in submission)

Hinton, V. J., Nereo, N. E., DeVivo, D. C., Goldstein, E., & Stern, Y. (2000). Poor verbal working memory across intellectual level in boys with Duchenne dystrophy. *Neurology, 54,* 2127–2132.

Hinton, V. J., Nereo, N. E., DeVivo, D. C., Goldstein, E., & Stern, Y. (2001). Selective deficits in verbal working memory associated with a known genetic etiology: The neuropsychological profile of Duchenne muscular dystrophy. *Journal of International Neuropsychological Society, 7,* 45–54.

Hinton, V. J., Nereo, N. E., Fee, R., & Cyrulnik, S. (2006). Social behavior problems in boys with Duchenne muscular dystrophy. *Journal of Developmental and Behavioral Pediatrics, 27,* 470–476.

Hoffman, E. P., Brown, R. H., & Kunkel, L. M. (1987). Dystrophin: The protein product of the Duchenne muscular dystrophy locus. *Cell, 51,* 919–928.

Hoffman, E. P., & Wang, J. (1993). Duchenne–Becker muscular dystrophy and the nondystrophic myotonias: Paradigms for loss of function and change of function of gene products. *Archives of Neurology, 50,* 1227–1237.

Holroyd, J., & Guthrie, D. (1986). Family stress with chronic childhood illness: Cystic fibrosis, neuromuscular disorders, and renal disease. *Journal of Clinical Psychology, 42,* 552–561.

Hyser, C. L., Province, M., Griggs, R. C., Mendell, J. R., Fenichel, G. M., Brooke, M. H., et al. (1987). Genetic heterogeneity in Duchenne dystrophy. *Annals of Neurology, 22,* 553–555.

Jancsik, V., & Hajos, F. (1998). Differential distribution of dystrophin in postsynaptic densities of spine synapses. *Neuroreport, 9,* 2249–2251.

Jones, K. J., Kim, S. S., & North, K. N. (1998). Abnormalities of dystrophin, the sarcoglycans, and laminin alpha2 in the muscular dystrophies. *Journal of Medical Genetics, 35*, 379–386.

Kaplan, L. C., Osborne, P., & Elias, E. (1986). The diagnosis of muscular dystrophy in patients referred for language delay. *Journal of Child Psychology and Psychiatry, 27*, 545–549.

Kimura, S., Abe, K., Suzuki, M., Ogawa, M., Yoshioka, K., Yamamura, K., & Miike, T. (1997). 2.1 kb 5′-flanking region of the brain type dystrophin gene directs the expression of lacZ in the cerebral cortex, but not in the hippocampus. *Journal of Neurological Science, 147*(1), 13–20.

Koenig, M., Hoffman, E. P., Bertelson, C. J., Monaco, A. P., Feener, C., & Kunkel, L. M. (1987). Complete cloning of the Duchenne muscular dystrophy (Duchenne) cDNA and preliminary genomic organization of the Duchenne gene in normal and affected individuals. *Cell, 50*, 509–517.

Koenig, M., Monaco, A. P., & Kunkel, L. M. (1988). The complete sequence of dystrophin predicts a rod-shaped cytoskeletal protein. *Cell, 53*, 219–226.

Komoto, J., Usui, S., Otsuki, S., & Terao, A. (1984). Infantile autism and Duchenne muscular dystrophy. *Journal of Autism and Developmental Disorders, 14*, 191–195.

Lederfein, D., Levy, Z., Augier, N., Mornet, D., Morris, G., Fuchs, O., et al. (1992). A 71-kilodalton protein is a major product of the Duchenne muscular dystrophy gene in brain and other nonmuscle tissues. *Proceedings of the National Academy of Sciences, U.S.A., 89*, 5346–5350.

Lee, J. S., Pfund, Z., Juhasz, C., Behen, M. E., Muzik, O., Chugani, D. C., et al. (2002). Altered regional brain glucose metabolism in Duchenne muscular dystrophy: A PET study. *Muscle Nerve, 26*, 506–512.

Leibowitz, D., & Dubowitz, V. (1981). Intellect and behaviour in Duchenne muscular dystrophy. *Developmental Medicine and Child Neurology, 23*, 577–590.

Lidov, H. G., Byers, T. J., Watkins, S. C., & Kunkel, L. M. (1990). Localization of dystrophin to postsynaptic regions of central nervous system cortical neurons. *Nature, 348*, 725–728.

McDonald, C., Abresch, R., Carter, G., Fowler, W., Johnson, E. R., Kilmer, D., & Sigford, B. (1995). Profiles of neuromuscular diseases: Duchenne muscular dystrophy. *American Journal of Physical Medicine and Rehabilitation, 74*(5), 70–92.

Mehler, M. F. (2000). Brain dystrophin, neurogenetics and mental retardation. *Brain Research—Brain Research Reviews, 32*, 277–307.

Mendell, J. R., Buzin, C. H., Feng, J., Yan, J., Serrano, C., Sangi, D. S., et al. (2001). Diagnosis of Duchenne dystrophy by enhanced detection of small mutations. *Neurology, 57*, 645–650.

Mendell, J. R., Province, M., Moxley, R. T., III, Griggs, R. C., Brooke, M. H., Fenichel, G. M., et al. (1987). Clinical investigation of Duchenne muscular dystrophy: A methodology for therapeutic trials based on natural history controls. *Archives of Neurology, 44*, 808–811.

Monaco, A. P., Neve, R. L., Colletti-Feener, C., Bertelson, C. J., Kurnit, D. M., & Kunkel, L. M. (1986). Isolation of candidate cDNAs for portions of the Duchenne muscular dystrophy gene. *Nature, 323*, 646–650.

Moxley, R., Ashwal, S., Pandya, S., A., Connolly, F. J., Mathews, K., et al. (2005). Practice parameters: Corticosteroid treatment of Duchenne dystrophy. *Neurology, 64*, 13–20.

Muntoni, F., Torelli, S., & Ferlini, A. (2003). Dystrophin and mutations: One gene, several proteins, multiple phenotypes. *Lancet Neurology, 2*, 731–740.

Nereo, N. E., Fee, R., & Hinton, V. J. (2003). Parental stress in mothers of children with Duchenne muscular dystrophy. *Journal of Pediatric Psychology, 28*, 473–484.

Ogasawara, A. (1989). Downward shift in IQ in persons with Duchenne muscular dystrophy compared to those with spinal muscular atrophy. *American Journal of Mental Retardation, 93*, 544–547.

Prosser, E. J., Murphy, E. G., & Thompson, M. W. (1969). Intelligence and the gene for Duchenne muscular dystrophy. *Archives of Disabled Child, 44*, 221–230.

Rahbek, J., Werge, B., Madsen, A., Marquardt, J., Steffensen, B. F., & Jeppesen, J. (2005). Adult life with Duchenne muscular dystrophy: Observations among an emerging and unforeseen patient population. *Pediatric Rehabilitation, 8*(1), 17–28.

Reid, D. T., & Renwick, R. M. (2001). Relating familial stress to the psychosocial adjustment of adolescents with Duchenne muscular dystrophy. *International Journal of Rehabilitation Research, 24*(2), 83–93.

Rodius, F., Claudepierre, T., Rosas-Vargas, H., Cisneros, B., Montanez, C., Dreyfus, H., et al. (1997). Dystrophins in developing retina: Dp260 expression correlates with synaptic maturation. *Neuroreport, 8*, 2383–2387.

Smith, R. A., Sibert, J. R., & Harper, P. S. (1990). Early development of boys with Duchenne muscular dystrophy. *Developmental Medicine and Child Neurology, 32*, 519–527.

Sollee, N. D., Latham, E. E., Bresnan, D. J., & Kindlon, M. J. (1985). Neuropsychological impairment in Duchenne muscular dystrophy. *Journal of Clinical and Experimental Neuropsychology, 7*, 486–496.

Soutter, J., Hamilton, N., Russel, P., Russel, C., Bushby, K., Sloper, P., & Bartlett, K. (2004). The Golden Freeway: A preliminary evaluation of a pilot study advancing information technology as a social intervention for boys with Duchenne muscular dystrophy and their families. *Health Social Care Community, 12*(1), 25–33.

Thompson, R. J., Zeman, J. L., Fanurik, D., & Sirotkin-Roses, M. (1992). The role of parent stress and coping and family functioning in parent and child adjustment to Duchenne muscular dystrophy. *Journal of Clinical Psychology, 48*, 11–19.

Tian, M., Jacobson, C., Gee, S. H., Campbell, K. P., Carbonetto, S., & Jucker, M. (1996). Dystroglycan in the cerebellum is a laminin alpha 2-chain binding protein at the glial-vascular interface and is expressed in Purkinje cells. *European Journal of Neuroscience, 8*, 2739–2747.

Tracey, I., Scott, R. B., Thompson, C. H., Dunn, J. F., Barnes, P. R., Styles, P., et al. (1995). Brain abnormalities in Duchenne muscular dystrophy: Phosphorus-31 magnetic resonance spectroscopy and neuropsychological study. *Lancet, 345*, 1260–1264.

Uchino, M., Teramoto, H., Naoe, H., Miike, T., Yoshioka, K., & Ando, M. (1994a). Dystrophin and dystrophin-related protein in the central nervous system of normal controls and Duchenne muscular dystrophy. *Acta Neuropathologica, 87*, 129–134.

Uchino, M., Teramoto, H., Naoe, H., Yoshioka, K., Miike, T., & Ando, M. (1994b). Localisation and characterisation of dystrophin in the central nervous system of controls and patients with Duchenne muscular dystrophy. *Journal of Neurology, Neurosurgery, and Psychiatry, 57*, 426–429.

Ueda, H., Kobayashi, T., Mitsui, K., Tsurugi, K., Tsukahara, S., & Ohno, S. (1995). Dystrophin localization at presynapse in rat retina revealed by immunoelectron microscopy. *Investigative Ophthalmology and Visual Science, 36*, 2318–2322.

Whelan, T. B. (1987). Neuropsychological performance of children with Duchenne muscular dystrophy and spinal muscle atrophy. *Developmental Medicine and Child Neurology, 29*, 212–220.

Wicksell, R. K., Kihlgren, M., Melin, L., & Eeg-Olofsson, O. (2004). Specific cognitive deficits are common in children with Duchenne muscular dystrophy. *Developmental Medicine and Child Neurology, 46*, 154–159.

Wilton, S. D., Honeyman, K., Fletcher, S., & Laing, N. G. (1998). Snapback SSCP analysis: Engineered conformation changes for the rapid typing of known mutations. *Human Mutation, 11*, 252–258.

Worden, D. K., & Vignos, P. J. (1962). Intellectual function in childhood progressive muscular dystrophy. *Pediatrics, 29*, 968–977.

Wu, J. Y., Kuban, K. C., Allred, E., Shapiro, F., & Darras, B. T. (2005). Association of Duchenne muscular dystrophy with autism spectrum disorder. *Journal of Child Neurology, 20*, 790–795.

Zellweger, H., & Hanson, J. W. (1967). Psychometric studies in muscualr dystrophy type 3a (Duchenne). *Developmental Medicine and Child Neurology, 9*, 576–581.

Zwaigenbaum, L., & Tarnopolsky, M. (2003). Two children with muscular dystrophies ascertained due to referral for diagnosis of autism. *Journal of Autism and Developmental Disorders, 33*, 193–199.

5 Neurofibromatosis

John M. Slopis and Bartlett D. Moore, III

History

Neurofibromatosis (NF) is a family of genetic disorders originally grouped together by virtue of common features of benign nerve sheath tumors. These disorders include NF type 1 (NF-1), NF type 2 (NF-2), and multiple schwannomatosis, each with distinctly different genetic mutations and pathologic bases. The original term "neurofibromatosis" was derived at the turn of the last century, but it is also called von Recklinghausen's disease. Severely disfigured individuals with this disorder were depicted in literature and art as early as the 16th century, but not until the late 1800s was the condition described clinically and scientifically by Friedrich Daniel von Recklinghausen (Crump, 1981; Viskochil et al., 1990; Cawthon et al., 1990) over 70 years before the distinguishing clinical features and molecular genetic basis of each were discovered. NF-1 was localized to chromosome 17 in 1990 by two teams of investigators (Wallace et al., 1990; Viskochil et al., 1990). NF-2 was localized to chromosome 22 shortly thereafter (Trofatter et al., 1993; Rouleau et al., 1993).

Virtually all organ systems can be affected in some fashion by mutations in the NF-1 gene and so this disorder was originally called "peripheral NF." NF-2 is a disorder of multiple Schwann cell tumors of the spine and brain stem, and so NF-2 was originally called "central NF." The hallmark of NF-2 is the presence of schwannomas of the acoustic nerves. NF-2 is a highly penetrant gene with far less variability than that seen in NF-1. Multiple schwannomatosis presents with painful spinal schwannomas pathologically similar to those seen in NF-2, but without involvement of the brainstem. The molecular genetic basis of multiple schwannomatosis remains to be determined.

John Merrick, the so-called "Elephant Man," was perhaps the most famous individual to be diagnosed with NF-1, although recent reports suggest that a more likely diagnosis for Mr. Merrick is Proteus syndrome, an unrelated condition that resembles NF-1 externally but that arises from a genetic mutation on a different chromosome (Ablon, 1995).

Epidemiology

NF-1 has an incidence of approximately 1 in 4,000 (North, 2000). NF-2 is far less common with an incidence of approximately 1 in 50,000. Although NF has been postulated to have as many as eight different forms (Riccardi & Eichner, 1986), this classification system has not been widely adopted. NF-1 and NF-2 are the most commonly described disorders. Multiple schwannomatosis is thought to occur with an incidence similar to that of NF-2, but only 15% of cases are reported to be familial in nature (Antinheimo et al., 2000).

NF-1 is an autosomal dominant genetic disorder with an incidence more common than muscular dystrophy, Tay-Sachs, and Huntington's diseases combined. Despite its high frequency of occurrence, NF-1 has caused a great deal of confusion among clinicians over the years because the symptoms and clinical outcome of the disorder are highly variable from individual to individual. Approximately 50% of all cases result from a spontaneous mutation in the NF-1 gene region, and so only half of all known cases are familial. The phenotype of NF-1 is highly variable between unrelated individuals and even within affected families (von Deimling, Krone, & Menon, 1995), despite the fact the gene produces near complete penetrance. There is no known ethnic, racial, or gender predominance in NF-1. Careful clinical observations have greatly refined definition of the phenotypic profile of NF-1 over the last century, but the first great breakthrough in contemporary genetic studies did not occur until the gene was localized to chromosome 17 (Wallace et al., 1990).

The phenotypic variability of NF-1 results in many individuals who live normal lives and experience relatively little impact from the condition, often unaware that they even carry the NF-1 gene. The presence of these mildly affected individuals calls into question the accuracy of the incidence and prevalence estimates of NF-1. Other individuals with NF-1 have chronic, progressive, and debilitating morbidity, including severely disfiguring physical stigmata or significant and even life-threatening medical complications such as cancer. These complications of the disorder in clinically affected individuals generally become more prevalent and severe with advancing age, and, consequently, NF-1 is also associated with a somewhat shortened life span (Riccardi, 1981). We have selected six cases (near the end of this chapter) to illustrate this variability of phenotypic expression and behavioral/cognitive profile. These cases are arranged to show that a child with severe clinical disease can nevertheless have normal learning, behavioral, and emotional functioning. Conversely, a child with mild clinical expression can have severe, debilitating problems in learning, behavior, or emotional functioning.

Table 5.1
Diagnostic criteria for neurofibromatosis type 1 (NF-1)

1. Six or more cafe-au-lait spots greater than 5 mm in diameter in prepubertal children or greater than 15 mm in diameter in postpubertal individuals

2. Two or more neurofibromas of any form or one plexiform neurofibroma

3. Freckling in the axillary or inguinal regions

4. Optic glioma

5. Two or more Lisch nodules (iris hamartomas)

6. A distinctive osseous lesion such as sphenoid dysplasia or thinning of long bone cortex with or without pseudoarthrosis

7. A first-degree relative with NF-1 by the above criteria

Note: The presence of 2 or more criteria constitutes a definitive diagnosis in an individual. If an individual has a first-degree relative with NF-1, then only one additional criterion is required for the diagnosis.

Clinical Features: The NF-1 Phenotype

Symptoms of NF-1 evolve with age, and early diagnosis is often problematic, especially in cases of spontaneous mutation. NF-1 can present with congenital anomalies that are obvious at birth or with clinical features conspicuous within the first few years of life, unlike NF-2 and multiple schwannomatosis, where morbidity develops in late adolescence or early adulthood. NF-1 is a generalized systemic disorder that includes characteristic patterns of cutaneous features and cognitive impairment that are not seen in NF-2 or multiple schwannomatosis.

To date, the most reliable approach to the diagnosis of NF-1 remains assessment of clinical features. The diagnostic criteria for NF-1 (see table 5.1) are based on a consensus statement developed by the National Institutes of Health (NIH) in 1988 (NIH, 1988) and reaffirmed in 1997 (Gutmann et al., 1997). These diagnostic criteria represent the most frequent clinical features of NF-1. The diagnosis of NF-1 is established with greater than 99% confidence when two or more features from this list are identified in the patient.

The hallmark of NF-1 is the presence of the characteristic benign tumor known as the "neurofibroma," meaning fibrous tissue of neural origin. Neurofibromata develop sporadically in any region of the body from dysplastic overgrowth of the myelin/connective tissue sheath encasing myelinated peripheral nerve fibers. These lesions arise from cutaneous, subcutaneous, and deep nerve fibers. Nodular neurofibromas develop in subcutaneous patterns along large nerve fibers. Plexiform neurofibromas are complex structures that grow as regions of dysplastic tissue both within the epidermis and dermis or immediately beneath the epidermis. Neurofibromas that develop within cutaneous structures rarely undergo malignant transformation. Deep neurofibromas are at risk for malignant conversion to neurofibrosarcomas at a lifetime risk of 5%–10% (Evans, 2003).

The most succinct list of clinical features of NF-1 is contained within the diagnostic criteria. However, in addition to those features, many other clinical signs and symptoms are associated with NF-1, including vascular abnormalities, cosmetic disfigurement, seizures, headaches, macrocephaly, dysarthria, spinal anomalies, and chest wall anomalies. Hypertrophy within single or multiple segments of the body, short stature, and constipation also are common (Riccardi & Eichner, 1986). The frequencies of the following "minor disease features" have been estimated within one hospital population as follows: macrocephaly (52.9%), short stature (24.7%), hypertelorism (63.5%), and thorax abnormalities (37.6%). The authors reporting these findings suggest that they are considered to be reliable clinical signs of NF-1 within the first 6 years of life and may also aid in predicting the ultimate diagnosis of NF-1 by adulthood (Cnossen et al., 1998).

The phenotype of NF-1 is also characterized by a high incidence of learning disabilities (LDs), behavioral problems such as attention deficit/hyperactivity disorder (ADHD), and neurocognitive deficits in visual–spatial abilities. The cognitive phenotype is considered to be a similarly important predictor of the early diagnosis by some investigators and will be discussed in detail later.

Enhancing Early Diagnosis

The diagnosis of NF-1 is easily made on the basis of the clinical features presented in table 5.1, but early recognition of these symptoms is not always possible. For children with NF-1 resulting from a spontaneous mutation (no family history), this diagnosis is especially problematic. Although some of the clinical features used to diagnose NF-1 (especially café-au-lait spots, neurofibromas, Lisch nodules, and freckling in the armpit and groin) are first evident between birth and 10 years of age, they may be subtle and go unnoticed by the child's family or pediatrician. However, for a parent with NF-1, there is about a 50% chance that each child born will have the mutation, and the family and pediatrician will therefore be more vigilant. Even so, because these and other diagnostic features generally increase with age, a definitive diagnosis may still take several years. Even with advanced age, not all of the clinical features become evident in all individuals with NF-1, but Lisch nodules are present in almost 100% of individuals by young adulthood, making it a strong diagnostic predictor in adults (table 5.2). Optic gliomas, which occur in about 15% of individuals with NF-1 (Listernick, Charrow, Greenwald, & Mets, 1994), are usually present by 6 year of age, but because only about 20% of these ever become symptomatic, this clinical feature may not be noticed unless the child has a magnetic resonance imaging (MRI) scan of the brain. Presence of any of the "minor disease features" mentioned above should alert clinicians to the possible diagnosis of NF-1 (Cnossen et al., 1998). Magnetic resonance (MR) hyperintensities as an incidental finding on MRI of the

Table 5.2

Prevalence of characteristic clinical and behavioral signs and symptoms of neurofibromatosis (NF) and prevalence of NF type 1 (NF-1) in these conditions

Characteristic	Percentage of Patients with NF Exhibiting This Symptom	Percentage of General Population Exhibiting This Symptom Who Also Have NF
Clinical features		
Six or more café au lait spots	Up to 90[a]	Very high
Axillary or inguinal freckling	Up to 90[a]	Very high
Lisch nodules	Up to 95[a]	Very high
Optic glioma	15	50%–70
Plexiform neurofibroma	Up to 30[a]	Very high
Scoliosis	10	Low
First degree relative with NF-1	50	50
Magnetic resonance hyperintensities	40–50%	Very high
Behavioral features		
Learning disabilities	40	Low
Attention deficit/hyperactivity disorder	40–50%	Low
Visual–spatial impairment	60–70%	Increased
Mental retardation	6–8%	Increased

[a] Age dependent.

brain (e.g., for mild head injury or headaches) should also alert clinicians to the possible diagnosis of NF-1.

Because visual–spatial impairment is so prevalent in this population (approximately 60%–70%), additional information may be provided by performance on tests of visual–spatial abilities, especially when the diagnosis based on clinical characteristics is marginal (e.g., five, but not six, café au lait spots). Schools and entities testing large numbers of school-age children should be aware that a profile consisting of visual–spatial deficits, ADHD, and learning deficits in the context of intact intellectual abilities is often associated with NF-1. For medical personnel caring for children with diagnosed NF-1, a comprehensive neurocognitive evaluation should become part of their standard of care. Since tests of visual–spatial functioning are related to reading and academic abilities in general, tests of visual–spatial abilities should be included. A brief screening examination is even warranted for suspected NF-1 should school or medical personnel have suspicions of the diagnosis.

The NF-1 Gene

Description and Diagnostic Considerations

In this section we will examine how mutations of the Ras gene contribute to disorders of somatic growth and function, including implications for learning, behavior,

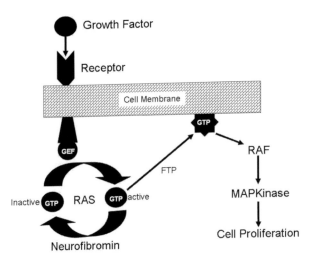

Figure 5.1
Growth regulatory pathways important for neurofibromatosis type 1 neurofibroma formation and progression. Abbreviations: GEF, guanine-nucleotide exchange factor; GTP, guanosine triphosphate; Ras, rat sar-
coma protein; FTP, famyseal transferase protein; Raf, receptor activation factor; MAP, mitogen-activated
protein.

and neurocognitive functioning. After the NF-1 gene was localized to human chromosome 17 in 1990, the product of the gene was identified and named "neurofibromin" (Wallace et al., 1990; Viskochil et al., 1990). This protein product is now
recognized to have a central role in signal transduction in the Ras system that regulates cellular growth in Schwann cells as well as numerous other cell types. The role
of the protein neurofibromin was discovered through study of juvenile myelomonocytic leukemia, a disorder seen in disproportionately high frequency in persons with
NF-1 (Niemeyer et al., 1997).

The Ras "oncogene" is linked to extracellular receptors that bind various "first
messenger" hormones including human growth hormone and nerve growth factors
(figure 5.1). The Ras system serves as the "second messenger" in the signal pathway
by induced phosphorylation, changing configuration and binding to the inner cell
membrane through cytoskeletal bonds. These bonds are promoted by the process of
farnesylation via the intracellular enzyme system farnesyl transferase. Neurofibromin
is a constituent component of the reversible phosphorylation enzyme GTPase, accel-
erating the process to proceed forward toward cell growth and activation.

The enzyme system farnesyl transferase has been the subject of intense investigation as a potential target to interrupt dysregulated growth and cellular activation in
NF-1. Pharmacologic agents known as farnesyl transferase inhibitors are currently
under clinical trial to inhibit growth of the benign Schwann cell tumors called neuro-

fibromas in NF-1, and these agents may ultimately play a role in treatment of neuro-fibromas that undergo malignant transformation.

Mutations in the gene coding region produce mutated or "truncated" copies of the protein neurofibromin leading to defective Ras signaling and uncontrolled Schwann cell growth seen in neurofibromas. Mutations in the NF-1 gene are highly variable among affected individuals, leading to the tremendous variability in the phenotypic expression of NF-1. Currently, several hundred distinct mutations in the NF-1 gene have been reported from clinically affected individuals using contemporary DNA sequencing methods. DNA genotype/clinical phenotype correlation studies are under way, but to date little reliable information is available to confirm genotype/phenotype relationships. In time, this body of information will provide useful prognostic information to predict relative risks and outcomes, including neurocognitive morbidity, for individuals who carry the NF-1 gene.

Early attempts to develop laboratory-based diagnostic probes for NF-1 include studies that assess the protein sequence of circulating neurofibromin obtained from blood samples. The abnormal neurofibromin protein found in affected individuals is referred to as "truncated protein product." These studies carry relatively high false positive and negative rates, rendering them of limited diagnostic value compared to conventional diagnostic techniques based on clinical features. These studies provide no prognostic value at this time.

Systemic Impact

Focal Growth Dysregulation in Benign Tumors   Neurofibromas are complex benign tumors containing multiple tissue elements, including neural tissue, connective tissue, and vascular components. Researchers have long recognized the abnormal patterns of growth in these various tissues, suggesting that the influence of the NF-1 gene is widespread. Neurofibromin now been identified in multiple tissues that are derived from virtually all embryonic tissue lines including mesoderm, ectoderm, neuroecto-derm, and neural crest. The gene product has been isolated from fetal ectoderm tissues as early as the first few weeks of gestation. This early presentation suggests that the NF-1 gene is a critical factor in embryonic development and therefore is a clue to the widespread systemic nature of the disorder, including impact on brain development.

Systemic Impact on Somatic Growth   Systemic growth derangement may also occur in a highly generalized fashion in NF-1. Precocious puberty is reported to occur in children with NF-1 in association with tumors of the optic chiasm abutting the hypo-thalamus. Short stature may be seen in over 20% of children with NF-1. While the mechanism of precocious puberty in NF-1 remains unclear, endocrine studies of short stature reveal evidence that human growth hormone/insulin related growth factor levels may be normal in many cases of short stature, implicating defective cellular receptor responses to stimulation by these circulating hormones (Vassilopoulou-Sellin, Klein, & Slopis, 2000).

Systemic Influences on Function   The impact of the NF-1 gene appears to extend far beyond the promotion of growth of benign nerve sheath fibromas. The goal of clinical trials of farnesyl-transferase inhibitors is to interrupt intercellular transmission of the growth message and so to inhibit the growth of benign neurofibromas. Of perhaps greater interest, however, is the recent demonstration that these agents have a positive impact upon learning deficits in NF-1 knock-out mice (Costa et al., 2002). Knock-out mice that are haploinsufficient for the NF-1 gene demonstrate deficits in spatial learning that model human NF-1 LDs in a limited way. These mice were studied in a Morris water maze system and found to have significant visual–spatial learning impairments. The mice were then treated with a farnesyl-transferase inhibitor, which led to significant reductions in learning time and improvement in overall learning efficiency (Costa et al., 2002). Since deficits in visual–spatial ability are considered a hallmark of NF-1, this represents a valid model to develop pharmacological agents for the treatment of learning disabilities associated with NF-1 in humans. However, the visual–spatial deficits in humans with NF-1 are perceptual in nature and do not involve spatial learning as exhibited by NF-1 knock-out mice.

The role of the NF-1 gene has also been studied in NF-1 haploinsufficient Drosophila. The Drosophila NF-1 protein is highly conserved, showing 60% identity with human neurofibromin (Guo, Tong, Hannan, Luo, & Zhong, 2000b). The fruit fly depends heavily upon olfaction for survival, so models of learning must distinguish between behavioral patterns that include or exclude olfaction. These models include olfactory guided avoidance, olfactory guided learning, and electric shock avoidance. Studies indicate that Drosophila NF-1 protein acts both as a Ras-GAP and as a regulator of the cyclic-AMP pathway that involves the *rutabaga* (*rut*)-encoded adenylyl cyclase. G-protein-activated adenylyl cyclase activity in the fruit fly appears to occur in NF-1 dependent and NF-1 independent mechanisms. The mechanism of NF-1 dependent activation of the Rut adenylyl cyclase pathway is essential for Drosophila learning and memory (Guo, Tong, Hannan, Luo, & Zhong, 2000a).

The implications of these animal studies are far-reaching with respect to learning disabilities in humans with NF-1. The functionally disordered GTPase of the Ras signaling system could potentially be present as a common defective second messenger in numerous signaling systems throughout the body including the brain. These animal studies suggest that abnormal cell signaling in brain leads to defects in neurotransmission and subsequent LDs that may respond to pharmacological intervention.

Influences on Central Nervous System Morphology

The NF-1 gene appears to influence central nervous system development during embryogenesis to produce malformations of spine and brain in animal models and in humans.

Spine Congenital dystrophic spinal malformation in NF-1, which occurs during embryonic development, has been recognized for many years. These spinal anomalies present as scoliosis or other anomalous curvature of the spine. Spinal meningocoels may be present early or later in development. These malformations frequently present without associated paraspinal neurofibroma formation, although paraspinal neurofibromata usually develop in time. These complex spinal anomalies are among the most frequent causes of morbidity in adults with NF-1. Recent studies have revealed that the NF-1 gene may produce abnormal bone development patterns by encoding abnormal bone-specific GTPase in a fashion analogous to the Ras 21 signaling defects described above (Abdel-Wanis & Kawahara, 2001).

Brain The most recognized brain malformation in NF-1 is aqueductal stenosis, which is seen in approximately 15% of children. The mechanism of this malformation remains unclear, although low-grade glioma or hamartoma may appear within the brain stem as age progresses (see Case 2). Benign macrocephaly, another common clinical feature of NF-1, also implies impact of the NF-1 gene upon the brain during embryogenesis. Volumetric MRI studies indicate significantly elevated gray matter volumes in children with NF-1 compared to children without NF-1 (Moore, Slopis, Jackson, De Winter, & Leeds, 2000), while morphologic studies demonstrate features of abnormal development of the corpus callosum (Kayl, Moore, Slopis, Jackson, & Leeds, 1999). Disorders of normal developmental apoptosis have been suggested to produce increased gray matter volumes. Disorders of normal oligodendrogliocyte myelin production have been proposed as the etiology of focal white matter anomalies (see the following discussion for details of MR hyperintensities). These developmental anomalies remain unexplained at this time, but they strongly implicate the NF-1 gene as a contributor to the production of abnormalities in gray matter and white matter volume development in the brain, which in turn are implicated in the cognitive phenotype of NF-1.

Frontal brain structural malformation (including forebrain fusion and holoprosencephaly) has been modeled in mice using multiple specific gene knock-out animals developed and studied in conjunction with an additional NF-1 knock-out. The NF-1 gene appears to have a significant influence on neuronal migration and frontal cortical formation (Zhu et al., 2001) in these models. These models predict the presence of the cortical malformations reported in NF-1 and human clinical descriptions. Gross malformations of cortex have also been reported in humans with NF-1

(Balestri et al., 2003). Brain scans defined right hemispheric cortical dysplasia with overlying pachygyria and polymicrogyria in these individuals. These major brain malformations seem a certain cause of the mental retardation and seizures in these three individuals, but they are not common features of NF-1. More significant is the fact that these malformations result from different pathological mechanisms, supporting the early role of neurofibromin in brain development (Balestri et al., 2003).

In contrast, minor malformations in cortical development may occur with greater frequency. Minor malformation of frontal cortical development has been studied in NF-1 as an associated feature with reading disability. MRI-based anatomical studies of individuals with dyslexia in the general population reveal specific patterns of cortical gyral formation in humans within the inferior frontal gyrus. MRI-based analysis of dyslexic individuals who also have NF-1 demonstrates a similar occurrence of these pathologic patterns within the inferior frontal gyrus, suggesting an approximate 40% rate of occurrence of these minor malformations (Billingsley, Schrimsher, Jackson, Slopis, & Moore, 2002).

Common clinical experience in the management of NF-1 also supports the concept that aberrant cell signaling with disordered neurotransmission occurs. Approximately 40%–60% of children with NF-1 demonstrate behavioral features of ADHD. This frequency is five- to sixfold greater than the general population. Dopamine reuptake inhibitor stimulant therapy is commonly used effectively in this population for the pharmacologic management of ADHD. Whether this high incidence of ADHD is a consequence of a neuropharmacologic disorder or frontal/callosal dysmorphism (Kayl et al., 1999), or both, remains uncertain at this time. Future studies of the impact of farnesyl transferase inhibitors and the statin drugs (agents that block hypercholesterolemia and coincidentally block cKit, an alternate signaling pathway) will provide further insight into mechanisms of signal transduction disorders in NF-1.

Neurocognitive Status of Children with NF-1

From a neuropsychological standpoint, NF-1 is an exceptionally interesting genetic disorder. Children and adolescents with NF-1 have much higher incidences of LDs, neurocognitive deficits, behavioral problems, and brain tumors in comparison with the general population. In addition, they have the neuroanatomical abnormalities discussed above, and most also have areas of high signal intensity viewed on MRI scans. Coupled with these structural abnormalities, neuropsychological studies of children and adolescents with NF-1 have revealed a wide range of cognitive sequelae associated with the disorder. Visual–spatial deficits and LDs are two of the most commonly reported problems, but difficulties with speech articulation, expressive and receptive language, and motor coordination are also typical features (Moore & Denckla, 1999; Eldridge et al., 1989; Eliason, 1986; Hofman, Harris, Bryan, &

Denckla, 1994; Moore, Ater, Needle, Slopis, & Copeland, 1994a; North et al., 1997; Brewer, Moore, & Hiscock, 1997).

Intellectual Functioning

It was once widely believed that NF-1 was associated with a high incidence of mental retardation. This idea has been widely discounted by numerous studies that have instead found a slight downward shift of the distribution of IQ and only a slightly elevated incidence of mental retardation over population estimates (Eldridge et al., 1989; Moore et al., 1994a; North et al., 1997). The NF-1 Cognitive Disorders Task Force reviewed 10 studies with a total or 416 patients with NF-1. Of the 6 studies that reported data on incidence of mental retardation ($n = 350$), the average rate (defined as IQ < 70) was 7.1% with a range from 4.8%–11.2%. This is higher than the estimated rate in the general population of 2%–3%, but not as high as once believed. The average full scale IQ was 92.9 in the 9 studies ($n = 389$) with objective standardized measures of IQ with a range from 88.6–94.8. Whereas the ranges of average IQ reported in these studies are somewhat similar, it is important to note that children with NF-1 cover the entire range of intellectual abilities that is seen in the general population (see figure 5.2).

Learning and Academic Achievement Profile

Difficulties with academic performance are often reported to be the most significant morbidity associated with childhood NF-1 (Coude, Mignot, Lyonnet, & Munnich,

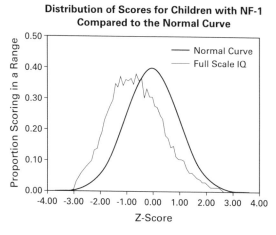

Figure 5.2
Full Scale IQ distribution in 84 children with neurofibromatosis type 1 (NF-1) compared to the normal curve.

2004). The NF Consensus Task Force reported variable rates of LDs with an average rate of 44.3% and a range from 30% to 61% in the six studies reporting this information (North et al., 1997). However, not all studies used the same criteria for defining what constituted an LD. The Diagnostic and Statistical Manual of Mental Disorders (4th ed.) does not list "learning disability" per se but describes disorders in reading, mathematics, and written expression. The criteria for a disorder in one of these areas is that academic achievement, as measured by standardized tests, must be substantially below expectations for the child's chronological age, intelligence, and age-appropriate education. This is the standard discrepancy model of LDs and, while controversial and in need of change, is what most school districts currently use. However, in most studies of NF-1, formal criteria for LDs have not been applied when arriving at incidence levels. Many children are in special classes or have repeated a grade and are thus thought to have LDs even when they may not meet strict diagnostic criteria.

Because visual–spatial deficits are reported to be a common characteristic of children with NF-1 (Moore, Slopis, Jackson, De Winter, & Leeds, 2000; Mazzocco et al., 1995; Varnhagen et al., 1988; Eldridge et al., 1989; Eliason, 1986), some have speculated that children with NF-1 suffer from nonverbal LDs (Varnhagen, 1988). Some studies reported a discrepancy between verbal and performance intellectual abilities favoring Verbal abilities (Eliason, 1986; Eliason, 1988; Wadsby, Lindehammar, & Eeg-Olofsson, 1989). This added to the belief that the LDs in NF-1 are similar to the reported classic nonverbal LD syndrome (Rourke, 1989). In their review of eight studies for which both Verbal and Performance IQ data were reported, the NF-1 Cognitive Disorders Task Force found no significant trend for verbal or performance intellectual advantage or disadvantage (North et al., 1997). Learning disabilities in this population, however, are not exclusively nonverbal in nature, as more recent studies have shown that verbal deficits are also common. Mazzocco and colleagues (Mazzocco et al., 1995) found a higher incidence of reading disability in children with NF-1 (53%) compared to their nonaffected siblings (26%). Children with NF-1, in comparison to their siblings without NF-1, have weaknesses in vocabulary and phonetic abilities, reading, and mathematics, in addition to their visual–spatial deficits (Mazzocco et al., 1995). Cutting (Cutting, Koth, & Denckla, 2000) compared the cognitive profiles of children with NF-1 to those of an LDs clinic population and found that while both groups performed more poorly than participants with noknown disability on sight reading and reading comprehension measures, the children with NF-1 had more global language impairments compared to the LD clinic group. Cutting also found that children with NF-1 scored significantly lower than the LD group on visual–spatial measures, indicating that children with NF-1 also have visual–spatial deficits that are not representative of the broader reading disabled population (Cutting et al., 2000).

When taken together, reports of cognitive deficits in children and adolescents with NF-1 show that this disorder is characterized by a complex range of both verbal and visual–spatial deficits and does not lead to the notion of a strictly nonverbal LDs syndrome, insofar as this syndrome has been described in other populations (Rourke, 1989).

Others have also suggested that the academic profile does not seem to fit the typical types of LDs. For example, Descheemaeker reported that half of a relatively small sample ($n = 17$) of children with NF-1 had learning disabilities, a figure in keeping with other reports. Of those with documented LDs ($n = 8$), half had spelling deficits but only one had a pure arithmetic deficit (Descheemaeker, Ghesquiere, Symons, Fryns, & Legius, 2005).

Brewer and colleagues used cluster analysis to document the neurocognitive profile in a large cohort ($N = 105$) of children with NF-1 (Brewer et al., 1997). Out of this group of 105, 72 children were found to have academic difficulties. Of these 72, three groups emerged; one group had a typical neurocognitive profile (39%), one had general academic deficits (47%), and the third had primarily visual spatial/motor deficits (14%). The low incidence of visual-spatial deficits was surprising given the often reported high incidence of deficits in this area. However, this study did not include the Judgment of Line Orientation task (Lindgren & Benton, 1980), which is often reported as the test leading to the most impaired performance of visual perceptual skills in this population (Schrimsher, Billingsley, Slopis, & Moore, 2003b).

Visual–Spatial and Neurocognitive Profile

Visual–Spatial Processing   In the general population, readers with dyslexia have deficits in the rapid processing of visual stimuli (Temple et al., 2000; Eden Van-Meter, Rumsey, et al., 1996; Eden, VanMeter, Rumsey, & Zeffiro, 1996c). Deficiencies in the rapid identification of letters may also contribute to reading problems in children and adolescents with NF-1. Visual–spatial processing problems, including the rapid identification of objects (Cutting et al., 2000) and the accurate identification of similar lines and angles (Eldridge et al., 1989; Moore, Slopis, Schomer, Jackson, & Levy, 1996), have been identified children and adolescents with NF-1, as well as in poor readers without NF-1 (Eden, Stein, Wood, & Wood, 1996).

Although performance by children on the Judgment of Line Orientation task (Lindgren et al., 1980), which is a purely visual-spatial task, is impaired in most children with NF-1, not *all* areas of visual perceptual processing are affected in children with NF-1. For example, the ability to discriminate among two-dimensional drawings of similar geometric figures is not impaired (figure 5.3) relative to ability in children without NF-1.

Children with NF-1 have visual–spatial deficits that are not representative of the broader LDs population (Cutting et al., 2000) but may be related to deficits in

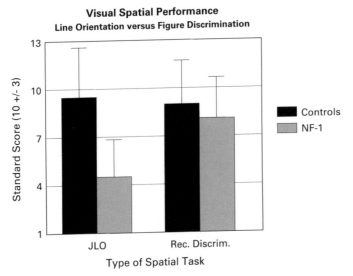

Figure 5.3
Visual–spatial performance on the Judgment of Line Orientation (JLO) versus the Recognition Discrimination tasks.

reading. However, the role of visual–spatial deficits in the learning deficits of children with NF-1 is far from clear (Brewer et al., 1997). We have found that the deficit
in visual–spatial abilities is somewhat specific rather than general. For example, the
Judgment of Line Orientation test is almost impaired in approximately 70% of children with NF-1. And, it bears a strong relation with academic performance in general (figure 5.4).

Schrimsher and colleagues (Schrimsher, Billingsley, Slopis, & Moore, 2003a)
reported that the multivariate combination of four visual–spatial/motor tasks (Judgment of Line Orientation, Block Design, Recognition Discrimination Test, Beery
Visual–Motor Integration Test) was highly discriminate of the NF-1 diagnosis in
that it correctly identified 90% of individuals with clinically diagnosed NF-1
($p = .0000004$). Two of these tests are purely visual–spatial, and two are visual–
perceptual/motor. The Judgement of Line Orientation test (Lindgren & Benton,
1980; a purely visual–spatial task) by itself, but not the other tests, was still highly
predictive of NF-1 diagnostic status.

Brain Structure/Function Correlates

As discussed in a previous section, NF-1 presents with a unique combination of brain
features, including white matter abnormalities, MR hyperintensities, low-grade or
sometimes malignant brain tumors, and abnormalities in gross and fine brain mor-

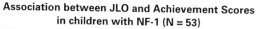

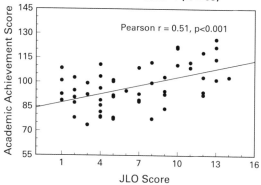

Figure 5.4

Correlation between standard score on the Judgment of Line Orientation (JLO) test and general academic achievement in children with NF-1. Individuals scoring zero on the JLO are excluded.

phology. These morphological differences can be seen in both gross and regional brain development and have been widely investigated for their role in the neuropsychological and learning deficits seen in NF-1. The relation between brain MR hyperintensities, brain tumors, and macrocephaly with neuropsychological functioning in NF-1 is an area of intense interest.

Brain Tumors In addition to MR hyperintensities, 15% of children and adolescents with NF-1 will be diagnosed with a brain tumor, usually an optic glioma (Listernick, Charrow, Greenwald, & Easterly, 1989). Of these, only about 20% are symptomatic. Although optic gliomas in NF-1 are usually benign and are often left untreated, one might surmise that an optic glioma is still a pathological condition of the central nervous system and, therefore, a potential marker of abnormality that might help explain the common learning and cognitive difficulties. We found, however, that the severity of cognitive and learning deficits in children with NF-1 was not exacerbated by the presence of a brain tumor unless cranial radiation therapy is given (De Winter, Moore, Slopis, Ater, & Copeland, 1999; Moore, Ater, Needle, Slopis, & Copeland, 1994b).

MR Hyperintensities Areas of hyperintense signal on T2-weighted and, more conspicuously, on fluid attenuation inversion recovery MRI sequences are observed in the brain of most children and adolescents with NF-1. These "MR hyperintensities," as we refer to them, are benign, do not appear to occupy space, and may occur in multiple regions in the same individual. Their most common locations are the basal ganglia, cerebellum, brainstem, and diencephalon. Uncertainty continues with regard to the makeup and clinical significance of MR hyperintensities in children with NF-1. One report of three children with NF-1 seen at autopsy documented that MR hyperintensities consisted of spongiotic tissue with fluid-filled vacuoles, which accounts for their appearance on MRI (DiPaolo et al., 1995). Because of their uncertain nature, these areas of MR hyperintensity have been informally referred to as "unidentified bright objects." However, because they are bright only on MRI, and because they are not space-occupying objects, we refer to them as MR hyperintensities. It has been estimated that between 50% and 70% of children and adolescents with NF-1 have MR hyperintensities, leading some to predict that they are markers for more extensive, albeit unobservable, white matter abnormalities (North et al., 1994; Moore et al., 1996). Several studies have reported that MR hyperintensities disappear or diminish in size with advancing age (Sevick et al., 1992; Aoki et al., 1989; Itoh et al., 1994), strengthening the case that they are an anomaly of the normal developmental process of myelination.

Neuropsychological studies of MR hyperintensities have generally been disappointing, however, because few consistent relations with cognitive functioning have been observed. Early studies failed to find a significant association between learning disabilities and MR hyperintensities in the brain (Dunn & Roos, 1989; Duffner, Cohen, Seidel, & Shucard, 1989; Ferner, Chaudhuri, Bingham, Cos, & Hughes, 1993). More recent studies have reported significant associations between the presence (North et al., 1994), number (Hofman et al., 1994; Denckla et al., 1996), and location (Moore et al., 1996) of MR hyperintensities and neurocognitive functioning. These conflicting results suggest that MR hyperintensities *are not consistent predictors* of cognitive deficits or learning disabilities across samples of the NF-1 population but may represent a neurocognitive burden if found in sufficient numbers and in certain locations. MR hyperintensities in the thalamus have been reported in one study to be associated with lower scores on tests of visual–spatial and memory ability (Moore et al., 1996). Goh (Goh, Khong, Leung, & Wong, 2004) also found an association between neurocognitive functioning and MR hyperintensity location. When located in the thalamus, MR hyperintensities were associated with lower IQ, and when in the globus palladus, lower attention scores were obtained.

Macrocephaly Macrocephaly occurs in 30%–50% of individuals with NF-1 (Bale, Amos, Parry, & Bale, 1991) and is associated with greater clinical and physical severity (Zvulunov, Weitz, & Metzker, 1998) but not greater neuropsychological impairment (Ferner, Hughes, & Weinman, 1996). The relationship between macrocephaly and learning disabilities in NF-1 has been a focus of several recent studies using quantitative volumetric imaging techniques. Said and colleagues reported greater overall brain volume, specifically white matter volume, using quantitative imaging techniques (Said et al., 1996). Our group, however, found significantly larger overall brain volumes, due to gray but not white matter differences (Moore et al., 2000).

Greenwood studied regional morphology of the brain in 39 children with NF-1 and reports larger volumes of both gray and white matter with greater increases in white matter relative to children without NF-1 (Greenwood et al., 2005). In another study, a higher gray-to-white-matter ratio and significantly larger corpus callosa was found (Kayl, Moore, Slopis, Jackson, & Leeds, 2000; Moore et al., 2000). Greater volume of gray matter and size of the corpus callosum was positively correlated with the degree of IQ–academic achievement discrepancy in children with NF-1 but not in children without NF-1. The differences between the findings in these studies may be related to the selection of brain structures included in the volumetric calculations (Moore et al., 2000).

Congenital Malformation   Studies of brain morphology have provided insight in understanding the differences in brain development associated with cognitive and learning disorders in general (Lyon & Rumsey, 1996). The planum temporale is an area of the brain in the superior temporal lobe that is associated with reading. In healthy children with normal reading ability, there is usually a left-greater-than-right hemispheric asymmetry in the planum temporale, but in children with dyslexia (without NF-1), this asymmetry is absent (Habib, 2000). In a study of 24 children and adolescents with NF-1, Billingsley reported that boys but not girls with NF-1 showed the lack of asymmetry commonly seen in children with dyslexia (Billingsley et al., 2002). Intelligence-based discrepancy scores of reading and math achievement, commonly used to define LDs, were significantly related to planum temporale asymmetry in the NF-1 group.

Functional Imaging Studies

Structural neuroanatomy is an important approach to studying neurocognitive impairment in disorders such as NF-1 because of the high incidence of abnormalities in brain morphology in children with this disorder (discussed above). However, this approach has limitations because there is not always a strict correlation between structure and function. In other words, just because an organ appears abnormal does not mean that it functions abnormally. Structural abnormalities may only be an indirect indication of function.

A more complete understanding of LDs in NF-1 requires methods that can associate underlying neuronal activity with cognitive operations in a time-linked fashion. Hemodynamic imaging methods, such as functional MRI (fMRI), provide a way to analyze regional brain function that is temporally linked to cognitive processing. Functional MRI detects blood-oxygen-level-dependent (BOLD) responses in the brain during cognitive activity. BOLD responses are temporally linked to changes in underlying neuronal activity resulting from cognitive activity.

Neuroimaging studies of visual–spatial processing of letters and other stimuli in healthy individuals have shown significant activity in bilateral inferior parietal and posterior–superior parietal cortex, as well as in lateral frontal and extrastriate cortex (Alivisatos & Petrides, 1997; Greenlee, Magnussen, & Reinvang, 2000; Booth et al., 2000). Functional MRI has also been used to study reading and visual–spatial processing associated with LDs, including dyslexia, in healthy individuals as well as a variety of populations with known neurological disorders (Shaywitz et al., 1998; Temple et al., 2001; Billingsley, McAndrews, Crawley, & Mikulis, 2001; Eden, Van-Meter, Rumsey, et al., 1996; Paulesu et al., 1996).

Developmental reading impairments involve difficulty in learning to relate visual input to phonological representations. Phonological discrimination, which requires an individual to identify distinct sounds that make up words and letters, has been shown to be a core component of learning to read (Fletcher et al., 1994; Stanovich, 1988). fMRI studies in other populations have implicated inferior frontal, dorsolateral prefrontal, and temporal cortices in phonological processing skills (Pugh et al., 1996; Temple et al., 2001; Shaywitz et al., 1998). Previous fMRI investigations of phonological processing in poor readers who do not have NF-1 have shown differential neural responses to phonological stimuli (Temple et al., 2001; Temple et al., 2000). Children with dyslexia were found to have reduced neural activity in left temporal–parietal cortex during a phonological decision task that required them to determine whether two letters rhymed. Activity in left inferior frontal cortex, a region that has been identified as critical to phonological processing in neurologically normal individuals (Pugh et al., 1996) was similar in dyslexic children compared to children without dyslexia (Temple et al., 2001).

Phonological processing in children with NF-1 follows a similar pattern of activation as described above for children with dyslexia but without NF-1 except that it was dependent on task modality. In comparing 15 children with NF-1 to 15 healthy children without NF-1, Billingsley (Billingsley et al., 2003) reported greater activation of inferior frontal cortex during an auditory phonetic processing task in participants with NF-1 than in those without NF-1. There was greater activation of the inferior frontal region compared to middle temporal cortex, especially in the right hemisphere during the auditory task. However, during a rhyming task presented orthographically on a monitor screen, children with NF-1 showed relatively less inferior frontal activation compared to middle temporal activation.

Billingsley also studied visual–spatial processing in children with NF-1 using fMRI (Billingsley et al., 2004). In healthy individuals, visual–spatial processing in a mental rotation task activates bilateral parietal and frontal cortex. Comparison participants in this study showed higher or equal activation of frontal areas in comparison to the parietal and occipital areas. Children with NF-1, however, showed the opposite pattern with greater activation of middle temporal, parietal, and occipital areas relative to frontal cortex.

The results of these two studies of brain function suggest that children with NF-1 do not utilize the same patterns of activation of cortical areas as comparison partic-

Table 5.3
Case vignettes

Neurocognitive/Behavioral Morbidity	Clinical Manifestations	
	Severe	Minimal
Normal	Case 5.1: Paige	Case 5.4: Trevor
Learning disorder	Case 5.2: Russell	Case 5.5: Ursula
Psychiatric/emotional	Case 5.3: Sara	Case 5.6: Xavier

ipants. These differences in activation, with the morphological differences in areas critical for reading, suggest that differences in brain development result in abnormal patterns of cortical processing and activation in activities related to learning to read in children with NF-1.

Clinical Case Studies

The following case studies (see also table 5.3) are presented to illustrate mechanisms by which NF-1 was first identified and to illustrate the extreme variability in the types and severity of clinical and behavioral manifestations found in children with NF-1. They also demonstrate the lack of concordance between the severity of the disorder and the presence and types of neurocognitive and behavioral morbidity exhibited. (Note that the fictitious names have been assigned by the volume editors.)

Case 5.1: Paige   Paige is a 10-year-old White female with NF-1 diagnosed at age 4 years following an unusual low-impact fracture of her left tibia. Pediatric orthopedic surgeons who recognized abnormal bone growth evaluated her noted bowing and pathologic thickening of the tibial bone cortex (figure 5.5). These features raised suspicion of NF-1 after the tibia failed to heal with casting. Multiple attempts to treat the fracture failed, including placement of internal rods within the bone. An Ilizarov internal fixation device was placed to stimulate growth of the tibia, and a bone strut graft was transplanted from the fibula (figure 5.5). Bone morphogenic protein was employed to stimulate and strengthen the graft. She is now walking with a simple external brace after multiple surgical procedures over 5 years.

Paige's additional physical findings include nine faint café au lait spots on the trunk and extremities, bilateral axillary freckles, and short stature. Her ocular examination revealed Lisch nodules by age 10 years, although none were noted at presentation at age 5 years. She has mild idiopathic hypertension, and, of interest, her "un-affected" sibling is also hypertensive with bilateral duplicated renal pelvises. Her family history is otherwise negative for features of NF-1.

Paige is in the fourth grade, where she is performing at average levels. Intellectually, she is in the average range with significantly higher verbal abilities (high average) compared to performance abilities (low average). She is above average on all tests of academic achievement, especially written math calculations, which are in the superior range. Reading and spelling are above average. Paige was diagnosed with mild attention and concentration problems in the past and now takes Strattera. On tests of attention, she now is in the average range. Visual spatial abilities are low average.

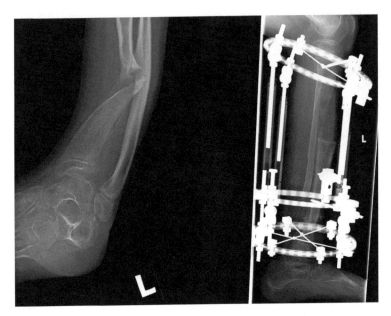

Figure 5.5
Low-impact fracture of left tibia with bowing and pathologic thickening of the tibial bone cortex (left).
Ilizarov external fixation device was placed to stimulate growth of the tibia (right).

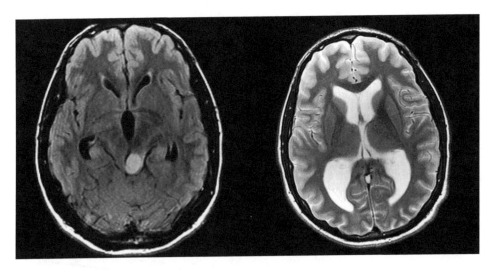

Figure 5.6
Aqueductal stenosis and enlargement of a previously noted signal abnormality within the brainstem (left)
resulting in progressive ventriculomegaly (right).

Case 5.2: Russell Russell is a 17-year-old White male who was diagnosed with NF-1 at age 4 months due to presence of multiple café au lait spots noted by his pediatrician.

The spots were very faint initially but slowly became more pronounced over the next year. A geneticist confirmed the clinical diagnosis. The initial MRI scan revealed multiple T2 signal hyperintensities in the cerebellum and basal ganglia as well as a pachygyral malformation in the left frontal cortex. A follow-up MRI scan at age 5 years revealed thickening of the right optic nerve extending into the optic chiasm consistent with optic nerve glioma. Repeat MRI scans revealed no progression of the optic nerve thickening and Russell did not develop visual deficits, so no intervention was needed. Russell's parents and teachers reported "daydreaming," staring spells, eye flutter, and distractiblilty. Electroencephalogram revealed spike and slow wave abnormalities from the left frontal lobe leading to the diagnosis of complex partial seizure. Russell's staring spells responded to treatment with Valproic acid although multiple motor tics were noted. Anticonvulsant treatment was discontinued after two years and followup electroencephalogram normalized. Motor tics persisted and vocal tics developed leading to the diagnosis of Tourette syndrome.

By age 14 years, follow-up MRI revealed progressive ventriculomegaly due to aqueductal stenosis and enlargement of a previously noted signal abnormality within the brain stem (figure 5.6). Russell underwent endoscopic third ventriculostomy to treat hydrocephalus without shunt placement. By age 15 years, Russell developed idiopathic gynecomastia with normal hormone levels for a pubertal male. In the same year, he developed left knee pain due to growth of a plexiform neurofibroma of the peroneal nerve. The nerve sheath tumor was resected without complication, and pathology revealed only benign tissue.

Russell is in the eleventh grade; he has consistently had difficulties with school performance and keeping up with his peers. Intellectually, he is in the high-average to superior range with slightly higher verbal than performance abilities. On tests of academic achievement Russell scores in the average range, but because of the discrepancy with IQ and in light of his academic underachievement, this meets diagnostic criteria for an LD. Russell also meets criteria for ADHD and takes Strattera as well as medications for mood control and for Tourette's syndrome. His visual–spatial ability is average.

Case 5.3: Sara Sara is a 23-year-old White female who was originally diagnosed with NF-1 at age 11 years after evaluation for progressive scoliosis. Her initial diagnosis was not established until she underwent surgical resection of a cervical dumbbell tumor. Pathology revealed benign neurofibroma. MRI of the cervical spine revealed the mass as well as congenital anomalies of the cervical vertebral bodies. Surgical treatment included placement of bone graft to stabilize the cervical spine (figure 5.7). MRI of the brain revealed multiple T2 signal hyperintensities in the basal ganglia as well as minor malformations of frontal cortical folding.

Sara's physical findings include multiple café au lait spots, axillary and groin freckling, multiple small cutaneous neurofibromata, Lisch nodules, and mild scoliosis. Sara recovered well from her spinal surgery but later developed multiple behavioral and psychiatric symptoms, leading to hospitalization in a psychiatric facility. Features of bipolar disorder, psychosis, and substance abuse complicated Sara's clinical course. Ultimately, she was married and has given birth to two children, both of whom have features of ADHD and NF-1. She experienced significant growth of her cutaneous fibromata during both pregnancies.

Sara's intellectual status has been assessed four times, between the ages of 11 and 16, and has remained in the average to low-average range. Academic skills have been commensurate with intellectual abilities, and math has been her weakest subject. Both motor coordination and visual–spatial abilities were severely compromised.

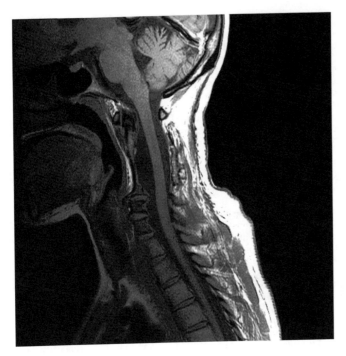

Figure 5.7
After surgical treatment and placement of bone graft for cervical spinal neurofibroma.

Case 5.4: Trevor Trevor is a 22-year-old White male who was noted to have five faint café au lait spots at age 5 years. Based on these findings, his pediatrician suspected NF-1 and referred him to genetics for evaluation. The diagnosis was not confirmed due to absence of other features of NF-1. Trevor was noted to have some minor discipline problems during school, and his pediatrician considered the diagnosis of attention deficit disorder (ADD). Treatment trials with stimulant agents did not improve his school performance significantly. Trevor developed bilateral leg pain during football practice, and x-ray studies revealed benign nonossifying fibromata in both tibias. Pain resolved without intervention. Trevor developed two small cutaneous neurofibromata on his trunk and left arm by age 17 years, and ocular examination revealed Lisch nodules that were not previously noted.

Trevor has had eight neuropsychological evaluations between the age of 8 and 15 years. Intellectually, Trevor has consistently demonstrated high-average skills in both verbal and nonverbal areas. His academic skills have remained in the average range, and at his last follow-up he planned to enter college the next year. Motor coordination was above average, but visual–spatial abilities were severely impaired.

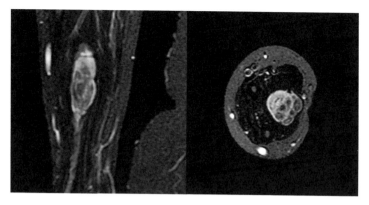

Figure 5.8
Coronal (left) and axial (right) magnetic resonance imaging of forearm showing a large, deep neuro-fibroma of ulnar nerve origin.

Case 5.5: Ursula Ursula is a 17-year-old Hispanic girl who was adopted shortly after birth. She was evaluated for short stature at age 5 years with all endocrine studies normal with the exception of stimulated release of growth hormone. The pediatric endocrinologist was concerned that growth hormone levels were not sufficiently low to account for Ursula's degree of short stature, and she suspected the diagnosis of NF-1 after noting axillary freckling. Ursula was treated with growth hormone but attained only minimal additional growth. Her current height remains at less than the 10th percentile for age. Ursula's additional physical findings are minimal, including absence of Lisch nodules and café au lait spots. Ursula developed numbness and tingling in her right fourth and fifth fingers in association with a painful small subcutaneous nodule proximal to the right wrist. Evaluation by electromyography was unremarkable, but MRI of the wrist revealed multiple nodular fibromata along the ulnar nerve extending below the carpal tunnel (figure 5.8). These fibromata were resected without complication, and pathology was benign neurofibroma, confirming the diagnosis of NF-1.

Ursula has been evaluated a total of 12 times between the ages of 5 and 17 years. As a young child, she demonstrated intellectual abilities in the average range with significantly stronger verbal than quantitative abilities. Her academic achievement scores were approximately 2 SDs below her intellectual level. Ursula's fine motor coordination was age appropriate, but her visual–spatial abilities were severely compromised. These performance patterns have remained stable across time. Ursula was diagnosed with ADD and has received special education throughout her school years.

Case 5.6: Xavier Xavier is a 19-year-old White male with NF-1. He was noted to have extreme hypertension in the 4th year of life, and evaluation by pediatric nephrologists revealed no obvious etiology beyond elevations in plasma rennin levels. Investigation for pheochromocytoma was negative. Renal angiogram was normal initially, but repeat studies revealed anomalous small renal arterial branching vessels. Xavier developed several small café au lait spots and small cutaneous neurofibromata on the trunk and extremities between the ages of 4 and 10 years, confirming the diagnosis of NF-1. Xavier's clinical course was complicated by significant developmental delay with features of pervasive developmental delay, oppositional behavior, hyperactivity, and insomnia. Xavier's hypertension resolved spontaneously by mid-adolescence without intervention. Several members of his own family considered Xavier autistic, but he followed an uncharacteristic pattern of developmental progression through school age. MRI of the brain was normal with no T2 signal abnormalities or obvious cortical malformation. Xavier's ocular examination revealed no Lisch nodules during childhood, but Lisch nodules were noted by age 19 years.

When first assessed at age 5 years, Xavier had a mental age of 3 years, 10 months, verbal abilities were in the low-average range, and letter–word knowledge was in the average range, but number knowledge and motor abilities were deficient. He has had a total of 10 annual neuropsychological evaluations, and his intellectual status has remained fairly stable with verbal abilities (generally average to low average) always significantly stronger than nonverbal abilities (generally borderline to deficient). His academic skills have remained stable as well, with spelling and reading in the low-average range and math in the severely deficient range. While in the 12th grade, Xavier's reading is at the 9th-grade level, but his math is between the 1st- and 3rd-grade levels. Fine motor coordination and visual–spatial abilities remain severely impaired. Behaviorally, Xavier does not give the impression of borderline mental deficiency, as he is quite conversational with age-appropriate vocabulary. Nevertheless, he continues to show signs of pervasive developmental disorder (PDD) and is quite impulsive and prone to fits of rage and self-injurious behavior.

Summary

NF-1 is far more common than many high-profile disorders such as muscular dystrophy and Huntington's disease and yet remains virtually unknown to the public, despite the fact that it was first described more than a century ago. Advances in understanding of the NF-1 gene mutation have led to insights into specific tumor suppressor gene function as well as insights into general impact of growth dysregulation upon embryonic development, including brain structural and functional development.

The vast size and complexity of the NF-1 gene results in a broad spectrum of distinct human NF-1 mutations, and so the disorder is expressed with variable manifestations of physical and behavioral phenotypes. Individuals with mild symptoms are often unaware that they carry the disordered gene, delaying diagnosis and possible interventions or surveillance that could reduce future morbidity. This is a particular problem in childhood, as the morbidity of NF-1 increases with age. The variability in the clinical phenotype is matched by variability in the behavioral phenotype, and the two are not highly correlated; severity in clinical manifestations does not mean there will be severity in behavioral manifestations, and vice versa. We have selected six cases of children with NF-1 to illustrate this broad range of clinical and behavioral expression. Our case studies illustrate that children with severe disease can nevertheless excel in school and be without behavior or emotional difficulties. On the other hand, a child with mild clinical manifestations can have severe, debilitating learning, behavioral, and emotional morbidity.

The neurocognitive phenotype of NF-1 consists of average or slightly below average intellectual abilities, difficulties in school performance, visual–spatial processing deficits, ADHD, and frequent low self-esteem. Some children with NF-1 have none of these neurocognitive features, a fact that demonstrates the variability of the phenotype. The neurocognitive phenotype ranges from severe mental deficiency to superior intellect, and yet any individual with NF-1 may suffer LD and academic underachievement. The NF-1 population includes children who struggle in special education hoping to graduate from high school and children who graduate at the top of their class and go on to success in college and career despite competition from their non-NF-1 peers. Whether LD is a cause of social dysfunction and failure in personal achievement remains to be studied, but one could argue that LD is the greatest morbidity of school-age children with NF-1.

The reasons for the high incidence of LD in the NF-1 population remain largely unknown. MRI-based morphologic studies of the brain of children with NF-1 have revealed both gross and fine structural abnormalities of brain development similar to abnormalities seen in idiopathic dyslexia and ADHD. Undoubtedly, mutation of the NF-1 gene plays a role in these specific disorders of neural development in children with NF-1 and thereby indirectly influences their learning and neurocognitive profile. Genetically engineered mouse and insect models bearing NF-1 mutations provide surrogates that mimic the human conditions of learning deficits. NF-1 haplosufficient mice model deficits in spatial learning (Costa et al., 2002; Silva et al., 1997), while NF-1 haplosufficient Drosophila models deficits in olfactory learning and independent mechanisms of memory. These models provide behavioral platforms for pharmacologic trials with a direct molecular genetic window into correlative studies of signal transduction in the brain. In this way, the ubiquitous nature of the NF-1 gene provides a rare opportunity to study neural signal transduction in models that correlate a specific genotype with stereotyped behavioral and developmental patterns.

References

Abdel-Wanis, M. E., & Kawahara, N. (2001). Aetiology of spinal deformities in neurofibromatosis: I. New hypotheses. *Medical Hypotheses, 56,* 400–404.

Ablon, J. (1995). "The Elephant Man" as "self" and "other": The psycho-social costs of a misdiagnosis. *Social Science & Medicine, 40,* 1481–1489.

Alivisatos, B., & Petrides, M. (1997). Functional activation of the human brain during mental rotation. *Neuropsychologia, 35,* 111–118.

Antinheimo, J., Sankila, R., Carpen, O., Pukkala, E., Sainio, M., & Jaaskelainen, J. (2000). Population-based analysis of sporadic and type 2 neurofibromatosis-associated meningiomas and schwannomas. *Neurology, 54,* 71–76.

Aoki, S., Barkovich, A. J., Nishimura, K., Kjos, B. O., Machida, T., Cogen, P., et al. (1989). Neurofibromatosis types 1 and 2: Cranial MR findings. *Radiology, 172,* 527–534.

Bale, S. J., Amos, C. I., Parry, D. M., & Bale, A. E. (1991). Relationship between head circumference and height in normal adults and in the nevoid basal cell carcinoma syndrome and neurofibromatosis type I. *American Journal of Medical Genetics, 40,* 206–210.

Balestri, P., Vivarelli, R., Grosso, S., Santori, L., Farnetani, M. A., Galluzzi, P., et al. (2003). Malformations of cortical development in neurofibromatosis type 1. *Neurology, 61,* 1799–1801.

Billingsley, R. L., Jackson, E. F., Slopis, J. M., Swank, P. R., Mahankali, S., & Moore, B. D. (2003). Functional magnetic resonance imaging of phonologic processing in neurofibromatosis 1. *Journal of Child Neurology, 18,* 731–740.

Billingsley, R. L., Jackson, E. F., Slopis, J. M., Swank, P. R., Mahankali, S., & Moore, B. D. (2004). Functional MRI of visual–spatial processing in neurofibromatosis, type I. *Neuropsychologia, 42,* 395–404.

Billingsley, R. L., McAndrews, M. P., Crawley, A. P., & Mikulis, D. J. (2001). Functional MRI of phonological and semantic processing in temporal lobe epilepsy. *Brain, 124,* 1218–1227.

Billingsley, R. L., Schrimsher, G. W., Jackson, E. F., Slopis, J. M., & Moore, B. D. (2002). Significance of planum temporale and planum parietale morphologic features in neurofibromatosis, type I. *Archives of Neurology, 59,* 616–622.

Booth, J. R., MacWhinney, B., Thulborn, K. R., Sacco, K., Voyvodic, J. T., & Feldman, H. M. (2000). Developmental and lesion effects in brain activation during sentence comprehension and mental rotation. *Developmental Neuropsychology, 18,* 139–169.

Brewer, V. R., Moore, B. D., & Hiscock, M. (1997). Learning disability subtypes in children with neurofibromatosis. *Journal of Learning Disabilities, 30,* 521–533.

Cawthon, R. M., Weiss, R., Xu, G. F., Viskochil, D., Culver, M., Stevens, J., et al. (1990). A major segment of the neurofibromatosis type 1 gene: cDNA sequence, genomic structure, and point mutations [published erratum appears in *Cell, 62,* following 608]. *Cell, 62,* 193–201.

Cnossen, M. H., Moons, K. G., Garssen, M. P., Pasmans, N. M., de Goede-Bolder, A., Niermeijer, M. F., et al. (1998). Minor disease features in neurofibromatosis type 1 (NF1) and their possible value in diagnosis of NF1 in children ≤ 6 years and clinically suspected of having NF1. Neurofibromatosis team of Sophia Children's Hospital. *Journal of Medical Genetics, 35,* 624–627.

Costa, R. M., Federov, N. B., Kogan, J. H., Murphy, G. G., Stern, J., Ohno, M., et al. (2002). Mechanism for the learning deficits in a mouse model of neurofibromatosis type 1. *Nature, 415,* 526–530.

Coude, F. X., Mignot, C., Lyonnet, S., & Munnich, A. (2004). Academic impairment is the most frequent complication of neurofibromatose type-1 (NF1) in children. *Behavior Genetics, 34,* 635.

Crump, T. (1981). Translation of case reports in *Ueber die miltiplen Fibrome der Haut und ihre Beziehung zu den multiplen Neuromen* [On multiple fibromas of the skin and their relationship to multiple neuromas] by F. v. Recklinghausen. In V. M. Riccardi & J. Mulvihill (Eds.), *Neurofibromatosis (von Recklinghausen disease): Genetics, cell biology, and biochemistry* (Vol. 23, pp. 259–275). New York: Raven Press.

Cutting, L. E., Koth, C. W., & Denckla, M. B. (2000). How children with neurofibromatosis type 1 differ from "typical" learning disabled clinic attenders: Nonverbal learning disabilities revisited. *Developmental Neuropsychology, 17,* 29–47.

De Winter, A. E., Moore, B. D., Slopis, J. M., Ater, J., & Copeland, D. R. (1999). Brain tumors in children with neurofibromatosis: Additional neuropsychological morbidity? *Neuro Oncology, 1,* 275–281.

Denckla, M. B., Hofman, K., Mazzocco, M. M., Melhem, E., Reiss, A. L., Bryan, R. N., et al. (1996). Relationship between T2-weighted hyperintensities (unidentified bright objects) and lower IQs in children with neurofibromatosis-1. *American Journal of Medical Genetics, 67,* 98–102.

Descheemaeker, M. J., Ghesquiere, P., Symons, H., Fryns, J. P., & Legius, E. (2005). Behavioural, academic and neuropsychological profile of normally gifted neurofibromatosis type 1 children. *Journal of Intellectual Disability Research, 49,* 33–46.

DiPaolo, D. P., Zimmerman, R. A., Rorke, L. B., Zackai, E. H., Bilaniuk, L. T., & Yachnis, A. T. (1995). Neurofibromatosis type 1: Pathologic substrate of high-signal-intensity foci in the brain. *Radiology, 195,* 721–724.

Duffner, P., Cohen, M., Seidel, F., & Shucard, D. (1989). The significance of MRI abnormalities in children with neurofibromatosis. *Neurology, 39,* 373–378.

Dunn, D. W., & Roos, K. L. (1989). Magnetic resonance imaging evaluation of learning difficulties and incoordination in neurofibromatosis. *Neurofibromatosis, 2*, 1–5.

Eden, G. F., Stein, J. F., Wood, H. M., & Wood, F. B. (1996). Differences in visuospatial judgement in reading-disabled and normal children. *Perceptual and Motor Skills, 82*, 155–177.

Eden, G. F., VanMeter, J. W., Rumsey, J. M., Maisog, J. M., Woods, R. P., & Zeffiro, T. A. (1996). Abnormal processing of visual motion in dyslexia revealed by functional brain imaging [see comments]. *Nature, 382*, 66–69.

Eden, G. F., VanMeter, J. W., Rumsey, J. M., & Zeffiro, T. A. (1996). The visual deficit theory of developmental dyslexia. *Neuroimage, 4*, S108–S117.

Eldridge, R., Denckla, M. B., Bien, E., Myers, S., Kaiser-Kupfer, M. I., Pikus, A., et al. (1989). Neurofibromatosis type 1 (Recklinghausen's disease): Neurologic and cognitive assessment with sibling controls. *American Journal of Diseases of Children, 143*, 833–837.

Eliason, M. J. (1986). Neurofibromatosis: Implications for behavior and learning. *Neurofibromatosis, 7*, 175–179.

Eliason, M. J. (1988). Neuropsychological patterns: Neurofibromatosis compared to developmental learning disorders. *Neurofibromatosis, 1*, 17–25.

Evans, D. G. R. (2003). Malignant peripheral nerve sheath tumours in neurofibromatosis 1. *Journal of Medical Genetics, 40*, 304.

Ferner, R. E., Chaudhuri, R., Bingham, J., Cos, T., & Hughes, R. A. C. (1993). MRI in neurofibromatosis 1: The nature and evolution of increased intensity T2 weighted lesions and their relationship to intellectual impairment. *Journal of Neurology, Neurosurgery, and Psychiatry, 56*, 492–495.

Ferner, R. E., Hughes, R. A., & Weinman, J. (1996). Intellectual impairment in neurofibromatosis 1. *Journal of the Neurological Sciences, 138*, 125–133.

Fletcher J. M., Shaywitz, S. E., Shankweiler, D. P., Katz, L., Liberman, I. Y., Stuebing, K. K., et al. (1994). Cognitive profiles of reading disability: Comparisons of discrepancy and low achievement definitions. *Journal of Educational Psychology, 85*, 1–18.

Goh, W. H. S., Khong, P. L., Leung, C. S. Y., & Wong, V. C. N. (2004). T-2-weighted hyperintensities (unidentified bright objects) in children with neurofibromatosis 1: Their impact on cognitive function. *Journal of Child Neurology, 19*, 853–858.

Greenlee, M. W., Magnussen, S., & Reinvang, I. (2000). Brain regions involved in spatial frequency discrimination: Evidence from fMRI. *Experimental Brain Research, 132*, 399–403.

Greenwood, R. S., Tupler, L. A., Whitt, J. K., Butt, A., Dombeck, C. B., Harp, A. G., et al. (2005). Brain morphometry, T2-weighted hyperintensities, and IQ in children with neurofibromatosis type 1. *Archives of Neurology, 62*, 1904–1908.

Guo, H. F., Tong, J. Y., Hannan, F., Luo, L., & Zhong, Y. (2000). A neurofibromatosis-1-regulated pathway is required for learning in Drosophila. *Nature, 403*, 895–898.

Gutmann, D. H., Aylsworth, A., Carey, J. C., Korf, B. R., Marks, J., Pyeritz, R. E., et al. (1997). The diagnostic evaluation and multidisciplinary management of neurofibromatosis 1 and neurofibromatosis 2. *Journal of the American Medical Association, 278*, 51–57.

Habib, M. (2000). The neurological basis of developmental dyslexia: An overview and working hypothesis. *Brain, 123*, 2373–2399.

Hofman, K. J., Harris, E. L., Bryan, R. N., & Denckla, M. B. (1994). Neurofibromatosis type 1: The cognitive phenotype. *Journal of Pediatrics, 124*, S1–S8.

Itoh, T., Magnaldi, S., White, R. M., Denckla, M. B., Hofman, K., Naidu, S., et al. (1994). Neurofibromatosis type 1: The evolution of deep gray and white matter MR abnormalities. *American Journal of Neuroradiology, 15*, 1513–1519.

Kayl, A., Moore, B. D., Slopis, J., Jackson, E., & Leeds, N. (1999). Quantitative morphology of the corpus callosum in children with neurofibromatosis and attention-deficit hyperactivity disorder. *Journal of Child Neurology, 15*, 90–96.

Kayl, A. E., Moore, B., Slopis, J. M., Jackson, E. F., & Leeds, N. E. (2000). Quantitative morphology of the corpus callosum in children with neurofibromatosis and attentin deficit hyperactivity disorder. *Journal of Child Neurology, 15,* 90–96.

Lindgren, S. D., & Benton, A. L. (1980). Developmental patterns of visuospatial judgment. *Journal of Pediatr Psychology, 5,* 217–225.

Listernick, R., Charrow, J., Greenwald, M., & Mets, M. (1994). Natural history of optic pathway tumors in children with neurofibromatosis type 1: A longitudinal study [see comments]. *Journal of Pediatrics, 125,* 63–66.

Listernick, R., Charrow, J., Greenwald, M. J., & Easterly, N. B. (1989). Optic gliomas in children with neurofibromatosis type 1. *Journal of Pediatrics, 114,* 788–792.

Lyon, G. R., & Rumsey, J. (1996). Application of neuroimaging methods to the understanding of childhood disorders. In G. R. Lyon & J. Rumsey (Eds.), *Neuroimaging: A window to the neurological foundations of learning and behavior in children* (pp. 53–54). Baltimore: Paul H. Brookes.

Mazzocco, M. M., Turner, J. E., Denckla, M. B., Hofman, K. J., Scanlon, D. C., & Vellutino, F. R. (1995). Language and reading deficits associated with neurofibromatosis type 1: Evidence for a not-so-nonverbal learning disability. *Developmental Neuropsychology, 11,* 503–522.

Moore, B. D., & Denckla, M. B. (1999). Neurofibromatosis. In K. Yeates, M. Ris, & H. Taylor (Eds.), *Pediatric neuropsychology: Research, theory, and practice* (pp. 149–170). New York: Guilford Publications.

Moore, B. D., III, Ater, J. L., Needle, M. N., Slopis, J., & Copeland, D. R. (1994b). Neuropsychological profile of children with neurofibromatosis, brain tumor, or both. *Journal of Child Neurology, 9,* 368–377.

Moore, B. D., Slopis, J. M., Jackson, E. F., De Winter, A. E., & Leeds, N. (2000). Brain volume in children with neurofibromatosis, type 1: Relation to neuropsychological status. *Neurology, 54,* 914–920.

Moore, B. D., Slopis, J. M., Schomer, D., Jackson, E. F., & Levy, B. M. (1996). Neuropsychological significance of areas of high signal intensity on brain MRIs of children with neurofibromatosis. *Neurology, 46,* 1660–1668.

Niemeyer, C. M., Arico, M., Basso, G., Biondi, A., Rajnoldi, A. C., Creutzig, U., et al. (1997). Chronic myelomonocytic leukemia in childhood: A retrospective analysis of 110 cases. *Blood, 89,* 3534–3543.

National Institutes of Health. (1988). National Institutes of Health Consensus Development Conference: Neurofibromatosis conference statement. *Archives of Neurology, 45,* 575–578.

North, K. (2000). Neurofibromatosis type 1. *American Journal of Medical Genetics, 97,* 119–127.

North, K., Joy, P., Yuille, D., Cocks, N., Mobbs, E., Hutchins, P., et al. (1994). Specific learning disability in children with neurofibromatosis type 1: Significance of MRI abnormalities [see comments]. *Neurology, 44,* 878–883.

North, K. N., Riccardi, V., Samango-Sprouse, C., Ferner, R., Moore, B., Legius, E., et al. (1997). Cognitive function and academic performance in neurofibromatosis. 1. Consensus statement from the NF1 Cognitive Disorders Task Force. *Neurology, 48,* 1121–1127.

Paulesu, E., Frith, U., Snowling, M., Gallagher, A., Morton, J., Frackowiak, R. S., et al. (1996). Is developmental dyslexia a disconnection syndrome? Evidence from PET scanning. *Brain, 119,* 143–157.

Pugh, K. R., Shaywitz, B. A., Shaywitz, S. E., Constable, R. T., Skudlarski, P., Fulbright, R. K., et al. (1996). Cerebral organization of component processes in reading. *Brain, 119,* 1221–1238.

Riccardi, V., & Eichner, J. (1986). *Neurofibromatosis: Phenotype, natural history, and pathogenesis.* Baltimore: John Hopkins University.

Riccardi, V. M. (1981). Von Recklinghausen neurofibromatosis. *New England Journal of Medicine, 305,* 1617–1627.

Rouleau, G. A., Merel, P., Lutchman, M., Sanson, M., Zucman, J., Marineau, C., et al. (1993). Alteration in a new gene encoding a putative membrane-organizing protein causes neurofibromatosis type-2. *Nature, 363,* 515–521.

Rourke, B. P. (1989). *Nonverbal learning disabilities.* New York: Guilford Press.

Said, S. M., Yeh, T. L., Greenwood, R. S., Whitt, J. K., Tupler, L. A., & Krishnan, K. R. (1996). MRI morphometric analysis and neuropsychological function in patients with neurofibromatosis. *Neuroreport, 7,* 1941–1944.

Schrimsher, G. W., Billingsley, R. L., Slopis, J. M., & Moore, B. D. (2003a). Visual–spatial performance deficits in children with neurofibromatosis type-1. *American Journal of Medical Genetics, 120A,* 326–330.

Sevick, R. J., Barkovich, A. J., Edwards, M. S., Koch, T., Berg, B., & Lempert, T. (1992). Evolution of white matter lesions in neurofibromatosis type 1: MR findings. AJR. *American Journal of Roentgenology, 159,* 171–175.

Shaywitz, S. E., Shaywitz, B. A., Pugh, K. R., Fulbright, R. K., Constable, R. T., Mencl, W. E., et al. (1998). Functional disruption in the organization of the brain for reading in dyslexia. *Proceedings of the National Academy of Sciences, U.S.A., 95,* 2636–2641.

Silva, A. J., Frankland, P. W., Marowitz, Z., Friedman, E., Lazlo, G., Cioffi, D., et al. (1997). A mouse model for the learning and memory deficits associated with neurofibromatosis type I. *Nature Genetics, 15,* 281–284.

Stanovich, K. E. (1988). Explaining the differences between the dyslexic and the garden-variety poor reader: The phonological-core variable-difference model. *Journal of Learning Disabilities, 21,* 590–604.

Temple, E., Poldrack, R. A., Protopapas, A., Nagarajan, S., Salz, T., Tallal, P., et al. (2000). Disruption of the neural response to rapid acoustic stimuli in dyslexia: Evidence from functional MRI. *Proceedings of the National Academy of Sciences, U.S.A., 97,* 13907–13912.

Temple, E., Poldrack, R. A., Salidis, J., Deutsch, G. K., Tallal, P., Merzenich, M. M., et al. (2001). Disrupted neural responses to phonological and orthographic processing in dyslexic children: An fMRI study. *Neuroreport, 12,* 299–307.

Trofatter, J. A., Maccollin, M. M., Rutter, J. L., Murrell, J. R., Duyao, M. P., Parry, D. M., et al. (1993). A novel moesin-like, ezrin-like, radixin-like gene is a candidate for the neurofibromatosis-2 tumor suppressor. *Cell, 72,* 791–800.

Varnhagen, C. K., Lewin, S., Das, J. P., Bowen, P., Ma, K., & Klimek, M. (1988). Neurofibromatosis and psychological processes. *Journal of Developmental and Behavioral Pediatrics, 9,* 257–265.

Vassilopoulou-Sellin, R., Klein, M. J., & Slopis, J. K. (2000). Growth hormone deficiency in children with neurofibromatosis type 1 without suprasellar lesions. *Pediatric Neurology, 22,* 355–358.

Viskochil, D., Buchberg, A. M., Xu, G., Cawthon, R. M., Stevens, J., Wolff, R. K., et al. (1990). Deletions and a translocation interrupt a cloned gene at the neurofibromatosis type 1 locus. *Cell, 62,* 187–192.

von Deimling, A., Krone, W., & Menon, A. G. (1995). Neurofibromatosis type 1: Pathology, clinical features and molecular genetics. *Brain Pathology, 5,* 153–162.

Wadsby, M., Lindehammar, H., & Eeg-Olofsson, O. (1989). Neurofibromatosis in childhood: Neuropsychological aspects. *Neurofibromatosis, 2,* 251–260.

Wallace, M. R., Marchuk, D. A., Andersen, L. B., Letcher, R., Odeh, H. M., Saulino, A. M., et al. (1990). Type 1 neurofibromatosis gene: Identification of a large transcript disrupted in three NF1 patients [published erratum appears in *Science, 250,* 1749]. *Science, 249,* 181–186.

Zhu, Y., Romero, M. I., Ghosh, P., Ye, Z., Charnay, P., Rushing, E. J., et al. (2001). Ablation of NF1 function in neurons induces abnormal development of cerebral cortex and reactive gliosis in the brain. *Genes Development, 15,* 859–876.

Zvulunov, A., Weitz, R., & Metzker, A. (1998). Neurofibromatosis type 1 in childhood: Evaluation of clinical and epidemiologic features as predictive factors for severity. *Clinical Pediatrics (Phila.), 37,* 295–299.

6 Cognitive and Behavioral Characteristics of Children with Chromosome 22q11.2 Deletion Syndrome

Tony J. Simon, Merav Burg-Malki, and Doron Gothelf

Enhancing Early Identification

In this initial section we will present information with the aim of increasing early identification of the chromosome 22q11.2 deletion syndrome. We will begin with a definition of the syndrome and its nomenclature and the current best estimates of its incidence. We then discuss some of the features that have the highest specificity or sensitivity for detection of the syndrome, both in terms of physical manifestations and behavioral or psychiatric disorders. We will then briefly discuss similar disorders that might be confused with or diagnosed instead of the chromosome 22q11.2 deletion syndrome. Finally, we will describe two diagnostic cases that together illustrate the range or variability of signs and symptoms that need to be considered when identifying this disorder

Definition

The chromosome 22q11.2 deletion syndrome (hereafter DS22q11.2) is considered to be the most common microdeletion syndrome known in humans (Botto et al., 2003). The syndrome was described clinically by Angelo DiGeorge during the 1960s and by Robert Shprintzen during the 1970s (Kirkpatrick & DiGeorge, 1968; Shprintzen et al., 1978). The DiGeorge syndrome was defined as being composed of immunologic deficiencies secondary to thymus hypoplasia, hypocalcemia secondary to hypoparathyroidism, and congenital cardiac anomalies (Kirkpatrick & DiGeorge, 1968). The Shprintzen syndrome, later renamed velocardiofacial syndrome (VCFS), expresses major features that are suggested by its acronym and include palate anomalies ("velo"), congenital cardiovascular defects ("cardio") and mild facial dysmorphism ("facial"; Shprintzen et al., 1978). In the early 1990s it was discovered that both the DiGeorge syndrome and VCFS were caused by a microdeletion in the long (q) arm of chromosome 22 at band 22q11.2 (Carey et al., 1992; Driscoll, Budarf, & Emanuel, 1992; Driscoll, Spinner et al., 1992). This region is depicted in figure 6.1. Since then, the clinical diagnosis of DS22q11.2 has been verified by a cytogenetic

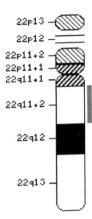

Figure 6.1
Ideogram of chromosome 22 and the deleted region of q11.22. From National Center for Biotechnology Information (http://www.ncbi.nlm.nih.gov).

test called "fluorescence in situ hybridization" (FISH; Driscoll et al., 1993). An example of the results of such a test is depicted in figure 6.2. It has also been established that, besides the above-mentioned signs and symptoms, the phenotypic spectrum of DS22q11.2 is extremely wide and includes over 180 possible congenital anomalies, learning disabilities, and psychiatric manifestations (Shprintzen, 2000). It is now widely recognized that several other previously identified syndromes also result from chromosome 22q11 deletions, including conotruncal anomaly face syndrome (Burn et al., 1993) and some cases of Cayler cardiofacial syndrome (Giannotti, Digilio, Marino, Mingarelli, & Dallapiccola, 1994) and Opitz G/BBB syndrome (McDonald-McGinn et al., 1995). This has led to some confusion about what label to use for cases in which the deletion is detected (e.g., see Wulfsberg, Leana-Cox, & Neri, 1996). Therefore, we shall adopt the most inclusive term of "chromosome 22q11.2 deletion syndrome."

Incidence

The exact incidence of DS22q11.2 is not known at this time. This is because exact incidence can be determined only if all infants born are screened for the deletion. As the FISH test is expensive, such a population-based screening would be too costly. Thus, currently there are only minimum incidence estimates based on cases referred to cardiologic clinics, genetic clinics, or registries of congenital defects. Based on studies of various ethnic backgrounds, the minimum incidence of DS22q11.2 is between 1 in 5,900 and 1 in 9,700 live births (for a review, see Botto et al., 2003). The actual incidence of DS22q11.2 is probably much higher, as the phenotypic expression of the syndrome is frequently mild and can be easily missed. In addition, cases are

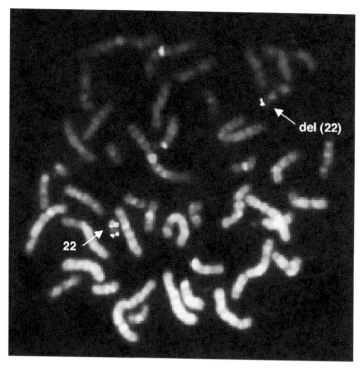

Figure 6.2
Image of fluorescence in situ hybridization test of one copy of chromosome with deleted (del) region.

missed because most clinicians are not aware of the full spectrum of the syndrome's manifestations.

In our view, a good way to efficiently increase the rate of diagnosis of DS22q11.2 is to emphasize the signs and symptoms that have high specificity and/or sensitivity for the diagnosis of the syndrome. In this light, we will now describe the physical and psychiatric manifestations of the syndrome followed by examples from two case vignettes. Then we will describe in greater detail the cognitive features of the DS22q11.2 in children and discuss some of the implications for academic achievement.

Physical Manifestations

Table 6.1 summarizes the rate of major physical diseases in the DS22q11.2 population and the rate of the chromosome 22q11.2 deletion found in all cases with the specified disease. As can be seen in table 6.1, the likelihood of the disease's being part of DS22q11.2 is dependent on its specific type. For example, the types of cardiovascular anomalies listed in table 6.1 are highly associated with DS22q11.2. Other

Table 6.1
Prevalence of characteristic physical signs and symptoms in chromosome 22q11.2 deletion syndrome
(DS22q11.2) and prevalence of DS22q11.2 in these conditions

Physical Disease	% of Cases in All Individuals with DS22q11.2	% of DS22q11.2 within All Cases of Specified Disease
Cardiovascular anomalies	75	very low[a]
Tetralogy of Fallot	15–35	10–15
Ventricular septal defect with pulmonary atresia	15–30	20–50
Persistent truncus arteriosus	5–10	30–35
Interrupted aortic arch type B	5–20	60–80
Palatal anomalies	40–75	0–8
Overt cleft palate	10	
Bifid uvula	5	
Submucosal cleft palate	15	
Velopharyngeal insufficiency	30	
Facial dysmorphism	75	very low[a]
Hypocalcemia	10–30	very low[a]

[a] To the best of our knowledge was not tested.

cardiovascular anomalies, like the atrial septal defect and the transposition of great vessels are far less common in DS22q11.2 (Marino, Mileto, Digilio, Carotti, & Di Donato, 2005). The palatal anomalies are manifested in hypernasal speech. It is important to remember that in most cases the palate anomaly is not overt and can only be detected by a nasendoscopic evaluation (Shprintzen & Golding-Kushner, 1989). As mentioned previously, DS22q11.2 can affect many of the body's organs, such as the eyes, ears, limbs, and kidneys. One of the most common manifestations is the characteristic but subtle facial appearance. This can include increased vertical length of the face, even at early ages, nasal changes such as increased height and bulbous nasal tip, hooded upper eyelids, ears that are small, cupped, or overfolded, and retrusion of the lower jaw (McDonald-McGinn et al., 1999; Shprintzen, 2005). It has been reported (C. A. Morris, personal communication) that identification of the syndrome can be significantly increased when any of the above features, or abnormal movement of the palate, in combination with hypernasal speech are used to initiate testing for the deletion. Examples of the craniofacial characteristics of individuals with chromosome 22q11.2 deletions are depicted in figure 6.3. A few diseases, such as the cardiovascular anomalies listed in table 6.1, are very specific to DS22q11.2. However, in most diseases that are a possible manifestation of the syndrome, DS22q11.2 is only rarely present (see table 6.1). Therefore, referring to a FISH test based on a single symptom is probably not very cost effective (Shprintzen, 2000). We recommend testing for DS22q11.2 when two of the major physical signs listed in the table are present because a DS22q11.2 diagnosis in these cases is far more likely.

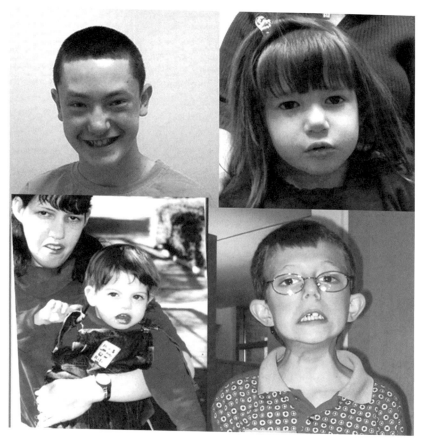

Figure 6.3
Pictures of four children (and one adult) with chromosome 22q11.2 deletion syndrome.

Psychiatric Disorders

A series of studies has shown that individuals with DS22q11.2 have very high rates of psychiatric morbidity and abnormal behaviors (Arnold, Siegel-Bartelt, Cytrynbaum, Teshima, & Schachar, 2001; Feinstein, Eliez, Blasey, & Reiss, 2002; Fine et al., 2005; Gothelf et al., 2003; Gothelf et al., 2004; Papolos et al., 1996; Prinzie et al., 2002; Shprintzen, 2000; Swillen, Devriendt, Ghesquiere, & Fryns, 2001). Starting from childhood, abnormal behaviors and increased rate of psychiatric disorders are already present in individuals with DS22q11.2. Children with DS22q11.2 tend to be shy, withdrawn, stubborn, emotionally labile, and afflicted with social and communication impairments (Swillen et al., 2001). Children and adolescents with DS22q11.2 have a high rate of nonpsychotic psychiatric disorders, including attention deficit/

hyperactivity disorder (ADHD), oppositional defiant disorder, anxiety and affective disorders, and autism spectrum disorders (Arnold et al., 2001; Feinstein et al., 2002; Fine et al., 2005; Gothelf et al., 2003; Gothelf et al., 2004; Papolos et al., 1996). It seems that most psychiatric disorders found in individuals with DS22q11.2 are also common in individuals with non-DS22q11.2 developmental disabilities. Feinstein et al. (2002) compared the rate of psychiatric disorders in children and adolescents with DS22q11.2 with that of matched IQ controls and found similar rates in both groups for all psychiatric disorders. Swillen et al. (2001) compared parents' and teachers' reports of the behavior of school-age children with DS22q11.2 with reports of matched age and IQ controls with speech and language impairments but without DS22q11.2. The results indicated that both groups exhibited similar degrees of abnormal behaviors. The only differences found were that children with DS22q11.2 were more withdrawn and controls were more aggressive. It is not surprising that children with developmental disabilities have similarly high rates of behavioral problems and psychiatric disorders because they share common risk factors for psychopathology, such as social isolation and rejection, impairments in social and daily living skills, low self-esteem, and overprotectiveness by parents. These factors could predispose them to psychiatric morbidity. Other factors include general CNS functional differences, executive function and other cognitive impairments, and we shall discuss those below.

During late adolescence and early adulthood, about 25% of individuals with DS22q11.2 develop schizophrenia-like psychotic disorders (Bassett et al., 2003; Bassett et al., 1998; Murphy, Jones, & Owen, 1999; Pulver et al., 1994). The clinical characteristics of the DS22q11.2 psychotic disorder are similar to those of non-DS22q11.2 schizophrenia patients. Higher rates of chromosome 22q11.2 deletions were found in children and adults with schizophrenia (Karayiorgou et al., 1995). This rate is especially high in schizophrenia patients with one (20%; Gothelf et al., 1997) or two (53%; Bassett et al., 1998) major physical symptoms of DS22q11.2. The strong association between DS22q11.2 and schizophrenia-like psychosis does indeed seem to be specific because the rate of schizophrenia in DS22q11.2 is about 25 times more common than in the general population and about 10 times more common than in individuals with developmental disabilities (Turner, 1989).

Infants and toddlers who suffer from severe physical diseases are usually identified by clinicians and referred for genetic testing at infancy and during the preschool years. Those children who are only mildly physically affected are easily missed, and only those that manifest marked cognitive limitations and psychiatric disorders, especially schizophrenia, are referred for genetic testing during adolescence or even adulthood.

Case 6.1—Diagnosis at preschool: Yagil Yagil was born to healthy parents after an uneventful pregnancy and labor. A few hours after the delivery, he became cyanotic and required mechanical respiration. Echocardiography demonstrated ventricular septal defect and interrupted aortic arch type B. At the age of 6 days he underwent cardiac corrective surgery. During the surgery, it was noticed that Yagil did not have any thymus tissue. After surgery, Yagil had seizures due to severe hypocalcemia. At that stage, the diagnosis of DS22q11.2 was suspected and Yagil was referred to a FISH test that confirmed the diagnosis. In addition to the aforementioned medical problems, he also suffered from recurrent ear and pulmonary infections during the first 2 years of life due to low IgG2 levels. He also had surgical repair of an inguinal hernia. On the Bayley developmental test, his development was delayed both on the mental and motor scales. He started walking at 19 months, produced his first words at 22 months, and was not yet toilet trained at the age of 4 years. His speech is hypernasal and difficult to comprehend due to occult submucous cleft palate, and his language is delayed for his age. Yagil's parents report that Yagil is stubborn and is very shy with people who are not part of his family.

Yagil is an example of a child with DS22q11.2 who is severely affected. The classical medical problems associated with the disease were manifested since infancy, including typical cardiovascular anomalies, hypocalcaemia, and recurrent infections. He also had an inguinal hernia; global developmental delays with significant speech delays; and shy, stubborn behavior, and although these findings are common in DS22q11.2, they are not specific to the syndrome.

Case 6.2—Diagnosis at adolescence: Zoe Zoe, a 17-year-old female, was hospitalized at a psychiatric inpatient unit after threatening to commit suicide and becoming physically violent toward her parents. On psychiatric evaluation, she reported delusions of reference, thinking that her classmate and even strangers in the street were saying "nasty things" about her. She also reported that figures from the TV were telling her how ugly she was. Zoe also reported that she heard voices telling her to commit suicide, and her parents noted that she was talking to herself loudly as if arguing with someone. The psychiatrist diagnosed Zoe with schizoaffective disorder, depressive type.

Zoe is otherwise a relatively physically healthy adolescent. She was born with mild ventricular septal defect (VSD) that closed spontaneously. Her attainment of developmental milestones was slightly delayed but within the normal range, and she had mild hypotonia as a young child. Her speech was mildly hypernasal. At elementary school, she had difficulties with mathematics and reading comprehension. Cognitive testing showed that Zoe's IQ score was 78. At elementary school, Zoe was also diagnosed with ADHD inattentive type and suffered from anxiety disorders. She used to cling to her parents and refused to go on a trip or to visit friends without being accompanied by her parents. At the age of 12 years, she also started having compulsions in which she repetitively touched her eye to make sure she would not develop strabismus and she compulsively hoarded paper, magazines, and advertisements and would not let anyone touch the collection. The combination of her psychiatric symptoms with a history of ventricular septal defect, hypernasal speech, and mild dysmorphic facial features raised her psychiatrist's suspicion that Zoe might have DS22q11.2. Zoe was referred for a FISH test, and the result was positive for the 22q11.2 deletion.

Zoe is an example of a physically healthy child with mild developmental delay but with severe psychiatric symptomatology. Zoe's psychiatric disorders were first noticed in elementary school and gradually escalated. Initially, ADHD developed, followed by separation anxiety disorder and obsessive–compulsive disorder (OCD), culminating at the age of 17 years with a psychotic disorder. Since Zoe's physical symptoms were very mild and included only a VSD and hypernasal speech, her diagnosis could have been easily missed. Of the myriad psychiatric symptoms that Zoe had, the schizophrenia-like symptoms were the ones that were relatively specific to DS22q11.2. Thus, it was the combination of psychotic symptoms, the few physical symptoms characteristic of the syndrome, and the borderline intelligence that raised the clinical suspicion that Zoe may be affected with DS22q11.2.

Cognitive and Academic Manifestations

In the following section we review the main findings concerning the manner in which the DS22q11.2 phenotype is expressed in terms of mental functioning. Having dealt above with psychiatric issues, we will focus here on the implications of DS22q11.2 for a child's ability to process information relating to everyday cognitive tasks and to specific academic domains like reading or arithmetic. Since the focus of this volume is on how the phenotypes of neurogenetic developmental disorders are expressed in children, we will include very little data gathered from adults with DS22q11.2. Also, given the increasing variety of research methods that are being used in the study of genotype/phenotype relationships of individuals with neurogenetic disorders, especially with respect to biobehavioral implications, we thought it valuable to initially make some distinctions between the types of data we will review, the means by which they were collected, and the interpretive strengths or weaknesses of each approach.

The majority of investigations concerning the cognitive and behavioral profiles of individuals with DS2211.2 have been carried out with two complementary sets of tools, namely, neuropsychological testing and cognitive experimentation. We will briefly review the characteristics of these two approaches and will then discuss in more detail the overall pattern of results that each has generated so far.

The most extensive set of results so far has resulted from neuropsychological testing studies. Here, a collection, or "battery," of standardized neuropsychological tests is designed in order to generate a broad profile of the individual's abilities. Tests are usually focused on the intellectual, academic, and behavioral domains. The tests used are referred to as "standardized" because large numbers of individuals have had the tests administered to them by testers trained to present and interpret them in a reliable fashion. Standardized tests also have their scores transformed from the actual score achieved by the individual to a score that represents that individual's competence with respect to the general population of the same chronological age. This yields a measure of "mental age" for the domain in question using "norms," which are the average scores of a large number of individuals at specific ages from a given population (usually typically developing). In this way, each individual can be scored within a percentile range so that his or her abilities on the test can be compared both *between* individuals, that is, to the normed population to determine relative advantage or disadvantage in that domain, and *within* the individual to determine domains of particular strength or weaknesses that exist.

Because of this standardization, results from neuropsychological testing studies have the advantage of being interpretable by a range of professionals, including teachers and educational psychologists, and they are often used to form the basis for an individualized educational or other remediation program for the individual concerned. They also have the advantage of being able to produce such results in a broad range of domains from a single testing session of several hours' duration. In this sense they are immensely valuable to parents, support professionals, clinicians, and researchers alike. However, one disadvantage of neuropsychological testing studies, from the perspective of researchers at least, is that they are primarily quantitative and descriptive. Despite being based on theory and evidence, these tests primarily generate what we might term "how well can you do" information. This indicates that an individual may be very good or very bad at a particular task or in a given intellectual domain but cannot directly explain why that profile is observed. By the same token, the behavior measured by such tests has, at best, a rather loose relationship to the underlying cognitive and neurobiological substrates that generate it. In other words, they reveal little about the mental representations being used, the manner in which they are processed, the brain circuits upon which those computations depend, the neurotransmitters involved, and so forth.

By contrast, there is currently only a small number of published research reports based on cognitive experimentation studies. Instead of a test battery, researchers using cognitive experimentation studies develop small sets of experiments, usually in the form of computer-based "games," carefully designed in order to test specific hypotheses about how particular cognitive functions work and the nature of the representations that they process. Results are then interpreted as a test of the hypotheses by determining whether or not the predicted performance patterns were observed. Typically, new, more detailed hypotheses emerge from such analyses, further experiments are designed, and the process progresses toward an ever more highly specified explanatory account. Informed mostly by the fields of cognitive psychology and cognitive neuroscience, many individual tests, known as "trials," are generated in order to create related sets, or "conditions," in which predictions of the speed, accuracy, and characteristics of performance can be made based on hypotheses of how information is processed, which brain circuits are involved, and how these interact.

A simple example would be an experiment that examines the processing required to find a target object (like a letter O) in a set of distracting objects (usually other letters). In this "visual search" experiment, the participant is required to press a button as soon as he or she detects a single letter O while ignoring the distractor objects, here letter Xs. There could be an O and a single X on one trial and an O and up to as many as 10 Xs on other trials. There might be 10 such examples of each trial, whose results can be averaged together to ensure that no single unusual response is taken as the performance capabilities of the individual. These 100 trials would constitute a condition that would be called "disjunctive search." The label reflects the fact that there are no features (like shape, angle, size, or even meaning) shared by the letters O and X. It has been shown in such experiments that the targets and distractors can be detected rather independently by the visual and attention systems of the human brain. Thus, we would predict, based on existing knowledge, that detection of the O would be fast, that it would be accurate, and that the time taken would be little affected by the number of Xs. The O almost appears to "pop out" of the field of Xs and so requires no real search on the part of the participant's visual and attention systems. Another condition, referred to as "conjunctive search," would also have 100 trials with 10 examples each of a single O but now placed among 1 to 10 letter Qs. This condition would be called "conjunctive search" since the letters O and Q share, or contain "conjunctions" of, many features. We would predict not only that detection would be slower and less accurate but that the time taken to find the O would be directly related to the number of distractors (Qs) in the display. This is because cognitive studies have revealed the different kinds of search patterns that take place in pop-out and conjunctive search conditions. Here the participant would need to examine each letter in turn, try to decide if it is an O or a Q, and respond when the target is found. Given that a good deal is known, at least in adults at present, about which brain circuits are involved in these processes, we might also predict that individuals with known disorders to those circuits would do more poorly under certain conditions, like conjunctive search. We might also infer that should one type of performance be much worse than is usually expected, or much worse than that of a group of comparison participants in the experiment, then the circuits concerned may be expected to be dysfunctional.

Because of the knowledge required to design and interpret results from cognitive experimentation studies, they are not easily interpretable by many professionals besides the researchers themselves and so cannot immediately be used to form the basis of remedial programs in the way that neuropsychological testing results can. Furthermore, because of the complexity involved in developing and interpreting cognitive experimentation studies, they typically only produce such results in a narrow range of domains but they do so in great detail. Their main strength, however, is that they are primarily explanatory and generate what we might term "how did you do it" information. By focusing on the mental representations being used, the manner in which they are processed, and the hypothesized brain circuits and neurotransmitters upon which those computations depend, they can generate a great deal of precise qualitative information about which mental computations were involved in producing the observed behavior. This can then be used to form the basis of detailed explanations for observed behavior and so should provide critical information for the design of specific cognitive processing interventions that potentially could change the way in the which the mind and the brain work together.

However, overly simple mappings from brain structure to cognitive function should be avoided in general—and when one is considering development, especially atypical development, they are particularly dangerous. As pointed out by Johnson et al. (Johnson, Halit, Grice, & Karmiloff-Smith, 2002), since brain development is a process of the incremental tuning and specialization of multiple areas connected as circuits, assumptions about functional impairment based on changes to single regions are likely to be inaccurate. Furthermore, due to this interactive process and the converging roles of genetics, brain activity, and environmental input, functional circuits are certain to change during development, and so any assumptions about the stability of a structure–function mapping would also be unwise when one is studying childhood. Finally, that interaction also means that brain change is being affected in a bidirectional manner, with circuitry influencing the behavioral repertoire and the behaviors influencing the changing nature of the connections.

Below we will review what has been and continues to be learned from neuropsychological testing studies of DS22q11.2 and then will review recent results emerging from cognitive experimentation studies. Then we will briefly review the current knowledge about possible relationships between those findings and changes in the brains of individuals with DS22q11.2 and also in some relevant genes. Because of the broad and descriptive capabilities neuropsychological testing studies offer, they have been able to provide a profile of both strengths and weaknesses. In contrast, the limited number of cognitive experimentation studies carried out so far has tended to focus on attempting to explain the nature of the impairments exhibited by children with DS22q11.2 in a small range of cognitive processing domains.

Overview and Typicality of Neuropsychological Profile

While the goal of this section is to focus on areas of *relative* strength and weakness, it is fairly clear that the global intellectual profile of children with DS22q11.2 is one of weakness relative to the level expected based on chronological age. On general intelligence measures, Verbal IQ (VIQ) at around 75–80, is typically higher than Performance (nonverbal) IQ, at around 70–75, and is often a little higher than Full Scale

IQ (FSIQ), although even this pattern is not universal (see Moss et al., 1999). Shprintzen (2000) suggested that overall competence appeared to drop from IQ scores in the mid 80s when preschoolers were tested to the mid 70s in the early school years. The former scores were measured using the Leiter and Stanford Binet tests while the latter came from the Wechsler tests. Shprintzen suggested that this change might be less a factor of increasing developmental delay than a factor of the differences in the tests, which focus increasingly on abstract learning for older children. Gerdes, Solot, Wang, McDonald-McGinn, and Zackai (2001) assessed 112 children under the age of 6 years using the Bayley scale (Bayley, 1969) and Wechsler Preschool and Primary Scale of Intelligence—Revised. They reported that, in this preschool group, 34% were assessed in the average range with FSIQ scores in the >85 range, 32% were in the mildly delayed range (FSIQ = 70–84), and 33% were in the significantly delayed range (FSIQ < 70). Thus, the pattern is more likely one of considerable variability, even early in life, with less complex areas of cognition showing relative strength initially. We will examine the overall pattern in more detail below.

By the early school years, most children with the deletion are experiencing fewer problems in domains related to language than in nonverbal domains. In one example of many similar reports, Moss and colleagues (1999) found that, in a group of 33 individuals with DS22q11.2, FSIQ was 71.2 ± 12.8 (mean ± standard deviation), VIQ was 77.5 ± 14.9, and Performance IQ (PIQ) was 69.1 ± 12.0. While it has been pointed out several times (e.g., Campbell & Swillen, 2005; Wang, Woodin, Kreps-Falk, & Moss, 2000) that not every individual with the deletion exhibits exactly the same Verbal IQ higher than PIQ profile, general intellectual performance tends to be around 10–25 points below the "normal" or average value of 100. At least two published reports of case studies, however, have pointed to some alternate patterns of manifestation. One extreme case, reported by Kozma (1998), describes a 22-year-old female with a confirmed chromosome 22q11.2 deletion who had an FSIQ of 13 and language skills of between 1 and 8 months' developmental age. She had also been given a diagnosis of autism at 3 years of age. Whether or not this unusual pattern was due to injury or insult secondary to the chromosome 22q11.2 deletion is unclear. A more extensive report of a 7-year-old boy (Stiers et al., 2005) describes a profile where the FSIQ of 73 revealed no significant differences between verbal and nonverbal subtest performance, an overall lack of visuospatial processing impairments, and some relative strengths in the area of attention and memory span. This pattern appears to be consistent with a minority of the children reported by Wang et al. (see figure 1 in Wang et al., 2000) and suggests that the profile of significantly stronger verbal than nonverbal skills is not specific to or highly diagnostic of DS22q11.2 and that more detailed examination of the cognitive profile, as discussed below, is necessary.

Areas of Relative Strength from Neuropsychological Testing Studies

The cognitive profile of DS22q11.2 has often been described as fitting the profile of a "nonverbal learning disorder" (e.g., Swillen et al., 1999), which suggests that verbal abilities are greater than nonverbal ones. As stated above, in the most general sense this is true of the majority of the population of children with DS22q11.2. However, the story concerning language and communication is a somewhat complex one of both strengths and weaknesses.

Language As stated above, abilities in the verbal domain are typically, but not always, superior to those in the nonverbal domain. Within the verbal domain, receptive language is generally the strongest component (e.g., Moss et al., 1999). However, this pattern is generally true of language learning in general and so may be less an indication of a significant dysfunction in neurocognitive basis of language expression than the manifestation of a typically functioning system that is slow in maturing due to a more global developmental delay. Either or both of these conditions might be true depending on the child in question, and so, clearly, further research is needed in order to examine this question. In one counterexample to the typical pattern (Glaser et al., 2002), stronger expressive than receptive language was found in a group of 27 children and adolescents with DS22q11.2. The authors suggest that the profile was due either to the therapeutic effects of speech therapy on expressive abilities or the progressively handicapping effects of abstract thinking impairments on expressive language abilities that require more abstraction and complexity. However, the age range in their sample was very large and included individuals from as young as 6 to as old as 19 years. There is, of course, considerable change in language abilities during that developmental window. Thus, it is unclear whether the profile would have been the same had they analyzed the youngest and oldest participants separately. Indeed, it might have been the inclusion of the older individuals that produced their reversed pattern, since that is the major difference from the other studies that have reported the more typical pattern of language development. Those studies instead focused on younger children in a smaller age range. Evidence for this interpretation comes from a larger study carried out by Solot et al. (2001) of 79 children with DS22q11.2 in two age ranges: 7 to 66 months and 5.9 to 16.7 years of age. In this study, the preschool children (7–66 months) were analyzed separately from the school-age ones (5–16 years). Solot et al. reported that receptive language scores were significantly higher than expressive scores for the younger children but that the pattern was reversed for the older ones. Some aspects of language and communication, however, are seriously impaired or delayed, and we will examine those below.

Reading and Spelling In a large study (Woodin et al., 2001) of 81 children with DS22q11.2, 50 of whom were school-age (6–17 years), it was reported that broad reading and spelling abilities were relative strengths at a similar level, both in the low-average range. The findings were slightly different from those in an earlier study (Moss et al., 1999) that included some of the same individuals. In the earlier study, scores for reading comprehension and single-word reading were similar; however, Woodin et al. found that word reading was better developed than was comprehension.

Memory   Rote verbal memory, which is the ability to repeat back after a delay a list of verbally presented items, was found to be at the level expected for chronological age, and thus not impaired, in a small study of school-age children (Swillen et al., 1999). In a larger study (Woodin et al., 2001), 50 children with DS2q11.2 ages 6–17 years of age were assessed with a variety of standardized tests of memory. The authors report a remarkable area of strength on tests of memory that required reproduction of lists of unrelated words and of categorically related words (such as those found in a shopping list). In fact 72% of the group scored in the low-average to very superior range despite 62% of the group having scored in the borderline to moderately deficient range on overall IQ scores! As part of a broader study, Wang and colleagues (2000) found that two thirds of a group of 36 children with DS22q11.2 ages 5 to 12 years scored within normal limits on a memory test requiring them to recall lists of numbers. Furthermore, a related study (Bearden et al., 2001) reported similar results for memory of objects made up from everyday shapes. In a small study of 9 children with DS22q11.2, Lajiness-O'Neill et al. (2005) found that, on the standardized Test of Memory and Learning (Reynolds & Kamphaus, 1992), performance on verbal memory tasks was in the low-average range. Unexpectedly, and inconsistently with other studies (e.g., Woodin et al., 2001), they found that performance on memory for stories was the same as that of controls. Also, their delayed recall abilities (which included verbal and nonverbal material) were at the high end of the low-average range, presumably due to the relative strength in verbal memory.

Areas of Relative Weakness from Neuropsychological Testing Studies

Language   While some aspects of language do represent an area of relative strength, as described above, there are also aspects of language that are far weaker. Specifically, the relative strength of receptive language reflects a relative weakness in expressive language. In a short-term longitudinal study of four children with DS22q11.2 ages 6 to 30 months, both aspects were found to be impaired by the age of 12 months. The authors concluded that the developmental delay in expressive language was greater than what would be predicted by the overall delays experienced by the children in the study (Scherer, D'Antonio, & Kalbfleisch, 1999). However, the almost total lack of a vocabulary and several restrictions in speech sounds led the authors to conclude that the children with DS22q11.2 "were essentially non-oral through 30 months of age" (p. 721). Evidence that the receptive/expressive imbalance appears to persist (Gerdes et al., 1999; Moss et al., 1999; Solot et al., 2000) suggests that a specific language problem exists rather than the pattern being due to a simple slowing of typical development where expressive language gradually catches up with receptive abilities. Shprintzen (2000) suggested that the receptive/expressive difference

demonstrates that speech intelligibility is likely to be at the root of the problem. Expressive language output tends to dramatically increase after four years of age when both speech therapy and surgery have often been applied to resolve the speech disorder. (p. 144)

While there is clear merit to this view, it does not rule out a more "central" delay in neurocognitive development related to expressive language, which includes the development of circuits linking the slowly developing frontal lobes and neocerebellum (Diamond, 2000). In fact, Solot et al.'s larger study (Solot et al., 2000) of 53 children with DS22q11.2 ages 7–66 months found a persisting and significant expressive language deficit, and language scores tended to follow the pattern of overall intelligence scores. By 4 years of age, 30% of the sample was still nonverbal or not speaking in sentences.

Reading and Spelling   As mentioned above, while spelling and early reading are relative strengths, reading comprehension is considerably impaired in children with DS22q11.2. Woodin et al. (2001) reported that, although broad reading scores were in the low-average range, there was a significant difference between the much better developed word reading skills of children with DS22q11.2 and their much poorer reading comprehension abilities.

Memory   In contrast to the surprising strength on rote verbal memory reported by Woodin et al. (2001), their participants with DS22q11.2 showed a significant impairment on a more complex memory task, which involved the delayed recall of story details. Here, performance was in the borderline range (between average and mild "mental retardation"). The same children also showed considerable weakness on a visual–spatial design memory test that is quite characteristic of their overall visuo-spatial difficulties. This study involved a larger sample than the one reported on by Wang et al. (2000), where a different test of spatial memory produced below average performance. Another subsample was also evaluated on several other tests, and Bearden et al. (2001) reported a significant discrepancy between the near average scores found on verbal memory tests and significantly lower scores on tests of memory for locations of dots on a grid, a measure of visuospatial memory. Furthermore, the results showed that the difference was due to the nature of the to-be-remembered information, since scores on memory for the shape of objects were similar to those for verbal memory and significantly higher than for those involving the locations of dots. Similar patterns of results where verbal memory was better than visual–spatial memory using different tests have been reported by other recent studies (Lajiness-O'Neill et al., 2005; Sobin, Kiley-Brabeck, Daniels et al., 2005).

Executive Function and Working Memory Few neuropsychological testing based studies have focused explicitly on executive function. However, Woodin et al. (2001) reported a significant impairment on the B subtest of the Trail Making test on the Wechsler Intelligence Scale for Children (3rd ed; WISC–III) when compared to the A subtest. This task requires the child to find and connect with a pencil line a series of sequentially labeled locations (e.g., A, B, C or 1, 2, 3) that are spatially distributed on the page. The difference between the A and B versions is that the latter adds inhibitory and working memory loads, since children have to not just connect up locations denoted by letters in sequence (e.g., A then B then C) but have to switch between letters and numbers (e.g., A then 1 then B then 2 ...). Working memory, which requires not just storage but also computation of intermediate results or application of rules, was also found by Sobin, Kiley-Brabeck, Daniels et al. (2004, 2005) to be an area of specific impairment.

Attention As measured by neuropsychological testing based studies, attention is a rather broadly defined domain of functioning. As we shall see below in our presentation of results from the Attentional Networks Test (ANT), attention can be decomposed into rather specific types of functions that are deployed in the service of very different goals and that are known, in adults at least, to depend on very different neural circuits. However, neuropsychological testing studies tend to give a rather more general view of attentional function. As discussed elsewhere in this chapter, there is an elevated rate of attention deficit disorders, mainly ADHD, in children with DS22q11.2, but this is a clinical diagnosis and not a specification of which attentional functions are impaired. ADHD diagnoses focus on three domains of symptoms—inattention, motor hyperactivity, and behavioral impulsivity—and so do suggest that certain measurable functions are likely to be worse in affected children than in controls. Consistent with this, Woodin et al. (2001) reported that scores on the Freedom from Distractibility index from the WISC–III test were significantly lower than those on the Verbal Comprehension index in their sample of 50 school-age children with DS22q11.2. Similarly, Sobin, Kiley-Brabeck, Daniels et al. (2005) found that, on the NEPSY (Korkman, Kirk, & Kemp, 1998) Visual Attention subtest, scores for omissions (indicating visual inattention) indicated an area of relative weakness for children with DS2211.2.

Motor Abilities A very common feature of children with DS22q11.2 is low muscle tone, and this can certainly negatively affect gross motor skills. However, some motor skills are better indicators of functioning levels in the neural system than the musculoskeletal system, and those tend to be the ones measured by neuropsychological testing studies. Tasks that require fine motor manipulation, sequenced actions, reaching for specific targets, and timed actions are particularly good examples. In Sobin, Kiley-Brabeck, Daniels et al.'s (2005) study, several such tests were included. Scores on tests of motor dexterity (Finger Tapping), kinesthetic/tactile awareness (Imitating Hand Positions) and graphomotor control (Visuomotor Precision) from the NEPSY battery were all at least 1 *SD* below average, the criterion used for an area of relative weakness. It is likely that one component of the weak performance on some of these tasks is the particular weakness in visual–spatial tasks that children with DS22q11.2 have.

Summary of Strengths and Weaknesses from Neuropsychological Testing Studies

The pattern revealed by the studies just reviewed is quite consistent, though not to the extent that those with slightly different profiles should not be considered to have DS22q11.2. Verbal abilities are usually stronger than nonverbal, but this is not always the case. Language abilities are strongest in the receptive mode, and the expression of early, concrete concepts and early word reading and spelling are also strong. They are weak in the expressive mode, with many children being essentially nonoral in the early speech years, though expression does improve in later childhood. In contrast to the effective decoding and understanding of individual words in early reading, most children with DS22q11.2 show marked impairments in the integration of patterns and relationships of meanings between words as is necessary in reading comprehension, and this negatively impacts a wide range of academic activities. Children with DS22q11.2 show remarkable strengths in simple verbal memory tasks like storing and retrieving strings of related or unrelated items or even objects. They have significant problems again when the spatial relationships between items have to be remembered and, just as with reading comprehension, when complex semantic sequences or relationships must be remembered in story memory tasks. Executive Function and Attention tests show impairments of several types. One example is for concurrent storage and manipulation of memory items, which is necessary for most working memory tasks and for "applied" tasks like arithmetic or reading comprehension. Another is when rules must be held and used to alter behavior (as in the Trails B task), and another is when suppression or inhibition of irrelevant or distracting information is required. Weaknesses are also found in finely tuned or timed visually guided motor tasks, which is consistent with a general weakness in the visual–spatial domain.

Areas of Relative Weakness from Cognitive Experimentation Studies

As stated earlier, and demonstrated above, neuropsychological testing studies provide us with a broad descriptive profile of both strengths and weaknesses in the cognitive phenotype of DS22q11.2. They also provide some clue as to the neurocognitive basis of that profile, although they are not able to generate explanations for the level of performance observed. We will turn now to the smaller number of cognitive experimentation studies that have been designed in order to try to explain some of the impairments just described. Necessarily, this complementary approach is much narrower in focus because groups rather than individuals have to be tested. This is because the measures these tests generate are not normed or standardized. Instead, performance measures from groups of individuals are analyzed for patterns of average performance and variability. Well-designed studies, however, reveal the "how it works" information underlying the impairments observed and can be used to generate hypotheses about the neural substrate that might be involved. So far, the focus of these studies has only been on areas of weakness for individuals with DS22q11.2 because the goal has largely been to explain the impairment in the interest of eventually developing remedial interventions. Perhaps the most comprehensive such program of experimental work with the DS22q11.2 population so far has come from studies directed by one of us (Tony J. Simon). The details of many of the studies are described elsewhere (Bish, Ferrante, McDonald-McGinn, Zackai, & Simon, 2005; Simon, Bearden, McDonald-McGinn, & Zackai, 2005; Simon, Bish et al., 2005), and so we will review just the main points here.

The cognitive experimental work in those studies is strongly motivated by a theoretical hypothesis influenced by a great deal of work in cognitive psychology, cognitive neuroscience, and clinical neuropsychology. Most of the preceding results were generated from studies of adults, and so, bearing in mind the caveats about atypical neurocognitive development discussed earlier, we had to be aware that predictions based on our hypothesis would not be likely to exactly match the adult patterns. The organizing principle behind the hypotheses is that relatively complex and varied cognitive abilities or impairments might be explained in terms of the function of a small set of "lower level" broadly applicable functions. These are then "co-opted" by new tasks or problems that are presented during development. In this way, they act as the building blocks for the construction of these higher level processes and abilities. A good example is how basic abilities for the representation of objects can form the foundation for simple numerical abilities (e.g., Simon, 1997). This is because simple comparison, estimation, and counting are, at root, tasks requiring the determination of how many objects exist in a set or in each of several sets. These necessarily involve processes related to the representation of objects and searching among sets of objects or locations, among others. The main hypothesis that emerged from our analyses was that many of the key cognitive nonverbal impairments (and to some extent the behavioral and psychiatric ones also) seen in children with DS22q11.2 are, at their most basic level, due to dysfunctions in various aspects of the visual attention system. That is because visual attention is involved in searching for and selecting objects and locations (for a more detailed discussion of this, see Simon, Bish et al., 2005). There is now much evidence (e.g., Corbetta, 1998; Posner & Petersen, 1990) from studies with adults that this system seems to depend primarily on neural circuits in the parietal and frontal lobes of the brain (and somewhat on the cerebellum also) that are referred to as the "frontoparietal network." A small amount of much more recent evidence from studies with children (e.g., Bunge, Dudukovic et al., 2002; Rueda, Posner et al., 2004) suggests that this network also supports the same functions in children, though likely not in exactly the same way, to the same extent, or with the same degree of exclusivity as it does in adults. Therefore, we designed experiments to test the ability of 7- to 14-year-old children with DS22q11.2 and typically developing controls to carry out several tasks that we thought should tap into different functions of this network to a greater or lesser degree. We will discuss each of the domains of processing below.

Visual–Spatial Attention   Our most basic task was one specifically designed to assess a key function of the attention system, namely, the ability to detect objects in the visual environment in the presence of helpful or confusing cues about their location. This is considered the lowest level task in our set of experiments because it requires little or no conceptual information and most directly taps into the workings of the spatial attention system. In the "Cueing" task children saw a central stimulus (a solid black diamond) on either side of which was a square box. Targets were black-and-white diamond checkerboards appearing inside the boxes, and their appearance was cued by a white triangle appearing within the black diamond, pointing either left or right. A valid cue pointed in the same direction as the subsequent appearance of the target, while an invalid cue pointed in the opposite direction (see figure 6.4 for an example). Neutral cues were white diamonds that almost filled the whole black diamond, thus pointing both ways and providing no location information about the upcoming target. The child's task was to press the left button on a button box when a target was detected on the left and the right button for a target on the right (for full task details see Simon, Bearden et al., 2005). Most of the cues correctly predicted the

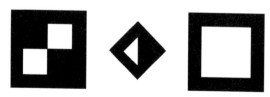

Figure 6.4
Example of stimuli from Cueing task showing valid cue (left-pointing white triangle in center diamond) and checkerboard target on left.

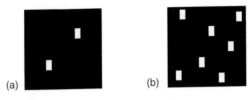

Figure 6.5
Example stimuli from enumeration task for (a) small (subitizing range) and (b) large (counting range) set sizes. (Actual stimuli were green squares on red background.)

target's location, but a small percentage were invalid and required disengagement from the (incorrectly) cued location and reorienting to the correct location of the target. Adults with damage to the posterior parietal lobes (PPLs) have particular difficulty when this disengage function is required. Thus, we predicted that, since that function depends on PPL in adults, it would be likely to produce poorer performance in children with DS22q11.2 on the invalid trials if our frontoparietal network hypothesis was correct. That pattern was exactly what we found and led us to conclude that the "results suggest that children with DS22q11.2. are significantly impaired at navigating the visuospatial environment in the absence of specific indications of where to direct their attention. They are particularly handicapped under conditions where previously allocated attentional resources need to be disengaged and reallocated to other locations in a self-directed fashion" (Simon, Bish et al., 2005).

Enumeration   Our "Enumeration" task (see figure 6.5) related Cueing to numerically related cognition because evidence from adults shows some cognitive processes are common to both tasks. This task is considered higher level than the Cueing task because it requires some conceptual (the number list) and procedural (how to count) knowledge. Regardless of the number of target items presented for enumeration, each must be detected and represented uniquely, designated as a target for enumeration, and subjected to further processing. When the number of items is very small (e.g., fewer than four), children and adults appear to be able to carry out the individuation process rather effortlessly (e.g., Chi & Klahr, 1975; Trick & Pylyshyn, 1993, 1994), just like in our earlier O and Xs example. However, for larger sets it appears that most, if not all, of the targets are processed one at a time or in a series of small groups, just as in our earlier O and Qs example. Each item is chosen as the current target, attention is directed to it, a record is made of having processed it, the next counting word is retrieved, and the total of items processed so far is incremented. The process is repeated until the child decides that all of the items have been dealt with. Counting has been shown, again primarily in adults, to depend on the frontoparietal network, while subitizing, or enumeration of very small sets of items, does not (Piazza, Giacomini, Le Bihan, & Dehaene, 2003; Sathian et al., 1999).

In the task, children were required to respond by speaking into a microphone, as quickly as possible, the number of objects (1–8) that were presented on a computer display. Targets were small bright green squares presented on a red background square (Simon, Bearden et al., 2005). We predicted that subitizing performance would not differ between the groups because we would not expect it to depend on fronto-parietal function, while counting, which we hypothesized would depend on the fron-toparietal network, would be expected to produce poorer performance in children with DS22q11.2 than in controls. That is precisely the pattern that we found, leading us to conclude that the "results again illustrate that self-directed navigation of the visuospatial environment, this time in the service of obtaining a count of the number of items presented, is a particularly difficult and error prone task for children with DS22q11.2" (Simon, Bish et al., 2005).

Magnitude Estimation and Mathematical Reasoning   To further probe the hypothesis that the relationship between space and quantity would be disturbed in children with DS22q11.2 and that this would impair numerical reasoning, we added a magnitude comparison task. This is the highest level in our set of experiments because of the knowledge of quantities and their relationships to one another, as well as some basic reasoning capabilities that are required. We used a numerical "distance effect" task in which children were required to judge whether a set of dots or an Arabic numerical had a value "greater than" or "less than" five. The stimuli consisted of the values "one," "four," "six," and "nine" (for more details, see Simon, Bearden et al., 2005). To respond in the distance effect task, one must first determine the value associated with the stimulus and then retrieve the value of the comparison. Both values are then typically represented as if on a mental "number line" for comparison with the nu-merical "distance" between the two values on the scale determining the difficulty of the comparison. In adults, such tasks appear to be primarily dependent on posterior parietal regions (e.g., Dehaene, Spelke, Pinel, Stanescu, & Tsivkin, 1999; Göbel, Walsh, & Rushworth, 2001; Pinel et al., 1999). Therefore, we predicted that children with DS22q11.2 should perform less well than control children if our hypothesis about frontoparietal dysfunction was correct. Our results indicated that children with DS22q11.2 could not perform as well or accurately as control children when making relative magnitude judgments. We concluded that

this may be due to difficulty in navigating the visuospatial environment (as reported for the cueing task), and in using visuospatial searches to determine numerical quantities (as reported for the enumeration task), which may indicate an anomalous mapping of quantity and space. Those impairments could conceivably create atypical spatial representations of relative magni-tude or "symbolic distance." (Simon, Bish et al., 2005)

In a newer version of this task, we asked children to simply choose the larger of a pair of objects, either bars varying in length differences of 1 to 7 cm or Arabic numbers varying in numerical differences of 1 to 7. Our results, as yet unpublished, show that children with DS22q11.2 require differences between the two values to be much greater than do control children before they find them easy to distinguish from one another. Given that both versions of the task had the same effect, we can conclude the impairment is not one of visual discrimination but one more dependent on the conceptual representation and comparison of quantity. It is as if the visuospatial impairments described above produce a representation system for magnitude that has poorer resolution, that is, with less detail represented, than that of unaffected children, so that subtle distinctions are harder to make. Therefore, much greater differences are required before children with DS22q11.2 can tell two values apart. This, of course, can handicap many aspects of numerical development. Further evidence for this comes from a recently published paper on the perception of time durations in individuals with DS22q11.2 (Debbane, Glaser, Gex-Fabry, & Eliez, 2005). Forty-two affected individuals ages 6–32 years were compared to 35 controls on two tasks. In one, each participant was asked to tap first one and then both index fingers in time with a string of tones. When the tones were stopped, the participants' task was to continue tapping at the same rate. Spacing between tones was varied on different trials. The results showed that individuals with DS22q11.2 consistently tapped more quickly, that is, they estimated the durations between tones to be much shorter than they really were. This was not done by the controls. In the second task, two sounds were presented consecutively and the task was to determine which was longer. Here, just as in our two-option numerical magnitude comparison task, individuals with DS22q11.2 required a much greater difference between the two tones than did controls in order to tell them apart. The fact that Debanné et al. found significant correlations between performance on both of the tasks led them to conclude that "an underlying temporal perception mechanism [was] common to both tasks" (p. 1758).

Our interpretation goes further to concur with an emerging view (e.g., Walsh, 2003) that a common representational and processing system is likely to underlie a large range of magnitude-related tasks (concerning time, space, quantity, intensity, etc). Indeed, there is now a growing body of neuroimaging data from adults that supports this view and that points to the posterior parietal cortex as a critical brain region (e.g., Cohen Kadosh et al., 2005). Further evidence comes from a study of mathematical reasoning carried out using functional magnetic resonance imaging (fMRI) with children who have DS22q11.2 (Eliez, Blasey, Menon et al., 2001). They performed more poorly on simple math problems than those without the deletion and showed less activation than did controls in a posterior parietal brain region, the angular gyrus, that is typically activated by adults during such tasks. They also showed an unusual brain response by showing more activation than controls of the supramarginal gyrus, which is a much less typically activated parietal region when adults carry out such tasks. This suggests that individuals with the deletion may develop an atypical and less effective neural circuit to support mathematical reasoning than do unaffected children and that this may partly explain their struggles in that academic domain. Thus, the data we have reviewed here lead us to conclude that there is considerable evidence in support of our frontoparietal impairment hypothesis and that general magnitude processing, which appears in adults to depend heavily on PPL processing, is an area of particular difficulty for children, and indeed adults too, with DS22q11.2.

Executive Function and Inhibition   We turn now to experimental analysis of executive function, which also plays an important role in the processing required by the spatial and numerical tasks described above. We described earlier how neuropsychological testing studies had showed weaknesses in tests of so-called executive function such as the Trails B. The focus in our experiments was on one aspect of executive function, specifically, children's responses to conflicting information in terms of inhibitory function. In order to test this, we used an adaptation of the ANT previously altered for use with children (Rueda, Fan et al., 2004). It is a single task that tests three related attentional functions: alerting, spatial cueing, and executive control. The ANT requires participants to identify the orientation (left or right) of a specific target, here a friendly green alien in an arrow-shaped spacecraft, either alone (the single condition) or in the presence of two identical characters (referred to as "flankers") on each side that face in the same direction (the congruent condition) or in the opposite direction (the incongruent condition) as the target. (See figure 6.6 for example stimuli). The predicted executive control problems in children with DS22q11.2 were evaluated in two ways using the ANT. First, we investigated whether children with DS22q11.2 demonstrated difficulty with trials containing increasing amounts of conflicting information, that is, a comparison of trials with no flankers, congruent flankers, or incongruent flankers. Slowed response time (RT)

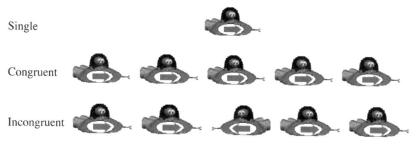

Figure 6.6
Example stimuli from Attentional Networks Test showing single target (top), central target with congruent flankers (center), and central target with incongruent flankers (bottom).

and/or errors on incongruent trials indicate problems with focusing on and processing only task-relevant information and "filtering out" irrelevant information. Second, we investigated dynamic adaptation to conflicting information by examining the Gratton effect (Gratton, Coles, & Donchin, 1992). The Gratton effect is a pattern of more efficient performance (i.e., RT is reduced and accuracy is high) on consecutive identical trials (e.g., two congruent flanker trials in a row) than when the amount of conflicting information changes from trial to trial (e.g., a congruent flanker trial followed by an incongruent flanker trial). Essentially, the Gratton effect measures the ability of the child to benefit from the already established allocation of attentional resources. Processing for tasks like the executive function component of the ANT appears to depend mainly on the anterior portions of the frontoparietal network, particularly the dorsolateral prefrontal cortex as well as the anterior cingulate, though posterior parietal cortex can be involved also (Bish et al., 2005; Bunge et al., 2002). For the flanker trials, we found that both children with DS22q11.2 and controls had significantly more difficulty with incongruent than congruent flankers but that children with DS22q11.2 showed a significantly greater impairment than did controls. This result was essentially a replication of one published using a different variant of the same task (Sobin et al., 2004). Our interpretation was that this indicated "dysfunction of the executive control network, in that children with DS22q11.2 were less able to inhibit the processing of irrelevant information such that it negatively affected their performance" (Simon, Bish et al., 2005). Our further, unexpected, finding that children with DS22q11.2 showed a benefit in performance rather than a cost from the presence of the congruent flankers suggested that they may be unable to narrow the focus of attention to the target item and so processed all the stimuli to the same degree (Bish et al., 2005).

We also found an atypical pattern of conflict monitoring in children with DS22q11.2 on the Gratton effect. Instead of benefiting from inhibition generated in response to incongruent flankers when an identical trial followed and thus performing more efficiently on the following trial, children with DS22q11.2 failed to benefit and their performance was even more negatively affected by the second trial's conflicting information. This led to poorer performance, unlike the controls, who showed the opposite and more typical pattern. We concluded that the results indicate "an inability on the part of children with DS22q11.2 to dynamically respond to a flow of facilitatory or conflicting information and to adjust their attentional resources accordingly, particularly when presented with incongruent distracting stimuli" (Simon, Bish et al., 2005). Patterns similar to this have been observed in individuals with schizophrenia (e.g., van Veen & Carter, 2002), and so it may be the case that individuals with the poorest performance on such tasks could be identified, along with a great deal of related data, as being those with increased risk for psychiatric disorders later in life.

Another similar cognitive measure of this sort tests a behavior known as prepulse inhibition (PPI). This is a psychophysiological measure of what is referred to as "sensorimotor gating". It is so labeled because, when a startle-eliciting stimulus like a loud noise is preceded by a warning signal, frontal brain circuits act to inhibit the startle circuit's response to the noise, probably serving a protective function by suppressing extreme neural signals. As such, it is a good measure of inhibitory function, and studies have shown that it is reduced in children with disorders like Tourette's and fragile X syndromes that are associated with inhibitory impairments. Sobin, Kiley-Brabeck, and Karayiorgou (2005) found that children with DS22q11.2, especially boys, produced a significantly reduced PPI compared with the sibling comparison group, and they interpreted this as indicating impairments in inhibitory function. In some exploratory analyses, they also found that, for children with DS22q11.2, those who had early indicator symptoms associated with schizophrenia had a significantly reduced PPI compared to others without such symptoms.

Another psychophysiologic measure that is also markedly altered in individuals with impairments to executive function or who have schizophrenia is the mismatch negativity (MMN) signal. This is a clear and consistent electrophysiological signal elicited by a discriminable change within a repetitive sequence of auditory stimuli. Possibly the first functional imaging study ever carried out with children who would now be diagnosed with DS22q11.2 (Cheour et al., 1997) showed this signal to be much reduced in 11 affected children ages 6 to 10 years. More recently, a larger study of older children and young adults with DS22q11.2 (Baker, Baldeweg, Sivagnanasundaram, Scambler, & Skuse, 2005) showed a significantly reduced MMN signal in the frontal lobes in those with DS22q11.2 when the dimension of change in the stimuli was its duration but not pitch or a combination of the two. This result not only provides further evidence for executive function impairment but, because the only significant dimension of impaired response was duration, it also links back to problems in DS22q11.2 with the magnitude judgment system. The authors, who were interested in MMN as a signal for schizophrenia risk, also showed a relationship between a reduced MMN signal and the methionine (Met) variant of the COMT gene in their participants with DS22q11.2. However, it should be noted that Met is not the variant that is usually thought to contribute to increased risk for schizophrenia.

Thus, several cognitive experimentation studies of individuals with DS22q11.2 have found different and related impairments in executive function that are also seen in individuals with schizophrenia and so raise the possibility that this kind of measurable cognitive dysfunction could conceivably be a contributing factor to the emergence of schizophrenia later in life. Clearly, impairment on such a task should *not* be taken as any kind of indication that schizophrenia will necessarily follow, but measures such as these, along with a range of other behavioral, biological, and psychophysical observations, might be valuable as a means of assessing very early risk for such psychiatric problems later in life. This might then enable early treatment and follow-up strategies to be developed and evaluated with respect to their effectiveness in suppressing the debilitating symptoms of such disorders.

Summary of Strengths and Weaknesses from Cognitive Experimentation Studies

An increasing number of experimental studies have shown impairments in children with DS22q11.2 that appear to be consistent with the hypothesis of dysfunction in the frontoparietal neural network. Tasks at different levels of complexity that are thought to depend more on the posterior parietal regions, such as visual-attentional orienting or search for objects or locations, simple enumeration, and simple magnitude judgment, all showed characteristic impairments in children with DS22q11.2. Although not every child's performance is identical, difficulties on tasks such as these appear to be particularly consistent in children with the deletion. However, the fact that they are also common in many other populations with so-called "nonverbal learning disorders" means that they are not specific to or diagnostic of the deletion. Tasks that are thought to be more dependent on frontal aspects of the network, such as cognitive control, inhibition of irrelevant information of inappropriate responses, or sensorimotor gating, all showed impairments too. Since there are fewer studies of this sort, the early indications of slightly greater variability in these tasks than those thought to be more dependent on posterior circuits may not be warranted in the long term. However, since many impairments of these so called "frontal" tasks share some characteristics found in populations of people with psychiatric disorders that are more common in the DS22q11.2 population, performance on these tasks and analysis of that variability may serve as an important component of the important task of trying to assess early risk for those disorders.

Neural and Genetic Correlates

Several brain development anomalies characteristic of DS22q11.2 have been noted in recent years due to the increasing availability of magnetic resonance imaging (MRI) scanners for research studies. Developing a clearer picture of what these are might enable researchers to use other data to develop explanatory accounts of anomalous neurocognitive development in DS22q11.2. Some features are easily seen from a clinical scan, while others have been described only as the result of detailed analytical research methods. Examples of the former include enlargements in the sylvian fissure and ventricular spaces (particularly the lateral ventricles) and reductions in the cerebellar vermis. Examples of the latter include reductions in posterior gray and white matter and changes to corpus callosum or other neural connectivity as measured in

Table 6.2
Major brain differences reported in children with chromosome 22q11.2 deletion syndrome

Brain Region	Major Findings	Reference
Sylvian fissure	Increased anterior interopercular distance (left) Reduced gray matter, increased CSF (right)	(Bingham et al., 1997) (Simon, Ding et al., 2005)
Posterior fossa	Reduced fossa and cerebellar vermis Reduced cerebellar vermis, midbrain, and pons Reduced cerebellar vermis, midbrain, and pons	(Mitnick et al., 1994) (Eliez, Schmitt et al., 2001) (Simon, Ding et al., 2005)
Ventricles	Enlarged ventricular spaces (especially lateral ventricles)	(Simon, Ding et al., 2005)
Temporal lobes	Reduced superior temporal gray matter (left) Reduced temporal gray matter (right)	(Eliez, Blasey et al., 2001) (Simon, Ding et al., 2005)
Basal ganglia	Enlarged caudate head (left > right)	(Eliez et al., 2002)
Corpus callosum	Increased fractional anisotropy in posterior corpus callosum to occipital lobes. Increased fractional anisotropy in posterior corpus callosum, parietal, and occipital lobes. Enlarged isthmus Enlarged callosum and all regions but genu	(Barnea-Goraly et al., 2003) (Simon, Ding et al., 2005) (Shashi et al., 2004) (Antshel et al., 2005)

terms of fractional anisotropy, an indirect measure of fiber tract orientation measured with the use of diffusion tensor MRI. Table 6.2 presents the most reliably reported findings in both categories along with representative publications.

We should stress that, at this time, the significance of these neurodevelopmental anomalies remains unclear, especially with respect to their effect on cognition and behavior. However, careful interpretation and use of data from cognitive neuroscience studies, as is done in the cognitive experimentation method, can be a very powerful means of generating hypotheses about the neural substrate of the observed cognitive impairments, so long as the caveats discussed earlier are borne in mind. Thus, while it is important to build up an increasingly sophisticated picture of brain development in children with DS22q11.2, at present the diagnostic implications of that pattern can, at best, only be a contributing factor to explaining the DS22q11.2 phenotype, and it is unlikely that any one feature or pattern of features will be specific enough to be used diagnostically.

Although the precise genetic basis of DS22q11.2 has been described in terms of the size and location of the deletion, there is currently little knowledge about the role of specific genes in the physical or behavioral manifestations of the disorder. However, specific gene variants, both within and outside the chromosome 22q11 region, have also been related to elevated risk of disorders such ADHD, schizophrenia, OCD, and bipolar disorder in the general population, as well as specifically in those with DS22q11.2 (e.g., Karayiorgou et al., 1995; Lachman et al., 1997; Liu et al., 2002; Papolos et al., 1996; Swanson et al., 2001). As discussed above, a good deal of attention has been paid to the role of one gene in particular in the cognitive and behavioral profile of DS22q11.2. The gene coding for the enzyme catechol-O-methyltransferase (COMT) is of particular interest with respect to cognition and behavior to DS22q11.2, given its location in the deleted region of the chromosome in patients with the disorder (Grossman, Emanuel, & Budarf, 1992), and its known role in metabolic degradation of synaptic dopamine and norepinephrine (Lachman et al., 1996), which are critical neurotransmitters in terms of their relation to executive function and disorders related to inhibitory behavior (e.g., Egan et al., 2001). The COMT gene contains a functional polymorphism (Val^{158}Met) that determines high and low activity, respectively, of this enzyme (Lachman et al., 1996). Homozygosity for (i.e., carrying only) the low-activity methionine (Met) allele is associated with a three- to fourfold reduction of COMT enzyme activity compared with those carrying only the high-activity valine (Val) variant, resulting in reduced degradation of synaptic catecholamines in individuals with the Met allele. Although results are somewhat inconsistent, probably due to the ethnicity, ages, and IQ levels of the participants tested, there is evidence to suggest that the Val variant of COMT may be associated in adults with both a slightly increased risk for schizophrenia (Glatt, Faraone, & Tsuang, 2003) and poorer performance on cognitive tasks known to depend on the prefrontal cortex, such as attention, working memory, and executive functions (Bilder et al., 2002; Egan et al., 2001; Malhotra et al., 2002).

Because of this, and of COMT haploinsufficiency (i.e., the absence of one copy of the COMT gene) due to the chromosome 22q11.2 deletion, several authors have linked COMT to some of the behavioral impairments and the elevated incidence of psychosis in DS22q11.2 (Graf et al., 2001; Henry et al., 2002). In the first prospective longitudinal study of this suspected link, Gothelf et al. (2005) demonstrate a clear relationship between the Met allele and increased incidence of psychotic symptoms and more severe decline in VIQ and language abilities and gray matter prefrontal volumes during adolescence. Our own studies (Bearden et al., 2005; Bearden et al., 2004) have shown a link between COMT, executive function, and behavioral symptomatology. The Val allele was associated with poorer performance on a composite executive function measure and with increased scores for behavior problems, especially internalizing and externalizing, on the Child Behavior Checklist (CBCL; Achenbach, 1984). However, the MMN study by Baker et al. (2005), described earlier, showed that their 8 participants with DS22q11.2 who had the Met allele had poorer working memory and expressive language abilities as well as a reduced MMN signal.

A similar, though less fully investigated, relationship to schizophrenia and sensorimotor gating has been proposed for the proline dehydrogenase gene (see Stevens & Murphy, 2005), though Gothelf and colleagues (2005) did not find a similar relationship to the one they reported for COMT. At this point, however, little is really known about the roles of other genes from the chromosome 22q11.2 region in the

DS22q11.2 neurocognitive phenotype. Some further aspects of this relationship are, however, beginning to be discussed (for one example, see Simon, Bish et al., 2005). As is the case with brain structure and function, no single gene or pattern of gene expression differences is currently known to be diagnostic of the DS22q11.2 phenotype, though it is certainly possible that in the near future, a genetic basis for some of the typical and specific features may be found.

Summary

DS22q11.2 is the most commonly occurring microdeletion syndrome known in humans and is one of the most common genetic causes of developmental disability. However, because of (a) the relatively recent characterization of the precise genetic basis of the syndrome and (b) the fact that a large proportion of children with the deletion are only mildly physically affected, the syndrome has a low rate of identification in the general medical community. Furthermore, the cognitive and behavioral implications are still poorly understood. Identification is further complicated by the fact that over 180 physical and behavioral anomalies have been associated with the disorder, and the precise presentation of each individual is a variable combination of those. The lack of a single diagnostic label for individuals with the deletion has only added to the confusion. Of the many signs and symptoms associated with the syndrome, only relatively few are specific to it. Because of this, we have tried in this chapter to identify those and to distinguish them from the nondiagnostic ones. We have also attempted to present typical patterns of the many nonspecific characteristics that may be used to increase the chances of identifying the syndrome, and we have alerted the reader to the variations in those patterns. The first section of the chapter presented the physical diseases that are most diagnostic and then discussed the issue of psychiatric disorders. The two diagnostic case studies described how differently the syndrome can present. Some children can be severely affected with physical disorders and have mild behavioral problems that are common to a range of childhood disorders. Other children can appear quite healthy and even well-adjusted but manifest serious psychiatric disorders, especially as they approach late childhood and early adulthood.

In almost every case of a child with the syndrome there is likely to be some degree of developmental delay, but the pattern is not uniform nor is it specific to DS22q11.2. In fact, children with the deletion are frequently described as having a "nonverbal learning disorder," and this profile is characteristic of children with other neurogenetic disorders with differing behavioral profiles and varying levels of overall intellectual ability (such as Turner, fragile X, and Williams Beuren syndromes) as well as many children with no known disease. Rather, too much attention has been paid to the advantage of verbal over nonverbal abilities that is characteristic of nonverbal learning disorder and typically used to describe most children with DS22q11.2. As shown by several studies described above, this pattern is not manifested by every child with the deletion and is even reversed in a minority of cases, such as the one reported by Stiers et al. (2005). There are also cases of individuals who have the deletion and who present with a radically different behavioral profile, such as the profoundly handicapped female described by Kozma (1998). However, it is likely that in most cases such presentations are due to some insult or injury that is independent of DS22q11.2.

While no behavioral and cognitive profile specifically diagnostic of children with DS22q11.2 exists, neuropsychological testing and cognitive experimentation studies have generated competence patterns that can be used to increase the likelihood of detecting the deletion when considered in conjunction with other features in the physical presentation. One of the most typical patterns is as follows. A marked delay in initial word use is apparent with the child being essentially nonverbal late into his or her second year. The problem often persists in the form of very limited expressive language abilities until at least age 4. Simple rote memory and word reading are in the average range in the early school years, but complex memory (e.g., for stories) and reading comprehension are impaired. These weaknesses are also somewhat persistent beyond that age. In general, a child with the deletion shows significant impairments in all tasks with a spatial component. These include memory for spatial locations (as opposed to details of objects) and tasks involving spatial reasoning (such as the relative locations of objects), visuomotor construction (such as the WISC Block Design task), or any task that requires representing and mentally manipulating the spatial relationships between the parts of an object or between the locations of multiple objects in relation to other objects, or to the child himself or herself. Most aspects of attention will also be impaired, especially the spatial component of attention where the visual field must be scanned or navigated in order to select specific items. Complementary aspects of attention, particularly the "executive" component that helps to control such searches and that is involved in the inhibition or ignoring of irrelevant information, will also show impairments. In the behavioral domain, the child may well show some combination of the inattentive or combined (as opposed to the hyperactive) type of ADHD and shy, stubborn behavior. Such a profile, along with some of the specific and characteristic physical manifestations, will be a strong indication of the presence of the deletion.

Of course, there are many children in whom not all of these difficulties are equally expressed and a minority who even show relative strengths in domains where the majority show weaknesses. This makes the task of identifying the syndrome more complex. In the behavioral domain, less common clues, though ones that occur at a much higher rate than in the general population, include symptoms associated with schizophrenia. However, these are rarely observed before late adolescence. In short,

DS22q11.2 is a complex disorder with considerable variability and changes during development. There are few medical or behavioral symptoms that are specific to the disorder, and so identification is complex. We have attempted in this chapter to broadly describe the most characteristic presentations and to illustrate some of the variations also. If used together, these should help clinicians and other professionals to more easily determine whether a given child is a candidate for the FISH test, which can definitively determine whether or not a diagnosis of DS22q11.2 should be made. A positive result can often be a relief to parents in search of an explanation for their child's constellation of problems and should be used to ensure that the child receives all the medical, behavioral, and cognitive/academic interventions and services to enable the fulfillment of his or her individual potential.

Acknowledgments

First and foremost, we would like to thank the families that have participated in our research programs and those of others whose work we have referenced. Tony J. Simon would also like to thank the team at the 22q and You Center at Children's Hospital of Philadelphia for their support and recruitment of study participants. This work was funded by National Institutes of Health Grant R01HD42974 (Tony J. Simon), an Israel President Ph.D. Stipend (Merav Burg-Malki), and the Keren Shalem Fund for the Development of Services for the Retarded in the Local Councils and Reut Foundation (Doron Gothelf).

References

Achenbach, T. M. (1984). *Child Behavior Checklist*. Burlington: University of Vermont, Department of Psychiatry.

Antshel, K. M., Conchelos, J., Lanzetta, G., Fremont, W., & Kates, W. R. (2005). Behavior and corpus callosum morphology relationships in velocardiofacial syndrome (22q11.2 deletion syndrome). *Psychiatry Research, 138*, 235–245.

Arnold, P. D., Siegel-Bartelt, J., Cytrynbaum, C., Teshima, I., & Schachar, R. (2001). Velo–cardio–facial syndrome: Implications of microdeletion 22q11 for schizophrenia and mood disorders. *American Journal of Medical Genetics, 105*, 354–362.

Baker, K., Baldeweg, T., Sivagnanasundaram, S., Scambler, P., & Skuse, D. (2005). COMT Val108/158 Met modifies mismatch negativity and cognitive function in 22q11 deletion syndrome. *Biological Psychiatry, 58*, 23–31.

Barnea-Goraly, N., Menon, V., Krasnow, B., Ko, A., Reiss, A. L., & Eliez, S. (2003). Investigation of white matter structure in velocardiofacial syndrome: A diffusion tensor imaging study. *American Journal of Psychiatry, 160*, 1863–1869.

Bassett, A. S., Chow, E. W., AbdelMalik, P., Gheorghiu, M., Husted, J., & Weksberg, R. (2003). The schizophrenia phenotype in 22q11 deletion syndrome. *American Journal of Psychiatry, 160*, 1580–1586.

Bassett, A. S., Hodgkinson, K., Chow, E. W., Correia, S., Scutt, L. E., & Weksberg, R. (1998). 22q11 deletion syndrome in adults with schizophrenia. *American Journal of Medical Genetics, 81*, 328–337.

Bayley, N. (1969). *Bayley Scales of Infant Development*. New York: Psychological Corporation.

Bearden, C. E., Jawad, A. F., Lynch, D. R., Monterossso, J. R., Sokol, S., McDonald-McGinn, D. M., et al. (2005). Effects of COMT genotype on behavioral symptomatology in the 22q11.2 deletion syndrome. *Child Neuropsychology, 11,* 109–117.

Bearden, C. E., Jawad, A. F., Lynch, D. R., Sokol, S. M., Kanes, S. J., McDonald-McGinn, D., et al. (2004). Effects of a functional COMT polymorphism on prefrontal cognitive function in the 22q11.2 deletion syndrome. *American Journal of Psychiatry, 161,* 1700–1702.

Bearden, C. E., Woodin, M. F., Wang, P. P., Moss, E., McDonald-McGinn, D., Zackai, E., et al. (2001). The neurocognitive phenotype of the 22q11.2 deletion syndrome: Selective deficit in visual–spatial memory. *Journal of Clinical and Experimental Neuropsychology, 23,* 447–464.

Bilder, R. M., Volavka, J., Czobor, P., Malhotra, A. K., Kennedy, J. L., Ni, X., et al. (2002). Neurocognitive correlates of the COMT Val(158)Met polymorphism in chronic schizophrenia. *Biological Psychiatry, 52,* 701–707.

Bingham, P., Zimmerman, R., McDonald-McGinn, D. M., Driscoll, D. A., Emmanuel, B. S., & Zackai, E. H. (1997). Enlarged sylvian fissures in infants with interstitial deletion of chromosome 22q11.2. *American Journal of Medical Genetics (Neuropsychiatric Genetics), 74,* 538–543.

Bish, J. P., Ferrante, S., McDonald-McGinn, D., Zackai, E., & Simon, T. J. (2005). Maladaptive conflict monitoring as evidence for executive dysfunction in children with chromosome 22q11.2 deletion syndrome. *Developmental Science, 8,* 36–43.

Botto, L. D., May, K., Fernhoff, P. M., Correa, A., Coleman, K., Rasmussen, S. A., et al. (2003). A population-based study of the 22q11.2 deletion: Phenotype, incidence, and contribution to major birth defects in the population. *Pediatrics, 112,* 101–107.

Bunge, S. A., Dudukovic, N. M., Thomason, M. E., Vaidya, C. J., & Gabrieli, J. D. (2002). Immature frontal lobe contributions to cognitive control in children: Evidence from fMRI. *Neuron, 33,* 301–311.

Bunge, S. A., Hazeltine, E., Scanlon, M. D., Rosen, A. C., & Gabrieli, J. D. (2002). Dissociable contributions of prefrontal and parietal cortices to response selection. *NeuroImage, 17,* 1562–1571.

Burn, J., Takao, A., Wilson, D., Cross, I., Momma, K., Wadey, R., et al. (1993). Conotruncal anomaly face syndrome is associated with a deletion within chromosome 22. *Journal of Medical Genetics, 30,* 822–824.

Campbell, L., & Swillen, A. (2005). The cognitive spectrum in velo–cardio–facial syndrome. In K. C. Murphy & P. J. Scambler (Eds.), *Velo–cardio–facial syndrome: A model for understanding microdeletion disorders* (pp. 147–164). Cambridge, England: Cambridge University Press.

Carey, A. H., Kelly, D., Halford, S., Wadey, R., Wilson, D., Goodship, J., et al. (1992). Molecular genetic study of the frequency of monosomy 22q11 in DiGeorge syndrome. *American Journal of Human Genetics, 51,* 964–970.

Cheour, M., Haapanen, M. L., Hukki, J., Ceponiene, R., Kurjenluoma, S., Alho, K., et al. (1997). The first neurophysiological evidence for cognitive brain dysfunctions in children with CATCH. *Neuroreport, 8,* 1785–1787.

Chi, M. T. H., & Klahr, D. (1975). Span and rate of apprehension in children and adults. *Journal of Experimental Child Psychology, 19,* 434–439.

Cohen Kadosh, R., Henik, A., Rubinsten, O., Mohr, H., Dori, H., van de Ven, V., et al. (2005). Are numbers special? The comparison systems of the human brain investigated by fMRI. *Neuropsychologia, 43,* 1238–1248.

Corbetta, M. (1998). Frontoparietal cortical networks for directing attention and the eye to visual locations: Identical, independent or overlapping neural systems? *Proceedings of the National Academy of Sciences, 95,* 831–838.

Debbane, M., Glaser, B., Gex-Fabry, M., & Eliez, S. (2005). Temporal perception in velo–cardio–facial syndrome. *Neuropsychologia, 43,* 1754–1762.

Dehaene, S., Spelke, E. S., Pinel, P., Stanescu, R., & Tsivkin, S. (1999). Sources of mathematical thinking: Behavioral and brain imaging evidence. *Science, 284,* 970–974.

Diamond, A. (2000). Close interaction of motor development and cognitive development and of the cerebellum and prefrontal cortex. *Child Development, 71,* 44–56.

Driscoll, D. A., Budarf, M. L., & Emanuel, B. S. (1992). A genetic etiology for DiGeorge syndrome: Consistent deletions and microdeletions of 22q11. *American Journal of Human Genetics, 50,* 924–933.

Driscoll, D. A., Salvin, J., Sellinger, B., Budarf, M. L., McDonald-McGinn, D. M., Zackai, E. H., & Emanuel, B. S. (1993). Prevalence of 22q11 microdeletions in DiGeorge and velocardiofacial syndromes: Implications for genetic counselling and prenatal diagnosis. *Journal of Medical Genetics, 30,* 813–817.

Driscoll, D. A., Spinner, N. B., Budarf, M. L., McDonald-McGinn, D. M., Zackai, E. H., Goldberg, R. B., et al. (1992). Deletions and microdeletions of 22q11.2 in velo–cardio–facial syndrome. *American Journal of Medical Genetics, 44,* 261–268.

Egan, M. F., Goldberg, T. E., Kolachana, B. S., Callicott, J. H., Mazzanti, C. H., Straub, R. E., et al. (2001). Effect of COMT Val108/158 Met genotype on frontal lobe function and risk for schizophrenia. *Proceedings of the National Academy of Sciences, 98,* 6917–6922.

Eliez, S., Barnea-Goraly, N., Schmitt, E. J., Liu, Y., & Reiss, A. L. (2002). Increased basal ganglia volumes in velo–cardio–facial syndrome (deletion 22q11.2). *Biological Psychiatry, 52,* 68–70.

Eliez, S., Blasey, C. M., Menon, V., White, C. D., Schmitt, J. E., & Reiss, A. L. (2001). Functional brain imaging study of mathematical reasoning abilities in velocardiofacial syndrome (del22q11.2). *Genetics in Medicine, 3,* 49–55.

Eliez, S., Blasey, C. M., Schmitt, E. J., White, C. D., Hu, D., & Reiss, A. L. (2001). Velocardiofacial syndrome: Are structural changes in the temporal and mesial temporal regions related to schizophrenia. *American Journal of Psychiatry, 158,* 447–453.

Eliez, S., Schmitt, J. E., White, C. D., Wells, V. G., & Reiss, A. L. (2001). A quantitative MRI study of posterior fossa development in velocardiofacial syndrome. *Biological Psychiatry, 49,* 540–546.

Feinstein, C., Eliez, S., Blasey, C., & Reiss, A. L. (2002). Psychiatric disorders and behavioral problems in children with velocardiofacial syndrome: Usefulness as phenotypic indicators of schizophrenia risk. *Biological Psychiatry, 51,* 312–318.

Fine, S. E., Weissman, A., Gerdes, M., Pinto-Martin, J., Zackai, E. H., McDonald-McGinn, D. M., & Emanuel, B. S. (2005). Autism spectrum disorders and symptoms in children with molecularly confirmed 22q11.2 deletion syndrome. *Journal of Autism and Developmental Disorders, 35,* 461–470.

Gerdes, M., Solot, C., Wang, P. P., McDonald-McGinn, D. M., & Zackai, E. H. (2001). Taking advantage of early diagnosis: Preschool children with the 22q11.2 deletion. *Genetics in Medicine, 3,* 40–44.

Gerdes, M., Solot, C. B., Wang, P. P., Moss, E. M., LaRossa, D., Randall, P., et al. (1999). Cognitive and behavior profile of preschool children with chromosome 22q11.2 deletion. *American Journal of Medical Genetics, 85,* 127–133.

Giannotti, A., Digilio, M. C., Marino, B., Mingarelli, R., & Dallapiccola, B. (1994). Cayler cardiofacial syndrome and del 22q11: Part of the CATCH22 phenotype. *American Journal of Medical Genetics, 53,* 303–304.

Glaser, B., Mumme, D. L., Blasey, C., Morris, M. A., Dahoun, S. P., Antonarakis, S. E., et al. (2002). Language skills in children with velocardiofacial syndrome (deletion 22q11.2). *Journal of Pediatrics, 140,* 753–758.

Glatt, S. J., Faraone, S. V., & Tsuang, M. T. (2003). Association between a functional catechol O-methyltransferase gene polymorphism and schizophrenia: Meta-analysis of case-control and family-based studies. *American Journal of Psychiatry, 160,* 469–476.

Göbel, S., Walsh, V., & Rushworth, M. F. S. (2001). The mental number line and the human angular gyrus. *NeuroImage, 14,* 1278–1289.

Gothelf, D., Eliez, S., Thompson, T., Hinard, C., Penniman, L., Feinstein, C., et al. (2005). COMT genotype predicts longitudinal cognitive decline and psychosis in 22q11.2 deletion syndrome. *Nature Neuroscience, 8,* 1500–1502.

Gothelf, D., Frisch, A., Munitz, H., Rockah, R., Aviram, A., Mozes, T., et al. (1997). Velocardiofacial manifestations and microdeletions in schizophrenic inpatients. *American Journal of Medical Genetics, 72,* 455–461.

Gothelf, D., Gruber, R., Presburger, G., Dotan, I., Brand-Gothelf, A., Burg, M., et al. (2003). Methylphenidate treatment for attention-deficit/hyperactivity disorder in children and adolescents with velocardiofacial syndrome: An open-label study. *Journal of Clinical Psychiatry, 64,* 1163–1169.

Gothelf, D., Presburger, G., Zohar, A. H., Burg, M., Nahmani, A., Frydman, M., et al. (2004). Obsessive–compulsive disorder in patients with velocardiofacial (22q11 deletion) syndrome. *American Journal of Medical Genetics, 126B,* 99–105.

Graf, W. D., Unis, A. S., Yates, C. M., Sulzbacher, S., Dinulos, M. B., Jack, R. M., et al. (2001). Catecholamines in patients with 22q11.2 deletion syndrome and the low-activity COMT polymorphism. *Neurology, 57,* 410–416.

Gratton, G., Coles, M. G. H., & Donchin, E. (1992). Optimizing the use of information: Strategic control of activation of responses. *Journal of Experimental Psychology: General, 121,* 480–506.

Grossman, M. H., Emanuel, B. S., & Budarf, M. L. (1992). Chromosomal mapping of the human catechol-O-methyltransferase gene to 22q11.2. *Genomics, 12,* 822–825.

Henry, J. C., van Amelsvoort, T., Morris, R. G., Owen, M. J., Murphy, D. G., & Murphy, K. C. (2002). An investigation of the neuropsychological profile in adults with velo–cardio–facial syndrome (VCFS). *Neuropsychologia, 40,* 471–478.

Johnson, M. H., Halit, H., Grice, S. J., & Karmiloff-Smith, A. (2002). Neuroimaging of typical and atypical development: A perspective from multiple levels of analysis. *Developmental Psychopathology, 14,* 521–536.

Karayiorgou, M., Morris, M. A., Morrow, B., Shprintzen, R. J., Goldberg, R., Borrow, J., et al. (1995). Schizophrenia susceptibility associated with interstitial deletions of chromosome 22q11. *Proceedings of the National Academy of Sciences, 92,* 7612–7616.

Kirkpatrick, J. A., Jr., & DiGeorge, A. M. (1968). Congenital absence of the thymus. *American Journal of Roentgenology, Radium Therapy, and Nuclear Medicine, 103,* 32–37.

Korkman, M., Kirk, U., & Kemp, S. (1998). *NEPSY: A neurodevelopmental neuropsychological assessment.* San Antonio, TX: Psychological Corporation.

Kozma, C. (1998). On cognitive variability in velocardiofacial syndrome: Profound mental retardation and autism. *American Journal of Medical Genetics, 81,* 269–270.

Lachman, H. M., Kelsoe, J. R., Remick, R. A., Sadovnick, A. D., Rapaport, M. H., Lin, M., et al. (1997). Linkage studies suggest a possible locus for bipolar disorder near the velo–cardio–facial syndrome region on chromosome 22. *American Journal of Medical Genetics, 74,* 121–128.

Lachman, H. M., Papolos, D. F., Saito, T., Yu, Y. M., Szumlanski, C. L., & Weinshilboum, R. M. (1996). Human catechol-O-methyltransferase pharmacogenetics: Description of a functional polymorphism and its potential application to neuropsychiatric disorders. *Pharmacogenetics, 6,* 243–250.

Lajiness-O'Neill, R. R., Beaulieu, I., Titus, J. B., Asamoah, A., Bigler, E. D., Bawle, E. V., & Pollack, R. (2005). Memory and learning in children with 22q11.2 deletion syndrome: Evidence for ventral and dorsal stream disruption? *Child Neuropsychology, 11,* 55–71.

Liu, H., Heath, S. C., Sobin, C., Roos, J. L., Galke, B. L., Blundell, M. L., et al. (2002). Genetic variation at the 22q11 PRODH2/DGCR6 locus presents an unusual pattern and increases susceptibility to schizophrenia. *Proceedings of the National Academy of Sciences, 99,* 3717–3722.

Malhotra, A. K., Kestler, L. J., Mazzanti, C., Bates, J. A., Goldberg, T., & Goldman, D. (2002). A functional polymorphism in the COMT gene and performance on a test of prefrontal cognition. *American Journal of Psychiatry, 159,* 652–654.

Marino, B., Mileto, F., Digilio, M. C., Carotti, A., & Di Donato, R. (2005). *Congenital cardiovascular disease and velo–cardio–facial syndrome.* Cambridge, England: Cambridge University Press.

McDonald-McGinn, D. M., Driscoll, D. A., Bason, L., Christensen, K., Lynch, D., Sullivan, K., et al. (1995). Autosomal dominant "Opitz" GBBB syndrome due to a 22q11.2 deletion. *American Journal of Medical Genetics, 59,* 103–113.

McDonald-McGinn, D. M., Kirschner, R., Goldmuntz, E., Sullivan, K., Eicher, P., Gerdes, M., et al. (1999). The Philadelphia Story: The 22q11.2 deletion: Report on 250 patients. *Genetic Counselling, 10,* 11–24.

Mitnick, R. J., Bello, J. A., & Shprintzen, R. J. (1994). Brain anomalies in velo–cardio–facial sydrome. *American Journal of Medical Genetics (Neuropsychiatric Genetics), 54,* 100–106.

Moss, E. M., Batshaw, M. L., Solot, C. B., Gerdes, M., McDonald-McGinn, D. M., Driscoll, D. A., et al. (1999). Psychoeducational profile of the 22q11.2 microdeletion: A complex pattern. *Journal of Pediatrics, 134,* 193–198.

Murphy, K. C., Jones, L. A., & Owen, M. J. (1999). High rates of schizophrenia in adults with velo–cardio–facial syndrome. *Archives of General Psychiatry, 56,* 940–945.

Papolos, D. F., Faedda, G. L., Veit, S., Goldberg, R., Morrow, B., Kucherlapati, R., & Shprintzen, R. J. (1996). Bipolar spectrum disorders in patients diagnosed with velo–cardio–facial syndrome: Does a hemizygous deletion of chromosome 22q11 result in bipolar affective disorder? *American Journal of Psychiatry, 153,* 1541–1547.

Piazza, M., Giacomini, E., Le Bihan, D., & Dehaene, S. (2003). Single trial classification of parallel preattentive and serial attentive processing using functional magnetic resonance imaging. *Proceedings of the Royal Society of London, Series B: Biological Sciences, 270,* 1237–1245.

Pinel, P., Le Clec'H, G., van de Moortele, P., Naccache, L., Le Bihan, D., & Dehaene, S. (1999). Eventrelated fMRI analysis of the cerebral circuit for number comparison. *Neuroreport, 10,* 1473–1479.

Posner, M. I., & Petersen, S. E. (1990). The attention system of the human brain. *Annual Review of Neuroscience, 13,* 25–42.

Prinzie, P., Swillen, A., Vogels, A., Kockuyt, V., Curfs, L., Haselager, G., et al. (2002). Personality profiles of youngsters with velo–cardio–facial syndrome. *Genetic Counseling, 13,* 265–280.

Pulver, A. E., Nestadt, G., Goldberg, R., Shprintzen, R. J., Lamacz, M., Wolyniec, P. S., et al. (1994). Psychotic illness in patients diagnosed with velo–cardio–facial syndrome and their relatives. *Journal of Nervous and Mental Disease, 182,* 476–478.

Reynolds, C. R., & Kamphaus, R. W. (1992). *Manual for behavior assessment system for children.* Circle Pine, MN: AGS.

Rueda, M. R., Fan, J., McCandliss, B. D., Halparin, J. D., Gruber, D. B., Lercari, L. P., & Posner, M. I. (2004). Development of attentional networks in childhood. *Neuropsychologia, 42,* 1029–1040.

Rueda, M. R., Posner, M. I., Rothbart, M. K., & Davis-Stober, C. P. (2004). Development of the time course for processing conflict: An event-related potentials study with 4 year olds and adults. *BMC Neuroscience, 5*(1), 39.

Sathian, K., Simon, T. J., Peterson, S., Patel, G. A., Hoffman, J. M., & Grafton, S. T. (1999). Neural evidence linking visual object enumeration and attention. *Journal of Cognitive Neuroscience, 11,* 36–51.

Scherer, N. J., D'Antonio, L. L., & Kalbfleisch, J. H. (1999). Early speech and language development in children with velocardiofacial syndrome. *American Journal of Medical Genetics, 88,* 714–723.

Shashi, V., Muddasani, S., Santos, C. C., Berry, M. N., Kwapil, T. R., Lewandowski, E., & Keshavan, M. S. (2004). Abnormalities of the corpus callosum in nonpsychotic children with chromosome 22q11 deletion syndrome. *NeuroImage, 21,* 1399–1406.

Shprintzen, R. J. (2000). Velo–cardio–facial syndrome: A distinct behavioral phenotype. *Mental Retardation & Developmental Disability Research Reviews, 6,* 142–147.

Shprintzen, R. J. (2005). Velo–cardio–facial syndrome. In S. B. Cassidy & J. E. Allanson (Eds.), *Management of Genetic Syndromes* (second ed., pp. 615–631): Wiley-Liss.

Shprintzen, R. J., Goldberg, R. B., Lewin, M. L., Sidoti, E. J., Berkman, M. D., Argamaso, R. V., & Young, D. (1978). A new syndrome involving cleft palate, cardiac anomalies, typical facies, and learning disabilities: Velo–cardio–facial syndrome. *Cleft Palate Journal, 15,* 56–62.

Shprintzen, R. J., & Golding-Kushner, K. J. (1989). Evaluation of velopharyngeal insufficiency. *Otolaryngologic Clinics of North America, 22,* 519–536.

Simon, T. J. (1997). Reconceptualizing the origins of number knowledge: A "non-numerical" approach. *Cognitive Development, 12,* 349–372.

Simon, T. J., Bearden, C. E., McDonald-McGinn, D. M., & Zackai, E. (2005). Visuospatial and numerical cognitive deficits in children with chromosome 22q11.2 deletion syndrome. *Cortex, 41,* 145–155.

Simon, T. J., Bish, J. P., Bearden, C. E., Ding, L., Ferrante, S., Nguyen, V., et al. (2005). A multiple levels analysis of cognitive dysfunction and psychopathology associated with chromosome 22q11.2 deletion syndrome in children. *Development and Psychopathology, 17,* 753–784.

Simon, T. J., Ding, L., Bish, J. P., McDonald-McGinn, D. M., Zackai, E. H., & Gee, J. (2005). Volumetric, connective, and morphologic changes in the brains of children with chromosome 22q11.2 deletion syndrome: An integrative study. *NeuroImage, 25,* 169–180.

Sobin, C., Kiley-Brabeck, K., Daniels, S., Blundell, M., Anyane-Yeboa, K., & Karayiorgou, M. (2004). Networks of attention in children with the 22q11 deletion syndrome. *Developmental Neuropsychology, 26,* 611–626.

Sobin, C., Kiley-Brabeck, K., Daniels, S., Khuri, J., Taylor, L., Blundell, M., et al. (2005). Neuropsychological characteristics of children with the 22q11 deletion syndrome: A descriptive analysis. *Child Neuropsychology, 11,* 39–53.

Sobin, C., Kiley-Brabeck, K., & Karayiorgou, M. (2005). Lower prepulse inhibition in children with the 22q11 deletion syndrome. *American Journal of Psychiatry, 162,* 1090–1099.

Solot, C. B., Gerdes, M., Kirschner, R. E., McDonald-McGinn, D. M., Moss, E., Woodin, M., et al. (2001). Communication issues in 22q11.2 deletion syndrome: Children at risk. *Genetics in Medicine, 3,* 67–71.

Solot, C. B., Knightly, C., Handler, S. D., Gerdes, M., McDonald-McGinn, D. M., Moss, E., et al. (2000). Communication disorders in the 22Q11.2 microdeletion syndrome. *Journal of Communication Disorders, 33,* 187–203; quiz 203–204.

Stevens, A. F., & Murphy, K. C. (2005). Behavioral and psychiatric disorder in velo–cardio–facial syndrome. In K. C. Murphy & P. Scambler (Eds.), *Velo–cardio–facial syndrome: A model for understanding microdeletion disorders* (pp. 135–146). Cambridge, England: Cambridge University Press.

Stiers, P., Swillen, A., De Smedt, B., Lagae, L., Devriendt, K., D'Agostino, E., et al. (2005). Atypical neuropsychological profile in a boy with 22q11.2 deletion syndrome. *Child Neuropsychology, 11,* 87–108.

Swanson, J., Posner, M., Fosella, J., Wasdell, M., Sommer, T., & Fan, J. (2001). Genes and attention deficit hyperactivity disorder. *Current Psychiatry Reports, 3,* 92–100.

Swillen, A., Devriendt, K., Ghesquiere, P., & Fryns, J. P. (2001). Children with a 22q11 deletion versus children with a speech–language impairment and learning disability: Behavior during primary school age. *Genetic Counseling, 12,* 309–317.

Swillen, A., Vandeputte, L., Cracco, J., Maes, B., Ghesquiere, P., Devriendt, K., & Fryns, J. P. (1999). Neuropsychological, learning and psychosocial profile of primary school aged children with the velo–cardio–facial syndrome (22q11 deletion): Evidence for a nonverbal learning disability? *Child Neuropsychology, 5,* 230–241.

Trick, L. M., & Pylyshyn, Z. W. (1993). What enumeration studies can tell us about spatial attention: Evidence for limited capacity preattentive processing. *Journal of Experimental Psychology: Human Perception and Performance, 19,* 331–351.

Trick, L. M., & Pylyshyn, Z. W. (1994). Why are small and large numbers enumerated differently? A limited capacity preattentive stage in vision. *Psychological Review, 101,* 80–102.

Turner, T. H. (1989). Schizophrenia and mental handicap: An historical review, with implications for further research. *Psychological Medicine, 19,* 301–314.

van Veen, V., & Carter, C. S. (2002). The anterior cingulate as a conflict monitor: fMRI and ERP studies. *Physiology & Behavior, 77,* 477–482.

Walsh, V. (2003). A theory of magnitude: Common cortical metrics of time, space and quantity. *Trends in Cognitive Sciences, 7,* 483–488.

Wang, P. P., Woodin, M. F., Kreps-Falk, R., & Moss, E. M. (2000). Research on behavioral phenotypes: Velocardiofacial syndrome (deletion 22q11.2). *Developmental Medicine & Child Neurology, 42,* 422–427.

Woodin, M. F., Wang, P. P., Aleman, D., McDonald-McGinn, D. M., Zackai, E. H., & Moss, E. M. (2001). Neuropsychological profile of children and adolescents with the 22q11.2 microdeletion. *Genetics in Medicine, 3,* 34–39.

Wulfsberg, E. A., Leana-Cox, J., & Neri, G. (1996). What's in a name? Chromosome 22q abnormalities and the DiGeorge, velocardiofacial, and conotruncal anomalies face syndromes. *American Journal of Medical Genetics, 65,* 317–319.

7 Williams Syndrome

Carolyn B. Mervis and Colleen A. Morris

Williams syndrome is a complex multisystem disorder caused by a ~1.6-Mb deletion of chromosome 7q11.23, containing ~25 genes (Hillier et al., 2003; Osborne, 2006). The prevalence of Williams syndrome is 1/7,500 (Strømme et al., 2002). The Williams syndrome deletion results in a recognizable pattern of physical characteristics including distinctive facial features, supravalvar aortic stenosis (SVAS), connective tissue abnormalities such as hernia or diverticuli of the bladder and colon, and growth deficiency (Morris, 2006b). The articles that led to the syndrome's name (Williams syndrome or Williams–Beuren syndrome) were published by cardiologists reporting on patients who, in addition to SVAS and mental retardation (MR), had similar facial features (J. P. C. Williams et al., 1961; Beuren et al., 1962). Infants and young children with Williams syndrome have developmental delay (DD); older children typically have mild to moderate MR or learning difficulties. Williams syndrome is associated with a specific cognitive profile of relative strength in verbal short-term memory and language and severe weakness in visuospatial construction (Mervis et al., 2000) and an unusual personality profile characterized by overfriendliness, anxiety, and empathy (Klein-Tasman & Mervis, 2003). The personality profile was one of the first to be described as a diagnostic clue (Bennett et al., 1978; Cassidy & Morris, 2002). As shown in table 7.1, all aspects of the Williams syndrome phenotype are variable in expression. In the remainder of this chapter, we describe the physical, medical, and psychological characteristics of children with Williams syndrome and genotype–phenotype correlations in the Williams syndrome critical region (WSCR), stressing both commonalities and individual differences.

Physical Features, Medical Needs, and Diagnosis of Williams Syndrome

In this section, we briefly describe the physical features and medical problems associated with Williams syndrome and the suggested therapeutic interventions. (See also Morris, 2005; Kaplan, 2006; and American Academy of Pediatrics Committee on Genetics, 2001; available at http://aappolicy.aappublications.org/cgi/content/full/

Table 7.1
Prevalence of characteristic medical, cognitive, and behavioral symptoms in children with Williams syndrome (WS) and prevalence of WS among persons with clinical presentation of these symptoms

Symptom	% of Children with WS Who Have This Symptom	% of Children with MR/DD with This Symptom Who Also Have WS*
Medical characteristics		
Cardiovascular disease[a]	80	1–2
Supravalvar aortic stenosis (SVAS)	75	90
Peripheral pulmonic stenosis	50	Low
High blood pressure	50	Low
Urinary tract malformation	35	Low
Hypercalcemia	15	Unknown
Early puberty	50	Low
WS facial gestalt ($\geq 9/17$ features)	100	100
Microcephaly	16	Low
Hypothyroidism	10	Low
Short stature	70	Low
Feeding difficulties	70	Low
Failure to thrive	70	Low
Hoarse voice	95	75
Inguinal hernia	40	Low
Joint laxity	90	Low
Joint limitation	50	Low
Neurological symptoms		
Hyptotonia	80	Low
Chiari I malformation	10	Unknown
Hyperreflexia or spasticity of lower extremities	75	Low
Strabismus	50	Low
Cognitive characteristics		
Developmental delay	100	Very low
Mental retardation	75	3
WS Cognitive Profile[b]	85	~20
Severe visuospatial construction deficit	95	Unknown
Relative strength in verbal short-term memory	90	Unknown
Relative strength in language	90	Unknown
Concrete vocabulary much better than abstract/relational vocabulary	99	Unknown but very low
Reading skills stronger than math skills	>90	Unknown but very low
Behavioral characteristics		
WS Personality Profile[c]	>90	~15
Overly friendly, inappropriate approach	>90	Unknown
Highly empathic	>90	Unknown
DSM–IV anxiety disorder	57[e]	~14[f]
Specific phobia	54[e]	~20[f]
Generalized anxiety disorder	12[e,g]	~20[h]
DSM–IV ADHD	65[e]	~20[f]
Autism spectrum disorder[d]	Low but not insignificant[e]	<1[h]

Table 7.1
(continued)

Note: Percentages in the third column are based on the assumption that 6% of children with mental retar-dation/developmental disability (MR/DD) of genetic etiology have WS (see Strømme et al., 2002) and that 50% of children with MR/DD have a genetic etiology (so, 3% of children with MR/DD have WS). These assumptions are combined with specificity (Sp) information (when available) or percentages for the general intellectual disability (ID) population of children (when available) to yield the percentages or descriptors provided.
[a] For cardiovascular disease entries, comparison group is children who have cardiovascular disease (includes both children with normal intellectual development and children with MR/DD).
[b] Based on specific pattern of performance on Differential Ability Scales or Mullen Scales of Early Learn-ing (Mervis, 2004; Mervis et al., 2000).
[c] Based on specific pattern of parental ratings on Multidimensional Personality Profile or Children's Behav-ior Questionnaire (Klein-Tasman & Mervis, 2003).
[d] Based on the Autism Diagnostic Observation Schedule (ADOS) and the Autism Diagnostic Interview—Revised (ADI-R) combined with clinical judgment.
[e] Leyfer et al. (2006). Percentages are for children ages 4–16 years.
[f] Prevalence for ID child population from Dekker and Koot (2003).
[g] Percentage increases significantly with age: 0% for ages 4–6 years, 13% for ages 7–10 years, 23% for ages 11–16 years (Leyfer et al., 2006).
[h] Prevalence for ID child population from Emerson (2003).

pediatrics;107/5/1192.) Finally, we make suggestions for increasing the likelihood of early diagnosis of Williams syndrome.

Physical Features

One of the cardinal features of Williams syndrome is the unique appearance of the face. An experienced examiner will recognize the facial features in early infancy; by age 12 months, the facial gestalt is evident to many casual observers. All children with Williams syndrome have at least 9 of the following 17 facial features (see figure 7.1): broad brow, bitemporal narrowing, periorbital fullness, epicanthal folds, stellate or lacy iris pattern, strabismus, short upturned nose, full or bulbous nasal tip, malar hypoplasia, long philtrum, full prominent lips (especially the lower lip), full cheeks, wide mouth, small jaw, small and widely spaced teeth, dental malocclusion, and prominent earlobes (Morris, 2006b). Children with Williams syndrome may appear to be younger than chronological age (CA) because they are short, their facial fea-tures seem small relative to head size, and the full cheeks typical of infancy persist (Dilts et al., 1990). The postpubertal child no longer has a low nasal root or full cheeks but develops a prominent supraorbital ridge, the appearance of a long neck, and sloping shoulders. Any of these individual craniofacial features may appear in other conditions associated with DD, but only Williams syndrome is associated with 9 or more.

Medical Problems and Therapeutic Recommendations

Infants with Williams syndrome typically have multiple medical problems. Approxi-mately 50% of neonates are small based on standard growth curves; even those in the

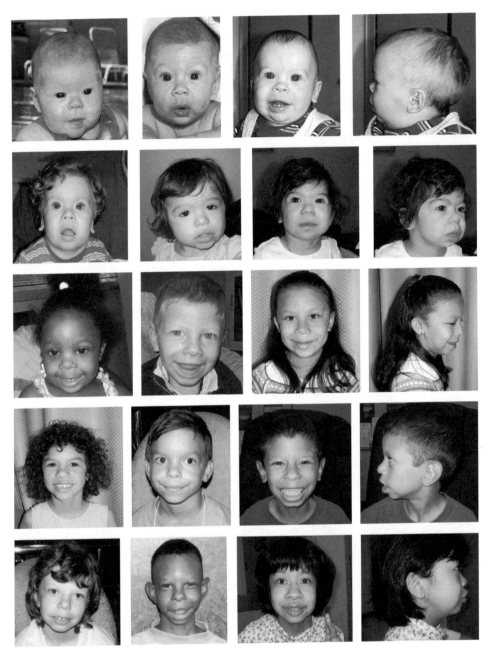

Figure 7.1
Photographs of children with Williams syndrome (WS). All of the children pictured have classic WS deletions. The ages of the children are as follows (from left to right): Row 1, 3 months, 4 months, 9 months;
Row 2, 16 months, 19 months, 19 months; Row 3, 2 years, 3 years, 6 years; Row 4, 5 years, 7 years, 7
years; Row 5, all 11 years.

normal range tend to be small for family background. Microcephaly (small head circumference) is observed in 16% (Morris et al., 1988). The infant is often irritable and typically has feeding difficulties secondary to hypotonia, incoordination of suck and swallow, and tactile defensiveness. Inguinal hernias are present in 40% and are treated surgically. Gastroesophageal reflux (GERD), prolonged colic, and constipation are quite common. Hypercalcemia, which causes irritability and constipation, is likely underdiagnosed; 15% of infants with Williams syndrome who are tested at the appropriate age have high serum calcium. This combination of feeding and gastrointestinal problems leads to failure to thrive in 70% (Morris et al., 1988). Intervention includes both medical treatment and feeding therapy. Mild hypercalcemia may be successfully treated by reducing the amount of calcium in the diet as directed by the pediatrician and monitored by a nutritionist; low-calcium formula is available. Infants with severe or refractory hypercalcemia may be treated with oral steroids or pamidronate infusion (Cagle et al., 2004; Oliveri et al., 2004). Vitamin D supplements are not recommended in infancy or childhood. Though hypercalcemia is most commonly observed in infancy, it can occur at any age. Yearly calcium monitoring is recommended for those who had hypercalcemia in infancy (Kaplan, 2006). If baseline calcium studies in blood and urine are normal, then serum calcium levels should be checked every 2 years in the absence of symptoms (Morris, 2006c). In addition to a yearly urinalysis, random urine calcium to creatinine ratio should be determined.

The growth pattern in Williams syndrome is characterized by prenatal growth deficiency, poor linear growth and weight gain in the first 4 years, a growth rate that is 70% of normal in childhood, and a brief pubertal growth spurt. Stature is short for family background. There is an increased incidence of endocrine problems including hypothyroidism, early puberty, and diabetes mellitus. Growth should be carefully monitored; Williams syndrome–specific growth charts are available (Morris et al., 1988; Pankau et al., 1992; see also http://www.williams-syndrome.org/fordoctors/growthcharts.html). If a child's linear growth decelerates, then an endocrine evaluation is indicated. Thyroid function tests should be obtained every 2–4 years in asymptomatic children.

Most children with Williams syndrome have either normal vision or hyperopia (farsightedness). Strabismus is common, occurring in 30%. Patching will be successful for 50%; the others will require surgical correction. Stereoacuity is often impaired (Sadler et al., 1996). Nevertheless, the significant visual–motor problems associated with Williams syndrome are not due to a primary visual abnormality (Atkinson et al., 2003). Ophthalmologic evaluation is recommended for all children with Williams syndrome.

Chronic otitis media is a problem in 50% of children with Williams syndrome, and half of those are treated with tympanotomy tubes. Recent studies have shown an increased incidence of sensorineural hearing loss in school-age children with Williams syndrome (Gothelf et al., 2006; Marler et al., 2005); this loss is likely progressive

(Marler et al., 2005). Hearing should be routinely tested. Hypersensitivity to sound is reported in ~80% of children with Williams syndrome (Levitin et al., 2005; Van Borsel et al., 1997), and 28% have a specific phobia of loud noise (Leyfer et al., 2006). Auditory training is not recommended. The voice is typically hoarse or deep (Vaux et al., 2003).

Dental problems include missing permanent teeth, microdontia, and malocclusion that usually responds well to orthodontic treatment (Axelsson et al., 2003; Hertzberg et al., 1994). Because there are significant problems with fine motor skills, most children with Williams syndrome require adult assistance with brushing and flossing to maintain dental hygiene. Dental examination and cleaning is recommended every 3 months.

Clinical neuroimaging studies rarely demonstrate structural abnormalities, though researchers employing advances in imaging technology are discovering differences in brain morphology that correlate with functional deficits (Meyer-Lindenberg et al., 2004, 2005, 2006). Chiari I malformation has been reported in a few children and is thought to be due to a mismatch between the size of the posterior fossa and the cerebellum (Kaplan, 2006). Infants with Williams syndrome are hypotonic, and a central hypotonia often persists. The hypotonia and joint laxity contribute to delayed attainment of gross motor milestones, although most children with Williams syndrome walk by age 24 months.

Older children with Williams syndrome typically develop hypertonicity of the lower extremities manifested by increased deep tendon reflexes, tightening of the Achilles tendon contributing to toe walking, and tight hamstrings. Early joint laxity typically resolves, but joint contractures develop in childhood in 50% (Kaplan et al., 1989). The neuromuscular abnormalities lead to the development of compensatory postures to maintain stability. The resultant lordosis, kyphosis, bent knee, and out-toeing culminate in a stiff and awkward gait in older children and adolescents. There is an increased risk for kyphoscoliosis due to central hypotonia complicated by the connective tissue abnormality caused by diminished elastin protein. Children with rapid progression of a spinal curve typically require surgery to avoid cardiopulmonary compromise. Easy fatigability is a common complaint, and leg cramps often occur at night. Supporting the ankles and knees with elastic bandages during times of high physical activity decreases the frequency of leg cramps (Morris, 2005).

Many individuals with Williams syndrome have difficulty navigating curbs, stairs, and transitions from one surface to another. Activities that require fine motor skills, such as tool use, handwriting, and clothes fastening (buttons, shoelaces, zippers), are also challenging. Abnormalities of cerebellar function such as dysmetria, dysdiadokinesis, and ataxia, are often demonstrable on neurological examination (Pober & Szekely, 1999). Early and continued physical and occupational therapy are important to treat these problems. Physical therapy goals initially address walking and balance and later address maintaining joint range of motion and posture. Occupational therapy is useful to address feeding and sensory integration issues in young children and is also necessary for attainment of daily living skills as well as written communication in older children.

Elastin arteriopathy is responsible for the greatest morbidity and mortality in Williams syndrome. The medial layer of the arteries consists of concentric rings of muscle and elastic fibers (lamellar units) that are important for normal blood flow. Due to the deficiency of elastin protein production, there is a compensatory increase in the number of lamellar units in the aorta, resulting in thickening of the arterial wall (Li et al., 1998). Increased pressure is required to pump the blood through narrowed sections, which can lead to hypertrophy of cardiac muscle, heart failure, and death if untreated. The most clinically significant area of narrowing occurs above the aortic valve, and is called supravalvar aortic stenosis (SVAS). SVAS occurs in 75% of individuals with Williams syndrome and requires surgical correction in 30% (Bruno et al., 2003; Kececioglu et al., 1993). Peripheral pulmonic stenosis (PPS), the most common cardiovascular problem in infancy, usually improves over time. The cardiovascular condition is quite variable (Lacro & Smoot, 2006). Children with more significant heart disease come to medical attention at a younger age, and the syndrome is diagnosed earlier. Males are more likely to have severe cardiovascular disease than females (Sadler et al., 2001). Neurovascular abnormalities are rarely reported but may result in stroke (Ardinger et al., 1994; Soper et al., 1995). Hypertension is more common in Williams syndrome and occurs at a younger age than in the general population (Eronen et al., 2002; Giordano et al., 2001). Blood pressure should be checked in both arms at each physician visit and, if elevated, treated medically. Each child with Williams syndrome should be evaluated and monitored by a pediatric cardiologist.

Abdominal pain is a common complaint in children with Williams syndrome. Potential causes include GERD, chronic constipation, hypercalcemia, bowel ischemia secondary to mesenteric artery stenosis, colonic diverticulitis, and celiac disease. GERD is most commonly treated medically, though some children require fundoplication. Constipation should be treated aggressively at all ages. Celiac disease has been reported in 9.6% of children with Williams syndrome compared to 0.5% in the general population and is treated with gluten-restricted diet (Giannotti et al., 2001). Severe abdominal pain should be evaluated promptly to determine if diverticulitis is present. Because arterial supply to the bowel is redundant, mesenteric artery stenosis is rarely symptomatic, but surgical intervention has been required in some cases (Lacro & Smoot, 2006). Rectal prolapse and hemorrhoids occur in children with Williams syndrome and are associated with the chronic constipation.

Urinary tract malformations occur in 35% of children with Williams syndrome. Renal ultrasound is recommended at the time of diagnosis. Bladder diverticuli occur in 40% and may be diagnosed at any age. Bladder capacity is reduced, and over-activity of the detrusor is present in 60% (Sammour et al., 2006), leading to urinary frequency. These difficulties contribute to late toilet training and enuresis. The likelihood of chronic urinary tract infections increases with age and is higher for females.

As described later in the chapter, the incidence of attention deficit/hyperactivity disorder (ADHD) and anxiety is significantly increased in Williams syndrome. Temperament is often difficult; parents may benefit from training in parenting skills for children with special needs. Medication has been successful in treating children with Williams syndrome who have ADHD, anxiety, and specific phobia (Bawden et al., 1997; Dykens, 2003; Power et al., 1997). Sleep is often disturbed, and periodic limb movements, restless legs syndrome, and sleep disordered breathing have been noted (Mason & Arens, 2006). Overnight polysomnography is indicated if there is a history of abnormal sleep; results will direct appropriate treatment.

Enhancing Early Diagnosis

Prior to the availability of a diagnostic test, the mean age of diagnosis of Williams syndrome was 6 years (Morris et al., 1988). The delay in diagnosis is not due to lack of medical attention because the frequency and severity of early medical problems necessitate multiple physician visits in the first year (Morris et al., 1988). If SVAS is discovered, then the diagnosis of Williams syndrome will be considered because although nonsyndromic SVAS is possible, most individuals with SVAS have Williams syndrome (see table 7.1). SVAS may initially be mild, which may delay the appearance of signs or symptoms leading to its detection.

The most common cardiovascular manifestation in early infancy is PPS, a narrowing of the peripheral pulmonary arteries that also occurs in other syndromes, in pre-term infants, and even in typically developing (TD) infants under 6 months of age. PPS typically improves over time. PPS that is associated with failure to thrive, facial features different from the family background, and/or DD should prompt an evaluation for a syndrome diagnosis.

After the first year, as the child's health improves, DD in an undiagnosed child with Williams syndrome may be mistakenly ascribed to early and multiple medical problems. Eventually, the developmental problems will result in a referral for early intervention services, so it is important that therapists be able to recognize the distinctive facial features of Williams syndrome. Another clue to early diagnosis is the striking Williams syndrome behavioral trait of staring intensely at faces (Mervis et al., 2003a). Children with DD and dysmorphic facial features, with or without known birth defects, should always be referred for a genetics evaluation. The diagnosis of Williams syndrome should be suspected in individuals with physical features, medical complications, cognitive profile, and personality profile characteristic of the syndrome.

Box 7.1
Case reports for three 2-year-olds with Williams syndrome*

Case 7.1: Arlene A sonogram at 16 weeks gestation detected intrauterine growth retardation and right-sided cardiac enlargement. Coarctation of the aorta was suspected on a subsequent ultrasound study. The ductus arteriosis closed prematurely at 38 weeks gestation, necessitating a caesarian section. Problems in infancy included right ventricular hypertrophy, irritability, difficulty feeding, and failure to thrive. At age 5 months, cardiac catheterization showed a narrow right outflow tract, moderate hypoplasia of the main pulmonary artery, hypoplasia of the branch pulmonary arteries, and narrowing of the proximal ascending aorta. Arlene was found to have hypercalcemia and mild nephrocalcinosis detected by ultrasound at age 9 months and was treated with low-calcium formula. She was diagnosed with Williams syndrome at age 10 months. She has a history of chronic constipation. Arlene's height, weight, length, and head circumference measurements are all below the 2nd percentile for typically developing children, and her weight is below the 2nd percentile for Williams syndrome. At age 2 years, she continues to be irritable. She has a typical Williams syndrome facies, a hoarse voice, grade III/VI systolic murmur at the upper sternal borders, decreased subcutaneous fat, acrocyanosis, an extra sacral crease, and hypertonicity of the lower extremities.

Arlene's developmental milestones were delayed. She sat independently at 14 months, began to crawl at 15 months, and was not walking at 2 years. On the Mullen Scales of Early Learning (Mullen, 1995), Arlene scored at floor, with severe delays in nonverbal reasoning, fine motor skills, and receptive and expressive language. At 28 months, her mother reported that Arlene produced only 1 word ("woof-woof," said in response to "What does the doggy say?") and understood 28 others. She has no interest in stuffed animals or dolls. Arlene has no fear of strangers; she approaches people she doesn't know indiscriminately. Arlene's mother reported that Arlene has a very difficult temperament; she is quite irritable and has severe behavior problems, including temper tantrums, which make taking her out in public almost impossible.

Case 7.2: Bernice Bernice's mother became pregnant after treatment with fertility drugs. The pregnancy was complicated by preeclampsia. An amniocentesis done for advanced maternal age was normal, 46,XX. Bernice was born by caesarian section at 38 weeks gestation due to fetal distress. She was small for gestational age. Bernice was hospitalized at age 6 weeks for failure to thrive and at that time was found to have branch pulmonary artery stenosis. At age 10 weeks, an echocardiogram detected mild SVAS and mild hypoplasia of the ascending and transverse aorta, and the diagnosis of Williams syndrome was made. Bilateral inguinal herniorrhaphy (hernia repair) was performed. A mildly elevated serum ionized calcium level was detected, but subsequent calcium studies were normal and treatment for hypercalcemia was never required. By age 11 months, Bernice's pulmonary arteries were normal, but the narrowing of the proximal ascending aorta had worsened. At age 23 months, a cardiac catheterization showed restriction of the aortic valve leaflets secondary to a supravalvar ring of the aorta. She had heart surgery to resect a 3-mm section of her aorta, and the aorta was repaired with patches of donor tissue. On the typical growth curves, Bernice's height and weight are at the 5th percentile and her head circumference is at the 10th percentile. She has a typical Williams syndrome facies, systolic ejection murmur and opening click, mild hypotonia, joint laxity, and difficulty with balance.

Bernice's motor milestones were delayed; she began walking at 24 months. Overall, Bernice has mild developmental delay, with a moderate delay in fine motor skills. At $2\frac{1}{2}$ years, she talks in single-word utterances but is able to sing several songs on key. (Both of her parents sing in choirs.) Bernice is very interested in stuffed animals and has a favorite that she carries with her. For the most part, Bernice is very easy going. She is highly social but prefers adults to children. According to her parents, Bernice has never shown any stranger anxiety.

Case 7.3: Cara Cara was born at 39 weeks gestation after an uncomplicated pregnancy. A murmur was noted shortly after birth; the echocardiogram showed a small atypical ventricular septal defect (which subsequently closed spontaneously), patent ductus arteriosis, and possible pulmonic stenosis. Subsequent cardiac evaluation at 6 weeks revealed pulmonary valve stenosis, peripheral pulmonic stenosis, and SVAS, and Cara was diagnosed with Williams syndrome. As an infant,

Box 7.1
(continued)

Cara had chronic otitis media, failure to thrive, and strabismus. At age 18 months, the peripheral pulmonic stenosis had improved, but the SVAS had worsened. Tympanotomy tubes were placed to treat the chronic otitis media. Cara had rectal prolapse as a consequence of constipation and is now treated with Lactulose. On the typically developing curves Cara is at the 10th percentile for height, 25th for weight, and 50th for head circumference. She has a typical Williams syndrome facies, grade II/VI systolic murmur heard best at the upper sternal borders, puffy feet, hyperreflexia in her lower extremities, and mild hypotonia.

Cara's developmental milestones were slightly delayed. She walked at 17 months. On the Mullen, Cara scores in the average range for a typically developing child on all subtests. She is able to stack several blocks and enjoys doing puzzles. At 28 months, Cara has a receptive vocabulary of ~300 words and an expressive vocabulary of ~240 words. She often produces word combinations, including statements such as "I want more sushi please" and questions such as "Where is the binky?" She is starting to enjoy pretend play with toys, especially with a toy farm animal set. Cara is very flexible, likes trying new activities and new foods, and is easy to take out in public. She is very friendly with adults and is beginning to parallel play with typically developing toddlers. She interacts well with her baby brother.

*All names are pseudonyms.

Diagnostic scoring systems have been developed to help the clinician distinguish Williams syndrome from other disorders (American Academy of Pediatrics Committee on Genetics, 2001; Preus, 1984). In a study of 65 individuals who were referred with a previous clinical diagnosis of Williams syndrome but had no deletion demonstrated by fluorescence in situ hybridization (FISH) for any genes in the WSCR, phenotypic features that overlapped Williams syndrome included MR/DD (92%), attention deficit disorder (50%), short stature (30%), and congenital heart defects (25%; Morris et al., 1998). The differential diagnosis for Williams syndrome includes Noonan syndrome, Smith–Magenis syndrome, velocardiofacial syndrome (chromosome 22q11.2 deletion syndrome; see chapter 6), Kabuki syndrome, Coffin–Lowry syndrome, and fetal alcohol syndrome. Each of these has its own distinctive facial gestalt (more difficult to distinguish from Williams syndrome in infancy than in early childhood) but also has some traits that overlap with Williams syndrome (see table 1.1, Morris, 2006b). The diagnosis of Williams syndrome is confirmed by demonstration of a submicroscopic deletion of chromosome 7q11.23, typically by FISH (Lowery et al., 1995). Individuals who do not have a deletion of the WSCR do not have Williams syndrome.

Language, Cognition, Personality, and Behavior

In this section, we consider research on the language and cognitive abilities and personality and behavior characteristics of children with Williams syndrome. To help

Box 7.2
Case reports for three 4-year-olds with Williams syndrome

Case 7.4: Dori   Dori was born at 37 weeks after a pregnancy complicated by fetal growth failure at 28 weeks gestation. As a newborn, Dori had hypoglycemia and umbilical hernia. She also had colic for 4 months and severe constipation and was diagnosed with hypercalcemia (highest serum calcium level 18 mg/dl) at age 9 months, requiring treatment until age $2\frac{1}{2}$ years. Dori was diagnosed with Williams syndrome at age 10 months. She had difficulty with feeding and gaining weight. Dori continues to be a very fussy eater and, even at age 4 years, will only rarely agree to eat if someone other than her mother is feeding her. Dori has peripheral pulmonic stenosis, poor weight gain, constipation, and nephrocalcinosis. On standard growth curves, Dori's height, weight, and head circumference are all below the 2nd percentile, and her head circumference is below the 2nd percentile even on the Williams syndrome curve. Dori has a typical Williams syndrome craniofacies, except that she has occipital flattening resulting in a brachycephalic head shape. She has a grade I/VI systolic murmur, mild pectus excavatum, an umbilical hernia, and an extra sacral crease. Her feet are flat, and she has hyperextensibility of the small joints.

Developmental milestones were quite delayed. Dori began walking at age 28 months. Overall, she has severe developmental delay in all areas. At age 48 months, Dori has an expressive vocabulary size of 4 words (all used very rarely) and a receptive vocabulary size of 47 words; she also understands a number of phrases in context. She is a very sweet child who has a beautiful smile but rarely approaches other people. Dori enjoys cause-and-effect toys, especially if they make music. She also enjoys playing notes on the piano. (Her older brother plays the piano very well.) Dori is able to entertain herself for long periods of time. She was diagnosed with autism (based on the Autism Diagnostic Observation Schedule (ADOS), the Autism Diagnostic Interview—Revised, (ADI-R), and clinical impression) at age 45 months.

Case 7.5: Eileen   Eileen's prenatal ultrasound was normal and she was delivered vaginally at 41 weeks gestation. As an infant, Eileen had episodes of irritability and gagging. Discovery of a heart murmur at age 3 months led to the diagnosis of SVAS and supravalvar pulmonic stenosis. During the cardiac catherization, Eileen had a cardiac arrest requiring 29 minutes of resuscitation. The SVAS was repaired surgically. She was diagnosed with Williams syndrome at age 8 months. Eileen has had surgery for strabismus. She has problems with feeding due to difficulty with certain textures and has had constipation. Eileen requires continued medical management for hypertension. She has had a normal renal ultrasound and normal calcium studies. Eileen's height is at the 3rd percentile and head circumference is at the 25th percentile on the typical growth curves. She has a typical Williams syndrome facies, small widely spaced teeth, a grade V/VI holosystolic murmur heard best in the left upper sternal border and radiating to the left carotid artery, and a thrill in the suprasternal notch. She has mild lordosis and a wide-based gait. Her joints are not hyperextensible.

Eileen had delayed motor milestones. She has mild developmental delay overall, with moderate delay in fine motor skills. Her receptive concrete vocabulary is very good, but she has difficulty with conceptual/relational words. She talks in sentences most of the time. Eileen is highly sociable and very empathic but has mild difficulty maintaining an appropriate social distance. Eileen is inattentive and easily distracted, but she is also easy to redirect. She is very well behaved and enjoys being taken to new places.

Case 7.6: Flora   Flora was delivered vaginally at 40 weeks gestation after labor was induced due to lack of fetal movement. A prenatal ultrasound did not reveal any structural abnormalities, and an amniocentesis performed for advanced maternal age was normal 46,XX. On the first day of life, Flora had some respiratory distress that quickly resolved. As an infant, she had significant colic. She also had constipation that led to an episode of rectal prolapse. In addition, Flora had multiple episodes of otitis media. At age 3 months she was found to have peripheral pulmonic stenosis, which resolved over time.

Flora walked at 13 months, but her parents were concerned because she had difficulty with balance. She was evaluated for developmental delay, which led to a genetic assessment and the diagnosis of Williams syndrome at age 28 months. Her height is at the 5th percentile, weight at the 25th percentile, and head circumference at the 25th percentile on the growth curve for typically

Box 7.2
(continued)

> developing children. She has a typical Williams syndrome facies, an anterior crossbite, a high
> arched palate, husky voice, an extra sacral crease, hyperextensibility of the small joints and the
> knees, and flat feet. She does not have a cardiac murmur and has normal muscle tone for age.
>
> Flora's nonverbal reasoning, receptive language, and expressive language are in the average
> range for typically developing children. Her fine motor skills are in the low-average to mild-delay
> range. She swims very well for her age and also does well in gymnastics. Flora is highly social and
> highly empathic and plays well with typically developing children her age, although she prefers
> adults. Flora has hypersensitivity to loud noises and, likely related to the hypersensitivity, a specific
> phobia of sneezing and coughing; when someone sneezes or coughs loudly, Flora cries hysterically
> and is difficult to calm down even when her parents hold her and reassure her. She also has a short
> attention span and is distractible.
>
> *All names are pseudonyms.

convey both the typical pattern of strengths and weaknesses and the variability seen in Williams syndrome in medical, cognitive, and personality characteristics, we present a series of short case studies of children ages 2 years (box 7.1), 4 years (box 7.2), and 10 years (box 7.3). For each age, we describe three children: one at the lower end of the ability range for Williams syndrome, one in the middle, and one at the upper end. We then present data from our large-sample study of the performance of children with Williams syndrome on standardized assessments and provide a brief review of the literature on language, cognition, personality, and behavior of children with Williams syndrome.

Performance on Standardized Assessments

Standardized assessments provide important information about children's abilities relative to the abilities of same-CA peers. For this reason, an excellent method to begin to convey the variability among children with a particular syndrome is to describe the performance of large groups of children with that syndrome on a variety of standardized assessments. In this section, we consider the performance of the children with Williams syndrome on measures of intelligence, language, and adaptive behavior. Descriptive statistics are presented in table 7.2. To provide visual information regarding the variability in Williams syndrome, histograms for some of the assessments are presented in figures 7.2–7.4. The children included in table 7.2 have classic-length deletions (as do >95% of individuals with Williams syndrome) and have not been diagnosed with ASD; children with ASD or atypical deletions are discussed later in the chapter.

Kaufman Brief Intelligence Test (KBIT)   The KBIT (Kaufman & Kaufman, 1990) is the most widely used assessment of intellectual ability in studies of individuals

Box 7.3
Case reports for three 10-year-olds with Williams syndrome

Case 7.7: Gregory   Gregory was born at 34 weeks gestation after a pregnancy complicated by preterm labor. He was small for gestational age and had transient tachypnea of the newborn and hyperbilirubinemia. Gregory had bilateral inguinal hernias that were repaired. He had significant colic and hypercalcemia in infancy. He had a ventricular septal defect that closed spontaneously. Gregory was diagnosed with Williams syndrome at age $2\frac{1}{2}$ years. Gregory has had multiple orthopedic problems. He wore a brace for scoliosis for 4 years and required several surgical interventions (growing rods) for severe progressive scoliosis. He has an abnormal gait. Gregory's height is at the 10th percentile and his head circumference is at the 50th percentile on the typically developing curves. He is overweight. Gregory has a typical Williams syndrome facies with an especially thick bowed upper lip and an anterior open bite. He has a grade II/VI systolic ejection murmur. He has scoliosis and tight heel cords and hamstrings. Gregory has a bilateral intention tremor that is worse on the left, and he has an abnormal, stiff gait.

Gregory has moderate to severe mental retardation, with better verbal than visuospatial abilities. His adaptive skills are more severely delayed than expected for his intellectual abilities. He rocks repetitively. Gregory speaks in sentences but makes frequent grammatical errors. He is not able to read at all. Gregory is hypersocial and has no understanding of personal space. He has not yet learned to shake hands rather than hug someone as a greeting. Gregory has ADHD, is highly impulsive, and has severe externalizing behaviors; it is very difficult for his mother to manage him on her own. Despite all these difficulties, Gregory is very sweet natured.

Case 7.8: Henry   Henry was born by caesarean section due to fetal distress. An amniocentesis done for advanced maternal age had been normal 46,XY. As an infant, Henry had colic, multiple urinary tract and upper respiratory tract infections, and occasional bouts of otitis media. Coarctation of the aorta was repaired at age 11 months, at which time hypertension and diffuse hypoplasia of the descending aorta were detected. He has been treated for hypertension since infancy. Henry was diagnosed with Williams syndrome at 11 months. An echocardiogram at age 2 years showed discrete narrowing distal to the left subclavian artery, left ventricular hypertrophy, and SVAS. Calcium studies have been normal. Growth has proceeded along the 50th percentile for height, weight, and head circumference on the curves for typically developing children.

Henry's verbal short-term memory is in the average range for typically developing children; his verbal abilities and nonverbal reasoning abilities are in the borderline normal range. Henry's visuospatial construction abilities are considerably weaker. Henry enjoys reading. At the end of third grade, he passed the state competency exams in both reading and writing (using a computer to type his responses) but not in mathematics. He has somewhat limited adaptive skills, in part because his family has not prioritized working on these. He sings quite well; recently he and his younger sister were tested at school and both were found to have relative pitch. (His sister also is an excellent pianist.) Henry is very friendly and sociable and is easy to take places. He understands and respects social distance. The other children at school like him, but he has had a great deal of difficulty making and keeping friends. Henry often pesters his mother. He is a very picky eater. Henry has a specific phobia of loud noises, especially fire alarms. He is very interested in fire engines and firefighters.

Case 7.9: Isaac   Isaac's mother's pregnancy was complicated by poor fetal growth. He was diagnosed with Williams syndrome shortly after birth due to recognition of the facial features. Isaac was found to have mild SVAS and a mildly thickened aortic valve. At age 5 months he had colic and his calcium levels were at the upper level of the normal range. He had many episodes of recurrent otitis media requiring several sets of tympanotomy tubes. Tonsillectomy and adenoidectomy were performed. Isaac also had repair of bilateral inguinal hernias. At age 10 years, he has hypertension that rises in the evening and is treated with Atenolol. He has early signs of puberty. Recent calcium and thyroid studies are normal. Isaac has had a normal renal ultrasound and a normal CT scan of the head. Isaac has complained of abdominal pain. He has developed joint contractures of the lower extremities. Isaac's weight is at the 75th percentile and height is less than the 5th percentile on the typically developing curves; head circumference is at the 50th percentile. He has a

Box 7.3
(continued)

typical Williams syndrome facies. Isaac has a grade I systolic ejection murmur heard at the upper sternal border that radiates to both carotids. His back is straight. His heel cords are tight bilaterally. He has an intention tremor and has hyperreflexia of the lower extremities.

Isaac's verbal and nonverbal reasoning abilities are in the average range for the general population and are significantly stronger than expected for his IQ; his spatial construction abilities are mildly impaired and are significantly lower than expected for his IQ. Isaac's adaptive abilities are in the low-average range for his age; his parents have made achievement of self-help skills a high priority. Isaac has been able to tie his shoes for several years, although he still has difficulty fastening small buttons. He can count change and saves money to buy books about dinosaurs, a special interest of his; he knows more about dinosaurs than do most adults in the general population. Isaac has ADHD—predominantly inattentive type, which is treated with methylphenidate. He reads at grade level and performs slightly below grade level in mathematics. He is very friendly and highly approaching, but he maintains appropriate social distance. Isaac has several typically developing friends, including a best friend. Isaac enjoys going to new places and can be counted on to behave appropriately. He is not interested in music.

*All names are pseudonyms.

with Williams syndrome. The KBIT measures verbal ability and nonverbal reasoning ability but does not assess visuospatial construction, the area of greatest weakness in Williams syndrome. Out of 306 children, 47% earned KBIT composite IQs of 70 or higher and 1% scored 100 or higher. At the other extreme, 3% earned the lowest possible IQ (40). A histogram of the KBIT composite IQs of the 238 participants who completed the KBIT and the Peabody Picture Vocabulary Test (3rd ed.; PPVT–III; Dunn & Dunn, 1997) during the same testing session is shown in figure 7.2.

Differential Ability Scales (DAS)   The DAS (Elliott, 1990) is a full-scale measure of children's abilities that was designed to provide specific information about a child's strengths and weaknesses across a wide range of intellectual activities. The Preschool and School Age forms both yield a General Conceptual Ability (GCA) standard score (similar to IQ), and the Pattern Construction and Recall of Digits subtests are included in both forms. The Preschool DAS includes two clusters: Verbal and Nonverbal (including both nonverbal reasoning and visuospatial construction). The School Age DAS includes three clusters: Verbal, Nonverbal Reasoning, and Spatial. The separation of Nonverbal Reasoning ability from Spatial ability makes the DAS a preferred measure of intellectual ability for children with Williams syndrome, given the extreme weakness that most individuals with Williams syndrome have in visuospatial construction. Figure 7.3 indicates the distribution of GCA scores for the School Age DAS as well as the distribution of Cluster standard scores for each of the three clusters and the distribution of standard scores for the DAS Recall of Digits subtest, which is not included in any of the clusters. This figure makes clear the

Table 7.2
Descriptive statistics for standardized assessments of children and adolescents with Williams syndrome (all children have classic deletions and have not been diagnosed with autism spectrum disorder)

Measure	N	Chronological Age Range (in Years)	Mean Standard Score	SD	Standard Score Range
Kaufman Brief Intelligence Test					
IQ	306	4.01–17.98	69.32	15.35	40[a]–116
Vocabulary	306	4.01–17.98	71.35	16.15	40[a]–110
Matrices	306	4.01–17.98	72.47	16.94	40[a]–112
DAS Preschool and School Age					
General Conceptual Ability	211	4.00–17.77	58.57	12.31	24[a]–94
Pattern Construction T	252	4.00–17.94	23.75	5.39	20[a]–46
Recall of Digits T	286	4.00–17.98	31.78	8.80	20[a]–54
DAS School Age					
General Conceptual Ability	119	8.01–17.77	58.29	12.77	24[a]–94
Verbal Cluster	119	8.01–17.77	70.18	14.16	51[a]–111
Nonverbal Reasoning Cluster	119	8.01–17.77	67.43	11.44	52[a]–100
Spatial Cluster	119	8.01–17.77	55.54	6.86	50[a]–83
Mullen Scales of Early Learning					
Early Learning Composite	79	2.01–4.96	63.44	11.97	49[a]–109
Visual Reception T	79	2.01–4.96	30.46	10.94	20[a]–63
Fine Motor T	79	2.01–4.96	21.48	4.03	20[a]–48
Receptive Language T	79	2.01–4.96	31.81	10.50	20[a]–55
Expressive Language T	79	2.01–4.96	34.59	9.20	20[a]–54
Scales of Independent Behavior—Revised[b]					
Broad Independence	122	4.02–17.77	55.11	15.45	24[a]–95
Motor Skills	122	4.02–17.77	57.82	15.13	24[a]–88
Social Interaction and Communication Skills	122	4.02–17.77	73.16	14.72	30–110
Personal Living Skills	122	4.02–17.77	61.22	14.53	24[a]–98
Community Living Skills	122	4.02–17.77	57.35	17.20	24[a]–96
PPVT–III	238	4.00–17.98	79.85	13.63	40[a]–118
Expressive Vocabulary Test	206	4.00–17.98	70.11	19.03	40[a]–117
Test of Relational Concepts[c]	86	5.00–7.95	55.15	16.45	40[a]–97
Test for Reception of Grammar (2nd ed.)	110	5.00–17.29	70.25	16.33	55[a]–111

Note: For the general population, mean = 100 and SD = 15 for all measures not labeled "T." For measures labeled "T," mean = 50 and SD = 10.
Abbreviations: DAS, Differential Ability Scales; PPVT–III, Peabody Picture Vocabulary Test (3rd ed.).
[a] lowest possible standard score.
[b] Actual lowest possible Scales of Independent Behavior—Revised standard score is 0. All scores <24 were converted to 24, to match the lowest possible standard score for the DAS.
[c] Test of Relational Concepts standard score is usually expressed as a T score but was converted to mean = 100 and SD = 15 to match the standard score range for the PPVT–III. Actual lowest possible Test of Relational Concepts standard score is 0, but all scores <40 were converted to 40 (lowest possible PPVT–III standard score).

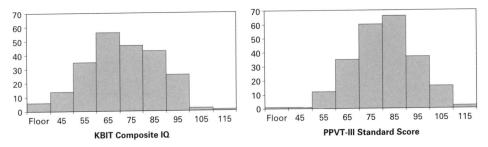

Figure 7.2
Kaufman Brief Intelligence Test (KBIT) IQ and Peabody Picture Vocabulary Test (3rd ed.; PPVT–III) standard scores for 238 children with Williams syndrome, ages 4–17 years, who completed the KBIT and PPVT–III as part of the same assessment. All children have classic deletions and have not been diagnosed with autism spectrum disorder.

extreme weakness in Spatial ability relative to other types of abilities for almost all children with Williams syndrome.

Mean GCA is considerably lower than mean KBIT IQ, and only 18% of children with Williams syndrome earned GCAs of 70 or above on the DAS. The discrepancy is due primarily to the inclusion of visuospatial construction subtests on the DAS. Mean GCA is not a valid indicator of intellectual ability for the majority of children with Williams syndrome; for 80%, Verbal Cluster standard score, Nonverbal Reasoning Cluster standard score, or both was significantly higher than expected for GCA (see also Meyer-Lindenberg et al., 2006); for 11%, both Verbal and Nonverbal Reasoning Cluster standard scores were significantly higher than expected for GCA, and Spatial Cluster standard score was significantly lower than expected. At the other extreme, 2% earned a significantly higher Spatial Cluster standard score than expected for GCA.

We (Frangiskakis et al., 1996; Mervis et al., 2000) used the pattern of performance of individuals with Williams syndrome on the DAS to quantify and test the Williams Syndrome Cognitive Profile (WSCP). Four specific criteria were proposed, focusing on the extreme weakness in visuospatial construction, relative strength in verbal short-term memory, and uneven nature of verbal memory and language abilities relative to visuospatial construction abilities even for individuals with low IQ. Based on a sample of 84 people with Williams syndrome and 56 with other forms of MR or learning disabilities, the WSCP was found to have a sensitivity of .88 and specificity of .92 (Mervis et al., 2000). Mervis et al. also considered the performance of 18 individuals who had been clinically diagnosed with Williams syndrome but later had a negative FISH test (no deletion) so do not actually have Williams syndrome. Only 2 fit the WSCP, yielding a specificity of .89 and providing further evidence that Williams syndrome is a genetic disorder of a single etiology.

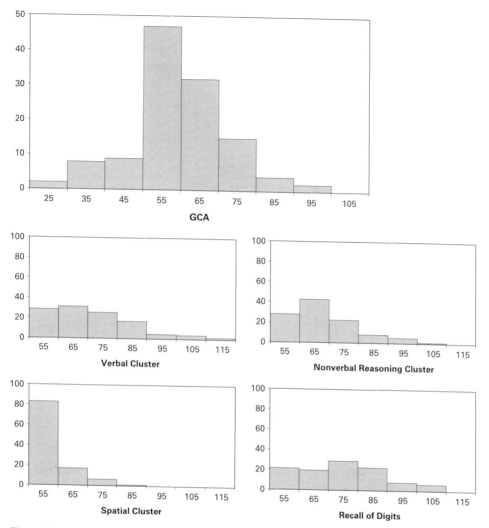

Figure 7.3
Differential Ability Scales (DAS) General Conceptual Ability (GCA) and Verbal Cluster, Nonverbal Reasoning Cluster, Spatial Cluster, and Recall of Digits standard scores for 119 children with Williams syndrome, ages 8–17 years, who completed the School-Age Level of the DAS. Recall of Digits T scores have been converted to the same scale as GCA and Cluster standard scores. All children have classic deletions and have not been diagnosed with autism spectrum disorder.

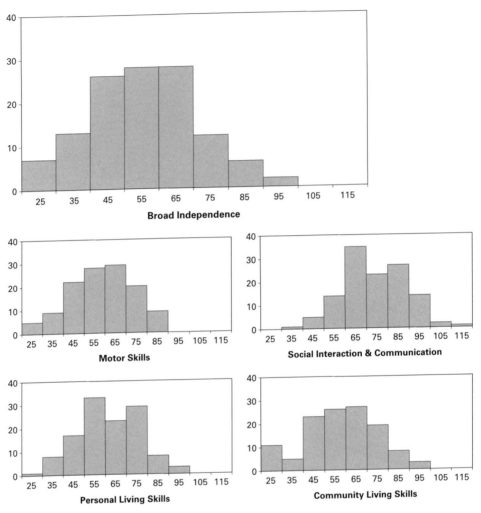

Figure 7.4
Scales of Independent Behavior—Revised Broad Independence, Motor Skills, Social Interaction and Communication Skills, Personal Living Skills, and Community Living Skills standard scores for 122 children with Williams syndrome, ages 4–17 years. All children have classic deletions and have not been diagnosed with autism spectrum disorder.

Mullen Scales of Early Learning (MSEL)   The MSEL (Mullen, 1995) provides a full-scale measure of intelligence for toddlers and preschoolers. As can be seen from the MSEL standard scores in table 7.2, the pattern of performance shown by school-age children with Williams syndrome is present by age 2 years. The area of greatest weakness was the Fine Motor Scale, which measures primarily visuospatial construction; 80% of children earned the lowest possible T score on this subtest. In contrast, children performed relatively well on the language subtests and on the Visual Reception subtest, which measures primarily nonverbal reasoning.

Scales of Independent Behavior—Revised (SIB–R)   The SIB–R (Bruininks et al., 1996) is a caregiver-interview measure of adaptive behavior. Four clusters are included. As is clear from table 7.2 and figure 7.4, there is a wide range of adaptive skills in children with Williams syndrome, with Broad Independence standard score similar to DAS GCA. Also similar to the DAS, performance on the verbally based cluster (Social Interaction and Communication) is considerably better than performance on the clusters for which either motor skills (Motor Skills, Personal Living Skills) or both motor skills and concepts of time and money (Community Living Skills) are critical. Results of earlier studies using the Vineland Adaptive Behavior Scales (Sparrow et al., 1984) indicated the same pattern, with verbally (including socially) based adaptive skills considerably stronger than motor-based adaptive skills (Greer et al., 1997; Mervis et al., 2001).

Adaptive behavior is perhaps the area where caregivers are most able to impact skill development. As described in Box 7.3, parents vary in how much emphasis they put on acquisition of self-help skills; this variation likely affects the child's long-term outcome, as successful employment and (semi-) independent living are heavily dependent on adaptive skills. In many cases, children with Williams syndrome who have normal intellectual abilities have very low adaptive skills because they have resisted learning these skills (which are much harder for them because of the fine motor component) and family members have acceded to the child's wishes.

Peabody Picture Vocabulary Test (3rd ed.; PPVT–III)   The PPVT–III (Dunn & Dunn, 1997) measures receptive single-word vocabulary, focusing on names of objects, actions, or attributes. On average, children with Williams syndrome earn their highest standard score on this measure. The distribution of PPVT–III standard scores for 238 children is shown in figure 7.2, along with the distribution of their KBIT IQs. The majority of children with Williams syndrome (78%) earned standard scores of 70 or higher on the PPVT–III, with 8% scoring at least 100; only one child (<1%) scored at floor.

Expressive Vocabulary Test (EVT)   The EVT (K. T. Williams, 1997) measures expressive single-word vocabulary. The child is asked either to name the object or action depicted in a picture or an attribute of the pictured item (early items) or to produce a synonym for a word provided by the researcher in the context of a picture illustrating the word. The EVT and PPVT–III were co-normed, making it easy to compare standard scores. Most children with Williams syndrome score higher on the PPVT–III than the EVT, most likely because the EVT has the added conceptual requirement of providing a synonym rather than simply naming a picture.

Test of Relational Concepts (TRC)   The TRC (Edmonston & Litchfield Thane, 1988) measures comprehension of five types of abstract relational concepts: temporal (e.g., before/after), quantitative (e.g., many/few), dimensional (e.g., tall/short), spatial (e.g., under/over), and other (e.g., same/different). On average, children with Williams syndrome perform worse on the TRC than on any other measure except those assessing visuospatial construction or self-help skills. All 86 children with Williams syndrome to whom we have administered the TRC scored lower on it than on the PPVT–III; mean difference was 29 points, or about 2 *SD*s. (The TRC yields a T score and has a minimum value of 0; to compare results to the PPVT–III, we have converted TRC T scores to a scale with $M = 100$ and $SD = 15$ and a minimum value of 40.) About 35% of the children earned a standard score of 40 on the TRC; in contrast, none scored less than 50 on the PPVT–III. The difficulty that children with Williams syndrome have with relational concepts is further discussed in the Semantics section later in this chapter.

Test for Reception of Grammar (2nd ed.; TROG–2)   The TROG–2 (Bishop, 2003) measures receptive understanding of grammar. The constructions tested range in difficulty from simple agent-action sentences to sentences containing center-embedded clauses. Mean standard score is similar to those for the EVT and the KBIT. However, this is somewhat misleading because the minimum standard score (earned by 31%) is 15 points higher on the TROG–2. The pattern of performance was similar to that reported by Karmiloff-Smith et al. (1997) for the TROG (Bishop, 1989). Karmiloff-Smith et al. identified particular difficulty for relative and embedded clauses. Zukowski (2004), while arguing that the task demands of the TROG lead to the measure's underestimating the grammatical knowledge of children with Williams syndrome, reported the same difficulty with relative and embedded clauses in an elicited production task.

Summary   Average performance for children with Williams syndrome is in the borderline to mild deficiency range for most measures of language and cognition. However, there is a great deal of variability, with some children performing in the average range for the general population and others performing in the range of severe deficiency. Performance on cognitive and language measures was best for concrete receptive vocabulary and most impaired for visuospatial construction and abstract/

relational language. Pattern of performance on the adaptive behavior measure was similar.

Language Acquisition

Based on her pioneering studies, Bellugi and her colleagues (1988, 1990, 1994) argued that despite severe MR, the language of adolescents with Williams syndrome was normal and showed an excellent command of vocabulary. Jackendoff (1994, p. 117) went further, stating that despite significant MR, the language of children with Williams syndrome "is if anything more fluent and advanced than that of their age-mates." Results of more recent research provide a more nuanced picture and suggest that the claim that the language of individuals with Williams syndrome is much more advanced than expected for people with significant MR was due to the incorrect assumptions that the language of individuals with Down syndrome (DS) could be taken as representative of the language of individuals with MR and that complex grammatical abilities required advanced cognitive abilities (Bates et al., 2001; Mervis, 2006; Mervis & Klein-Tasman, 2000). In the remainder of this section, we briefly review the literature on language development by children with Williams syndrome.

Early Language and Communicative Development Early language acquisition is delayed for almost all children with Williams syndrome. Mervis et al. (2003b) followed 13 children with Williams syndrome (all with classic deletions) longitudinally and found that for all 13, age of acquisition of a 10-word vocabulary was below the 5th percentile (the lowest percentile provided) for the norms for the 680-word Early Vocabulary Checklist included in the Words and Sentences form of the MacArthur Communicative Development Inventory (CDI; Fenson et al., 1993). Age of acquisition of 50- and 100-word vocabularies was below the 5th percentile for 12 of the 13 children. Mean age of acquisition of a 100-word vocabulary was 40.90 months (range: 26.24–68.05 months); the 5th percentile is 26 months for girls and 28 months for boys.

Nevertheless, 30-month-olds with Williams syndrome had significantly larger expressive vocabularies (mean: 132 words; range: 3–391) than CA-matched children with DS (mean: 79 words; range: 0–324), and two boys with Williams syndrome and classic deletions (excluded from the group comparisons because they were outliers) had expressive vocabularies at the 75th percentile on the CDI norms at age 24 months (Mervis & Robinson, 2000). Vicari et al. (2002) compared the early language development of Italian children with Williams syndrome to that of a mental age (MA)-matched but somewhat older DS group and found that the groups had equivalent expressive vocabulary sizes although they differed significantly in grammatical ability and verbal memory ability (see also Volterra et al., 2003).

Several links between specific aspects of early language acquisition and specific aspects of early communicative or cognitive development that previously have been shown to hold for both TD children and children who have DS (see Mervis & Bertrand, 1997) have also been found to hold for children with Williams syndrome. First, the onset of canonical babble (repetition of the same syllable two or more times, e.g., "dada" but not "da") occurs at about the same time as the onset of rhythmic hand banging (Masataka, 2001; Mervis & Bertrand, 1997). Masataka (2001) has argued that rhythmic hand banging may be a rate-limiting control parameter for the emergence of canonical babble. If so, the delay in onset of rhythmic hand banging may contribute to the delay in the onset of language for children with Williams syndrome. Second, the extension of children's early object labels corresponds to their pattern of play with these objects (Mervis, 2006; Mervis & Bertrand, 1997). For example, children in all three groups roll spherical objects, even if they are not balls, and both comprehend and produce "ball" in relation to these objects. These patterns occur even when parents try to correct their children. Third, all three groups begin to sort objects spontaneously at the same time as they begin to fast map object labels (Mervis, 2006; Mervis & Bertrand, 1997). Gopnik and Meltzoff (1987, 1992) argued that these should occur at the same time because they represent parallel insights: All objects belong to some category (cognitive insight) and all objects have a name (linguistic insight).

In contrast, a well-established link between an important early communicative ability (referential pointing) and early language acquisition does not hold for children with Williams syndrome. For TD children and children with DS, the onset of referential pointing occurs prior to the onset of referential language (Adamson, 1995; Mervis & Bertrand, 1997). This sequential ordering is one of the most robust findings in early language acquisition and presumably obtains because the cognitive manifestation of reference (pointing) provides the child with an especially useful way to determine the referents of words. Adults routinely use pointing to identify the referent of the label they provide, and preverbal TD infants and toddlers with DS use pointing to indicate interesting objects and to request labels. In contrast, almost all toddlers with Williams syndrome produce referential language well before they begin to produce or follow referential pointing gestures (Mervis, 2006; Mervis & Bertrand, 1997). Because joint attention to the referent is necessary for the child to acquire object labels, alternative methods of establishing joint attention must be used; Mervis and Bertrand (1997) identified three such methods.

This difficulty with nonverbal communication relative to verbal communication also was evident in two cross-sectional studies of young children with Williams syndrome. Laing et al. (2002) compared the performance of a group of young children with Williams syndrome to that of an MA-matched group of TD infants and toddlers on the Early Social Communication Scales (Mundy et al., 2003) and found that even though they had larger expressive vocabularies than the TD group, the Williams syndrome group was significantly less likely to follow or produce pointing gestures, or to engage in triadic joint attention (attention to both a communicative partner and an object). Rowe et al. (2005) compared the performance of toddlers with Williams syndrome or DS on the Behavior Sample of the Communication and Symbolic Behavior Scales, Developmental Profile (CSBS–DP–BS; Wetherby & Prizant, 2002). Ten toddlers with Williams syndrome were individually matched to toddlers with DS for CA, Developmental Quotient (DQ), and CDI expressive vocabulary size. The two groups did not differ on number of words used during the CSBS–DP–BS. However, there were large between-group differences in nonverbal communication. The children with Williams syndrome showed significantly fewer gaze shifts and significantly fewer episodes of triadic joint attention and used significantly fewer distal gestures (including pointing) or conventional gestures. Mean differences were often dramatic. For example, the mean number of episodes of joint attention was 0.6 (range: 0–4) for the Williams syndrome group but 6.1 (range: 0–18) for the DS group.

Semantics Studies of the semantic development of children with Williams syndrome beyond the preschool years have focused on spatial language and on semantic organization. The literature on these topics is reviewed briefly below.

Spatial language Because spatial language has been proposed to provide clues to nonverbal spatial representation (e.g., Bowerman, 1996), Bellugi et al. (2000) argued that people with Williams syndrome will have much more difficulty with spatial language than with other aspects of language. Bellugi et al. found that adolescents and adults with Williams syndrome made significantly more errors (11%) than an 11-year-old TD group (~0%) on a comprehension test of spatial prepositions. When the participant was asked to describe the spatial position of a colored object relative to a noncolored object, the Williams syndrome group again performed significantly worse. These errors often reflected figure–ground reversals (e.g., saying "The box is in the ball" rather than, "The ball is in the box."). Bellugi et al. interpreted these results as indicating that individuals with Williams syndrome have particular difficulty with spatial language. Landau et al. (2006b) offered a different interpretation, suggesting that these difficulties may instead be due to problems in the alignment of the components of a sentence during the process of sentence production.

The TRC measures several types of relational vocabulary, including spatial terms. Mervis et al. (2003b) compared the TRC performance of 45 5- to 7-year-olds with Williams syndrome and 43 TD 4- to 7-year-olds matched for PPVT–III vocabulary size. The between-groups difference in relational vocabulary size was significant and large. Mervis et al. then matched a Williams syndrome subgroup to a TD subgroup on relational vocabulary size. A comparison of performance on the four major types of relational concepts included in the TRC (spatial, temporal, quantitative, dimensional) indicated no between-group differences. Thus, the relational vocabularies of the two groups contained the same distribution of types of relational concepts, indicating that children with Williams syndrome have difficulty with relational vocabulary in general, rather than specifically with spatial words.

This pattern is consistent with Walsh's (2003) argument that spatial, temporal, and quantitative processing are all governed by a common magnitude system, the posterior section of which is centered in the inferior parietal cortex. Meyer-Lindenberg et al. (2004, 2006) have identified a structural abnormality in the intraparietal sulcus of normal-IQ adults with Williams syndrome (classic deletions) that serves as a roadblock to dorsal stream information flow (including information needed for visuospatial construction) from inferior-posterior to superior-anterior visual processing areas. Path analysis using data from functional magnetic resonance imaging (fMRI) studies indicated that the only difference between the Williams syndrome group and a CA- and IQ-matched group of TD adults was that the path from the intraparietal sulcus to the later dorsal stream region was significant only for the TD group. This finding, combined with Walsh's theory, suggests that individuals with Williams syndrome should have difficulty with spatial, temporal, and quantitative concepts, consistent with the TRC findings.

Landau and Zukowski (2003; Landau et al., 2006b) have also considered the question of the possible effect of difficulties with spatial representation on spatial language in Williams syndrome. They compared the spatial language of 12 children with Williams syndrome (mean CA = 9.6 years) to that of an MA-matched TD group (mean CA = 5.0 years) and a group of college students. Participants described what happened in a series of 80 video clips of events containing spatial relations. In describing figure–ground events, the children with Williams syndrome correctly encoded the figure (main character, typically subject of the sentence) and ground (typically, object of the preposition) more than 99% of the time, reversing the figure and ground less than 1% of the time. The three groups tended to use the same verbs, and the most common path descriptions (typically prepositional phrases) were the same for the three groups. However, the Williams syndrome group was significantly more likely to omit the path description. Landau and Zukowski concluded that children with Williams syndrome have good control over much of the language needed to describe spatial events, including the semantic–syntactic mapping between spatial representation of the event and linguistic structure. They argued that the difficulty with path description is due to spatial memory problems. A recent study of the use of spatial language by Hungarian children with Williams syndrome (Lukács et al., 2004) provides additional evidence that spatial memory problems contribute to the difficulty children with Williams syndrome have with certain types of path descriptions. It is unknown if this pattern of difficulty is restricted to children with Williams syndrome (or other syndromes involving difficulty with visuospatial construction) or is characteristic of MR more generally.

Semantic organization Semantic organization (how an individual cognitively relates the members of a category) is usually measured by word fluency tests in which a person is asked to list as many members of a category specified by the researcher as possible. Bellugi et al. (1994) compared the semantic organization of the category 'animal' for 6 adolescents with Williams syndrome, 6 adolescents with DS matched for IQ and CA, and a group of TD second-graders. The authors concluded that the semantic organization of individuals with Williams syndrome was deviant, based on the finding that they were more likely to name unusual (defined as low-frequency) animals.

The results of more recent studies suggest that semantic organization in Williams syndrome is appropriate. Mervis et al. (1999a) compared the responses of 12 9- and 10-year-olds with Williams syndrome to those of CA- and IQ-matched children with DS, MA-matched TD children, and CA-matched TD children. Children were asked to list all the animals that they could. On seven of the eight measures of semantic organization (including measures of word frequency and representativeness), the Williams syndrome, DS, and MA-matched TD groups performed equivalently. On the remaining measure—the representativeness of the least representative category member named by the child, the Williams syndrome and DS groups performed equivalently to the CA-matched TD group. Volterra et al. (1996) and Temple et al. (2002) also found that the semantic organization of children with Williams syndrome was similar to that of MA-matched TD groups. Levy and Bechar (2003) compared a small group of Israeli children with Williams syndrome to a CA- and IQ-matched group of children with MR of unknown etiology and an MA-matched TD group and found no differences between groups.

Grammatical Ability Grammatical ability often has been considered a particular strength of individuals with Williams syndrome. In fact, the ability of children and adolescents with Williams syndrome to comprehend and produce complex syntax was the primary basis for Bellugi et al.'s claim (1988, 1990, 2000) that Williams syndrome provides a compelling case for the independence of language from cognition. Bellugi et al. demonstrated that constructions such as passives, tag questions, and relative clauses were much more likely to be comprehended and produced by individuals with Williams syndrome than by CA- and IQ-matched individuals with DS. More recent studies comparing the grammatical abilities of English-speaking (Mervis et al., 2003b) and Italian-speaking (Vicari et al., 2004) children have confirmed Bellugi et al.'s findings. However, these results most likely reflect the inordinate difficulties that children with DS have with grammar rather than that children with Williams syndrome have unusually good grammatical abilities. When the contrast groups are either CA- and IQ-matched children with other forms of MR or younger MA-matched TD children, the results of studies of children acquiring English (Grant et al., 2002; Mervis et al., 2003b; Udwin & Yule, 1990; Zukowski, 2004), German (Gosch, Städing, & Pankau, 1994), and Italian (Volterra et al., 1996, 2003) have consistently indicated that the syntactic abilities of children with Williams syndrome are at the level of the comparison group.

Studies of the morphological abilities of English-speaking children with Williams syndrome have focused primarily on the acquisition of the past tense. Researchers agree that by late childhood, most individuals with Williams syndrome reliably mark the past tense correctly on regular verbs but often overregularize the past tense of irregular verbs (e.g., "eated"). Interpretation of these findings is the subject of vigorous debate between researchers favoring a dual-mechanism model of language (Clahsen & Almazan, 1998; Clahsen et al., 2003; Marshall & van der Lely, 2006) and those arguing for a single-mechanism model (M. S. C. Thomas et al., 2001; M. S. C. Thomas & Karmiloff-Smith, 2003). Results of studies of children with Williams syndrome acquiring languages with more complex morphology indicate that morphological ability is similar to or less advanced than those of younger TD children matched for MA (e.g., for French, Karmiloff-Smith et al., 1997; for Hebrew, Levy & Hermon, 2003; for Hungarian, Lukács et al., 2001, 2004).

Pragmatics An area of considerable concern for both parents of children with Williams syndrome and the professionals who serve them is pragmatics, the everyday use of language. Problems with inappropriate initiation of conversation, turn taking, conversational and topic maintenance, appropriate use of eye gaze (looking at the conversational partner rather than looking away), and stereotyped conversations are commonly reported, and improvements in these areas are often targeted as individualized education program (IEP) goals. Despite this concern, there has been little research on pragmatic development. The results of two studies of early communicative development were reported earlier. Two studies of older children and young adults have been conducted using the Children's Communication Checklist (CCC; Bishop, 1998) or the revised version (CCC–2; Bishop, 2002). The CCC and CCC–2 are parent-report measures. Laws and Bishop (2004) compared the pragmatic abilities of 19 children and young adults with Williams syndrome to those of children and adults with DS, children with specific language impairment (SLI), and TD children, as measured by the CCC. Fifteen of the 19 individuals with Williams syndrome scored in the range of pragmatic impairment. The Williams syndrome group evidenced significant difficulties in all five areas of pragmatics measured by the CCC. The use of stereotyped conversations and inappropriate initiation of conversations were particularly problematic. The Williams syndrome and DS groups were both more likely to rely on context to interpret what was said to them and to have difficulty with conversational rapport.

Peregrine et al. (2005) compared the CCC–2 standard scores of 53 6- to 12-year-olds with Williams syndrome to their TD siblings in the same CA range. The sibling group scored significantly higher than the Williams syndrome group ($p < .001$) on the four scales measuring pragmatics (Inappropriate Initiation, Stereotyped Language, Use of Context, Nonverbal Communication) as well as on the six remaining scales, one of which measures Social Relations. Particular difficulties included talking to people too readily; standing too close to people when talking to them; talking repetitively about topics not of interest to others; persisting in asking a question after the answer had been provided; missing the point of jokes, puns, or irony; being confused when a word is used with a different meaning from usual; and taking in only a few words from a sentence, leading to misunderstanding. These difficulties likely contribute to the problems children with Williams syndrome have in forming and maintaining reciprocal relationships with peers despite a strong desire for friendships.

Relations between Language and Cognitive Abilities   Bellugi et al. (1988, 1994) have argued that Williams syndrome is a paradigm case of the independence of language from cognition. In particular, individuals with Williams syndrome comprehend and produce complex syntax and have an unusual command of vocabulary, despite having severe MR. One of the primary pieces of evidence that Bellugi et al. provide for this position is that individuals with Williams syndrome comprehend and produce passive sentences—an ability that had been argued to depend on the ability to conserve (in a Piagetian sense)—yet most adolescents with Williams syndrome could not conserve. More recent research, however suggests both that more than 50% of adolescents and adults with Williams syndrome can conserve (Mervis et al., 2004) and that young TD children who cannot conserve nevertheless comprehend and produce passives (e.g., Allen & Crago, 1996; Brooks & Tomasello, 1999). These findings suggest that the original claim that passive constructions and conservation rely on the same underlying structures is incorrect. Furthermore, results of several studies suggest that rather than language being independent of cognition in Williams syndrome, relations between language and cognition may be even stronger for children with Williams syndrome than for TD children.

Mervis (1999) provided one of the first systematic examinations of the relations between language and cognition in Williams syndrome. In this study, correlations were computed among the raw scores (for memory measures, span length) of a sample of 50 children and adults with Williams syndrome on standardized assessments of vocabulary, grammar, verbal memory, nonverbal reasoning, and visuospatial construction, controlling for CA. All of the correlations were highly significant. Based on a series of additional partial correlations, Mervis found that the strong relations between language abilities and visuospatial construction abilities were mediated by verbal working memory and nonverbal reasoning.

More recent studies have focused on the relations between language and verbal memory and between verbal and nonverbal communication. For TD children and adults, verbal working memory is associated with both vocabulary acquisition (Gathercole & Baddeley, 1989, 1993) and grammatical ability (Kemper et al., 1989; Norman et al., 1992). For children with SLI, the nonword repetition task (measuring phonological short-term memory) has been proposed as a phenotypic marker (Bishop et al., 1996). Similar relations have been found for children with Williams syndrome; in some cases, the relations are stronger than for TD children. Robinson et al. (2003) compared the relations among memory abilities and grammatical abilities for 39 children with Williams syndrome (mean CA = 10.2 years; range: 4.5–16.7 years) and 32 younger TD children matched for TROG raw score. Results of a regression analysis for the children with Williams syndrome indicated that phonological memory contributed uniquely to variance in grammatical scores even after CA, rote memory span, and working memory span were taken into account. This finding is consistent with Grant et al.'s (1997) result that phonological working memory ability is significantly related to receptive vocabulary size in Williams syndrome. Verbal working memory accounted for the largest proportion of variance in grammatical ability, accounting for an additional 10% of the variance after CA, verbal rote memory, and phonological memory were controlled. Furthermore, even after controlling for CA, the correlation between verbal working memory and grammar was significantly stronger for the Williams syndrome group than the TD group, suggesting that children with Williams syndrome may need to rely more heavily than TD children on verbal working memory to puzzle out complex grammatical constructions. For TD children, much of the process of extracting meaning from context is effortless and therefore not limited by working memory capacity. However, for children with Williams syndrome, who have deficits in one or more of the domains necessary for the processing and integration of nonlinguistic cues, more time and effort are needed for meaning extraction, and therefore verbal working memory capacity might be more important for language acquisition. Karmiloff-Smith and her colleagues (e.g., 2003a) have raised the more general possibility that although language development in Williams syndrome may for the most part follow a normal but delayed path, the processes by which language abilities are acquired may not be the same as for TD children. The increased importance of verbal memory in language acquisition is consistent with this possibility.

Several additional studies provide further evidence of relations between memory ability and grammatical ability. Klein and Mervis (1999) compared the performance of 13 9- and 10-year-olds with Williams syndrome to that of CA- and MA-matched children with DS on the McCarthy Scales of Children's Abilities (McCarthy, 1972). The two groups performed equivalently on the verbal scales. However, there were large and significant differences between the groups on verbal memory ability. Consistent with this difference, there was a large difference in the proportion of children who spoke in complete, grammatical sentences: 9/13 of the children with Williams syndrome but only 4/13 of the children with DS. These children were selected from a larger sample; to obtain the matched sample, most of the high functioning children with Williams syndrome (who had the highest memory scores) were excluded as were most of the lowest functioning children with DS (who had the lowest memory scores). Comparison of the full samples revealed an even larger difference: 19/23 children with Williams syndrome but only 4/25 children with DS spoke in complete, grammatically correct sentences (Mervis, 2006). Pléh et al. (2002) considered the relation between verbal memory span and morphological ability for 15 Hungarian children and adolescents with Williams syndrome (mean CA = 13.2 years; range: 5.9–19.6 years). Results based on a median split of digit span indicated that the longer span group performed significantly better than the shorter span group on both regular plural nouns and regular accusative nouns (97% vs. 77%) and irregular plurals and accusatives (90% vs. 61%). The memory span effect remained even after controlling for CA. Digit span also was significantly negatively correlated with number of errors on both regular and irregular morphological forms. Vicari et al. (2002) found that CDI expressive vocabulary size was significantly and strongly correlated with sentence repetition ability for a group of 12 Italian-speaking preschool and early school-age children with Williams syndrome.

Summary   Overall, the language abilities of children with Williams syndrome are at the level expected for general cognitive ability. The apparent difficulty with spatial language is due to a more general difficulty with abstract/relational vocabulary relative to concrete vocabulary and may reflect limitations in spatial memory. Grammatical abilities may be more dependent on verbal working memory for children with Williams syndrome than for TD children.

Cognition

Studies of the nonlinguistic cognitive abilities of children and adolescents with Williams syndrome have focused on memory and spatial cognition. An additional topic on which there is relatively little research but a great deal of media attention is musicality. Research on these topics is reviewed below.

Memory   As we described previously, the cognitive profile for Williams syndrome is characterized by relative strength in verbal short-term memory (typically measured by forward digit recall) and language and severe weakness in visuospatial construction. Given this pattern, individuals with Williams syndrome would be predicted to have significantly better verbal memory than spatial memory. Individuals with Williams syndrome might also be expected to have significantly better verbal memory and significantly weaker spatial memory than CA- and IQ-matched individuals who have other forms of MR. In this section, we review studies in which the contrast groups were matched to the Williams syndrome group for CA and IQ. Many studies have used a contrast group of considerably younger TD children matched for MA. There are serious methodological problems with these studies that make the results very difficult to interpret. In particular, contrary to the assumptions on which this design is based, younger (TD) children who have the same MA (or level of verbal or nonverbal ability) as older children or adolescents with Williams syndrome (or any other form of MR) should be predicted to have better verbal memory abilities (see figure 1 in Mervis & Robinson, 2005) than the MR group. That is, the assumption that if groups of different CAs are matched for MA then they should be expected in principle to perform at the same level on any other cognitive or linguistic measure is incorrect (see discussion in Mervis & Robinson, 2005; Mervis & Klein-Tasman, 2004). For this reason, we have not included studies in which the contrast groups are not matched for CA. These studies are reviewed in Rowe and Mervis (2006), along with a discussion of methodological problems. Note that the problem with designs that do not match for CA and IQ applies to studies of all aspects of intellectual development, although the problem is particularly acute for studies of memory, as shown in figure 1 in Mervis and Robinson (2005).

Verbal memory   Most studies of the verbal memory abilities of children and/or adolescents with Williams syndrome have focused on forward digit recall (rote memory for strings of digits presented once, usually at a rate of 1 digit per second). Four of these studies included a CA- and MA- (or IQ-) matched group with DS (Edgin, 2003; Klein & Mervis, 1999; Vicari et al., 2004; P. P. Wang & Bellugi, 1994). The results were consistent: The Williams syndrome group had significantly better forward digit recall than the DS group. In a fifth study, the list-learning skills of adolescents with Williams syndrome were compared to those of CA-matched adolescents with DS (Nichols et al., 2004). The Williams syndrome group performed significantly better than the DS group on initial recall of both the first (target) list and the interference list.

Although these findings are typically interpreted as indicating a strength in verbal memory for individuals with Williams syndrome, another possible interpretation is that the apparent Williams syndrome advantage is an artifact of the unusual difficulty individuals with DS have with digit recall. Thus, comparisons of the memory abilities of individuals with Williams syndrome to those of well-matched individuals with other forms of MR are important. Two such studies have been conducted, one involving CA- and MA-matched children with MR of mixed etiology (ME; Udwin & Yule, 1991) and one involving CA- and IQ-matched adults with MR of unknown etiology (Devenny et al., 2004). In both studies, the Williams syndrome group had significantly better forward digit recall than the contrast group, indicating that forward digit recall is indeed a relative strength for individuals with Williams syndrome.

Devenny et al. (2004), Edgin (2003), and P. P. Wang and Bellugi (1994) also measured backward digit recall (repetition of the list of numbers provided by the researcher in reverse order). In all three studies, the Williams syndrome group performed better than the matched DS group, but the difference was not significant. Although this could be because of low statistical power, the contrasting finding of reliably significant between-group differences in the same studies for forward digit recall indicates that at a minimum, group differences are more reliable for forward digit recall, which does not require mental manipulation of items in memory, than for backward digit recall, which does require mental manipulation.

Spatial memory   The most common measure of spatial memory in studies that include a Williams syndrome group is the Corsi block-tapping task (Milner, 1971), which involves a board containing nine randomly arranged same-colored blocks. This task is parallel to digit recall tasks, except that rather than saying numbers, the researcher taps a sequence of blocks, and the participant's task is to tap the same blocks, in the same sequence. Participants in three of the studies testing verbal memory also completed the Corsi block-tapping task. P. P. Wang and Bellugi (1994) and Edgin (2003) found that the Williams syndrome group performed significantly worse than the DS group on the Corsi task. Vicari et al. (2004) also reported that the Williams syndrome group did not perform as well as the DS group; however, the difference was not significant. The only study of backward spatial recall was performed by Edgin (2003). The performance of the Williams syndrome and DS groups was almost identical.

In summary, the performance of individuals with Williams syndrome on forward Corsi recall was considerably weaker than the performance of matched groups of individuals with DS. In contrast, performance on backward Corsi recall was highly similar. Because three studies included measures of both forward digit recall and forward Corsi recall, researchers were able to compare performance across verbal and spatial memory tasks. Results consistently indicated that the Williams syndrome group performed significantly better on the verbal memory task than on the spatial memory task, paralleling findings that verbal abilities are considerably stronger than visuospatial constructive abilities for individuals with Williams syndrome.

Spatial Cognition   Research on the spatial cognitive abilities of children and adolescents with Williams syndrome has focused on drawing, visual perception, and visuospatial construction. Each topic is reviewed briefly below. For a more detailed summary, see Farran and Jarrold (2003).

Drawing Bellugi and her colleagues (e.g., Bellugi et al., 1988, 1994) have provided a number of illustrations of the difficulties children and adolescents with Williams syndrome have with drawing. When asked to draw an object (e.g., a bicycle or an elephant), the Williams syndrome group drew a series of parts scattered about the page; most of the parts were identifiable only if the participant provided a label (see figure 11.1 in Bellugi et al., 1988). When asked to copy a shape composed of small items of a different shape (e.g., a square [global shape] composed of small circles [local parts]), the Williams syndrome group typically drew several of the smaller shapes scattered over the page, whereas the DS group typically drew the outline of the larger shape (Bihrle et al., 1989). Bellugi et al. have argued that drawings like these indicate that individuals with Williams syndrome are local processors.

Research on very young TD children, however, has shown that such drawings are part of the normal process of learning to draw (e.g., Bertrand et al., 1997; Cox, 1934 [cited in Freeman, 1980]; Tada & Stiles-Davis, 1989). Results of a recent study of the geometric drawing abilities of 6- to 14-year-olds with Williams syndrome (Georgo-poulos et al., 2004) indicated that the quality of their drawings was similar to that of younger TD children matched for nonverbal MA. Two of the items were large shapes composed of smaller shapes; for these items, the children with Williams syndrome were more likely than the TD children to draw only the global (outline) shape; several children with Williams syndrome correctly represented both the local and the global aspects of the drawings. Bertrand et al. found that the order of difficulty of items on the Test of Visuomotor Integration (VMI; Beery, 1997) was similar for 9- to 10-year-olds with Williams syndrome and younger MA-matched TD children; both conformed to the order intended by Beery. Bertrand and Mervis (1996) reported 4-year follow-up data for 6 of the participants; all showed improvement on the VMI.

The participants in Bertrand et al. (1997) and Bertrand and Mervis (1996) were also asked to draw and then copy a flower, an elephant, and a house and to draw a bicycle (the same items as used by Bellugi et al., 1988, 1994). The flower drawings of the children with Williams syndrome were as likely to be recognized as the intended object (flower) or a related object (another kind of plant) as those of the MA-matched TD children. However, the house and elephant drawings of the TD group were considerably more likely to be recognizable than those of the Williams syndrome group. Nevertheless, clear improvement over a 4-year period was shown for all the children with Williams syndrome (Bertrand & Mervis, 1996). An example of considerable progress in drawing ability for a younger child with Williams syndrome is shown in figure 7.5. Overall, the development of drawing skills in Williams syn-

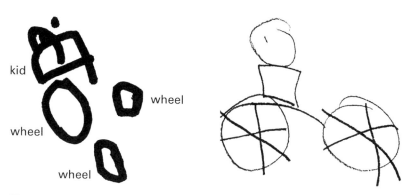

Figure 7.5
Two bicycles drawn by the same girl with Williams syndrome, at age 5 years 9 months (left) and 10 years 9 months (right). Both times, the child was given a blank piece of paper and asked to draw the best bicycle she could. The labels on the left drawing were provided spontaneously by the child.

drome, although considerably delayed, appears to follow the same developmental path as for TD children.

Pattern construction The severe difficulty that most individuals with Williams syndrome have with pattern construction (block design) is apparent in the standard score distribution for the DAS Pattern Construction subtest. As indicated in table 7.2, the mean T score is extremely low; furthermore, more than 50% earned the lowest possible T score. Bellugi et al. (e.g., 1988, 1994) noted that not only were the participants with Williams syndrome unable to copy even the simplest patterns on the Wechsler Intelligence Scale for Children—Revised (Wechsler, 1974) correctly they also did not maintain the overall 2×2 arrangement of the blocks, although they often selected the correct blocks. In contrast, the matched DS group maintained the overall configuration but did not select the correct blocks. These findings were again interpreted as indicating that individuals with Williams syndrome attended to the local elements at the expense of the global arrangement.

More recent results suggest that this conclusion was premature. Ashkoomoff and Stiles (1996) found that broken configurations are part of the normal sequence of learning to copy block patterns. Consistent with this result, Mervis et al. (1999b) found that adults with Williams syndrome were significantly less likely than children to produce broken configurations; the majority of adults did not produce any broken configurations for 2×2 patterns. Furthermore, the proportion of incorrect patterns produced by adults for which the correct block surfaces were used but placed in an incorrect orientation—the type of error closest to the correct pattern—was more than double that for the children. Mervis et al. (1999a) found that ability score on the DAS Pattern Construction subtest was correlated with CA, indicating improvement over time. Hoffman, Landau, and Pagani (2003), in an elegant analysis of the eye movements of 7- to 13-year-old children with Williams syndrome as they worked on a computerized pattern construction task, demonstrated that the difficulty children with Williams syndrome have with pattern construction is not due to executive function (planning and maintaining information in working memory) but rather to problems with spatial representation (incorrect encoding and manipulation of the spatial structure of individual blocks and the spatial relations among the blocks). In particular, the children with Williams syndrome showed the same pattern of checking their constructions against the model and initiating repairs as the MA-matched TD group. However, the Williams syndrome group had considerably more difficulty both in matching individual blocks for pattern and orientation and, if given the correct block, in placing it in the correct position in the copy space. Most of the errors for both groups involved choosing mirror images of blocks that are diagonally divided. The task used by Hoffman et al. minimized the visuomotor demands of pattern construction; blocks clicked into place when put near a possible location, and broken configurations were prevented; see Atkinson et al. (2003) for evidence regarding the impact of visuomotor demands on performance of children with Williams syndrome.

Visual perception   Overall, recent studies suggest that the difficulties children with Williams syndrome have with visuospatial construction, while quite severe, are characteristic also of younger TD children, that performance improves with age, and that the pattern of improvement is consistent with the normal sequence of development. At the same time, these findings suggest that an important part of the difficulty with visuospatial construction involves spatial representation of individual objects, especially those involving oblique representations. Atkinson et al. (2003) identified another type of difficulty with spatial representation: Most children with Williams syndrome have difficulty with perception of form from motion relative to perception of static form in visual noise. As the authors noted, this pattern is part of the normal sequence of development. They also reported a wide range of performance, from children whose responses on both tasks were at the level expected for CA to children who had great difficulty with both tasks.

In contrast, children with Williams syndrome perform relatively well on other types of visual perception tasks. Jordan et al. (2002) found that 9- to 15-year-olds with Williams syndrome were as good as MA-matched TD children at perceiving biological motion in moving point-light displays. Landau et al. (2006a) studied the object recognition abilities of 7- to 15-year-olds with Williams syndrome relative to those of MA- or CA-matched TD children. Color photographs or black-and-white line drawings of objects were presented either in canonical orientation or in an unusual orientation and were either clear or blurred. Performance of the Williams syndrome group was consistent with the MA-matched group in all conditions and with the CA-matched group in the blurred condition.

Musicality The position that Williams syndrome is associated with unusual music talent has emerged more strongly in recent years. For example, a program broadcast nationally in the United States was titled "Williams Syndrome: A Highly Musical Species" (Mons et al., 1996), and Levitin and Bellugi (1998) have suggested that musical ability is higher than cognitive ability in Williams syndrome and may even reflect an independent module of mind. The results of two parental-questionnaire studies indicate that individuals with Williams syndrome are highly interested in music. Levitin et al. (2004) compared the responses of parents of individuals with Williams syndrome, DS, TD, and autism to a questionnaire on musical ability and interest. The Williams syndrome group showed significantly more interest in, and significantly stronger emotional response to, music than the TD and autism groups; was significantly more likely to play rhythmical patterns and to play musical instruments than the autism group; and was more likely to reproduce music accurately and to play musical instruments more often than the DS group. Dykens et al. (2005) compared parental responses for Williams syndrome, DS, and Prader-Willi syndrome (PWS) groups and found that the Williams syndrome group spent significantly more time listening to music than the PWS group and significantly more time than either group playing a musical instrument. The groups did not differ in amount of time spent singing in a choir.

However, high interest in music and the existence of a small proportion of individuals who have musical talent does not indicate that as a group, individuals with Williams syndrome are musically gifted. Recently, concerns have been raised about this characterization (e.g., Carrasco et al., 2005). The results of the few systematic studies of the musical abilities of individuals with Williams syndrome are consistent with this concern. On Gordon's Primary Measures of Music Audiation (Gordon, 1980), performance of the Williams syndrome group on the Rhythm scale was consistent with that of a younger TD group matched for vocabulary age (VA; Don et al., 1999) but below that of a CA-matched TD group (Hopyan et al., 2001). On the Tonal scale, the Williams syndrome group performed significantly worse than both comparison groups. Hopyan et al. also administered the Music Aptitude Profile (Gordon, 1995). On this measure, the Williams syndrome and control groups performed equivalently on identifying which of two phrases sounded nicer and on the easier melodic imagery items. However, the control group performed better than the Williams syndrome group on the more difficult melodic imagery items. On a musical affect task, the Williams syndrome group was significantly less able to indicate the emotional resonance of a musical excerpt than the control group. The authors conclude that although individuals with Williams syndrome do not show special musical skills, they are "engaged by music as a form of spontaneous expression" (p. 49). The claim that individuals with a particular syndrome show unusual aptitude or love for music is not limited to Williams syndrome. For example, White et al. (2004) stated that many parents of children who have Kabuki syndrome reported that their children loved music and were more talented musically than other family members. Levitin et al. (2004) found no difference between the Williams syndrome and DS groups regarding interest in music or emotional response to music. In one of the first studies addressing the question of whether DS is associated with musical ability, Rabensteiner (1975) found that children with DS performed significantly better than children with MR of ME matched for CA and IQ on a test of musicality.

Social Behavior and Psychopathology

The paradoxical nature of social behavior and personality in Williams syndrome was aptly described by von Arnim and Engel (1964, p. 376) more than 40 years ago: "They show outstanding loquacity and a great ability to establish interpersonal contacts. This stands against a background of insecurity and anxiety." To better understand social behavior, personality, and psychopathology in Williams syndrome, researchers have used questionnaires, *Diagnostic and Statistical Manual of Mental Disorders (DSM)* based interviews, and experiments. The findings from each approach are described below. Finally, the occurrence of comorbid ASD in Williams syndrome is briefly addressed.

Questionnaire Studies of Personality and Temperament   The first extensive study of temperament in children with Williams syndrome was conducted by Tomc et al. (1990), who compared parental ratings for 204 children with Williams syndrome (ages 1–12 years) to the general population norms for the CA-appropriate version of a temperament questionnaire based on A. Thomas and Chess's (1977) model. The Williams syndrome group was rated significantly higher on approach, intensity, negative mood, and distractibility, and significantly lower on persistence and threshold of excitability.

Two studies comparing the personality characteristics of children with Williams syndrome to those of children with other syndromes have been reported. Gosch and Pankau (1996, cited in Gosch & Pankau, 1997) asked parents of children with Williams syndrome, DS, or Brachman–de Lange syndrome to rate their child on a series of personality characteristics. The Williams syndrome group was significantly more anxious, more tearful, more curious, and less reserved toward strangers. Van Leishout et al. (1998) compared the personality characteristics of children and adolescents with Williams syndrome to CA-matched TD, fragile X syndrome, and PWS groups using the California Q-set (Block & Block, 1980). The groups did not differ on Extroversion. The syndrome groups scored significantly lower on Emotional Stability and

Openness and significantly higher on Irritability than the TD group but did not differ among themselves. The Williams syndrome group scored significantly lower on Conscientiousness than the TD or fragile X groups and significantly higher on Agreeableness than the PWS group.

To quantify the Williams Syndrome Personality Profile (WSPP), Klein-Tasman and Mervis (2003) compared parental ratings of temperament on the long form of the Children's Behavior Questionnaire (CBQ; Rothbart & Ahadi, 1994) and on the parent-report version of the Multidimensional Personality Questionnaire (MPQ; Tellegen, 1985) for a group of 8- to 10-year-olds with Williams syndrome to a CA- and IQ-matched ME group. The Williams syndrome group was rated as significantly higher on the Empathy, Approach, and Sadness scales and significantly lower on Shyness. This pattern of characteristics (high empathy, high approach, low shyness—or high sociability) fits well with previous descriptions of the personality and behavior of children with Williams syndrome. Using a combination of the ratings for the Empathy, Approach, and Shyness subscales, Klein-Tasman and Mervis were able to correctly classify 21 of 22 children with Williams syndrome and 17 of 20 children in the ME group. Thus, the CBQ WSPP has a sensitivity (Se) of .96 and specificity (Sp) of .85. On the MPQ, the children with Williams syndrome were rated significantly higher on 5 items: gregarious, people-oriented, tense, sensitive, and visible. Using a combination of the ratings for these items, the authors correctly classified 21 of 22 children with Williams syndrome and 17 of 20 children in the ME group, yielding $Se = .96$ and $Sp = .85$ for the MPQ WSPP. Recent analyses of more than 100 additional MPQs we have collected for individuals with Williams syndrome indicated that $Se > .90$ for ages 5–20 years but then decreases considerably. Because a large enough contrast sample was not available, Sp could not be computed.

Doyle et al. (2004) administered the Salk Institute Sociability Questionnaire (Jones et al., 2000) to the parents of 64 1- to 12-year-olds with Williams syndrome and smaller samples of parents of TD children or children with DS. The Williams syndrome group was rated significantly higher that the TD group on all rating scales (Social Emotional, Approach Familiars, Approach Strangers) and on Global Sociability and significantly higher than the DS group on Global Sociability and the Social Emotional and Approach Strangers scales. There was a significant increase in Approach Strangers and in Global Sociability between the youngest (1–3 years) and middle (4–7 years) Williams syndrome groups.

Experimental Studies of Personality   Experimental studies of personality in children with Williams syndrome have focused on empathy, theory of mind (ToM), attention to faces, and interpreting facial expressions. The two studies that have addressed empathy in children with Williams syndrome have used the simulated-distress procedure (Sigman et al., 1992) in which a researcher pretends to injure herself and then displays appropriate facial and vocal expressions for about 30 s. Plesa-Skwerer and Tager-Flusberg (2006) compared the reactions of a group of children with Williams syndrome to a CA- and IQ-matched group of children with PWS. The Williams syndrome group showed significantly more empathy, as measured by expressions of sympathy and help, comforting behavior, and overall level of concern. M. L. Thomas et al. (2002) compared the reactions of a group of 4-year-olds with Williams syndrome to a CA- and DQ-matched ME group and a CA-matched TD group. The Williams syndrome group spent significantly more time looking at the injured researcher and showed significantly more concern than the other groups.

The initial studies of ToM were conducted by Karmiloff-Smith and her colleagues (1995) on individuals with Williams syndrome ages 9–23 years. The majority of participants passed first-order ToM tasks, and some also passed the second-order and higher order tasks, leading the authors to conclude that ToM is "an islet of relatively preserved ability" (p. 202). Tager-Flusberg and Sullivan (2000) questioned these findings on methodological grounds, including the CA of the Williams syndrome group and the lack of a matched comparison group.

Tager-Flusberg and Sullivan (2000) argued that ToM involves both a social–perceptual component (e.g., judging emotion from facial expression) and a social–cognitive component (e.g., understanding the mind as a representational system as judged by more traditional ToM tasks such as false belief). Based on a series of systematic studies, Tager-Flusberg and her colleagues concluded that individuals with Williams syndrome have significant difficulty with both components. To address the social–perceptual component, Plesa-Skwerer et al. (2006a) compared the performance of adolescents and adults with Williams syndrome to a CA- and IQ-matched group with learning or intellectual disabilities (LID) and a CA-matched TD group on the Diagnostic Analysis of Nonverbal Accuracy Scale (DANVA-2; Nowicki & Duke, 1994). The DANVA-2 is a standardized measure of emotion perception as measured by facial or vocal expression (paralanguage). The Williams syndrome and LID groups were both significantly less accurate than the TD group at identifying the emotion expressed by either a facial expression or paralanguage, and the Williams syndrome group was significantly less accurate than the LID group at recognizing emotions expressed by paralanguage. Between-group differences were due to differences in differentiating negative emotions (sad, angry, fearful); there were no group differences in identifying positive (happy) emotion. Overall, the Williams syndrome group correctly identified ~75% of the facial expressions and 61% of the vocal expressions. Plesa-Skwerer et al. (2006b) compared the ability of matched Williams syndrome, LID, and TD groups of adolescents and adults to identify emotions from a revised version of the Eyes task (Baron-Cohen et al., 2001), measuring perception of emotion from the eye region of the face, and from brief dynamic displays of emotion selected from the Mindreaders collection (Baron-Cohen & Tead, 2003). There were no differences between the Williams syndrome and LID groups, and both performed significantly worse than the TD group. Gagliardi et al. (2003) reported a similar pattern, with no differences between a Williams syndrome group (ages 5–32 years) and a MA-matched TD group on identification of emotion from brief dynamic displays; both groups performed significantly worse than a CA-matched TD group. Tager-Flusberg and Sullivan (2000) found that 4- to 8-year-olds with Williams syndrome were no better at matching facial expressions than CA-, IQ-, and VA-matched children with either PWS or MR of unknown etiology.

To address the social–cognitive component of ToM, Tager-Flusberg and her colleagues have conducted a series of studies. In the first, Tager-Flusberg et al. (1997) compared 14 children with Williams syndrome (ages 5–9 years) to a CA- and VA-matched PWS group on a location-change false belief task. Only 43% of the Williams syndrome group and 60% of the PWS group passed this task, which is easily passed by TD 4-year-olds. Tager-Flusberg and Sullivan (2000) compared the performance of a group of children with Williams syndrome (mean CA = 7 years; range: 4–8 years) to that of CA-, IQ-, and VA-matched groups of children with PWS or MR of unknown etiology on both a location-change task and an unexpected-contents task. The Williams syndrome group performed significantly worse than the contrast groups, with only about 25% passing these tasks. When asked to explain the actions of protagonists in short vignettes, children with Williams syndrome were no more likely to provide appropriate mental-state explanations than children in the contrast groups.

Sullivan and Tager-Flusberg (1999) compared the performance of CA-, IQ-, and VA-matched Williams syndrome (mean CA = 11.6 years; range: 8–17 years), PWS, and MR groups on second-order ToM tasks and again found no between-group differences. Only 45% of the Williams syndrome group passed the false belief questions. Sullivan et al. (2003) investigated higher order ToM by studying the understanding of the differences between lies and ironic jokes by adolescents with Williams syndrome (mean CA = 12.3 years; range: 8–16 years) and CA-, IQ-, and VA-matched PWS and MR groups. None of the participants with Williams syndrome and only 2 of the participants in each of the other groups could differentiate between lies and ironic jokes. The participants with Williams syndrome classified both as lies; that is, all statements that were not literally true were considered lies. As Sullivan et al. pointed out, this difficulty in differentiating between intentionally false statements meant as jokes and those meant to deceive (lies) is likely to lead to severe social problems with peers.

One of the most striking characteristics of the hypersocial behavior of young children with Williams syndrome is the unusual manner in which toddlers gaze at strangers, a gaze that is often described as, "It was like he [she] was boring his [her] eyes into me." The gaze is unnerving; people who are unfamiliar with it often respond with nervous laughter if they are not able to break the gaze. To address this pattern experimentally, Mervis et al. (2003a) compared the looking patterns of a 10-month-old girl ("Jenny") with Williams syndrome to those of CA-matched and MA-matched TD groups both when playing with their mother and when playing with a stranger. Jenny spent significantly longer looking at the stranger than at her mother, as did both of the TD groups. Jenny also spent significantly longer looking at both her mother and the stranger than did either of the TD groups. The most dramatic difference, however, was in the quality of Jenny's gaze at the stranger. Jenny's gaze was coded as intense for more than 70% of the time she spent looking at the stranger. In contrast, the TD groups looked intensely less than 1% of the time that they spent looking at the stranger. Mervis et al. (2003a) also compared the looking patterns of 31 infants and toddlers with Williams syndrome during an initial genetics exam to those of 273 infants and toddlers with DD due to other causes and 87 infants and toddlers who had genetic conditions not associated with DD. Looking behavior was coded during measurement of the child's hands and feet. Almost all of the 8- to 23-month-olds with Williams syndrome and most of the 24- to 33-month-olds with Williams syndrome looked intensely at the geneticist's face. In contrast, no one in the other groups looked at the geneticist's face intensely during this (or any other) part of the exam. Although older children with Williams syndrome no longer gaze intensely, they continue to spend a great deal of time looking at people.

Researchers have approached the question of hypersociability in Williams syndrome by asking whether the overly approaching behavior seen in Williams syndrome is due to differences in judgments of the approachability of strangers. Bellugi et al. (1999) reported that adults with Williams syndrome consistently rated faces of strangers as more approachable than did a CA-matched TD group and suggested this pattern may reflect amygdala dysfunction. Frigerio et al. (2006) compared the approachability ratings provided by adolescents and adults with Williams syndrome for a series of pictures illustrating happy, angry, disgusted, and fearful faces to those of MA- and CA-matched TD groups. A separate group of TD adults rated all the pictures, including those used by Bellugi et al. (1999), for approachability. Frigerio et al. found that the Williams syndrome group's ratings of approachability were significantly higher than the control groups' for "happy" faces but significantly lower (less approachable) than the control groups' for the remaining pictures. The authors noted that Bellugi et al.'s pictures were all rated similarly to the "happy" faces, which explains the different pattern of results.

Although Frigerio et al.'s (2006) findings suggest that there are many people who would be considered less approachable by a person with Williams syndrome than by a person in the general population, children and adolescents with Williams syndrome are much more likely than other groups to approach people indiscriminately. This indiscriminate approach may reflect disinhibition (Davies et al., 1998; Frigerio et al.,

2006), suggesting possible frontal lobe impairment. In fact, Meyer-Lindenberg et al. (2005, 2006) have reported a structural abnormality in the orbitofrontal cortex (OFC) of normal-IQ adults with Williams syndrome. In an fMRI study, the same individuals showed significantly reduced amygdala activation to angry or fearful faces but significantly increased amygdala activation to threatening or fearful scenes. This pattern is consistent with findings of indiscriminate approach to people combined with specific phobias of a nonsocial nature. It also suggests abnormal regulation of the amygdala in Williams syndrome. A path analysis indicated a deficiency in the OFC in the context of social processing; in particular, the OFC was not regulating the amygdala. Adolphs (2003) stated that OFC–amygdala interactions link sensory representations of stimuli with social judgments about them based on their motivational value. Meyer-Lindenberg et al. argued that lack of regulation of the amygdala by the OFC in Williams syndrome contributes to the social disinhibition, reduced reactivity to social cues, and increased tendency to approach other people, including strangers, that characterize Williams syndrome.

Questionnaire Studies of Problem Behaviors   Several research groups have used the Child Behavior Checklist (CBCL; Achenbach, 1991) to characterize the problem behaviors of children with Williams syndrome. Pagon et al. (1987) administered an earlier version of the CBCL to parents of 9 persons with Williams syndrome ages 10–20 years. Behavior identified as problematic included "acts too young for age," "can't concentrate or pay attention," "confused or seems in a fog," "talks too much," and "argues a lot." Dilts et al. (1990) administered the CBCL to parents of 48 children with Williams syndrome ages 4–16 years and reported that 67% scored above the 98th percentile on the Hyperactivity scale (which includes distractibility, which was the most frequent parental concern). Greer et al. (1997) provided CBCL data for 15 children with Williams syndrome ages 4–18 years and also identified significant levels of Attention Problems. Furthermore, 73% had significantly elevated Total Problems scores and another 14% had borderline elevations. Sarimski (1997) compared CBCL data for 14 school-age children with Williams syndrome, 13 with PWS, and 11 with fragile X. The Williams syndrome group differed significantly from both groups on several items, scoring significantly higher on "worries," "talks too much," and "does not eat well" and significantly lower on "self-conscious," "overeats," and "is overweight." Ten of the 14 children with Williams syndrome were considered significantly maladjusted. Fidler et al. (2002) compared CBCL data for groups of 20 children with Williams syndrome (ages 3–10 years), DS, or Smith–Magenis syndrome; 75% of the Williams syndrome group, 80% of the Smith–Magenis group, and only 10% of the DS group scored in the clinical range for Total Problems. Fidler et al. also assessed family stress using the Parent and Family Problems and Pessimism domains of the Questionnaire on Resources and Stress—

Friedrich edition (Friedrich et al., 1983). The stress levels of the families of children with Williams syndrome or Smith–Magenis syndrome were similar and significantly higher than for the families of children with DS. Significant predictors of family stress for the Williams syndrome group were child's age (higher stress associated with younger age) and maladaptive behavior as measured by the CBCL.

Einfeld and colleagues (Einfeld et al., 1997, 1999, 2001; Tonge & Einfeld, 2003) conducted a longitudinal study of the behavioral characteristics of children with Williams syndrome, using the Developmental Behavior Checklist (DBC; Einfeld & Tonge, 1995), a parent-report instrument for assessing behavioral and emotional disturbance in individuals with MR. The Williams syndrome group included 70 children (mean CA = 9.4 years) and was compared to an epidemiologically derived control group, with gender, CA, and level of MR statistically controlled (Einfeld et al., 1997). The Total Behavior Problems score for the Williams syndrome group was significantly elevated, and the Williams syndrome group had significantly more problems on the Communication Disturbance and Anxiety subscales. Twelve items were endorsed significantly more often for the Williams syndrome group than the control group, including "tense or anxious," "covers ears or avoids particular sounds," "short attention," "overly attention-seeking," and "doesn't mix with own age group/prefers adult company." At the 5-year follow-up (Einfeld et al., 1999, 2001), the between-group differences on Total Behavior Problems, the Anxiety and Communication Disturbance subscales, and 10 of the 12 items (including those listed above) remained significant. Although the Total Behavior Problems score for the Williams syndrome group decreased significantly at the 8-year follow-up (Tonge & Einfeld, 2003), it was still significantly higher than for the control group. The Williams syndrome group's score on the Anxiety subscale decreased significantly and no longer differed from that of the control group. However, the Communication Disturbance subscale score did not decrease and continued to be significantly higher than for the control group.

DSM Interview Studies of Psychopathology   Two interview studies of psychopathology in children with Williams syndrome have been conducted. Dykens (2003) interviewed parents of 51 persons with Williams syndrome ages 5–49 years (mean CA = 15.9 years) using the anxiety disorders domain of the *DSM–III*-based Diagnostic Interview Schedule for Children—Parent (Reich et al., 1991). Results for children and adults were not reported separately. Overall, 35% of individuals with Williams syndrome were diagnosed with specific phobia and 16% with overanxious disorder.

Leyfer et al. (2006) interviewed parents of 119 children with Williams syndrome ages 4–16 years using the Anxiety Disorders Interview Schedule—Parent (Silverman & Albano, 1996), a structured-interview measure that provides *DSM–IV* diagnoses for all anxiety and related disorders, including ADHD. The prevalence for any anxiety disorder was 57%, which is considerably higher than reported in the two population-based studies of psychopathology in children with intellectual disabilities (ID) that used *DSM–IV* or International Classification of Diseases (ICD–10) criteria (10.5% in Dekker and Koot, 2003, and 8.7% in Emerson, 2003).

Almost all of the children with Williams syndrome who had any anxiety disorder had specific phobia (54% of the entire sample). This is similar to the 50% prevalence Cherniske et al. (2004) reported based on *DSM–IV* parent interview measures for adults with Williams syndrome. The most common type of phobia was for loud noises (28% of the entire sample of children with Williams syndrome). Hypersensitivity to loudness of sound was reported by parents for 80% of the participants with Williams syndrome in Levitin et al.'s (2005) questionnaire study; in cases in which this hypersensitivity leads to both fear and adaptive impairment, the child will be diagnosed with specific phobia. This hypersensitivity and the sometimes resulting specific phobia may be related to sensorineural hearing loss, which Marler et al. (2005) found for 78% of 18 school-age children with Williams syndrome. The majority of children who had specific phobia of loud noise (61%) had at least one other specific phobia, usually medically related. The prevalence of specific phobia in children with Williams syndrome was much higher than in *DSM–IV*-based epidemiological studies of children in the general population (1.5%; Shaffer et al., 1996), or children with ID (Dekker & Koot, 2003: 6.8%; Emerson, 2003: 1.9%) or a *DSM–IV* based study of psychopathology in DS (Myers & Pueschel, 1991: 1.5%).

Generalized anxiety disorder (GAD) was diagnosed in 12% of the children with Williams syndrome. The prevalence of GAD changed significantly with age, with 0% prevalence in the 4- to 6-year-old group but 23% prevalence in the 11- to 16-year-old group. Although the pattern of increased prevalence in older children is consistent with that for the general population (Last et al., 1987; Strauss et al., 1988), the prevalence in Williams syndrome is considerably higher than in either the general population (3.2%; Shaffer et al., 1996) or children with ID (0% in Dekker & Koot, 2003; 1.5% in Emerson, 2003). Leyfer et al. (2006) argue that based on clinical experience, the *DSM–IV* criteria for GAD often do not capture the nature of the worrying in children with Williams syndrome. Most children with Williams syndrome worry in anticipation of both events they expect to dislike and events they expect to enjoy. The worry is perseverative and typically manifested by repeated questions about the upcoming activity, leading many parents to avoid telling their child about an upcoming event until the last possible moment. This anxiety typically takes up a significant amount of time and is consistently reported as impairing but is not captured by the *DSM–IV* GAD criteria.

ADHD, the most prevalent *DSM–IV* diagnosis for children with Williams syndrome, was diagnosed in 65%. There was no sex difference. Prevalence was significantly higher for the 7- to 10-year-old group than for the older or younger groups.

Most children diagnosed with ADHD had the predominantly inattentive type. The proportion diagnosed with ADHD—combined type decreased significantly with age. ADHD—predominantly hyperactive was very rare. Although the pattern is similar to that for the general population, prevalence in Williams syndrome was much higher than for children in the general population (3%–7%; American Psychiatric Association, 2000), children with ID (6.8%; Dekker & Koot, 2003), or children with DS (6.1%; Myers & Pueschel, 1991), although similar to the prevalence for boys with fragile X syndrome (72%; Backes et al., 2000).

Autism Spectrum Disorder and Williams Syndrome   Meyer-Lindenberg et al. (2006) note that although autism and Williams syndrome have often been seen as clinical opposites, there are overlapping nonverbal communication difficulties, especially in maintaining eye gaze during conversations, understanding and using gestures, and interpreting facial expressions. Some children with Williams syndrome show more serious limitations in communication and social interaction than are typical for the syndrome; many also show significant repetitive behaviors. Many of these children will meet criteria for autism or ASD based on the Autism Disorders Observation Schedule (ADOS; Lord et al., 2000), Autism Diagnostic Interview-Revised (ADI-R; Lord et al., 1994), and clinical impression. Leyfer et al. (2006) excluded 9 children from their sample because they met criteria for autism or ASD based on these criteria. Three of 29 preschoolers assessed by Klein-Tasman et al. (in press) using the ADOS met the autism cutoff; all 3 were subsequently diagnosed with autism based on further assessment. Klein-Tasman et al. raise the possibility that diagnostic overshadowing may lead to underdiagnosis of autism or ASD in Williams syndrome (e.g., only 6 prior cases reported in the literature; Gillberg & Rasmussen, 1994; Reiss et al., 1985), which in turn may prevent the child from receiving appropriate services. The reasons for the co-occurrence of Williams syndrome and autism or ASD are unknown. None of the genes deleted in Williams syndrome has been associated with autism or ASD. However, MR itself is a risk factor for autism and ASD (e.g., Fombonne, 2005). Children may also have familial genetic risk factors. For example, one 6-year-old with Williams syndrome recently diagnosed with Pervasive Developmental Disorder–Not Otherwise Specified (PDD–NOS) has a maternal first cousin with the same diagnosis. In addition, his mother talked late and has dyslexia and written language disabilities, and his younger sister talked late and is receiving speech therapy.

Genetics and Genotype–Phenotype Correlations

In this section, we address the mechanism by which Williams syndrome occurs, the variability in Williams syndrome, and the factors influencing that variability. In the context of discussing cardiovascular disease, deletion length, and weakness in visuo-spatial construction, we also consider genotype–phenotype correlations involving four of the deleted genes.

Williams Syndrome as a Genomic Disorder

Williams syndrome is a genomic disorder caused by a submicroscopic deletion of chromosome 7q11.23 that is mediated by the genomic structure of the region. The ~1.6-Mb deletion includes ~25 genes that comprise the WSCR. These genes are listed in table 7.3, along with their proposed function and possible relevance to the Williams syndrome phenotype. The WSCR is flanked by repetitive DNA elements called low copy repeats (LCRs). A genomic disorder results when there is non-allelic homologous recombination between chromosomes. These errors are common in areas of chromosomes that contain LCRs, because these repetitive regions composed of genes, pseudogenes, and gene clusters have greater than 95% sequence homology (Stankiewicz & Lupski, 2002). Because these genetically similar LCRs are relatively close to each other, unequal crossing over may occur, leading to either a deletion or duplication of the region between the LCRs. The Williams syndrome region is flanked by one block of LCRs on the centromeric side and two blocks on the telomeric side; these LCRs have high homology (98% identical), which facilitates recombination during meiosis (Bayes et al., 2003). This unequal crossing over may result in deletion (Williams syndrome), duplication (Somerville et al., 2005), or inversion (Bayes et al., 2003; Osborne et al., 2001). Hobart et al. (2004) reported that in a sample of 266 parents of individuals with Williams syndrome, 25% of the transmitting parents had an inversion of the Williams syndrome region, as did 7% of the non-transmitting parents. No phenotypic effect of the parental inversion on the individual with Williams syndrome has been reported. The size of the deletion depends on which blocks of LCRs are involved in the recombination. Deletion length is 1.55 Mb in 95% of people with Williams syndrome and 1.84 Mb in ~5% (Bayes et al., 2003). The only phenotypic difference between these two deletion lengths that has been reported is that the 1.84-Mb deletion is associated with a decreased risk for hypertension due to loss of a copy of *NCF1* (Del Campo et al., 2006). In addition to this variation in "classic" deletion size, a very small number of individuals with Williams syndrome have deletions that are either shorter or much longer.

Variability in the Williams Syndrome Phenotype

Variability has been reported for every aspect of the Williams syndrome phenotype, with each individual's expression of the genetic mutation being influenced by several factors. One obvious genetic variable is which genes are deleted (often referred to as "deletion size"). In Williams syndrome, genotypic variability in deletion size has resulted in phenotypic diversity that has informed genotype–phenotype correlations

Table 7.3
Genes deleted in Williams syndrome (WS)

Gene Name	Proposed Function	Possible Relevance to WS Phenotype
FKBP6	Stabilizes protein complexes	
FZD9	Functions in cell fate pathway	
BAZ1B	Binds vitamin D receptor	Transient hypercalcemia
BCL7B	Unknown	
TBL2	Unknown	
WBSCR14	Regulates lipogenic enzyme genes	Obesity, diabetes
WBSCR18	Molecular chaperone	
WBSCR22	Unknown	
STX1A	Mediates neurotransmitter release in brain and insulin release in pancreas	Diabetes, impaired glucose tolerance
WBSCR21	Unknown	
CLDN3	Cell-to-cell tight junction protein	
CLDN4	Cell-to-cell tight junction protein	
ELN	Elastin structural protein	Supravalvar aortic stenosis, abnormal connective tissue[a]
LIMK1	Regulates actin cytoskeleton in axon growth, dendritic spine development	Deficit in visuospatial construction
WBSCR1	Regulates other genes via binding RNA	
LAT2	May regulate mast cells	
RFC2	Cofactor for DNA replication	Growth deficiency
CYLN2	Microtubule binding	Impaired motor coordination, cerebellar dysfunction[b]
GTF2IRD1	Transcription activator	Facial asymmetry, fatigability
WBSCR23	Unknown	
GTF2I	Transcription factor	Mental retardation (lowered IQ)
NCF1[c]	Subunit of NADPH oxidase	Hypertension
GTF2IRD2[c]	Transcription factor	

Note: Genes are listed in centromere to telomere order. The information is based on Osborne (2006).
[a] Elastin deficiency has been shown to cause supravalvar aortic stenosis and connective tissue abnormalities (see Morris, 2006a, for a review).
[b] Hemizygous knockout mice show decreased contextual fear response (Hoogenraad et al., 2002).
[c] Deleted in only 5% of individuals with WS (Del Campo et al., 2006).

and advanced knowledge regarding the function of some of the genes in the region; the major findings from these studies are discussed below (see also Morris, 2006a). Other genetic factors that may influence the severity of a particular symptom are the function of the WSCR alleles on the intact chromosome 7 and the presence of mutations in other genes that are in the same metabolic pathway or developmental cascade. Environmental modifiers include prenatal exposures, nutritional status, socioeconomic background, educational opportunity, and treatment. Most phenotypic features also vary with time due to the effects of developmental processes and aging. Finally, epigenetic factors may influence gene expression. For instance, Sadler et al. (2001) and Bruno et al. (2003) found increased prevalence, severity, and earlier presentation of cardiovascular disease in males. Another potential genetic modifier is the parent of origin of the deletion. Multiple series have shown an even distribution between mothers and fathers (Ewart et al., 1993; Hobart et al., 2004; Perez Jurado et al., 1996). No phenotypic effect related to parent of origin has been identified (M. S. Wang et al., 1999; Wu et al., 1998).

Cardiovascular Disease, Connective Tissue Abnormalities, and *Elastin*

Williams syndrome is a contiguous gene syndrome; that is, the deletion of different genes in the WSCR contributes to different aspects of the phenotype. The *elastin* gene was the first to be identified (Ewart et al., 1993) and is the only gene whose role in the phenotype of Williams syndrome is definitively established. Absence of one *elastin* gene causes the cardiovascular and connective tissue manifestations of Williams syndrome.

Different genetic alterations affecting the *elastin* gene lead to SVAS or cutis laxa. SVAS can occur as a familial condition inherited in an autosomal dominant fashion or as part of a broader pattern of malformation, Williams syndrome. Most families with SVAS have point mutations in *ELN*, have normal intelligence, and do not fit the WSCP (Frangiskakis et al., 1996). The arterial pathology and the variability in severity of the cardiovascular disease is the same as for Williams syndrome, and hypertension is common in both familial SVAS and in Williams syndrome. Individuals with familial SVAS or Williams syndrome often have other connective tissue abnormalities including hoarse voice and hernias (Grimm & Wesselhoeft, 1980; Morris & Moore, 1991). Individuals with familial SVAS usually showed some of the Williams syndrome facial features at some point in their life span, though none had the classic Williams syndrome facies (≥ 9 scored facial features). The mutations that cause SVAS have occurred in the region between *elastin* exons 1 and 30 (Metcalfe et al., 2000). Frameshift mutations in *elastin* exons 30 and 32 lead to the autosomal dominant condition cutis laxa, whose phenotype is primarily observed in the skin, which is loose and soft but not hyperextensible or fragile (Tassabehji et al., 1998; Zhang et al., 1999).

Deletion Length

Long Deletions in the Williams syndrome Region and *HSP27* (*HSPB1*)   Although ~98% of individuals with Williams syndrome have classic-length deletions, some with shorter or longer deletions have been reported. In a series of 255 individuals we studied who had *elastin* deletion and clinical diagnosis of Williams syndrome, 250 had classic deletions, 3 had longer deletions, and 2 had shorter deletions. The cognitive strengths and weaknesses of the 5 individuals with atypical deletions were consistent with the WSCP. However, IQ was considerably and significantly lower for the 3 individuals with long deletions than for those with classic deletions, suggesting that there are one or more genes telomeric to the classic Williams syndrome region that are important for cognitive development. The gene *HSP27* was deleted in all 3 (Stock et al., 2003). Both *HSP27* and *LIMK1* (a gene in the classic deletion region) are important in actin dynamics. It is possible that neuronal migration, which depends on normal actin function, is more severely disturbed with *both* genes deleted. Several earlier cases of individuals with long deletions had been reported (see Zackowski et al., 1990). Although these individuals share the facial features and medical problems of classic Williams syndrome, they (especially if they have cytogenetically visible deletions) have additional disabilities, often including seizures, infantile spasms, and severe MR (Crawfurd et al., 1979; Mizugishi et al., 1998; Young et al., 1984; Wu et al., 1999).

Short Deletions

Intelligence and **GTF2I**   Short deletions of the WSCR occur in two clinical settings. The first is families with autosomal dominant SVAS; 7 such families have been reported. The second is individuals with a sporadic deletion that is shorter than the classic deletion. The sporadic deletions can be subdivided into two major genotypic categories, those that include the classic Williams syndrome telomeric breakpoint, and those that do not. Individuals with short deletions that include the usual Williams syndrome telomeric breakpoint, including deletion of *GTF2I*, have DD or MR (Botta et al., 1999; Heller et al., 2003; Morris et al., 2003). In contrast, most individuals whose deletions did not include *GTF2I* but did include the centromeric genes had normal intelligence (Doyle et al., 2004; Gagliardi et al., 2003; Hirota et al., 2003; Karmiloff-Smith et al., 2003b; Korenberg et al., 2000; Morris et al., 2003; Tassabehji et al., 1999, 2005). *GTF2I* is not deleted in any of the 7 SVAS families with short deletions. Morris et al. (2003) studied 5 of these families and found that the KBIT IQs of affected members were in the average range, 27 points higher than the Williams syndrome mean.

  GTF2I is a transcription factor that regulates gene expression both by activating other genes and repressing transcription (Hakimi et al., 2003). Alternative splicing of the gene results in four isoforms of the protein TFII-I (Hinsley et al., 2004); the gamma form is predominantly expressed in neurons and is strongly expressed in fetal brain (Perez-Jurado et al., 1998). A similar expression pattern is found in mice, suggesting evolutionary conservation of function. In embryonic mice, TFII-I is expressed throughout the brain, and in adult mice it is only present in neurons, with the highest levels of expression in cerebellar cells and hippocampal interneurons (Danoff et al., 2004).

Visuospatial construction and **LIMK1**   Studies of 6 of the 7 families have also focused more specifically on cognitive abilities. Tassabehji et al. (1999) reported two adult brothers with SVAS who had a deletion of *LIMK1* and *ELN* who had normal intelligence and did not fit the WSCP. Del Campo et al. (2002) reported a family with a deletion of *ELN* through *GTF2IRD1*. Affected family members reportedly had borderline IQ and the Williams syndrome personality; detailed cognitive and behavioral data were not published.

We have characterized the remaining 5 families. Affected members had normal intelligence but 19/21 still fit the WSCP (Frangiskakis et al., 1996; Morris et al., 2003). DNA sequence analysis of the region affected by the smallest deletion revealed only two genes, *ELN* and *LIMK1*, which encodes a novel protein strongly expressed in the brain (Frangiskakis et al., 1996). Because *ELN* mutations cause vascular disease but not cognitive abnormalities, these data implicate *LIMK1* hemizygosity in impaired visuospatial constructive cognition. Visuospatial construction ability is a heritable trait that varies in the general population, probably following a quantitative trait loci model (Mervis et al., 1999b). Thus, *LIMK1* is likely one of the genes contributing to visuospatial construction ability. The LIM kinase1 protein phosphorylates cofilin, a protein important in actin mechanics necessary for growth of neuronal axons. *LIMK1* hemizygous knockout mice have abnormal neuronal dendritic spines in the hippocampus, and homozygous knockouts have impaired spatial learning as demonstrated by their performance in the Morris water maze (Meng et al., 2002).

Other Genes Deleted in Williams syndrome That Are Expressed in the Brain

Only those genes that are dosage sensitive would be expected to play a role in the Williams syndrome phenotype. Prime candidate genes for other Williams syndrome phenotypic features include *BAZ1B*, *CYLN2*, *FZD9*, and *GTF2IRD1*. Clues to the possible roles of these genes come from expression studies and knockout mouse studies, as reviewed in Osborne (2006), Morris (2006a), and Meyer-Lindenberg et al. (2006).

In summary, research on genotype–phenotype correlations in Williams syndrome has identified a gene that is involved in the cardiovascular and connective tissue abnormalities in Williams syndrome and familial SVAS. In addition, candidate genes for MR or lowered IQ and for visuospatial construction difficulties in Williams syndrome have been identified. These genes likely also contribute to variability in intelligence and visuospatial constructive ability in the general population.

Conclusion

Williams syndrome is an autosomal multisystem disorder leading to a characteristic but variable physical, cognitive, and behavioral phenotype. Some of the primary features of Williams syndrome are evident in infancy. These include a distinctive facies, SVAS, the behavioral trait of staring intensely at faces, and DD. When early cognitive or motor delay is misinterpreted as secondary to medical complications, both intervention and diagnosis may be unnecessarily postponed. Familiarity with the physical and behavioral phenotypes and/or realization of the signs that indicate that any infant or child should be referred for genetics evaluation are critical for early diagnosis of Williams syndrome.

Williams syndrome is associated with a specific cognitive profile (WSCP) that differentiates most individuals with this syndrome from most persons with other forms of MR or learning disability on the basis of a pattern of DAS T scores: extreme weakness in pattern construction, relative strength in verbal short-term memory, and verbal memory and/or language abilities above the 1st percentile. For 80%, visuospatial construction difficulties are extreme enough to reduce the child's GCA (IQ) to a score significantly below that expected based on the child's verbal or nonverbal reasoning abilities. IQ scores on tests that include visuospatial construction average more than 10 points lower than on tests that do not. This pattern of performance demonstrates the extent to which test selection may influence the outcome of cognitive phenotype research.

Whereas early studies suggested *deviant* visuospatial construction processes in persons with Williams syndrome, more recent findings indicate that persons with Williams syndrome instead have considerable *delay* in the progression of visuospatial construction skills such as drawing and pattern construction. That is, the types of errors made by children with Williams syndrome are part of the normal pattern of acquiring visuospatial construction skills, and adults with Williams syndrome are much less likely than children to make these errors. Neuroimaging studies have identified differences in the neural substrate that likely lead to the extreme difficulty most people with Williams syndrome have with visuospatial construction

Descriptions of the verbal strengths initially associated with Williams syndrome have also been refined by more recent research. Earlier reports indicated age-appropriate vocabulary and grammatical ability in the context of severe MR. Recent studies have led to a more nuanced pattern: Although vocabulary and grammatical abilities of children with Williams syndrome typically are strong *relative to visuospatial construction skills,* comparisons with same-age children with forms of MR other than DS or with younger MA-matched TD children indicate that language abilities are delayed relative to CA and at a similar level to the matched comparison groups. Intellectual ability is typically in the moderate-MR to low-average range. Furthermore, although concrete vocabulary knowledge is usually the most advanced ability for children with Williams syndrome, abstract relational vocabulary (including spatial, quantitative, temporal, and dimensional terms) is among the weakest skills. Early language receives less support from nonverbal communicative skills for children with Williams syndrome than for TD children or children with DS. In general, verbal memory plays a stronger role in language acquisition for children with Williams syndrome than for TD children.

One finding noted in the earliest reports of children with Williams syndrome that continues to receive empirical support is the hypersociability and undercurrent of anxiety associated with the syndrome. These behaviors are included in the WSPP, along with empathy. Recent studies demonstrate increased prevalence of several comorbid disorders diagnosed according to *DSM–IV* criteria, including anxiety (especially specific phobia and GAD) and ADHD. Neuroimaging studies have begun to provide evidence of the neural substrate of some of the Williams syndrome personality characteristics.

Discrepancies in findings between different studies of children with Williams syndrome often are due to methodological differences. We stressed the importance of careful choice of contrast groups, of standardized assessments, and of research designs for advancing our understanding of both Williams syndrome and other developmental disorders. A solid understanding of the typical developmental path(s) for acquisition of particular cognitive abilities is critical for determining if development of a particular ability is delayed or deviant.

Williams syndrome is unique in its combination of physical, cognitive, and behavioral characteristics. Yet equally as impressive as this implied homogeneity is the variation with which phenotypic characteristics are expressed. This variability is due to differences between children with Williams syndrome in the remaining alleles of the ~25 missing genes, to genetic variation in the remainder of the child's genome, and to transactions between the child's genome and his or her environment. Genotype–phenotype studies of individuals who have Williams syndrome or who have unusual deletions in the Williams syndrome region have begun to make significant contributions to the understanding of genetic sources of variation in the physical, cognitive, and behavioral characteristics that together constitute the Williams syndrome phenotype, and major additional advances are likely in the next few years.

Acknowledgments

We are very grateful to the children and families who have participated so enthusiastically in our research. The authors' research and preparation of this chapter were supported by National Institute of Child Health and Human Development Grant R37 HD29957 and National Institute of Neurological Disorders and Stroke Grant R01 NS35102. We thank Joanie Robertson for computing the descriptive statistics for the psychological assessment standard scores and Steve LoMastro, Joanie Robertson, and Ella Peregrine for figure preparation. Michèle Mazzocco provided thoughtful comments on an earlier draft of this chapter.

References

Achenbach, T. M. (1991). *Child Behavior Checklist/4-18*. Burlington: University of Vermont.

Adamson, L. B. (1995). *Communication development during infancy*. Madison, WI: Brown & Benchmark.

Adolphs, R. (2003). Cognitive neuroscience of human social behaviour. *Nature Reviews: Neuroscience, 4*, 165–178.

Allen, S. E. M., & Crago, M. B. (1996). Early passive acquisition in Inuktitut. *Journal of Child Language, 23*, 129–155.

American Academy of Pediatrics Committee on Genetics. (2001). Healthcare supervision for children with Williams syndrome. *Pediatrics, 107*, 1192–1204.

American Psychiatric Association. (2000). *Diagnostic and statistical manual of mental disorders* (4th ed., text rev.). Washington, DC: Author.

Ardinger, R. H., Goertz, K. K., & Mattioli, L. F. (1994). Cerebrovascular stenosis with cerebral infarction in a child with Williams syndrome. *American Journal of Medical Genetics, 51*, 200–202.

Ashkoomoff, N. A., & Stiles, J. (1996). The influence of pattern type on children's Block Design performance. *Journal of the International Neuropsychological Society, 2*, 392–402.

Atkinson, J., Braddick, O., Anker, S., Curran, W., Andrew, R., Wattam-Bell, J., & Braddick, F. (2003). Neurobiological models of visuospatial cognition in Williams syndrome: Measures of dorsal-stream and frontal function. *Developmental Neuropsychology, 23*, 139–172.

Axelsson, S., Bjornland, T., Kjaer, I., Heiberg, A., & Storhaug, K. (2003). Dental characteristics in Williams syndrome: A Clinical and radiographic evaluation. *Acta Odontologica Scandinavica, 61*, 129–136.

Backes, M., Genc, B., Schreck, J., Doerfler, W., Lehmkuhl, G., & von Gontard, A. (2000). Cognitive and behavioral profile of fragile X boys: Correlations to molecular data. *American Journal of Medical Genetics, Part A, 95*, 150–156.

Baron-Cohen, S., & Tead, T. (2003). *Mind reading: The interactive guide to emotions* [Computer software]. Cambridge, England: Human Emotions.

Baron-Cohen, S., Wheelwright, S., Hill, J., Raste, Y., & Plumb, I. (2001). The "Reading the Mind in the Eyes" Test revised version: A study with normal adults, and adults with Asperger syndrome or high-functioning autism. *Journal of Child Psychology and Psychiatry, 42*, 241–251.

Bates, E., Tager-Flusberg, H., Vicari, S., & Volterra, V. (2001). Debate over language's link with intelligence. *Nature, 413*, 565–566.

Bawden, H. N., MacDonald, G. W., & Shea, S. (1997). Treatment of children with Williams syndrome with methylphenidate. *Journal of Child Neurology, 12*, 248–252.

Bayes, M., Magano, L. F., Rivera, N., Flores, R., & Perez Jurado, L. A. (2003). Mutational mechanisms of Williams–Beuren syndrome deletions. *American Journal of Human Genetics, 73*, 131–151.

Beery, K. E. (1997). *The Beery–Buktenica developmental test of visual–motor integration* (4th ed.). Parsippany, NJ: Modern Curriculum Press.

Bellugi, U., Adolphs, R., Cassady, C., & Chiles, M. (1999). Towards the neural basis for hypersociability in a genetic syndrome. *NeuroReport, 10,* 1653–1657.

Bellugi, U., Bihrle, A., Jernigan, T., Trauner, D., & Doherty, S. (1990). Neuropsychological and neuro-anatomical profile of Williams syndrome. *American Journal of Medical Genetics, 6,* 115–125.

Bellugi, U., Lichtenberger, L., Jones, W., Lai, Z., & St. George, M. (2000). The neurocognitive profile of Williams syndrome: A complex pattern of strengths and weaknesses. *Journal of Cognitive Neuroscience, 12*(Suppl. 1), 7–29.

Bellugi, U., Marks, S., Bihrle, A., & Sabo, H. (1988). Dissociation between language and cognitive functions in Williams syndrome. In D. Bishop & K. Mogford (Eds.), *Language development in exceptional circumstances* (pp. 177–189). London: Churchill Livingstone.

Bellugi, U., Wang, P., & Jernigan, T. L. (1994). Williams syndrome: An unusual neuropsychological profile. In S. H. Broman & J. Grafman (Eds.), *Atypical cognitive deficits in developmental disorders: Implications for brain function* (pp. 23–56). Hillsdale, NJ: Erlbaum.

Bennett, C., LaVeck, B., & Sells, C. J. (1978). The Williams elfin facies syndrome: The psychological profile as an aid in syndrome identification. *Pediatrics, 61,* 303–306.

Bertrand, J., & Mervis, C. B. (1996). Longitudinal analysis of drawings by children with Williams syndrome: Preliminary results. *Visual Arts Research, 22,* 19–34.

Bertrand, J., Mervis, C. B., & Eisenberg, J. D. (1997). Drawing by children with Williams syndrome: A developmental perspective. *Developmental Neuropsychology, 13,* 41–67.

Beuren, A. J., Apitz, J., & Harmjanz, D. (1962). Supravalvular aortic stenosis in association with mental retardation and a certain facial appearance. *Circulation, 27,* 1235–1240.

Bihrle, A. M., Bellugi, U., Delis, D., & Marks, S. (1989). Seeing either the forest or the trees: Dissociation in visuospatial processing. *Brain and Cognition, 11,* 37–49.

Bishop, D. V. M. (1989). *Test for Reception of Grammar.* Manchester, England: Chapel Press.

Bishop, D. V. M. (1998). Development of the Children's Communication Checklist (CCC): A method for assessing qualitative aspects of communicative impairment in children. *Journal of Child Psychology and Psychiatry, 39,* 879–891.

Bishop, D. V. M. (2002). *The Children's Communication Checklist* (2nd ed.). London: Psychological Corporation.

Bishop, D. V. M. (2003). *Test for Reception of Grammar, Version 2.* London: Psychological Corporation.

Bishop, D. V. M., North, T., & Dolan, C. (1996). Nonword repetition as a behavioural marker for inherited language impairment: Evidence from a twin study. *Journal of Child Psychology and Psychiatry, 37,* 391–403.

Block, J. H., & Block, J. (1980). The role of ego-control and ego-resiliency in the organization of behavior. In W. A. Collins (Ed.), *Development of cognition, affect, and social relations. Minnesota Symposia on Child Psychology* (Vol. 13, pp. 39–101). Hillsdale, NJ: Erlbaum.

Botta, A., Novelli, G., Mari, A., Novelli, A., Sabini, M., Korenberg, J., et al. (1999). Detection of an atypical 7q11.23 deletion in Williams syndrome patients which does not include the STX1A and FZD3 genes. *Journal of Medical Genetics, 36,* 478–480.

Bowerman, M. (1996). Learning how to structure space for language: A cross-linguistic perspective. In P. Bloom, M. A. Peterson, L. Nadel, & M. F. Garrett (Eds.), *Language and space* (pp. 385–436). Cambridge, MA: MIT Press.

Brooks, P. J., & Tomasello, M. (1999). Young children learn to produce passives with nonce verbs. *Developmental Psychology, 35,* 29–44.

Bruininks, R. H., Woodcock, R., Weatherman, R., & Hill, B. (1996). *Scales of Independent Behavior—Revised.* Chicago: Riverside.

Bruno, E., Rossi, N., Thuer, O., Cordoba, R., & Alday, L. E. (2003). Cardiovascular findings, and clinical course, in patients with Williams syndrome. *Cardiology in the Young, 13,* 532–536.

Cagle, A. P., Waguespack, S. G., Buckingham, B. A., Shankar, R. R., & Dimeglio, L. A. (2004). Severe infantile hypercalcemia associated with Williams syndrome successfully treated with intravenously administered pamidronate. *Pediatrics, 114,* 1091–1095.

Carrasco, X., Castillo, S., Aravena, T., Rothhammer, P., & Aboitiz, F. (2005). Williams syndrome: Pediatric, neurologic, and cognitive development. *Pediatric Neurology, 32,* 166–172.

Cassidy, S. B., & Morris, C. A. (2002). Behavioral phenotypes in genetic syndromes: Genetic clues to human behavior. *Advances in Pediatrics, 49,* 59–86.

Cherniske, E. M., Carpenter, T. O., Klaiman, C., Young, E., Bregman, J., Insogna, K., et al. (2004). Multisystem study of 20 older adults with Williams syndrome. *American Journal of Medical Genetics, A, 131,* 255–264.

Clahsen, H., & Almazan, M. (1998). Syntax and morphology in children with Williams syndrome. *Cognition, 68,* 167–198.

Clahsen, H., Ring, M., & Temple, C. (2003). Lexical and morphological skills in English-speaking children with Williams syndrome. *Essex Research Reports in Linguistics, 43,* 1–27.

Cox, J. W. (1934). *Manual skill: Its organization and development.* Cambridge, England: Cambridge University Press.

Crawfurd, M. D., Kessel, I., Liberman, M., McKeown, J. A., Mandalia, P. Y., & Ridler, M. A. (1979). Partial monosomy 7 with interstitial deletions in two infants with differing congenital abnormalities. *Journal of Medical Genetics, 16,* 453–460.

Danoff, S. K., Taylor, H. E., Blackshaw, S., & Desiderio, S. (2004). TFII-I, a candidate gene for Williams syndrome cognitive profile: Parallels between regional expression in mouse brain and human phenotype. *Neuroscience, 123,* 931–938.

Davies, M., Udwin, O., & Howlin, P. (1998). Adults with Williams syndrome: Preliminary study of social, emotional and behavioral difficulties. *British Journal of Psychiatry, 172,* 273–276.

Dekker, M. C., & Koot, H. M. (2003). *DSM–IV* disorders in children with borderline to moderate intellectual disability: I. Prevalence and impact. *Journal of the American Academy of Child and Adolescent Psychiatry, 42,* 915–922.

Del Campo, M., Antonell, A., Magano, L. F., Munoz, F. J., Flores, R., Bayes, M., & Perez-Jurado, L. A. (2006). Hemizygosity at the NCF1 gene in patients with Williams–Beuren syndrome decreases their risk for hypertension. *American Journal of Human Genetics, 78,* 533–542.

Del Campo, M., Magano, L., Martinez Iglesias, J., & Perez Jurado, L. (2002). Partial features of Williams–Beuren syndrome in a family with a novel 700 KB 7q11.23 deletion. *Proceedings of the Greenwood Genetic Center, 21,* 169.

Devenny, D. A., Krinsky-McHale, S. J., Kittler, P. M., Flory, M., Jenkins, E., & Brown, W. T. (2004). Age-associated memory changes in adults with Williams syndrome. *Developmental Neuropsychology, 26,* 691–706.

Dilts, C., Morris, C. A., & Leonard, C. O. (1990). A hypothesis for the development of a behavioral phenotype in Williams syndrome. *American Journal of Medical Genetics,* (Suppl. 6), 126–131.

Don, A. J., Schellenberg, G., & Rourke, B. P. (1999). Music and language skills of children with Williams syndrome. *Child Neuropsychology, 5,* 154–170.

Doyle, T. F., Bellugi, U., Korenberg, J. R., & Graham, J. (2004). "Everybody in the world is my friend" hypersociability in young children with Williams syndrome. *American Journal of Medical Genetics, 124A,* 263–273.

Dunn, L. E., & Dunn, L. E. (1997). *Peabody Picture Vocabulary Test* (3rd ed.). Circle Pines, MN: American Guidance Service.

Dykens, E. M. (2003). Anxiety, fears, and phobias in persons with Williams syndrome. *Developmental Neuropsychology, 23,* 291–316.

Dykens, E. M., Rosner, B. A., Ly, T., & Sagun, J. (2005). Music and anxiety in Williams syndrome: A harmonious or discordant relationship? *American Journal on Mental Retardation, 110,* 346–358.

Edgin, J. O. (2003). A neuropsychological model for the development of the cognitive profiles in mental retardation syndromes: Evidence from Down syndrome and Williams syndrome. *Dissertation Abstracts International, 64*(3), 1522B (UMI No. 3086381).

Edmonston, N. K., & Litchfield Thane, N. (1988). *TRC: Test of Relational Concepts.* Austin, TX: PRO-ED.

Einfeld, S. L., & Tonge, B. J. (1995). The Developmental Behavior Checklist: The development and validation of an instrument to assess behavioral and emotional disturbance in children and adolescents with mental retardation. *Journal of Autism and Developmental Disorders, 25,* 81–104.

Einfeld, S., Tonge, B., & Florio, T. (1997). Behavioral and emotional disturbance in individuals with Williams syndrome. *American Journal on Mental Retardation, 102,* 45–53.

Einfeld, S., Tonge, B., & Rees, V. (2001). Longitudinal course of behavioral and emotional problems in Williams syndrome. *American Journal on Mental Retardation, 106,* 73–81.

Einfeld, S., Tonge, B., Turner, G., Parmenter, T., & Smith, A. (1999). Longitudinal course of behavioural and emotional problems of young persons with Prader–Willi, fragile X, Williams and Down syndromes. *Journal of Intellectual & Developmental Disability, 24,* 349–354.

Elliott, C. D. (1990). *Differential Ability Scales.* San Antonio, TX: Psychological Corporation.

Emerson, E. (2003). Prevalence of psychiatric disorders in children and adolescents with and without intellectual disability. *Journal of Intellectual Disability Research, 47,* 51–58.

Eronen, M., Peippo, M., Hiippala, A., Raatikka, M., Arvio, M., Johansson, R., & Kahkonen, M. (2002). Cardiovascular manifestations in 75 patients with Williams syndrome. *Journal of Medical Genetics, 39,* 554–558.

Ewart, A. K., Morris, C. A., Atkinson, D., Jin, W., Sternes, K., Spallone, P., et al. (1993). Hemizygosity at the *elastin* locus in a developmental disorder, Williams syndrome. *Nature Genetics, 5,* 11–16.

Farran, E. K., & Jarrold, C. (2003). Visuospatial cognition in Williams syndrome: Reviewing and accounting for the strengths and weaknesses in performance. *Developmental Neuropsychology, 23,* 173–200.

Fenson, L., Dale, P. S., Reznick, J. S., Thal, D., Bates, E., Hartung, J. P., et al. (1993). *MacArthur Communicative Development Inventories: User's guide and technical manual.* San Diego, CA: Singular.

Fidler, D. J., Hodapp, R. M., & Dykens, E. M. (2000). Stress in families of young children with Down syndrome, Williams syndrome, and Smith–Magenis syndrome. *Early Education & Development, 11,* 395–406.

Fombonne, E. (2005). Epidemiology of autistic disorder and other pervasive developmental disorders. *Journal of Clinical Psychiatry, 66*(Suppl. 10), 3–10.

Frangiskakis, J. M., Ewart, A. K., Morris, C. A., Mervis, C. B., Bertrand, J., Robinson, B. F., et al. (1996). LIM-kinase1 hemizygosity implicated in impaired visuospatial constructive cognition. *Cell, 86,* 59–69.

Freeman, N. H. (1980). *Strategies of representation in young children: Analysis of spatial skills and drawing processes.* London: Academic Press.

Friedrich, W. N., Greenberg, M. T., & Crnic, K. (1983). A short-form of the Questionnaire on Resources and Stress. *American Journal on Mental Retardation, 88,* 41–48.

Frigerio, E., Burt, D. M., Gagliardi, C., Cioffi, G., Martelli, S., Perrett, D. I., & Borgatti, R. (2006). Is everybody always my friend? Perception of approachability in Williams syndrome. *Neuropsychologia, 44,* 254–259.

Gagliardi, C., Bonaglia, M. C., Selicorni, A., Borgatti, R., & Giorda, R. (2003). Unusual cognitive and behavioural profile in a Williams syndrome patient with atypical 7q11.23 deletion. *Journal of Medical Genetics, 40,* 526–530.

Gathercole, S. E., & Baddeley, A. D. (1989). Evaluation of the role of phonological STM in the development of vocabulary in children: A longitudinal study. *Journal of Memory and Language, 28,* 200–213.

Gathercole, S. E., & Baddeley, A. D. (1993). *Working memory and language.* Hillsdale, NJ: Erlbaum.

Georgopoulos, M.-A., Georgopoulos, A. P., Kurz, N., & Landau, B. (2004). Figure copying in Williams syndrome and normal subjects. *Experimental Brain Research, 157,* 137–146.

Giannotti, A., Tiberio, G., Castro, M., Virgilii, F., Colistro, F., Ferretti, F., et al. (2001). Coeliac disease in Williams–Beuren syndrome. *Journal of Medical Genetics, 38,* 767–768.

Gillberg, C., & Rasmussen, P. (1994). Brief report: Four case histories and a literature review of Williams syndrome and autistic behavior. *Journal of Autism and Developmental Disorders, 24,* 381–393.

Giordano, U., Turchetta, A., Giannotti, A., Digilio, M. C., Virgilii, F., & Calzolari, A. (2001). Exercise testing and 24-hour ambulatory blood pressure monitoring in children with Williams syndrome. *Pediatric Cardiology, 22,* 509–511.

Gopnik, A., & Meltzoff, A. N. (1987). The development of categorization in the second year and its relation to other cognitive and linguistic developments. *Child Development, 58,* 1523–1531.

Gopnik, A., & Meltzoff, A. N. (1992). Categorization and naming: Basic level sorting in eighteen-month-olds and its relation to language. *Child Development, 63,* 1091–1103.

Gordon, F. E. (1980). *Primary measures of music audiation* [Book and sound recording]. Chicago: G. I. A. Publications.

Gordon, F. E. (1995). *Musical Aptitude Profile* [Book and sound recording]. Boston: Houghton Mifflin.

Gosch, A., & Pankau, R. (1996). Psychologische aspekte beim Williams–Beuren syndrom. [Psychological aspects of Williams–Beuren syndrome.] *Forum Kinderarzt, 9,* 8–11.

Gosch, A., & Pankau, R. (1997). Personality characteristics and behaviour problems in individuals of different ages with Williams syndrome. *Developmental Medicine & Child Neurology, 39,* 527–533.

Gosch, A., Städing, G., & Pankau, R. (1994). Linguistic abilities in children with Williams–Beuren syndrome. *American Journal of Medical Genetics, 52,* 291–296.

Gothelf, D., Farber, N., Raveh, E., Apter, A., & Attias, J. (2006). Hyperacusis in Williams syndrome: Characteristics and associated neuroaudiologic abnormalities. *Neurology, 66,* 390–395.

Grant, J., Karmiloff-Smith, A., Gathercole, S. A., Paterson, S., Howlin, P., Davies, M., & Udwin, O. (1997). Phonological short-term memory and its relationship to language in Williams syndrome. *Cognitive Neuropsychiatry, 2,* 81–99.

Grant, J., Valian, V., & Karmiloff-Smith, A. (2002). A study of relative clauses in Williams syndrome. *Journal of Child Language, 29,* 403–416.

Greer, M. K., Brown, F. R., Pai, G. S., Choudry, S. H., & Klein, A. J. (1997). Cognitive, adaptive, and behavioral characteristics of Williams syndrome. *American Journal of Medical Genetics (Neuropsychiatric Genetics), 74,* 521–525.

Grimm, T., & Wesselhoeft, H. (1980). Zur Genetik des Williams-Beuren-Syndroms und der Isolierten Form der Supravalvularen Aortenstenose Untersuchungen von 128 Familien. [The genetic aspects of Williams–Beuren syndrome and the isolated form of supravalvar aortic stenosis: Investigation of 128 families.] *Zeitschrift fur Kardiologie, 69,* 168–172.

Hakimi, M. A., Dong, Y., Lane, W. S., Speicher, D. W., & Shiekhattar, R. (2003). A candidate X-linked mental retardation gene is a component of a new family of histone deacetylase-containing complexes. *The Journal of Biological Chemistry, 278,* 7234–7239.

Heller, R., Rauch, A., Luttgen, S., Schroder, B., & Winterpacht, A. (2003). Partial deletion of the critical 1.5 Mb interval in Williams–Beuren syndrome. *Journal of Medical Genetics, 40,* e99.

Hertzberg, J., Nakisbendi, L., Neddleman, H. L., & Pober, B. (1994). Williams syndrome—Oral presentation of 45 cases. *Pediatric Dentistry, 16,* 262.

Hillier, L. W., Fulton, R. S., Fulton, L. A., Graves, T. A., Pepin, K. H., Wagner-McPherson, C., et al. (2003). The DNA sequence of chromosome 7. *Nature, 424,* 157–164.

Hinsley, T. A., Cunliffe, P., Tipney, H. J., Brass, A., & Tassabehji, M. (2004). Comparison of TFII-I gene family members deleted in Williams–Beuren syndrome. *Protein Science, 13,* 2588–2599.

Hirota, H., Matsuoka, R., Chen, X. N., Salandanan, L. S., Lincoln, A., Rose, F. E., et al. (2003). Williams syndrome deficits in visual spatial processing linked to GTF2IRD1 and GTF2I on chromosome 7q11.23. *Genetics in Medicine, 5,* 311–321.

Hobart, H. H., Gregg, R. G., Mervis, C. B., Robinson, B. F., Kimberley, K. W., Rios, C. M., et al. (2004). *Heterozygotes for the microinversion of the Williams–Beuren region have an increased risk for affected offspring.* American Society of Human Genetics, Toronto, Ontario, Canada. Retrieved 10-2-06 from http://genetics.faseb.org/genetics/ashg/annmeet/2004/menu-annmeet-2004.shtml

Hoffman, J. E., Landau, B., & Pagani, B. (2003). Spatial breakdown in spatial construction: Evidence from eye fixations in children with Williams syndrome. *Cognitive Psychology, 46,* 260–301.

Hoogenraad, C. C., Koekkoek, B., Akhmanova, A., Krugers, H., Dortland, B., Miedema, M., et al. (2002). Targeted mutation of Cyln2 in the Williams syndrome critical region links CLIP-115 haploinsufficiency to neurodevelopmental abnormalities in mice. *Nature Genetics, 32,* 116–127.

Hopyan, T., Dennis, M., Weksberg, R., & Cytrynbaum, C. (2001). Music skills and the expressive interpretation of music in children with Williams–Beuren syndrome: Pitch, rhythm, melodic imagery, phrasing, and musical affect. *Child Neuropsychology, 7,* 42–53.

Jackendoff, R. (1994). *Patterns in the mind: Language and human nature.* New York: Basic Books.

Jones, W., Bellugi, U., Lai, Z., Chiles, M., Reilly, J., Lincoln, A., & Adolphs, R. (2000). Hypersociability in Williams syndrome. *Journal of Cognitive Neuroscience, 12*(Suppl.), 30–46.

Jordan, H., Reiss, J. E., Hoffman, J. E., & Landau, B. (2002). Intact perception of biological motion in the face of profound spatial deficits: Williams syndrome. *Psychological Science, 13,* 162–167.

Kaplan, P. (2006). The medical management of children with Williams–Beuren syndrome. In C. A. Morris, H. M. Lenhoff, & P. P. Wang (Eds.), *Williams–Beuren syndrome: Research, evaluation, and treatment* (pp. 83–106). Baltimore: Johns Hopkins University Press.

Kaplan, P., Kirschner, M., Watters, G., & Costa, M. T. (1989). Contractures in patients with Williams syndrome. *Pediatrics, 84,* 895–899.

Karmiloff-Smith, A., Brown, J. H., Grice, S., & Paterson, S. (2003a). Dethroning the myth: Cognitive dissociations and innate modularity in Williams syndrome. *Developmental Neuropsychology, 23,* 229–244.

Karmiloff-Smith, A., Grant, J., Berthoud, I., Davies, M., Howlin, P., & Udwin, O. (1997). Language and Williams syndrome: How intact is "intact"? *Child Development, 68,* 274–290.

Karmiloff-Smith, A., Grant, J., Ewing, S., Carette, M. J., Metcalfe, K., Donnai, D., et al. (2003b). Using case study comparisons to explore genotype–phenotype correlations in Williams–Beuren syndrome. *Journal of Medical Genetics, 40,* 136–140.

Karmiloff-Smith, A., Klima, E., Bellugi, U., Grant, J., & Baron-Cohen, S. (1995). Is there a social module? Language, face processing and theory of mind in individuals with Williams syndrome. *Journal of Cognitive Neuroscience, 7,* 196–208.

Kaufman, A. S., & Kaufman, N. L. (1990). *Kaufman Brief Intelligence Test.* Circle Pines, MN: American Guidance Services.

Kececioglu, D., Kotthoff, S., & Vogt, J. (1993). Williams–Beuren syndrome: A 30-year follow-up of natural and postoperative course. *European Heart Journal, 14,* 1458–1464.

Kemper, S., Kynette, D., Rash, S., & O'Brien, K. (1989). Life span changes to adults' language: Effects of memory and genre. *Applied Psycholinguistics, 10,* 49–66.

Klein, B. P., & Mervis, C. B. (1999). Cognitive strengths and weaknesses of 9- and 10-year-olds with Williams syndrome or Down syndrome. *Developmental Neuropsychology, 16,* 177–196.

Klein-Tasman, B. P., & Mervis, C. B. (2003). Distinctive personality characteristics of 8-, 9-, and 10-year-old children with Williams syndrome. *Developmental Neuropsychology, 23,* 271–292.

Klein-Tasman, B. P., Mervis, C. B., Lord, C., & Phillips, K. D. (in press). Socio-communicative deficits in young children with Williams syndrome: Performance on the Autism Diagnostic Observation Schedule. *Child Neuropsychology.*

Korenberg, J. R., Chen, X. N., Hirota, H., Lai, Z., Bellugi, U., Burian, D., et al. (2000). VI. Genome structure and cognitive map of Williams syndrome. *Journal of Cognitive Neuroscience, 1,* 89–107.

Lacro, R. V., & Smoot, L. B. (2006). Cardiovascular disease in Williams–Beuren syndrome. In C. A. Morris, H. M. Lenhoff, & P. P. Wang (Eds.), *Williams–Beuren syndrome: Research, evaluation, and treatment* (pp. 107–124). Baltimore: Johns Hopkins University Press.

Laing, E., Butterworth, G., Ansari, D., Gsödl, M., Longhi, E., Panagiotaki, G., et al. (2002). Atypical development of language and social communication in toddlers with Williams syndrome. *Developmental Science, 5,* 233–246.

Landau, B., Hoffman, J. E., & Kurz, N. (2006a). Object recognition with severe spatial deficits in Williams syndrome: Sparing and breakdown. *Cognition, 100,* 483–510.

Landau, B., Hoffman, J. E., Reiss, J. E., Dilks, D. D., Lakusta, L., & Chunyo, G. (2006b). Specialization, breakdown, and sparing in spatial cognition: Lessons from Williams–Beuren syndrome. In C. A. Morris, H. M. Lenhoff, & P. P. Wang (Eds.), *Williams–Beuren syndrome: Research, evaluation, and treatment* (pp. 207–236). Baltimore: Johns Hopkins University Press.

Landau, B., & Zukowski, A. (2003). Objects, motions, and paths: Spatial language in children with Williams syndrome. *Developmental Neuropsychology, 23,* 107–139.

Last, C. G., Strauss, C. C., & Francis, G. (1987). Comorbidity among childhood anxiety disorders. *Journal of Nervous and Mental Disorders, 175,* 726–730.

Laws, G., & Bishop, D. (2004). Pragmatic language impairment and social deficits in Williams syndrome: A comparison with Down's syndrome and specific language impairment. *International Journal of Language and Communication Disorders, 39,* 45–64.

Levitin, D. J., & Bellugi, U. (1998). Musical abilities in individuals with Williams syndrome. *Music Perception, 15,* 357–389.

Levitin, D. J., Cole, K., Chiles, M., Lai, Z., Lincoln, A., & Bellugi, U. (2004). Characterizing the musical phenotype in individuals with Williams syndrome. *Child Neuropsychology, 10,* 223–247.

Levitin, D. J., Cole, K., Lincoln, A., & Bellugi, U. (2005). Aversion, awareness, and attraction: Investigating claims of hyperacusis in the Williams syndrome phenotype. *Journal of Child Psychology and Psychiatry, 46,* 514–523.

Levy, Y., & Bechar, T. (2003). Cognitive, lexical, and morpho–syntactic profiles of Israeli children with Williams syndrome. *Cortex, 29,* 255–271.

Levy, Y., & Hermon, S. (2003). Morphological abilities of Hebrew-speaking adolescents. *Developmental Neuropsychology, 23,* 61–85.

Leyfer, O. T., Woodruff-Borden, J., Klein-Tasman, B. P., Fricke, J. S., & Mervis, C. B. (2006). Prevalence of psychiatric disorders in 4- to 16-year-olds with Williams syndrome. *American Journal of Medical Genetics, Part B, 141B,* 615–622.

Li, D. Y., Faury, G., Taylor, D. G., Davis, E. C., Boyle, W. A., Mecham, R. P., et al. (1998). Novel arterial pathology in mice and humans hemizygous for elastin. *The Journal of Clinical Investigation, 102,* 1783–1787.

Lord, C., Risi, S., Lambrecht, L., Cook, E., Leventhal, B., DiValore, P., et al. (2000). The Autism Diagnostic Observation Schedule—Generic: A standard measure of social and communication deficits associated with the spectrum of autism. *Journal of Autism and Developmental Disorders, 30,* 205–223.

Lord, C., Rutter, M., & Le Couteur, A. (1994). Autism Diagnostic Interview—Revised: A revised version of a diagnostic interview for caregivers of individuals with possible pervasive developmental disorders. *Journal of Autism and Developmental Disorders, 24,* 659–685.

Lowery, M. C., Morris, C. A., Ewart, A., Brothman, L., Xiao, L. Z., Leonard, C. O., et al. (1995). Strong correlations of *elastin* deletions, detected by FISH, with Williams syndrome: Evaluation of 235 patients. *American Journal of Human Genetics, 57,* 49–53.

Lukács, A., Pléh, C., & Racsmány, M. (2004). Language in Hungarian children with Williams syndrome. In S. Bartke & J. Siegmüller (Eds.), *Williams syndrome across languages* (pp. 187–220). Amsterdam: John Benjamins.

Lukács, A., Racsmány, M., & Pléh, C. (2001). Vocabulary and morphological patterns in Hungarian children with Williams syndrome: A preliminary report. *Acta Linguistica Hungarica, 48,* 243–269.

Marler, J. A., Elfenbein, J. L., Ryals, B. M., Urban, Z., & Netzloff, M. L. (2005). Sensorineural hearing loss in children and adults with Williams syndrome. *American Journal of Medical Genetics, A, 138,* 318–327.

Marshall, C. R., & van der Lely, H. K. (2006). A challenge to current models of past tense inflection: The impact of phonotactics. *Cognition, 100,* 302–320.

Masataka, N. (2001). Why early linguistic milestones are delayed in children with Williams syndrome: Late onset of hand banging as a possible rate-limiting constraint on the emergence of canonical babbling. *Developmental Science, 4,* 158–164.

Mason, T. B. A., & Arens, R. (2006). Sleep patterns in Williams–Beuren syndrome. In C. A. Morris, H. M. Lenhoff, & P. P. Wang (Eds.), *Williams–Beuren syndrome: Research, evaluation, and treatment* (pp. 294–308). Baltimore: Johns Hopkins University Press.

McCarthy, D. (1972). *McCarthy Scales of Children's Abilities.* New York: Psychological Corporation.

Meng, Y., Zhang, Y., Tregoubov, V., Janus, C., Cruz, L., Jackson, M., et al. (2002). Abnormal spine morphology and enhanced LTP in LIMK-1 knockout mice. *Neuron, 35,* 121–133.

Mervis, C. B. (1999). The Williams syndrome cognitive profile: Strengths, weaknesses, and interrelations among auditory short term memory, language, and visuospatial constructive cognition. In E. Winograd, R. Fivush, & W. Hirst (Eds.), *Ecological approaches to cognition: Essays in honor of Ulric Neisser* (pp. 193–227). Mahwah, NJ: Erlbaum.

Mervis, C. B. (2004). Cross-etiology comparisons of cognitive and language development. In M. L. Rice & S. F. Warren (Eds.), *Developmental language disorders: From phenotypes to etiologies* (pp. 153–186). Mahwah, NJ: Erlbaum.

Mervis, C. B. (2006). Language abilities in Williams–Beuren syndrome. In C. A. Morris, H. M. Lenhoff, & P. P. Wang (Eds.), *Williams–Beuren syndrome: Research, evaluation, and treatment* (pp. 159–206). Baltimore: Johns Hopkins University Press.

Mervis, C. B., & Bertrand, J. (1997). Developmental relations between cognition and language: Evidence from Williams syndrome. In L. B. Adamson & M. A. Romski (Eds.), *Communication and language acquisition: Discoveries from atypical development* (pp. 75–106). New York: Brookes.

Mervis, C. B., & Klein-Tasman, B. P. (2000). Williams syndrome: Cognition, personality, and adaptive behavior. *Mental Retardation and Developmental Disabilities Research Reviews, 6,* 148–158.

Mervis, C. B., & Klein-Tasman, B. P. (2004). Methodological issues in group-matching designs: Alpha levels for control variable comparisons and measurement characteristics of control and target variables. *Journal of Autism and Developmental Disorders, 34,* 7–17.

Mervis, C. B., Klein-Tasman, B. P., & Mastin, M. E. (2001). Adaptive behavior of 4- through 8-year-old children with Williams syndrome. *American Journal on Mental Retardation, 106,* 82–93.

Mervis, C. B., Morris, C. A., Bertrand, J., & Robinson, B. F. (1999a). Williams syndrome: Findings from an integrated program of research. In H. Tager-Flusberg (Ed.), *Neurodevelopmental disorders* (pp. 65–110). Cambridge, MA: MIT Press.

Mervis, C. B., Morris, C. A., Klein-Tasman, B. P., Bertrand, J., Kwitny, S., Appelbaum, L. G., & Rice, C. E. (2003a). Attentional characteristics of infants and toddlers with Williams syndrome during triadic interactions. *Developmental Neuropsychology, 23,* 245–270.

Mervis, C. B., & Robinson, B. F. (2000). Expressive vocabulary of toddlers with Williams syndrome or Down syndrome: A comparison. *Developmental Neuropsychology, 17,* 111–126.

Mervis, C. B., & Robinson, B. F. (2005). Designing measures for profiling and genotype/phenotype studies of individuals with genetic syndromes or developmental language disorders. *Applied Psycholinguistics, 26,* 41–64.

Mervis, C. B., Robinson, B. F., Bertrand, J., Morris, C. A., Klein-Tasman, B. P., & Armstrong, S. C. (2000). The Williams Syndrome Cognitive Profile. *Brain and Cognition, 44,* 604–628.

Mervis, C. B., Robinson, B. F., Rowe, M. L., Becerra, A. M., & Klein-Tasman, B. P. (2003b). Language abilities of individuals who have Williams syndrome. In L. Abbeduto (Ed.), *International review of research in mental retardation* (Vol. 27, pp. 35–81). Orlando, FL: Academic Press.

Mervis, C. B., Robinson, B. F., Rowe, M. L., Becerra, A. M., & Klein-Tasman, B. P. (2004). Relations between language and cognition in Williams syndrome. In S. Bartke & J. Siegmüller (Eds.), *Williams syndrome across languages* (pp. 63–92). Amsterdam, The Netherlands: John Benjamins Publishing.

Mervis, C. B., Robinson, B. F., & Pani, J. R. (1999b). Visuospatial construction. *American Journal of Human Genetics, 65,* 1222–1229.

Metcalfe, K., Rucka, A. K., Smoot, L., Hofstadler, G., Tuzler, G., McKeown, P., et al. (2000). Elastin: Mutational spectrum in supravalvular aortic stenosis. *European Journal of Human Genetics, 8,* 955–963.

Meyer-Lindenberg, A., Hariri, A. R., Munoz, K. E., Mervis, C. B., Mattay, V. S., Morris, C. A., & Berman, K. F. (2005). Neural correlates of genetically abnormal social cognition in Williams syndrome. *Nature Neuroscience, 8,* 991–993.

Meyer-Lindenberg, A., Kohn, P., Mervis, C. B., Kippenhan, J. S., Olsen, R., Morris, C. A., & Berman, K. F. (2004). Neural basis of genetically determined visuospatial construction deficit in Williams syndrome. *Neuron, 43,* 623–631.

Meyer-Lindenberg, A., Mervis, C. B., & Berman, K. F. (2006). Neural mechanisms in Williams syndrome: A unique window to genetic influences on cognition and behavior. *Nature Reviews: Neuroscience, 7,* 380–393.

Milner, B. (1971). Interhemispheric differences in the localization of psychological processes in man. *British Medical Bulletin, 27,* 272–277.

Mizugishi, K., Yamanaka, K., Kuwajima, K., & Kondo, I. (1998). Interstitial deletion of chromosome 7q in a patient with Williams syndrome and infantile spasms. *Journal of Human Genetics, 43,* 178–181.

Mons, A., Wilmowski, W. A., & Detweiler, C. (1996). *Williams syndrome: A highly musical species* [Film]. EO Productions International.

Morris, C. A. (2005). Williams syndrome. In S. B. Cassidy & J. E. Allanson (Eds.), *Management of genetic syndromes* (2nd ed., pp. 655–665). Hoboken, NJ: Wiley.

Morris, C. A. (2006a). Genotype–phenotype correlations in Williams–Beuren syndrome. In C. A. Morris, H. M. Lenhoff, & P. P. Wang (Eds.), *Williams–Beuren syndrome: Research, evaluation, and treatment* (pp. 59–82). Baltimore: Johns Hopkins University Press.

Morris, C. A. (2006b). The dysmorphology, genetics, and natural history of Williams–Beuren syndrome. In C. A. Morris, H. M. Lenhoff, & P. P. Wang (Eds.), *Williams–Beuren syndrome: Research, evaluation, and treatment* (pp. 3–17). Baltimore: Johns Hopkins University Press.

Morris, C. A. (2006c). Williams syndrome (WS). [*GeneClinics:* ™*Medical Genetics Knowledge Base* Web site]. Retrieved 10-2-06 from http://www.geneclinics.org/

Morris, C. A., Dilts, C., Demsey, S. A., Leonard, C. O., & Blackburn, B. (1988). The natural history of Williams syndrome: Physical characteristics. *The Journal of Pediatrics, 113,* 318–326.

Morris, C. A., Lu, X., & Greenberg, F. (1998). Syndromes identified in patients with a previous diagnosis of Williams syndrome who do not have *elastin* deletion. *Proceedings of the Greenwood Genetic Center, 17,* 116.

Morris, C. A., Mervis, C. A., Hobart, H. H., Gregg, R. G., Bertrand, J., Ensing, G. J. (2003). *GTF21* hemizygosity implicated in mental retardation in Williams syndrome: Genotype–phenotype analysis of 5 families with deletions in the Williams syndrome region. *American Journal of Medical Genetics, Part A, 123,* 45–59.

Morris, C. A., & Moore, C. A. (1991). The inheritance of Williams syndrome. *Proceedings of the Greenwood Genetics Center, 10,* 81–82.

Mullen, E. M. (1995). *Mullen Scales of Early Learning.* Circle Pines, MN: American Guidance Service.

Mundy, P., Delgado, C., Block, J., Venezia, M., Hogan, A., & Seibert, J. (2003). *A manual for the abridged Early Social Communication Scales (ESCS).* Coral Gables, FL: University of Miami Psychology Department. Retrieved 10-2-06 from http://www.psy.miami.edu/faculty/pmundy/ESCS.pdf

Myers, B. A., & Pueschel, S. M. (1991). Psychiatric disorders in persons with Down syndrome. *Journal of Nervous and Mental Disorders, 179,* 609–613.

Nichols, S., Jones, W., Roman, M. J., Wulfeck, B., Delis, D. C., Reilly, J., & Bellugi, U. (2004). Mechanisms of verbal memory impairment in four neurodevelopmental disorders. *Brain and Language, 88,* 180–189.

Norman, S., Kemper, S., & Kynette, D. (1992). Adult reading comprehension: Effects of syntactic complexity and working memory. *Journals of Gerontology, 47,* 258–265.

Nowicki, S., Jr., & Duke, M. P. (1994). Individual differences in the nonverbal communication of affect: The Diagnostic Analysis of Nonverbal Accuracy Scale. *Journal of Nonverbal Behavior, 18,* 9–35.

Oliveri, B., Mastaglia, S. R., Mautalen, C., Gravano, J. C., & Pardo Argerich, L. (2004). Long-term control of hypercalcaemia in an infant with Williams–Beuren syndrome after a single infusion of biphosphonate (Pamidronate). *Acta Paediatrica, 93,* 1002–1003.

Osborne, L. R. (2006). The molecular basis of a multisystem disorder. In C. A. Morris, H. M. Lenhoff, & P. P. Wang (Eds.), *Williams–Beuren syndrome: Research, evaluation, and treatment* (pp. 18–58). Baltimore: Johns Hopkins University Press.

Osborne, L. R., Li, M., Pober, B., Chitayat, D., Bodurtha, J., & Mandel, A. (2001). A 1.5 million-base pair inversion polymorphism in families with Williams–Beuren syndrome. *Nature Genetics, 29,* 321–325.

Pagon, R. A., Bennett, F. C., LaVeck, B., Stewart, K. B., & Johnson, J. (1987). Williams syndrome: Features in late childhood and adolescence. *Pediatrics, 80,* 85–91.

Pankau, R., Partsch, C.-J., Gosch, A., Oppermann, H. C., & Wessel, A. (1992). Statural growth in Williams–Beuren syndrome. *European Journal of Pediatrics, 151,* 751–755.

Peregrine, E., Rowe, M. L., & Mervis, C. B. (2005, April). *Pragmatic language difficulties in children with Williams syndrome.* Poster presented at the meeting of the Society for Research in Child Development, Atlanta, GA.

Perez Jurado, L. A., Peoples, R., Kaplan, P., Hamel, B. C., & Francke, U. (1996). Molecular definition of the chromosome 7 deletions in Williams syndrome and parent-of-origin effects on growth. *American Journal of Human Genetics, 59,* 781–792.

Perez Jurado, L. A., Wang, Y. K., Peoples, R., Coloma, A., Cruces, J., & Francke, U. (1998). A duplicated gene in the breakpoint regions of the 7q11.23 Williams–Beuren syndrome deletion encodes the initiator binding protein TFII-I and BAP-135, a phosphorylation target of BTK. *Human Molecular Genetics, 7,* 325–334.

Pléh, C., Lukács, A., & Racsmány, M. (2002). Morphological patterns in Hungarian children with Williams syndrome and the rule debates. *Brain and Language, 86,* 377–383.

Plesa-Skwerer, D., & Tager-Flusberg, H. (2006). Social cognition in Williams–Beuren syndrome. In C. A. Morris, H. M. Lenhoff, & P. P. Wang (Eds.), *Williams–Beuren syndrome: Research, evaluation, and treatment* (pp. 237–253). Baltimore: Johns Hopkins University Press.

Plesa-Skwerer, D., Faja, S., Schofield, C., Verbalis, A., & Tager-Flusberg, H. (2006a). Perceiving facial and vocal expressions of emotion in individuals with Williams syndrome. *American Journal on Mental Retardation, 111,* 15–26.

Plesa-Skwerer, D., Verbalis, A., Schofield, C., Faja, S., & Tager-Flusberg, H. (2006b). Social–perceptual abilities in adolescents and adults with Williams syndrome. *Cognitive Neuropsychology, 23,* 338–349.

Pober, B. R., & Szekely, A. M. (1999). Distinct neurological profile in Williams syndrome. *American Journal of Human Genetics Supplement, 65*(4), A70.

Power, T. J., Blum, N. J., Jones, S. M., & Kaplan, P. E. (1997). Response to methylphenidate in two children with Williams syndrome. *Journal of Autism and Developmental Disorders, 27,* 79–87.

Preus, M. (1984). The Williams syndrome: Objective definition and diagnosis. *Clinical Genetics, 25,* 422–428.

Rabensteiner, B. (1975). Sozialverhalten, musikalität und visuelle wahrnehmung bei mongoloiden kindern. [Social behavior, musicality and visual perception in mongoloid children.] *Pädiatrie und Pädologie Supplementum, 4,* 59–69.

Reich, W., Shayka, J. J., & Taibelson, C. (1991). *Diagnostic Interview Schedule for Children and Adolescents, parent version.* St. Louis, MO: Washington University.

Reiss, A., Feinstein, C., Rosenbaum, K., Borgengasser-Caruso, M., & Goldsmith, B. (1985). Autism associated with Williams syndrome. *The Journal of Pediatrics, 106,* 247–249.

Robinson, B. F., Mervis, C. B., & Robinson, B. W. (2003). Roles of verbal short-term memory and working memory in the acquisition of grammar by children with Williams syndrome. *Developmental Neuropsychology, 23,* 13–31.

Rothbart, M. K., & Ahadi, S. A. (1994). Temperament and the development of personality. *Journal of Abnormal Psychology, 103,* 55–66.

Rowe, M. L., & Mervis, C. B. (2006). Working memory in Williams syndrome. In T. P. Alloway & S. E. Gathercole (Eds.), *Working memory and neurodevelopmental conditions* (pp. 267–293). Hove, England: Psychology Press.

Rowe, M. L., Peregrine, E., & Mervis, C. B. (2005, April). *Communicative development in toddlers with Williams syndrome.* Poster presented at the meeting of the Society for Research in Child Development, Atlanta, GA.

Sadler, L. S., Pober, B. R., Grandinetti, A., Scheiber, D., Fekete, G., Sharma, A. N., & Urban, Z. (2001). Differences by sex in cardiovascular disease in Williams syndrome. *Journal of Pediatrics, 139,* 849–853.

Sadler, L. S., Olitsky, S. E., & Reynolds, J. D. (1996). Reduced stereoacuity in Williams syndrome. *American Journal of Medical Genetics, 66,* 287–288.

Sammour, Z. M., Gomes, C. M., Duarte, R. J., Trigo-Rocha, F. E., & Srougi, M. (2006). Voiding dysfunction and the Williams–Beuren syndrome: A clinical and urodynamic investigation. *Journal of Urology, 175,* 1472–1476.

Sarimski, K. (1997). Behavioural phenotypes and family stress in three mental retardation syndromes. *European Child and Adolescent Psychiatry, 6,* 26–31.

Shaffer, D., Fisher, P., Dulcan, M. K., Davies, M., Piacentini, J., Schwab-Stone, M. E., et al. (1996). The NIMH Diagnostic Interview Schedule for Children Version 2.3 (DISC–2.3): Description, acceptability, prevalence rates, and performance in the MECA Study. Methods for the Epidemiology of Child and Adolescent Mental Disorders Study. *Journal of the American Academy of Child and Adolescent Psychiatry, 35,* 865–877.

Sigman, M. D., Kasari, C., Kwon, K., & Yirmiya, N. (1992). Responses to the negative emotions of others by autistic, mentally retarded, and normal children. *Child Development, 63,* 796–807.

Silverman, W. K., & Albano, A. M. (1996). *The Anxiety Disorders Interview Schedule for DSM–IV: Parent interview schedule.* San Antonio, TX: Graywind Publications, a Division of the Psychological Corporation.

Somerville, M. J., Mervis, C. B., Young, E. J., Seo, E.-J., del Campo, M., Bamforth, S., et al. (2005). Severe expressive language delay related to duplication of the Williams–Beuren locus. *New England Journal of Medicine, 353,* 1694–1701.

Soper, R., Chaloupka, J. C., Fayad, P. B., Greally, J. M., Shaywitz, B. A., Awad, I. A., & Pober, B. R. (1995). Ischemic stroke and intracranial multifocal cerebral arteriopathy in Williams syndrome. *Journal of Pediatrics, 126,* 945–948.

Sparrow, S. S., Balla, D. A., & Cicchetti, D. V. (1984). *Vineland Adaptive Behavior Scales–Interview Edition.* Circle Pines, MN: American Guidance Service.

Stankiewicz, P., & Lupski, J. R. (2002). Genome architecture, rearrangements and genomic disorders. *Trends in Genetics, 18,* 74–82.

Stock, A. D., Spallone, P. A., Dennis, T. R., Netski, D., Morris, C. A., Mervis, C. B., & Hobart, H. H. (2003). Heat shock protein 27 gene: Chromosomal and molecular location and relationship to Williams syndrome. *American Journal of Medical Genetics, Part A, 120,* 320–325.

Strauss, C. C., Lease, C. A., Last, C. G., & Francis, G. (1988). Overanxious disorder: An examination of developmental differences. *Journal of Abnormal Child Psychology, 16,* 433–443.

Strømme, P., Bjørnstad, P. G., & Ramstad, K. (2002). Prevalence estimation of Williams syndrome. *Journal of Child Neurology, 17,* 269–271.

Sullivan, K., & Tager-Flusberg, H. (1999). Second-order belief attribution in Williams syndrome: Intact or impaired? *American Journal on Mental Retardation, 104,* 523–532.

Sullivan, K., Winner, E., & Tager-Flusberg, H. (2003). Can adolescents with Williams syndrome tell the difference between lies and jokes? *Developmental Neuropsychology, 23,* 85–103.

Tada, W. L., & Stiles-Davis, J. (1989). Children's analysis of spatial patterns: An assessment of their errors in copying geometric forms. *Cognitive Development, 4,* 177–195.

Tager-Flusberg, H., & Sullivan, K. (2000). A componential view of theory of mind: Evidence from Williams syndrome. *Cognition, 76,* 59–89.

Tager-Flusberg, H., Sullivan, K., & Boshart, J. (1997). Executive functions and performance on false belief tasks. *Developmental Neuropsychology, 13,* 487–493.

Tassabehji, M., Hammond, P., Karmiloff-Smith, A., Thompson, P., Thorgeirsson, S. S., Durkin, M. E., et al. (2005). GTF2IRD1 in craniofacial development of humans and mice. *Science, 310,* 1184–1187.

Tassabehji, M., Metcalfe, K., Hurst, J., Ashcroft, G. S., Kielty, C., Wilmot, C., et al. (1998). An *elastin* gene mutation producing abnormal tropoelastin and abnormal elastic fibres in a patient with autosomal dominant cutis laxa. *Human Molecular Genetics, 7,* 1021–1028.

Tassabehji, M., Metcalfe, K., Karmiloff-Smith, A., Carette, M. J., Grant, J., Dennis, N., et al. (1999). Williams syndrome: Use of chromosomal microdeletions as a tool to dissect cognitive and physical phenotypes. *American Journal of Human Genetics, 64,* 118–125.

Tellegen, A. (1985). Structures of mood and personality and their relevance to assessing anxiety, with an emphasis on self-report. In A. H. Tum & J. D. Maser (Eds.), *Anxiety and the anxiety disorders* (pp. 681–716). Hillsdale, NJ: Erlbaum.

Temple, C. M., Almazan, M., & Sherwood, S. (2002). Lexical skills in Williams syndrome: A cognitive neuropsychological analysis. *Journal of Neurolinguistics, 15,* 463–495.

Thomas, A., & Chess, S. (1977). *Temperament and development.* New York: Bruner/Mazel.

Thomas, M. L., Becerra, A. M., & Mervis, C. B. (2002, July). *Empathic behavior of 4-year-olds with Williams syndrome, other forms of developmental delay, or typical development.* Paper presented at the International Professional Meeting of the Williams Syndrome Association, Long Beach, CA.

Thomas, M. S. C., Grant, J., Barham, Z., Gsödl, M., Laing, E., Lakusta, L., et al. (2001). Past tense formation in Williams syndrome. *Language & Cognitive Processes, 16,* 143–176.

Thomas, M. S. C., & Karmiloff-Smith, A. (2003). Modeling language acquisition in atypical phenotypes. *Psychological Review, 110,* 647–682.

Tomc, S. A., Williamson, N. K., & Pauli, R. M. (1990). Temperament in Williams syndrome. *American Journal of Medical Genetics, 36,* 345–352.

Tonge, B., & Einfeld, S. (2003). Psychopathology and intellectual disability: The Australian Child to Adult Longitudinal Study. In L. M. Glidden (Ed.), *International review of research in mental retardation* (pp. 61–91). San Diego, CA: Elsevier Science.

Udwin, O., & Yule, W. (1990). Expressive language of children with Williams syndrome. *American Journal of Medical Genetics,* (Suppl. 6), 108–114.

Udwin, O., & Yule, W. (1991). A cognitive and behavioural phenotype in Williams syndrome. *Journal of Clinical and Experimental Neuropsychology, 13,* 232–244.

Van Borsel, J., Curfs, L. M. G., & Fryns, J. P. (1997). Hyperacusis in Williams syndrome: A sample survey study. *Genetic Counseling, 8,* 121–126.

Van Lieshout, C. F. M., De Meyer, R. E., Curfs, L. M. G., & Fryns, J.-P. (1998). Family contexts, parental behavior, and personality profiles of children and adolescents with Prader–Willi, fragile-X, or Williams syndrome. *Journal of Child Psychology and Psychiatry, 39,* 699–710.

Vaux, K. K., Wojtczak, H., Benirschke, K., & Jones, K. L. (2003). Vocal cord abnormalities in Williams syndrome: A further manifestation of elastin deficiency. *American Journal of Medical Genetics, 119A,* 302–304.

Vicari, S., Bates, E., Caselli, M. C., Pasqualetti, P., Gagliardi, C., Tonucci, F., & Volterra, V. (2004). Neuropsychological profile of Italians with Williams syndrome: An example of a dissociation between language and cognition? *Journal of the International Neuropsychological Society, 10,* 862–876.

Vicari, S., Caselli, M. C., Gagliardi, C., Tonucci, F., & Volterra, V. (2002). Language acquisition in special populations: A comparison between Down and Williams syndromes. *Neuropsychologia, 40,* 2461–2470.

Volterra, V., Capirci, O., Pezzini, G., Sabbadini, L., & Vicari, S. (1996). Linguistic abilities in Italian children with Williams syndrome. *Cortex, 32,* 663–677.

Volterra, V., Caselli, M. C., Capirci, O., Tonucci, F., & Vicari, S. (2003). Early linguistic abilities of Italian children with Williams syndrome. *Developmental Neuropsychology, 23,* 33–59.

von Arnim, G., & Engel, P. (1964). Mental retardation related to hypercalcaemia. *Developmental Medicine and Child Neurology, 6,* 366–377.

Walsh, V. (2003). A theory of magnitude: Common cortical metrics of time, space and quantity. *Trends in Cognitive Sciences, 7,* 483–488.

Wang, M. S., Schinzel, A., Kotzot, D., Balmer, D., Casey, R., Chodirker, B. N., et al. (1999). Molecular and clinical correlation study of Williams–Beuren syndrome: No evidence of molecular factors in the deletion region or imprinting affecting clinical outcome. *American Journal of Medical Genetics, 86,* 34–43.

Wang, P. P., & Bellugi, U. (1994). Evidence from two genetic syndromes for a dissociation between verbal and visual–spatial short-term memory. *Journal of Clinical and Experimental Neuropsychology, 16,* 317–322.

Wechsler, D. (1974). *Wechsler Intelligence Scale for Children—Revised.* New York: Psychological Corporation.

Wetherby, A. M., & Prizant, B. M. (2002). *CSBS DP manual: Communication and Symbolic Behavior Scales Developmental Profile, first normed edition.* Baltimore: Brookes.

White, S. M., Thompson, E. M., Kidd, A., Savarirayan, R., Turner, A., Amor, D., et al. (2004). Growth, behavior, and clinical findings in 27 patients with Kabuki (Niikawa–Kuroki) syndrome. *American Journal of Medical Genetics, 127A,* 118–127.

Williams, J. C. P., Barratt-Boyes, B. G., & Lowe, J. B. (1961). Supravalvular aortic stenosis. *Circulation, 24,* 1311–1318.

Williams, K. T. (1997). *Expressive Vocabulary Test.* Circle Pines, MN: American Guidance Service.

Wu, Y.-Q., Nickerson, E., Shaffer, L. G., Keppler-Noreuil, K., & Muilenburg, A. (1999). A case of Williams syndrome with a large, visible cytogenetic deletion. *Journal of Medical Genetics, 36,* 928–932.

Wu, Y.-Q., Reid Sutton, V., Nickerson, E., Lupski, J. R., Potocki, L., Korenberg, J. R., et al. (1998). Delineation of the common critical region in Williams syndrome and clinical correlation of growth, heart defects, ethnicity, and parental origin. *American Journal of Medical Genetics, 78,* 82–89.

Young, R. S., Weaver, D. D., Kukolich, M. K., Heerema, N. A., Palmer, C. G., Kawira, E. L., & Bender, H. A. (1984). Terminal and interstitial deletions of the long arm of chromosome 7: A review with five new cases. *American Journal of Medical Genetics, 17,* 437–450.

Zackowski, J. L., Raffel, L. J., Blank, C. A., & Schwartz, S. (1990). Proximal interstitial deletion of 7q: A case report and review of the literature. *American Journal of Medical Genetics, 36,* 328–332.

Zhang, M. C., He, L., Giro, M., Yong, S. L., Tiller, G. E., & Davidson, J. M. (1999). Cutis laxa arising from frameshift mutations in exon 30 of the *elastin* gene (ELN). *The Journal of Biological Chemistry, 274,* 981–986.

Zukowski, A. (2004). Investigating knowledge of complex syntax: Insights from experimental studies of Williams syndrome. In M. Rice & S. Warren (Eds.), *Developmental language disorders: From phenotypes to etiologies* (pp. 99–119). Cambridge, MA: MIT Press.

II COMPLEX ETIOLOGIES AND COMPLEX OUTCOMES

8 Congenital Hypothyroidism: Genetic and Biochemical Influences on Brain Development and Neuropsychological Functioning

Joanne F. Rovet and Rosalind Brown

Congenital hypothyroidism is a pediatric endocrine disorder affecting 1 in 3,000 to 1 in 4,000 children. Congenital hypothyroidism is caused by a lack of thyroid hormone (LaFranchi, 1999), which is essential for the developing brain (Zoeller & Rovet, 2004). Although congenital hypothyroidism can be readily treated with replacement hormone, this must be given right after birth to prevent subsequent brain damage.

The most common signs and symptoms of congenital hypothyroidism are a large protruding tongue, puffy face, umbilical hernia, prolonged jaundice, constipation, and lethargy (see figure 8.1). Unfortunately, because these features take time to appear, clinical diagnosis is often delayed. This used to mean that by the time a child with congenital hypothyroidism could be treated, extensive brain damage would have occurred, and congenital hypothyroidism was once a leading cause of mental retardation (Crome & Stern, 1972). However, since the advent of newborn screening for congenital hypothyroidism several decades ago, the diagnosis of congenital hypothyroidism is made much earlier with treatment being given before clinical symptoms even appear. As a consequence, the mental retardation previously associated with congenital hypothyroidism has now been eliminated (Brook, 1995). Nevertheless, because these children still undergo a brief period of thyroid hormone insufficiency, they are at risk for neurocognitive impairment (Rovet, 1999a). Research by us and others has been instrumental in characterizing the neuropsychological phenotype in screened children with congenital hypothyroidism and in pinpointing the factors contributing to variability.

Case 8.1: Jena (diagnosed with congenital hypothyroidism prior to newborn screening) Jena was 12 years of age and in fifth grade at the time of her neuropsychological assessment for problems at school. She was described as fidgety, easily distracted and confused, and unable to concentrate and finish assignments, and she had a long history of academic problems. Although she received in-class remedial help in the past and was now in a learning disabilities class, because of her poor performance, she was being considered for a slow learner class.

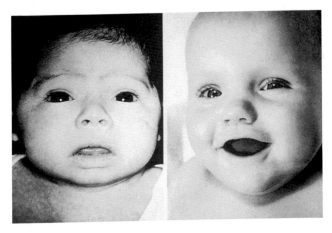

Figure 8.1
Infants with congenital hypothyroidism. The child on the left was diagnosed clinically after 3 months of age; the child on the right was diagnosed by newborn screening before 3 weeks of age.

Jena was born full-term in the last city hospital to enter the newborn screening program. Her mother described a normal pregnancy and unremarkable delivery. At birth, Jena weighed 8 lbs. and had a "bloated" appearance and jaundice. As an infant, she was a poor eater and very placid, seldom crying. At 3 months of age, she was clinically diagnosed with congenital hypothyroidism and treated with L-thyroxine. She sat at 6 months, crawled at 1 year, and walked and spoke her first words at age 2. She had a speech problem and was hypotonic, for which she received speech therapy and physiotherapy.

Jena's behavior during testing was described as anxious, unengaged, and immature, while her speech was unclear. Testing revealed an IQ of 80 with equivalent scores on the Verbal and Performance subscales and a particular strength on the Picture Completion subtest (SS = 11). Her scores were low on the Arithmetic (SS = 2), Digit Span (SS = 4), Coding (SS = 4), and Mazes (SS = 6) subtests, and she showed memory impairments for associative learning, recall of stories, recognition of faces, and reconstruction of figures. She also showed severe deficits in visual–motor integration and visual perception and was unable to draw a human figure, and her writing was extremely immature. Academically, Jena read at the 10th percentile, while her arithmetic was below the 1st percentile and reflected significant weaknesses with basic operations. She showed behavior problems related to attention and anxiety.

This chapter aims to delineate the characteristics of children with congenital hypothyroidism detected by newborn screening and examine how their disease and treatment factors contribute to variability in phenotypic expression. The first section deals with thyroid development and functioning; the next section provides a brief overview of thyroid hormone's influences on brain development; the next section summarizes the neuropsychological findings; the next section examines the influence of disease- and treatment-related factors on outcome and potential phenotype–genotype corre-

Table 8.1
Variants of thyroid dysgenesis and associated molecular defects

Variant of Congenital Hypothyroidism in Humans	Percentage of Cases	Severity of Hypothyroidism	Gene Defect
Agenesis	~20–40	Severe	TTF-2
Ectopia	~40–80	Mild	TTF-2
Hypoplasia	~ 5–10	Mild to moderate	TTF-1, PAX-8, and TSH receptors
Hemiagenesis	~0.5	Mild or none	SHH

lations; and the final section provides a summary and conclusions. It is hoped that upon completing this chapter, the reader will have gained an understanding of the complexity of this disease and its effects on long-term outcome as well as an appreciation of thyroid hormone's role in brain development.

The Etiologies of Congenital Hypothyroidism

The main etiologies of congenital hypothyroidism are (a) thyroid dysgenesis due to a missing, misplaced, or malformed thyroid gland; (b) thyroid dyshormonogenesis from a blockage in one of the many steps in thyroid hormone production; and (c) central hypothyroidism caused by a disruption in the negative feedback system involving the hypothalamus and pituitary. To understand how these etiologies arise, one must know about normal thyroid gland development and its physiology and regulation. The recent identification of genes associated with these various processes gives insight as to the factors accounting for the different etiologies (Gillam & Kopp, 2001; Moreno, de Vijlder, Vulsma, & Ris-Staplers, 2003).

Thyroid Dysgenesis

Thyroid morphogenesis follows a set schedule: Thyroid tissue is first evident at gestational day (GD) 20 to 22 as an outpouching of epithelial cells in the floor of the primitive pharynx; at GD 28, the fetal thyroid migrates downward reaching final position at the base of the neck at GD 45 to 50; the gland continues to proliferate and differentiate, and achieves a definite structure consisting of two lateral lobes separated by an isthmus by GD 70; at GD 70, low levels of thyroid hormones are produced; by midgestation, the gland starts to be regulated by hormones produced in the brain; the gland continues to grow and its production of hormones continues to increase through to term. Table 8.1 shows the molecular defects that have so far been identified with each of these variants of thyroid dysgenesis (Van Vliet, 2003; Grüters, Krude, & Bierbermann, 2004). However, because defects in this set of genes only account for about 10% of all congenital hypothyroidism cases, the picture is currently far from complete.

Thyroid agenesis (an absent thyroid gland), which is seen in approximately 20%–40% of congenital hypothyroidism cases due to thyroid dysgenesis, generally represents the most severe form of congenital hypothyroidism. Children with thyroid agenesis often exhibit hypothyroidism in utero as indicated by their severely delayed bone development at birth. Mutations of the TTF-2 (also known as FOXE8) have been associated with thyroid agenesis. TTF-2 mutations are often comorbid with spiky hair, cleft palate, bifid epiglottis, and choanal atresia (Grüters, 2004) and suggest a role for TTF-2 in midline development. Defects of the TTF-1 gene (also known as NKX2.1) are associated with developmental disabilities, severe neonatal respiratory distress, pulmonary problems, ataxia, and hypotonia. Surprisingly, in humans, unlike homozygous "knockout mice," the hypothyroidism is mild and agenesis has not been described, probably because a homozygous deletion of TTF-1 is incompatible with life.

Thyroid ectopy affects approximately 80% of children with congenital hypothyroidism due to thyroid dysgenesis and results from a failure in migration, with the gland remaining small and in a lingual or sublingual position in the throat. Children with ectopic glands usually have a milder form of congenital hypothyroidism because their glands initially produce a small amount of hormone until they eventually give out. In humans, thyroid ectopia has been associated rarely with the TTF-2 mutation (Van Vliet, 2003) and is associated with the same congenital anomalies described above.

Thyroid hypoplasia (a properly located but small gland) is seen in ~5%–10% of the remaining individuals with thyroid dysgenesis. Like with thyroid ectopy, these individuals have a mild to moderate form of congenital hypothyroidism. This etiology has been associated with mutations in the genes for TTF-1, TSH receptor, and, less commonly, mutations of PAX8 (Van Vliet, 2003).

In thyroid hemiagenesis, half the thyroid is present, and so this represents a mild condition, which can pass the newborn screening test and be undetected for years. In fact, a recent study of "healthy" Sicilian schoolchildren who underwent thyroid ultrasounds showed 1 in 2,000 had hemiagenesis (Maiorana et al., 2003). The sonic hedgehog (SHH) gene, which plays a role in symmetrical bilobation, has been implicated in this variant.

Thyroid Dyshormonogenesis

The thyroid gland produces two hormones: triodothyronine (T3) and thyroxine (T4). T3 is the biologically active form, while T4, which is far more abundant, is later converted to T3. Their synthesis, secretion, and transport represent a series of complex

Table 8.2
Genes involved in thyroid synthesis and secretion

Gene	Full Name	Process
PDS	Pendrin	Iodine transport
NIS	Sodium iodide symporter	Transport of iodide into thyroid
THOX1 & *THOX2*	Thyroid oxidase	Iodination of thyroglobulin
TPO	Thyroid peroxidase	Coupling of monoiodothyronine/diiodothyronine to form T3 and T4; iodination of thyroglobulin
Tg	Thyroglobulin	Protein precursor of thyroid hormone to which iodide is affixed

processes under the control of a number of genes (see table 8.2). A defect in any one of these genes can lead to thyroid dyshormonogenesis, which affects about 15% of congenital hypothyroidism cases. This etiology is heritable and often seen in siblings and across generations. To understand how the different kinds of thyroid dyshormonogenesis occur, one must know the different processes in the manufacture and transport of thyroid hormones.

Thyroid hormones are composed of a tyrosine couplet to which three (T3) or four (T4) iodide residues are affixed. Since the body does not produce its own iodide, this must be derived from dietary iodine, which is converted in the gut to iodide by enzymes. Iodide is transferred into the thyroid gland via a mechanism known as the sodium iodide symporter (NIS; Dohan & Carrasco, 2003), which, if defective, also causes congenital hypothyroidism. Within the thyroid, iodide is transported from the apical border to the colloid via a protein called pendrin (Brown & Huang, 2005), which, if defective, leads to Pendred syndrome and causes deafness and a large goiter. Iodide molecules are then affixed to the tyrosine residues stored in a large protein known as thyroglobulin. Monoiodothyronine (MIT) is created by binding one iodide molecule to tyrosine, and diiodothyronine (DIT), by binding two. The thyroid oxidases, *THOX1* and *THOX2* are also important in iodination of thyroglobulin and, if defective, lead to goiter and hypothyroidism (Moreno et al., 2002). Next, MIT and DIT are coupled to form T3, and two DITs are coupled to form T4. Both iodination and coupling are controlled by an enzyme known as thyroid peroxidase (TPO), which, if defective, leads to a moderate to severe form of congenital hypothyroidism. TPO mutations are by far the most common defect in thyroid dyshormonogenesis.

Once formed, T3 and T4 are stored in the thyroid colloid for later release. This release occurs in response to signals from thyroid-stimulating hormone (TSH), or thyrotropin, which is produced in the pituitary. Individuals with inactivating TSH receptor mutations also have congenital hypothyroidism (Kopp, 2001). After T3 and

T4 are released from the thyroid, they are transported to distant sites of action, including the brain, via binding proteins such as thyroxine-binding globulin or albumin. Thyroid hormones are taken up by target cells via several families of transporters, including the monocarboxylate transporters (MCT). A defect in the MCT-8 gene located on the X chromosome has been associated with a severe thyroid deficiency and mental retardation (Friesman et al., 2004).

Once in tissues, the T3/T4 balance is maintained by deiodinase enzymes, which serve to "clip" iodide residues from T4 to produce T3 inactive reverse T3 (Kester et al., 2004).

Central Hypothyroidism

Central hypothyroidism arises from disruption in the production of thyrotropin-releasing hormone (TRH) in the hypothalamus or from a disruption in the production of TSH produced in the pituitary. TRH and TSH serve to regulate thyroid hormone production and release via a negative feedback system: When circulatory thyroid hormone levels are high, less TRH and TSH are produced, leading to a slowdown in hormone synthesis, and, conversely, when thyroid hormone levels are low, more TRH and TSH are produced, in order to increase levels of thyroid hormone. This regulatory system develops at midgestation with first production of TSH at 22–30 weeks' gestation and TRH at 25 weeks. However, full maturity of the hypothalamic–pituitary–thyroid axis is not evident until birth (Brown & Huang, 2005).

Secondary congenital hypothyroidism arises from a disruption of TRH production, and tertiary congenital hypothyroidism, from a disruption of TSH production. These forms of congenital hypothyroidism are rare, affecting only about 1 in 50,000 to 100,000 children. Gene defects contributing to central hypothyroidism include (a) a loss-of-function mutation in the TRH receptor gene at the level of the pituitary, causing severe congenital hypothyroidism with short stature and mental retardation, and (b) a defect in TSH secretion due to Pit-1, Prop-1, and LHX3 gene, mutations, causing combined hypopituitarism and congenital hypothyroidism (Brown & Huang, 2005).

Thyroid Hormone Resistance

Thyroid hormones bind to nuclear transcription factors via receptors, which are temporally and spatially distributed in the brain (Bradley, Towle, & Young, 1992). There are four thyroid hormone receptors, located on chromosomes 3 and 17: TRα1 and TRα2 are ubiquitous, whereas TR β1 is found in the brain and the developing ear, and TR β2 is restricted to the pituitary. Individuals with a TR β1 gene defect have a condition known as thyroid hormone resistance, which affects about 1 in 50,000 persons. Thyroid hormone resistance contributes to high levels of serum thyroxine with thyroid-hormone deficiency at local sites and causes characteristic growth, cognitive, and behavioral abnormalities, including high risk of attention deficit/hyperactivity disorder (ADHD; Hauser et al., 1993).

Transient Hypothyroidism

A small proportion of newborns identified by newborn screening have a transient form of hypothyroidism. This can follow preterm birth, neonatal illness, and exposure to thyroid blocking agents (e.g., antithyroid medications used to treat maternal hyperthyroidism) or maternal blocking antibodies (Brown et al., 1996). Transient hypothyroidism is also associated with exposure to certain environmental contaminants, radiocontrasts, antiseptic solutions containing iodine, and excess iodine (which has suppressive effects). Although transient hypothyroidism usually resolves by 3 to 4 months of age, affected children may have cognitive deficits from low thyroid hormone levels during early life.

Other factors affecting thyroid hormone production include iodine deficiency and certain environmental chemicals and medications (Surks & Sievert, 1995). Because iodine is ascertained only through diet, iodine intake must always be sufficient to meet one's daily thyroid needs. Because many regions worldwide undergo a severe iodine deficiency, endemic cretinism is by far the most prevalent cause of congenital hypothyroidism. Since some iodine-sufficient regions—including the United States (Hallowell et al., 1998)—also experience declining iodine levels, this may be contributing to the growing incidence of subclinical hypothyroidism in the general population (Delange, de Benoist, Preteil, & Dunn, 2001). Because mild iodine deficiency has been associated with specific neurocognitive dysfunction including increased attention problems (Vermiglio et al., 2004), it is crucial to maintain adequate dietary iodine levels, particularly in pregnant and lactating women, whose needs for iodine are increased at this time.

Synthetic chemicals disrupt the various stages of thyroid hormone synthesis (Howdeshell, 2002). Perchlorates used in rocket fuel and propellants inhibit the sodium/iodide symporter; flame retardants or polybrominated diphenyl ethers (PBDE), which are used in the manufacture of fabrics, affect thyroid peroxidase action and impede iodination of tyrosine (Legler & Brouwer, 2003); mercury is associated with reduced iodination (Howedeshell, 2002); lead reduces T3/T4 synthesis by blocking deioidinase activity; and dioxins and PCBs block thyroid hormone transport and decrease availability of circulating thyroid hormones (Gauger et al., 2004). Since these chemicals cannot easily be disposed of and are accumulating in food production and the breast milk supply (Kirk et al., 2005), there is concern that they may be associated with the rising incidence of subclinical (and even clinical) hypothyroidism and are contributing to specific disabilities and behavior problems, including ADHD.

Table 8.3
Genes regulated by thyroid hormones in the central nervous system (see Chan & Rovet, 2003)

Site	Gene
Neurons and glia	Neurogranin (RC3)
	Connexin 43
	Neurospecific protein-A (NSP-A)
	Neural cell adhesion molecule (N-CAM)
	Basic transcription element-binding protein (BTEB)
	Transferrin
	Dab 1
	Oct-1
	Reelin
	ZAKI-4
Oligodendrocytes	Myelin basic protein (MBP)
	Proteolipid protein (PLP)
	Myelin-associated glycoprotein (MAG)
Cerebellar cells	Purkinje-cell Protein 2 (PCP-2)
	Calbindin
	Myo-inositol-triphosphate (IP3)
	Brain-derived neurotrophic factor (BDNF)
	Neurotropin 3 (NT-3)
	Hairless (hr)

Thyroid Hormone and Brain Development

Thyroid hormone is without a doubt one of the most important hormones—if not the most important hormone—in early brain development. Thyroid hormone acts by regulating critical brain genes that underlie fundamental neurodevelopmental processes. This regulation occurs in an exquisitely controlled and orderly sequence (Morreale de Escobar, Obregon, & Escobar del Rey, 2000; Bernal, Guadano-Ferraz, & Morte, 2003), with different genes having different periods of thyroid hormone dependency (see table 8.3).

Studies with Animals

Various experimental techniques have served to model congenital hypothyroidism in laboratory animals: thyroid ablation, exposure of the pregnant dam and neonate to antithyroid medications, and genetically engineered mutants. Research with these procedures has identified the abnormalities associated with insufficient thyroid hormone at different stages of development. Findings reveal thyroid hormone is essential for neurogenesis (Schapiro, 1976), neuronal migration (Auso et al., 2004), axon and dendrite formation (Legrand, 1984), synaptogenesis (Iniguez et al., 1996), myelination (Rosman, Malone, Helfenstein, & Kraft, 1972), and neurotransmitter production and release (Virgili, Saverino, Vaccari, Barnabei, & Contestabile, 1991). Rats rendered experimentally hypothyroid during early development demonstrated retarded development of the neuropil in the corpus callosum, stunting of dendritic arborization of Purkinje cells in the cerebellum, and significant migrational abnormalities (Ruiz-Marcos & Ipina, 1986).

The cerebellum, hippocampus, caudate, corpus callosum, anterior commissure, somatosensory cortex, auditory cortex, and visual cortex are particularly vulnerable to an early lack of thyroid hormone (Berbel, Guadanao-Ferraz, Angulo, & Ramon Cerezo, 1994; Gilbert & Paczkowksi, 2003; Morreale de Escobar, Obregon, & Escobar del Rey, 2004). Besides gross morphological structural changes in process growth and aberrant migration in the cortex, abnormal projections and altered networks have also been observed in projections emanating from the thalamus (Auso et al., 2001). Functional changes in synaptic regulation have been reported (Gilbert, 2004). Within the ear and eye, cochlear and retinal abnormalities lead to auditory and visual abnormalities (Rusch, Erway, Oliver, Vennström, & Forrest, 1998; Kelley, Thomas, & Reh, 1995; Roberts, Srinivas, Forrest, Morreale de Escobar, & Reh, 2006), including poor color vision (Ng et al., 2001). Finally, behavioral studies have established that thyroid-deficient rats and mice show impaired memory and sensorimotor abilities (Eayrs, 1966).

The specific effects of thyroid hormone insufficiency differ among brain structures depending on the timing of thyroid hormone insufficiency and when a particular brain region or subregion is undergoing its development. For example, because cerebellar Purkinje cells emerge earlier than cerebellar granule cells, the effects within the cerebellum and types of motor impairment differ if thyroid hormone is lacking early in gestation versus later. In the same way, because the CA1, CA3, and dendate gyrus regions of the hippocampus emerge at different times during gestation or early life, the timing of thyroid hormone loss has different manifestations in these substructures as well (Iniguez et al., 1996). Because timing of need for thyroid hormone is protracted in the forebrain (Gould & Butcher, 1989) but much earlier in visual and motor cortices (Ruiz-Marcos & Ipina, 1986), the effects on the cortex also depend on timing.

Studies with Humans

Studies based on fetal autopsy material have shown thyroid hormone receptors are present in human brain tissue throughout gestation—including the first two trimesters of pregnancy when the fetus is incapable or not fully capable of producing its own thyroid hormone (Kilby, Gittoes, McCabe, Verhaeg, & Franklyn, 2000). These findings signify that the fetal brain needs thyroid hormone early in pregnancy and, because of the relatively late development of the fetal thyroid system, the fetus has to depend on the maternal thyroid supply (Chan & Rovet, 2003). Indeed, maternal hormones were shown to be present in human coelomic fluid prior to 12 weeks' gestation and in amniotic fluid shortly thereafter (Lavado-Autric et al., 2003).

Following the animal findings showing different effects of a lack of thyroid hormone at different stages of gestation and early life on the brain, one would expect children with congenital hypothyroidism (identified by screening) who are lacking thyroid in late pregnancy and early life to show defective synaptogenesis and myelination. In addition, brain regions with protracted development (e.g., the hippocampus dentate gyrus, the frontal lobe), would be affected if diagnosis is late and/or treatment requires a long time to take effect.

To date, few neuroanatomic or neuroimaging studies have been conducted on children with congenital hypothyroidism. Autopsy reports indicate extensive neuropathology in children who either had late diagnosis or died for other reasons. A magnetic resonance imaging (MRI) study of five late-treated hypothyroid children from India reported mild cerebral atrophy in the frontal and parietal lobes as well as delayed myelination (Gupta, Bhatia, Poptani, & Gujral, 1995), whereas MRI findings on 11 infants with congenital hypothyroidism detected by newborn screening before replacement therapy showed no morphological brain abnormalities and no effects on myelination (Alves, Eidson, Engle, Sheldon, & Cleveland, 1989; Siragusa et al., 1997). In a structural MRI study of 16 children with congenital hypothyroidism and 18 typically developing children we recently conducted, we found an increased likelihood of abnormal scans in the group with congenital hypothyroidism compared with the group without congenital hypothyroidism (50% vs. 33%), who also differed as to type of abnormality. Whereas controls had mainly incidental findings (e.g., pineal cysts, mucosal disease), the group with congenital hypothyroidism had either T2 signal hyperintensities or structural abnormalities reflecting increased asymmetries, including asymmetry of the hippocampus.

A study using magnetic resonance spectroscopy (MRS) to compare brain constituents before and after thyroxine replacement found children with congenital hypothyroidism had elevated choline levels in the hypothyroid state but not when they were euthyroid (Gupta et al., 1995). Preliminary findings from our lab using MRS on 10-year-olds with congenital hypothyroidism diagnosed via newborn screening showed reductions in metabolites, particularly low levels of glutamine in the left hippocampus and low levels of glutamine, choline, and myoinositol in the right frontal lobe (Rovet, Desrocher, Williamson, Nash, Blaser, & Soreni, 2006).

Several studies have used electrophysiological techniques to study children with congenital hypothyroidism and have found abnormalities in several EEG parameters (Moschini et al., 1986), including abnormal visual evoked potentials in 64% of cases studied. Using an event-related EEG paradigm, we observed children with congenital hypothyroidism had attenuated P300 responses to a repeated stimulus relative to controls (Hepworth, Pang, & Rovet, 2006; see figure 8.2), suggestive of a short-term memory abnormality. The only functional MRI study conducted so far on congenital hypothyroidism has revealed reduced parietal but increased frontal activation relative to controls on a visuospatial task (Blasi et al., 2006).

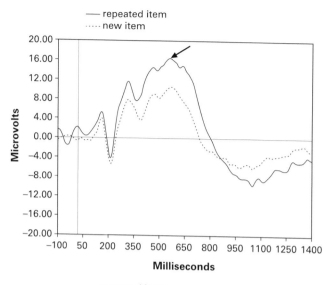

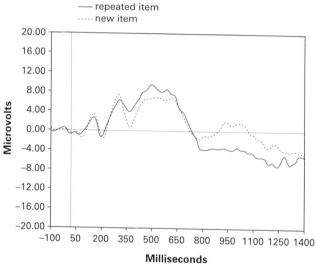

Figure 8.2
Event-related potential results using a repetition paradigm. Results in the upper panel show findings from an individual without congenital hypothyroidism (CH) and on the lower panel a child with CH. Note the P3 elevation for a repeated item in the child without CH (indicated by the arrow) but not in the individual with CH.

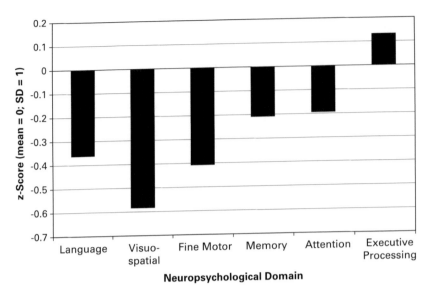

Figure 8.3
Results on neuropsychological domains. Results are presented as difference in *z* scores between children with congenital hypothyroidism and controls.

The Neuropsychological Profile in Children with Congenital Hypothyroidism

It is generally agreed that outcome will be normal in children with congenital hypothyroidism if the diagnosis is made early in life by newborn screening and they receive adequate therapy (Brook, 1995). However, several large-scale follow-up studies indicate selective deficits (Rovet, 2003a), which are far milder than those seen in children diagnosed clinically prior to newborn screening (see cases 8.2 to 8.4). The profiles of early treated children reveal visuospatial, language, and sensorimotor impairments and selective memory and attention deficits, while their executive function skills are usually spared. Figures 8.3 and 8.4 present our findings based on two cohorts of children with congenital hypothyroidism tested at different ages and with different tests. Figure 8.3 shows the findings at adolescence using a broad spectrum of multiple clinical neuropsychological tests, while figure 8.4 shows the findings for a later born cohort of children tested at 7–12 years of age with the NEPSY®. In both studies, differences between children with vs. without congenital hypothyroidism are clearly evident. Below we summarize the results of our work and the literature by specific domains.

Intelligence

The earliest studies of children with congenital hypothyroidism identified by newborn screening reported a low-to-nonexistent rate of mental retardation and IQs within

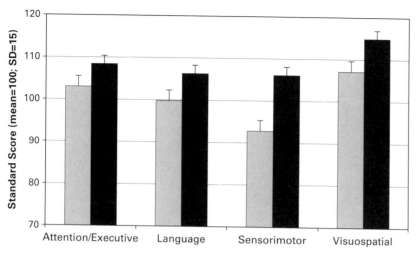

Figure 8.4
Results on four NEPSY scales by children with congenital hypothyroidism (striped bars) and controls (black bars).

the normal range but below expectation. A meta-analysis conducted on seven of the major studies at the time reported a 6.3-point IQ difference between children with congenital hypothyroidism and siblings or closely matched controls (Derksen-Lubsen & Verkerk, 1996). A recent extension of this paper comparing the results from 11 studies in the literature supported the earlier findings and showed that the IQ difference was maintained (Heyerdahl & Oerbeck, 2003) and seen in adults (Oerbeck, Sundet, Kase, & Heyerdahl, 2003; Kempers et al., 2006).

Because the above studies involved cases treated in the earliest years of newborn screening when age at therapy was slightly delayed and starting doses not always optimal, we recently culled the data from "second-generation" cohorts who were identified after 1990 and treated earlier and with higher starting dosages than first-generation cases. Our findings revealed a persisting 4- to 6-IQ-point difference between controls and congenital hypothyroidism, despite their early and effective therapy (Rovet, 2005). At a population level, this difference is not insignificant and has a high cost associated with it (Muir & Zegarac, 2001).

Differences in IQ between congenital hypothyroidism and non–congenital hypothyroidism groups persist, if not increase, with age and are observed on most of the IQ tests studied. The Bayley Scales of Infant Development appear to yield the smallest between-groups differences, whereas the Griffiths, which is also an infant test, shows large significant differences between congenital hypothyroidism and sibling comparison groups (Rovet, 1992) and is predictive of later outcome (Rovet, unpublished data).

Case 8.2: Kit (diagnosed with congenital hypothyroidism by newborn screening) Kit is a 7-year-old boy who was born in 1988 at 42 weeks' gestation following a normal pregnancy and delivery. He weighed 7.5 lbs. at birth, and was slightly jaundiced. His diagnosis and first treatment took place in the first week of life. He walked at 17 months, spoke his first words at 11 months, and spoke in sentences at 15 months. His vision was normal, but he suffered high-frequency hearing loss in both ears and was described as having relatively weak motor skills and being socially imma- ture. His parents, a magazine editor and a stockbroker, were concerned about hypersensitive be- havior and social problems at school.

During testing, he was friendly, compliant, and likable but seemed awkard and socially gauche. He would at times stare off into space. He engaged in normal conversation but hummed and sang while working and made silly remarks. Kit described himself as "really smart" and preferred to lead his own agenda, which included writing a lengthy and creative story about a mysterious babysitter.

Kit's overall level of intelligence was at the 50th percentile with equivalent scores on verbal and nonverbal indices. He showed some scatter on subtests with a score in the 91st percentile for Infor- mation; scores in the above-average range for Digit Span, Picture Completion, Arithmetic, and Coding; and a weak score on Mazes (SS = 7). On tests of language ability, Kit performed above average; visuospatial ability, average; and fine motor ability, below average. On a test of motor skills, he showed average catching and throwing ability but was weak in balance, jumping, and agility. He showed variable performance on a test of various memory skills with strength in recall- ing sequences and weakness in remembering picture locations. His attention and executive func- tioning were average. Academically, Kit was reading and writing above grade level, whereas his arithmetic was at par for grade.

Case 8.3: Lana (diagnosed with congenital hypothyroidism by newborn screening) Lana is a child who participated annually in our research program. She was diagnosed by newborn screening in 1982 and treated with 37.5 µg L-thyroxine at 18 days of age. Her father is a lawyer, and her mother is a housewife.

Testing at 12, 18, 24, 36, and 48 months revealed consistently above-average intelligence with slightly stronger verbal than nonverbal skills and no evidence of any major deficits. At age 6, Lana scored solidly average in intelligence but was weak in her general motor proficiency and scored below average on tests of balance and agility. At age 9, her IQ was 98 with slightly higher verbal than nonverbal ability, and she was particularly weak in assembling blocks and solving puz- zles. Her rote memory for numbers was also low. She indicated weak reading and arithmetic abili- ties for age. When tested at age 13 with a comprehensive battery of neuropsychological tasks, Lana exhibited difficulty on tests of mental rotation, visual memory, vigilance, and visuomotor integra- tion but performed at an average level on tests of language processing, working memory, and exec- utive functioning.

Cognitive Abilities

A variety of specific cognitive deficits have been described in children with congenital hypothyroidism, and the nature of their deficit appears to reflect the types of instru- ments and procedures used as well as factors relating to aspects of screening and treatment. Across studies, findings revealed (a) delays in speech acquisition and sub- sequently reduced verbal ability; (b) motor weakness and general clumsiness (see Kit and Lana, cases 8.2 and 8.3); (c) sensorimotor deficits; (d) visual, visuomotor, and visuospatial impairments; and (e) attention and memory problems (case 8.3). Among the various deficits, those in the visual domain appear to be most prominent and are seen as early as 1 year of age.

Language Skills   Children with congenital hypothyroidism show subtle speech and language deficits (Gottshalk, Richman, & Lewandowski, 1994). Among very young children, delayed speech development is not uncommon, particularly if the children have the athyrotic etiology. We observed significantly delayed speech acquisition, which was most evident at age 3, and catch-up thereafter (Rovet, 1992). Psychometric tests of language abilities indicated scores significantly below those of controls on the Reynell Expressive Language scale at age 3 ($p < .01$), the Reynell Receptive Language scale at 3 and 4 years of age ($p < .001$ and $p < .01$, respectively), the Peabody Picture Vocabulary Test ($p < .05$) but not NEPSY Comprehension of Instructions at age 5, NEPSY Speeded Naming and Comprehension of Instructions at 8–12 years of age ($p < .005$ and $p < .01$), and the Test of Language Development's Listening Vocabulary ($p < .01$) but not its Spoken Grammar subtest or on the Token test at 13 years. The discrepancy between age groups on the NEPSY Comprehension of Instructions subtest may be due to either the increasing demands on knowledge of grammatical complexity and working memory for the 8–12 versus 5-year age range or because the younger age group was drawn from a cohort born after 1995, whereas the older group born before 1995 was treated less optimally. Overall, these results suggest that the expression and comprehension of words may be more affected than grammar in children with congenital hypothyroidism. A recent study of language functioning in congenital hypothyroidism adults who were detected by newborn screening showed significantly lower scores on the Boston Naming Test than in sibling controls (Oerbeck, Sundet, Kase, & Heyredahl, 2005).

Visuospatial Abilities   The visuospatial area of cognitive functioning appears to be one of the most severely compromised abilities in children with congenital hypothyroidism (Rovet, 2003b). Differences from controls, which are consistently reported on Performance scales of intelligence tests, are evident from as early as 1 year of age (Rovet, 1992) through to adolescence (Rovet, 1999a, 1999b) and adulthood (Oerbeck et al., 2005; Kempers et al., 2006). This effect has been more strongly associated with initial disease severity than later treatment factors, suggesting the weakness in visuospatial processing was most likely if children had moderate to severe hypothyroidism at diagnosis.

In order to determine what aspects of visuospatial functioning are most vulnerable in congenital hypothyroidism, we contrasted performance on tasks that had primarily spatial demands and are thought to invoke the "where," or magnocellular, visual pathway versus those that had primarily visual demands and are thought to invoke

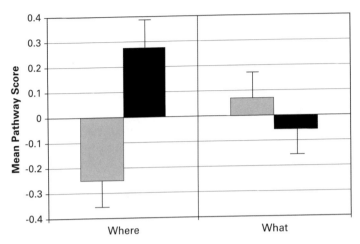

Figure 8.5
Scores on "where" versus "what" pathway visuospatial tasks by congenital hypothyroidism (striped bars) and control (black bars) groups. Results are presented as z scores for domain composites.

the "what," or parvocellular, visual pathway (see figure 8.5). Significant group effects were seen on "where" pathway tasks, which were correlated with initial disease severity factors, but not on "what" pathway tasks, which were correlated with demographic factors (Leneman, Buchanan, & Rovet, 2001).

We recently extended this line of research to identify the core visual processes affected in congenital hypothyroidism. Using electrophysiological techniques and advanced paradigms that assess specific visual functions, we showed that children with congenital hypothyroidism had reduced ability in distinguishing contrasts but normal visual acuity compared with controls (Mirabella et al., 2005). Given that contrast detection is thought to invoke thalamic magno cells, these findings provide further support that the magnocellular pathway may be disrupted in children with congenital hypothyroidism.

Motor Abilities   Children with congenital hypothyroidism detected early via newborn screening are prone to weak motor skills, particularly strength and balance, as seen in Kit and Lana, cases 8.2 and 8.3. In contrast, their age at acquisition of gross motor skills and coordination is largely unaffected. Their weak motor skills may also continue into adulthood (Oerbeck et al., 2005; Kempers et al., 2006). While these effects are subtle and not likely to impact daily functioning, they may nevertheless compromise their ability to partake in certain sports, an area that has never been explored in this population.

Given the major role of the cerebellum in motor skills and that this structure is highly vulnerable to thyroid hormone loss, Kooistra et al. (1994) assessed children with congenital hypothyroidism on tests that directly tap cerebellar functioning, namely, tasks of dysmetria, dysdiadochokinesia, and motor timing. Although the congenital hypothyroidism group clearly showed more atypical motor performance than controls, there was no evidence of a specific cerebellar motor problem.

Children and adults with congenital hypothyroidism also show selective fine motor deficits including weakness in visuomotor integration, manual dexterity, and ball throwing (Kempers et al., 2006). We found that on the NEPSY, the Sensorimotor domain was the most strongly affected in 7- to 12-year-old children with congenital hypothyroidism (see figure 8.4), reflecting their selective difficulties in hand and finger movements, while visuomotor precision was unaffected. Scores in this domain were negatively correlated with the postnatal duration of hypothyroidism and so suggest either an effect of the postnatal lack of thyroid hormone on primary motor cortex development, consistent with the animal literature, or an effect of reduced myelin in motor association areas given thyroid hormone's role in regulating myelin production.

Attention   Attention is another area of cognitive functioning compromised in congenital hypothyroidism. Our early results, based on parent-report questionnaires given when the children were 7 years of age, showed that attention was a primary concern of parents. Direct testing revealed the children with congenital hypothyroidism scored significantly below controls on clinical tests of attention, especially those requiring focused or sustained attention (Rovet & Alvarez, 1996; Rovet & Hepworth, 2001a, 2001b; Kooistra, van der Meere, Vulsma, & Kalverboer, 1996). Attention problems were correlated with both severity of initial hypothyroidism and thyroid hormone levels at time of testing, with children less able to attend having both elevated and depressed thyroid hormone levels (Rovet, 2003a). These findings suggest the need to maintain ambient levels of thyroid hormone in the normal range at all times to ensure optimal attention.

Direct comparisons between children with congenital hypothyroidism and ADHD revealed the congenital hypothyroidism group was less impulsive, was better able to concentrate, and had better search skills than the ADHD group (Rovet, 2003a; see figure 8.6). The children with congenital hypothyroidism were found to deploy different strategies than those with ADHD on a visual search task with the ADHD group terminating their searches early when the target was absent and the congenital hypothyroidism group being slower and having a weaker memory trace than controls (Rovet, Hepworth, & Lobaugh, 2006). On the Continuous Performance test, the congenital hypothyroidism group erred because they forgot what they were attending to, whereas the ADHD group was more impulsive in responding (Rovet & Hepworth, 2001b).

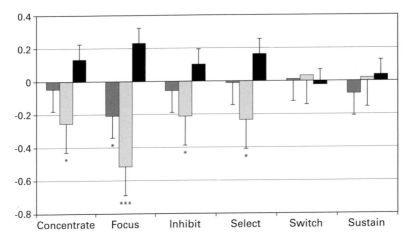

Figure 8.6
Comparison between groups of children with congenital hypothyroidism (striped bars), attention deficit/hyperactivity disorder (white bars), or neither disorder (black bars) on different components of attention. Results are presented as average composite scores per component in *z*-score units. Single asterisk represents *p* < .05, and triple asterisk, *p* < .001.

Case 8.4: Molly (diagnosed with congenital hypothyroidism by newborn screening) Molly is a 10-year-old girl seen for a clinical neuropsychological assessment due to parents' concerns about her school performance. She is currently in a modified program at a local private school and also receives home tutoring. Her father is an accountant, and her mother works for a philanthropic organization. Molly was born full term, weighing 5 lbs., following a normal pregnancy and delivery. She was diagnosed with congenital hypothyroidism at 12 days of age and started on a dose of 25 μg L-thyroxine. As an infant, Molly seldom cried, was quiet and content, and had a good appetite and slept well. She walked at 14 months and had normal speech and social development. She has excellent social skills and a large set of friends and is very outgoing and empathic. Molly is also very active in sports.

During testing, Molly was reported to be easily distracted and very fidgety, always in motion and talking or singing. She frequently had to be redirected to the task at hand and gave up easily.

Her test results revealed her IQ to be in the low-normal range (25th percentile) with stronger verbal comprehension and working memory skills than perceptual reasoning. Her processing speed was below normal. She was particularly weak at Coding (SS = 5), Block Design (SS = 6), and Picture Concepts (SS = 5). On tests of language she scored in the high-average range in comprehension of verbal instructions and average in her understanding of and ability to name common objects and concepts. She showed a personal weakness in generating words on demand and elaborating her ideas. Her visuomotor skills were well developed, but she had difficulty copying a complex figure.

Molly indicated variable memory skills, performing in the above-average range in recognizing the essential elements of a story, the average range in recalling a story, and the below-average range in learning new word-pair combinations or object locations. She failed to reproduce essential elements of the complex figure she had previously drawn. She was also weak on tests of working memory, number–letter sequencing, and vigilance, and her scores on a computerized attention test showed strong evidence of a clinically significant attention problem. Molly's parents report considerable difficulty with everyday and working memory but no other behavioral problems. Her teacher recognized problems with attention span and concentration. Academically, Molly is performing above average in reading and spelling but is slightly below average in arithmetic.

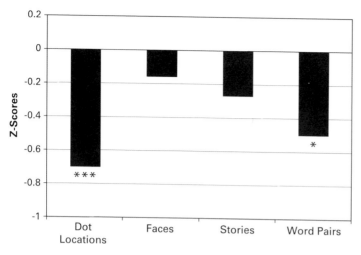

Figure 8.7
Results on individual Children's Memory Scale delayed recall subtests by groups of children with or without congenital hypothyroidism. Results are presented as difference scores in z-score units. Single asterisk represents $p < .05$, and triple asterisk, $p < .001$.

Memory   Memory is strongly compromised in children with congenital hypothyroidism who performed significantly below siblings on the McCarthy Memory scale (Rovet, 1992) and the Wechsler Intelligence Scale for Children Digit Span subtest, particularly on the Forward span task (Rovet, 1995), suggesting greater difficulty with short-term than working memory demands. On the Children's Memory Scale (CMS), children with congenital hypothyroidism were significantly outperformed by age- and gender-matched controls on the Global Memory Index (corrected for intelligence) as well as Dot Locations and Word Pairs subtests (Song, Daneman, & Rovet, 2001) but not Face and Story recall tasks (see figure 8.7). Recently, Hepworth et al. (2006) reported that on an event-related paradigm, children with congenital hypothyroidism showed less neural activation to previously seen stimuli than controls (see figure 8.2).

Because of the hippocampus's critical role in place and associative learning and its high need for thyroid hormone, we hypothesized that children with congenital hypothyroidism would show abnormal hippocampal development. Partial support for this hypothesis came from our findings of low scores on CMS Dot Locations and Word Pairs subtests and high scores on the Everyday Memory Questionnaire (EMQ), suggesting more problems. On the EMQ, which has been shown to reflect reduced hippocampal size and integrity (Vargha-Khadem et al., 1997), we found the congenital hypothyroidism children relative to controls showed a propensity to forget (a) recent events, (b) where things are kept, (c) what they were told, and (d) to do something (Rovet, 2003b). Furthermore, their EMQ scores were significantly corre-lated with time to achieve hormone normalization but not initial disease severity, suggesting that hippocampal dysfunction may arise from a lack of thyroid hormone later in infancy.

One aspect of memory that appears to be less affected in children with congenital hypothyroidism is working memory, which involves the frontal lobes. However, when children with congenital hypothyroidism were assessed with a working memory task that distinguished between storage and controlled attention components, we found the congenital hypothyroidism group was weaker in the storage aspect in con-trast to the ADHD group, who were weaker in the controlled attention component (Hepworth & Rovet, 2006).

Executive Function   Executive function skills are generally unaffected in children with congenital hypothyroidism if they are diagnosed promptly and treated early following newborn screening (Rovet, 1999b). We found these children performed comparably to controls on classic executive-function tasks such as Wisconsin Card Sorting, Stroop, Go–No Go, and Verbal Fluency. We proposed this was likely due to the fact that their early treatment occurred before the frontal lobes would have needed thyroid hormone. However, this is not the case in children whose diagnosis of congenital hypothyroidism is delayed due to missed screening. These children, in fact, show significant executive function deficits and have behavior problems sugges-tive of abnormal development of the frontal lobes.

School Achievement

Children with congenital hypothyroidism perform satisfactorily at school, but their levels are typically below those of siblings without congenital hypothyroidism, and they are also at greater risk of a learning disability. On tests of academic achieve-ment, children with congenital hypothyroidism scored below controls on tests of arithmetic (Rovet, 1995; Rovet & Ehrlich, 2000), a finding that has been maintained into adulthood (Oerbeck et al., 2005). While this effect is common, there are some children with congenital hypothyroidism who show unique and distinguished talents including gifted math abilities (see case 8.5).

At sixth grade, children with congenital hypothyroidism had difficulty in science and social studies, while their math difficulties appeared to diminish (Rovet & Ehr-lich, 2000). Adults with congenital hypothyroidism rated themselves lower than siblings in arithmetic and overall school functioning but not reading, writing, or physical education (Kempers et al., 2006). Children with congenital hypothyroidism were less likely than their siblings to graduate from senior high school with school completers differing from noncompleters in terms of initial dose of thyroxine.

The learning disability profile of children with congenital hypothyroidism is typically of the nonverbal learning disability variety (Rovet, 1995). Seldom, if ever, do children with congenital hypothyroidism indicate a verbal learning disability, unless they have a hearing deficit. In this case, we reported that children with congenital hypothyroidism who had a mild sensorineural hearing loss demonstrated difficulty in early reading processes, which relied heavily on good auditory information processing and phonological processing skills (Rovet, Walker, Bliss, Buchanan, & Ehrlich, 1997). However, these children later caught up in their reading ability (Rovet & Ehrlich, 2000).

Case 8.5: Neal (who has congenital hypothyroidism and shows atypical math abilities)   Neal is a 7-year-old boy who was seen as part of a research study in which he was assessed regularly between 12 months and 5 years of age. His mother requested the current assessment to evaluate whether he was eligible for a gifted placement at school. Neal was born with an ectopic thyroid and treated at 12 days of age with 50 μg L-thyroxine. He was a content, cuddly, and happy infant who achieved his speech and motor milestones at the appropriate age. He was presently described as a leader, independent and cooperative, and did not show any behavioral or academic problems.

Infant testing revealed Neal performed average relative to controls, while intelligence testing at age 5 indicated above-average intelligence with superior Perfomance IQ (96th percentile). Neal showed above average verbal and visuospatial abilities but was weak in his motor skills, particularly his fine motor coordination. His memory was above average, especially in the verbal domain, and his preschool reading and arithmetic skills were advanced.

Current testing revealed Neal's intelligence was at the 99th percentile and his abilities were outstanding in all domains. He performed in the superior range on tests of math achievement and showed unusual counting abilities (e.g., he could accurately and quickly count backwards by 3 and forwards by 4). Although advanced in his multidigit addition and subtraction skills and his simple multiplications problems, he could not compute multidigit multiplication or division problems (and told the examiner he was not taught this).

Behavior Problems

Behavior problems in children with congenital hypothyroidism include attention difficulties as well as introversion and social immaturity (Rovet, 2000; Kooistra, Stemerdink, van der Meere, Vulsma, & Kalverboer, 2001), while increased temperamental difficulty and elevated arousal levels and environmental sensitivity were seen in infants with congenital hypothyroidism (Rovet, Ehrlich, & Sorbara, 1989). A recent study of 5-year-olds with congenital hypothyroidism and closely matched controls using both parents' and teachers' ratings indicated moderately elevated scores on scales of oppositionality and attention problems, while teachers also saw them as generally more restless and emotionally labile (Rovet, 2005; see figures 8.8 and 8.9). However, children with congenital hypothyroidism were not at risk of any major behavior problems, and their patterns of attentional difficulty differed from those of children with ADHD.

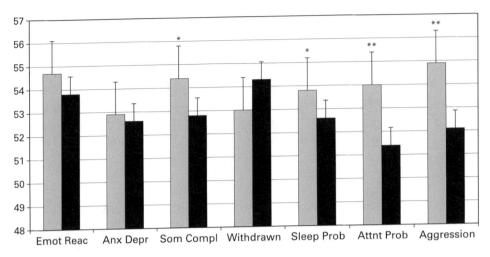

Figure 8.8
Child Behavior Checklist narrow-band scale results for children with congenital hypothyroidism (CH) (black bars) and children without CH (striped bars). Results are presented in *z*-score units.

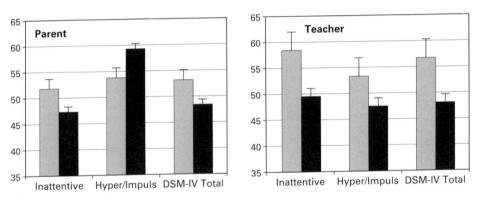

Figure 8.9
Results on selective Conners' Parent and Teacher rating scales for children with congenital hypothyroidism (CH) (black bars) and children without CH (striped bars).

Table 8.4
Factors influencing outcome in children with congenital hypothyroidism

Factor	Time of Effect
Etiology	Prenatal/postnatal
Age at onset	Prenatal/postnatal
Thyroid hormone levels at diagnosis	Postnatal (early)
Age at treatment onset	Postnatal (early)
Dose level	Postnatal (early/mid)
Time to normalization	Postnatal (mid/late)

Influence of Disease and Treatment-Related Variables

Despite consistent findings from the many follow-up investigations, wide variability does exist among the various cohorts studied. Table 8.4, which lists some of the major factors influencing variability and impacting outcome, also provides information on timing of these effects. Disease-related factors reflect etiology of congenital hypothyroidism and disease severity at diagnosis as measured by the thyroid hormone levels at that time as well as when the disease began. There is clear evidence that some children, particularly those with a total lack of a thyroid gland who showed clear evidence of hypothyroidism in utero, may be more affected than those whose disease began after delivery (Rovet, 1992; Rovet & Daneman, 2003). For example, Tillotson, Fuggle, Smith, Ades, and Grant (1994) reported that severity of disease at diagnosis was the strongest predictor of global outcome compared to other disease- and treatment-related factors. Generally, disease-related factors are associated with performance on tasks of visual, visuospatial, and visuomotor functioning and are seen in children with both permanent and transient hypothyroidism (Rovet & Daneman, 2003).

The major treatment-related factors are age at onset of therapy, starting dose, time to normalization of thyroid hormone levels, subsequent therapy, and compliance. With respect to age at start of treatment, there is no doubt that the earlier treatment begins, the better the outcome should be. Surprisingly, however, the data do not consistently support this interpretation (Hrystiuk, Gilbert, Logan, Pindoria, & Brook, 2002), in that significant negative correlations between treatment age and outcome have not usually been found (Heyerdahl & Oerbeck, 2003). According to Heyerdahl (2001), this lack of statistical correlation may be because the restricted ranges of treatment ages allow for little variability. Alternatively, it is possible that treatment age was confounded by other factors, such as earliest treated children being identified clinically in advance of the screening results due to their severe presentation or, conversely, to delayed treatment because of near normal thyroid hormone levels. Studies subgrouping samples by age of treatment onset have shown that earlier treated children indicate better outcome than later treated ones (Bongers-Schokking, Koot, Wiersma, Verkerk, & de Muinck Keizer-Schrama, 2000; Bongers-Schokking & de Muinck Keizer-Schrama, 2005). While outcome is also generally more favorable in children treated with higher starting dosages (Rovet & Ehrlich, 1995), it is not established what constitutes too high a dose, a topic of considerable debate (Oerbeck et al., 2005). Because skills such as language and memory seem to need thyroid hormone mainly in the postnatal period, one would expect these abilities to be more vulnerable to delays in treatment or establishing euthyroidism than other abilities (Rovet, 1992; Song et al., 2001). Finally, although executive function skills are typically unaffected in children treated early and adequately, deficits are seen in this domain if diagnosis and treatment are delayed, usually due to a missed diagnosis from laboratory, physician, or other error (see case 8.6).

Another variable of interest is thyroid hormone levels at time of testing, which can vary naturally or result from over- or undertreatment. For example, we found that children with both elevated and low levels of thyroid hormone at time of testing performed less adequately on tests of attention and memory than did children whose thyroid hormone levels were well within the normal range (Rovet, 2003b).

Further sources of variability include child's country of residence, ethnic and socioeconomic background, and age at assessment as well as when the study was conducted in relation to the established test norms and the type of data collected (Rovet & Daneman, 2003). Country of residence can refer to (a) similarity with the country on which test norms were developed; (b) ethnic makeup and mix of the sample, which can be restricted or vary considerably; and (c) average IQ, which can be higher for some countries than others (e.g., the Netherlands reports a higher general IQ than the United States and France, while Canadian children show a different distribution of IQ scores than do American children; Rovet, 2005). Testing in relation to when the test was developed can affect ultimate results given the Flynn effect, or upward skew of scores with the passing of time.

Case 8.6: Oliver (whose congenital hypothyroidism was missed by the newborn screening program)
Oliver is a 10-year-old boy with a dizygotic twin brother, Oscar. Their father is a firefighter and mother, a laboratory technician. Oliver was diagnosed at 10 weeks of age following emergency admission to a regional hospital for severe stomach distress. Mother's persistent complaints to the pediatrician that Oliver was frequently constipated and not developing at the same rate as his brother went unheeded. At time of admission, Oliver was jaundiced; was flaccid; and had an umbilical hernia, protruding tongue, and puffy face. His TSH was more than 1,000 mU/L, and he had a small lingual thyroid on ultrasound. He was treated at 72 days with 37.5 µg/kg L-thyroxine, and while his overt symptoms abated within several weeks, he lagged far behind his brother in all developmental milestones and was very uncoordinated and had an unusual gait. His speech was very delayed and unclear, necessitating speech therapy from 2 to 5 years of age.

Both boys were assessed at age 10. According to mother, Oliver was in a special needs class in a different school than Oscar, and Oliver needed to be bussed to this school, whereas Oscar walked to school. Oliver had no friends and experienced considerable anxiety at school and in strange places. Oliver's behavior was often considered odd and inappropriate (e.g., he could not be quieted in movie theaters and spoke his mind freely). Oscar, by contrast, had many friends and was active in team sports such as hockey, soccer, and baseball.

The examiner described Oliver as shy, silly, immature, distractible, and tangential in his conversation due to his frequent references to fire trucks and siren sounds. In contrast, Oscar was described as a typical outgoing and engaging boy whose behavior was age appropriate and who showed good attention throughout the assessment.

Oliver achieved a full scale IQ of 81, 30 points below Oscar's. Oliver's Performance IQ was 7 points higher than his Verbal IQ, and he scored particularly low in Vocabulary (SS = 3), Comprehension (SS = 4), Digit Span (SS = 4), and Mazes (SS = 2). Additional testing revealed Oliver showed strengths on tests of visuospatial processing (e.g., NEPSY Arrows, the Wide Range Assessment of Visuomotor Abilities Matching Subtest) and object recognition (NEPSY Faces) but experienced considerable difficulty on tests of working memory, and his fine motor skills were weak. Academically, Oliver was two grades behind in arithmetic and three grades behind in reading comprehension. Parent questionnaires revealed clinically significant concerns in socialization, thinking, attention, anxiety, and working memory. Oliver was particularly prone to forget where he puts his things, where he was, when he has to do something, and what he has just said.

Oscar showed no areas of cognitive deficit and no major behavior problems. He was achieving at grade level and excelled in physical education and art.

Phenotype–Genotype Correlations

Few attempts have been made at specifying the phenotypic–genotypic relationships among children with the various etiologies of congenital hypothyroidism. As a rule, most differences are attributed to the severity of the thyroid condition and timing of the hormonal deficiency rather than to the specific genetic determinant. Several exceptions are the characteristic behavioral and learning disability profile in resistance to thyroid hormone, association between goiter and deafness in Pendred syndrome, and the severe motor deficits and retardation in MCT deficiency. However, given the role of PAX8 and TTF-1 genes in brain development (Trueba et al., 2005), children with these specific gene defects may have brain as well as thyroid malformations.

We recently described a common profile among three children with rare forms of hypothyroidism: (a) a male with an isolated hypothalamic hypothyroidism, (b) a male with hypothyroidism secondary to hypopituitarism, and (c) a female with thyroid hormone resistance (Rovet, Daneman, & Huang, 2003). Results were similar for the three children, reflecting their low-normal IQ levels (81–83 range), impaired attention and memory, significant weakness in visuospatial and learning abilities, and low but less affected language and executive function skills. Academically, these children were impaired in math but had normal reading skills, and their teachers reported they had significant problems with attention and restlessness at school.

Summary and Conclusions

Without a doubt, children with congenital hypothyroidism detected by newborn screening and treated early show far improved outcome relative to children diagnosed clinically prior to the advent of newborn screening. Nevertheless, screened children with congenital hypothyroidism are still at risk for subtle neurocognitive and behavioral deficits that depend on when exactly their condition began and how long it lasted. Because brain development is progressive with different regions needing thyroid hormone at different times in utero or postnatally, it follows that the type of impairment manifested by children with congenital hypothyroidism depends on timing of deficiency and the adequacy of therapy. Thus, the congenital hypothyroidism phenotype reflects mainly factors associated with the disease and its management, while certain genotypes may be prone to specific additional phenotypic characteristics (e.g., Pendred syndrome and deafness, resistance to thyroid hormone and ADHD, MCT deficiency and motor weakness).

However, few genotype–phenotype correlational studies have been performed, and even though most instances of congenital hypothyroidism are genetically determined, the full spectrum of underlying gene defects has not as yet been identified. This is likely due to the rarity of some of the conditions and that this approach is relatively recent. As the different genetic causes of more cases become revealed, the greater the possibility that such correlations can be determined—provided the assessments the children receive are broad and not limited to IQ.

In conclusion, because of the critical windows of thyroid hormone–dependent brain development in different brain regions, congenital hypothyroidism represents an ideal model for studying events that take place in the human brain between the third trimester and first few months of life. Also because the various etiologies of congenital hypothyroidism are genetically mediated, congenital hypothyroidism represents a unique condition for studying the genetic determinants of specific learning disabilities and variability in human brain function. However, this work is just in its beginning stages, and clearly further detailed studies of this population are required. One area that begs further study is outcome in relation to the underlying gene defect causing hypothyroidism, independent of the effect of loss of thyroid hormone.

In closing, this chapter has described in detail the complexity of congenital hypothyroidism and its many causes and effects on children with different congenital hypothyroidism etiologies. By assuming a neuropsychological approach and by providing some of the latest neuroimaging findings, this chapter has elucidated some of the specific effects of a loss of thyroid hormone in the time window when children identified by screening, or missed by screening, are thyroid-hormone deficient. In addition, this chapter has revealed areas of research on this population that beg further study. We hope this chapter will inspire new researchers to address the outstanding issues in this area.

References

Alves, C., Eidson, M., Engle, H., Sheldon, J., & Cleveland, W. W. (1989). Changes in brain maturation detected by magnetic resonance imaging in congenital hypothyroidism. *Journal of Pediatrics, 115,* 600–603.

Auso, E., Cases, O., Fouquet, C., Camacho, M., Garcia-Velasco, J. V., Gaspar, P., & Berbel, P. (2001). Protracted expression of serotonin transporter and altered thalamocortical projections in the barrelfield of hypothyroid rats. *European Journal of Neuroscience, 14,* 1968–1980.

Auso, E., Lavado-Autric, R., Cuevas, E., Del Rey, F. E., Morreale De Escobar, G., & Berbel, P. (2004). A moderate and transient deficiency of maternal thyroid function at the beginning of fetal neocorticogenesis alters neuronal migration. *Endocrinology, 145,* 4037–4047.

Berbel, P., Guadanao-Ferraz, A., Angulo, A., & Ramon Cerezo, J. (1994). Role of thyroid hormones in the maturation of interhemispheric connections in rats. *Behavior & Brain Research, 64,* 9–14.

Bernal, J., Guadano-Ferraz, A., & Morte, B. (2003). Perspectives in the study of thyroid hormone action on brain development and function. *Thyroid, 13,* 1005–1012.

Blasi, V., Longaretti, R., Giovanettoni, C., Baldoli, C., Ponsesilli, S., Vigone, M. C., et al. (2006). *Visuo-spatial deficit in pediatric congenital hypothyroidism: Hypoactivity in left inferior parietal cortex.* Manuscript submitted for publication.

Bongers-Schokking, J. J., & de Muinck Keizer-Schrama, S. M. (2005). Influence of timing and dose of thyroid hormone replacement on mental, psychomeotor, and behavioral development in children with congenital hypothyroidism. *Journal of Pediatrics, 147,* 768–774.

Bongers-Schokking, J. J., Koot, H. M., Wiersma, D., Verkerk, P. H., & de Muinck Keizer-Schrama, S. M. P. (2000). Influence of timing and dose of thyroid hormone replacement on development in infants with congenital hypothyroidism. *Journal of Pediatrics, 136,* 292–297.

Bradley, D. J., Towle, H. C., & Young, W. S. (1992). Spatial and temporal expression of α- and β-thyroid hormone receptor mRNAs, including the β2-subtype in the developing mammalian nervous system. *The Journal of Neuroscience, 12,* 2288–2302.

Brook, C. (1995). The consequences of congenital hypothyroidism. *Clinical Endocrinology, 42,* 432–438.

Brown, R. S., & Huang, S. (2005). The thyroid and its disorders. In C. G. D. Brook, P. Clayton, & R. S. Brown (Eds.), *clinical pediatric endocrinology* (5th edition, pp. 218–253). Oxford: Blackwell.

Brown, R. S., Bellisario, R. L., Botero, D., Fourneir, L., Abrams, C. A., Cowger, M. L., et al. (1996). Incidence of transient congenital hypothyroidism due to maternal thyrotropin receptor-blocking antibodies in over one million babies. *Journal of Endocrinology and Metabolism, 81,* 1147–1151.

Chan, S., & Rovet, J. (2003). Thyroid hormones in fetal central nervous system. *Fetal and Maternal Medicine Review, 14,* 177–208.

Crome, L., & Stern J. (1972). *Pathology of mental retardation.* Edinburgh, Scotland: Churchill Livingstone.

Delange, F., de Benoist, B., Preteil, E., & Dunn, J. T. (2001). Iodine deficiency in the world: Where do we stand at the turn of the century? *Thyroid, 11,* 437–447.

Derksen-Lubsen, G., & Verkerk, P. H. (1996). Neuropsychologic development in early-treated congenital hypothyroidism: Analysis of literature data. *Pediatric Research, 39,* 561–566.

Dohan, O., & Carrasco, N. (2003). Advances in NA^+/I^- symporter (NIS) research in the thyroid and beyond. *Molecular and Cellular Endocrinology, 213,* 50–58.

Eayrs, J. T. (1966). Thyroid and central nervous development. *The Scientific Basis of Medicine Annual Review,* 317–339.

Friesema, E. C., Grueters, A., Biebermann, H., Krude, H., von Moers, A., Reeser, M., et al. (2004). Association between mutations in a thyroid hormone transporter and severe X-linked psychomotor retardation. *Lancet, 364,* 1435–1437.

Gauger, K. J., Kato, Y., Haraguchi, K., Lehmler, H. J., Robertson, L. W., Bansal, R., & Zoeller, R. T. (2004). Polychlorinated biphenyls (PCBs) exert thyroid hormone-like effects in the fetal rat brain but do not bind to thyroid hormone receptors. *Environmental Health Perspectives, 11,* 516–523.

Gilbert, M. E. (2004). Alterations in synaptic transmission and plasticity in area CA1 of adult hippocampus following developmental hypothyroidism. *Developmental Brain Research, 148,* 11–18.

Gilbert, M. E., & Paczkowski, C. (2003). Propylthiouracil (PTU)-induced hypothyroidism in the developing rat impairs synaptic transmission and plasticity in the dentate gyrus of the adult hippocampus. *Developmental Brain Research, 145,* 19–29.

Gillam, M. P., & Kopp, P. (2001). Genetic regulation of thyroid development. *Current Opinion in Pediatrics, 13,* 358–363.

Gottschalk, B., Richman, R., & Lewandowski, L. (1994). Subtle speech and motor deficits of children with congenital hypothyroidism treated early. *Developmental Medicine and Child Neurology, 36,* 216–220.

Gould, E., & Butcher, L. L. (1989). Developing cholinergic basal forebrain neurons are sensitive to thyroid hormone. *Journal of Neuroscience, 9,* 3346–3358.

Grüters, A., Krude, H., & Biebermann, H. (2004). Molecular genetic defects in congenital hypothyroidism. *European Journal of Endocrinology, 151,* U39–U44.

Gupta, R. K., Bhatia, V., Poptani, H., & Gujral, R. B. (1995). Brain metabolite changes on in vivo proton magnetic resonance spectroscopy in children with congenital hypothyroidism. *Journal of Pediatrics, 126,* 389–392.

Hallowell, J. G., Staehling, N. W., Hannon, W. H., Flanders, D. W., Gunter, E. W., Maberly, G. F., et al. (1998). Iodine nutrion in the United States. Trends and public health implications: Iodine excretion data from National Health and Nutrition Examination Surveys I and III (1971–1974 and 1988–1994). *Journal of Clinical Endocrinology and Metabolism, 83,* 3401–3408.

Hauser, P., Zametkin, A., Martinez, P., Vitiello, B., Matochik, J. A., Mixson, A. J., & Weintraub, B. (1993). Attention deficit-hyperactivity disorder in people with generalized resistance to thyroid hormone. *New England Journal of Medicine, 328,* 997–1001.

Hepworth, S., Pang, E., & Rovet, J. (2006). Word and Face Recognition in children with congenital hypothyroidism: An event-related potentials study. *Journal of Clinical and Experimental Neuropsychology, 28,* 509–527.

Hepworth, S., & Rovet, J. F. (2006). Memory function in early treated congenital hypothyroidism. *International Neuropsychological Society Meeting Abstracts, 222.*

Heyerdahl, S. (2001). Long-term outcome in children with congenital hypothyroidism. *Acta Paediatrica, 90,* 1220–1222.

Heyerdahl, S., & Oerbeck, B. (2003). Congenital hypothyroidism: Developmental outcome in relation to levothyroxine treatment variables. *Thyroid, 13,* 1029–1038.

Howdeshell, K. L. (2002). A model of the development of the brain as a construct of the thyroid system. *Environmental Health Perspectives, 110,* 337–348.

Hrytsiuk, K., Gilbert, R., Logan, S., Pindoria, S., & Brook, C. G. (2002). Starting dose of levothyroxine for the treatment of congenital hypothyroidism: A systematic review. *Archives of Pediatric and Adolescent Medicine, 156,* 485–491.

Iniguez, M. A., De Lecea, L., Guadano-Ferraz, A., Morte, B., Gerendasy, D., Sutcliffe, J. G., & Bernal, J. (1996). Cell-specific effects of thyroid hormone on RC3/neurogranin expression in rat brain. *Endocrinology, 137,* 1032–1041.

Kelley, M. W., Thomas, J., & Reh, T. A. (1995). Ligands of steroid/thyroid receptors induce cone photoreceptors in vertebrate retina. *Development, 121,* 3777–3785.

Kempers, M. J. E., van der Sluijs, L., VNijhuis-van der Sanden, M. W., Kooistra, L., Wiedijk, B. M., Faber, I., et al. (2006). Intellectual and motor development of young adults with congenital hypothyroidism diagnosed by neonatal screening. *Journal of Clinical Endocrinology and Metabolism, 91,* 418–424.

Kester, M. H., Martinez de Mena, R., Obregon, J. J., Marinkovic, D., Howatson, A., Visser, T. J., et al. (2004). Iodothyronine levels in the human developing brain: Major regulatory roles of iodothyonine deiodinases in different areas. *The Journal of Clinical Endocrinology and Metabolism, 89,* 3117–3128.

Kilby, M. D., Gittoes, N., McCabe, C., Verhaeg, J., & Franklyn, J. A. (2000). Expression of thyroid receptor isoforms in the human fetal central nervous system and the effects of intrauterine growth restriction. *Clinical Endocrinology, 53,* 469–477.

Kirk, A. B., Martinelango, P., Tian, K., Dutta, A., Smit, E. E., & Dasgupta, P. (2005). Perchlorate and iodide in dairy and breast milk. *Environmental Science & Technology, 39,* 2011–2017.

Kooistra, L., Laane, C., Vulsma, T., Schellekens, J. M., van der Meere, J. J., & Kalverboer, A. F. (1994). Motor and cognitive development in children with congenital hypothyroidism: A long-term evaluation of the effects of neonatal treatment. *Journal of Pediatrics, 124,* 903–909.

Kooistra, L., Stemerdink, N., van der Meere, J., Vulsma, T., & Kalverboer, A. F. (2001). Behavioural correlates of early-treated congenital hypothyroidism. *Acta Paediatrica, 90,* 1141–1146.

Kooistra, L., van der Meere, J. J., Vulsma, T., & Kalverboer, A. F. (1996). Sustained attention problems in children with early treated congenital hypothyroidism. *Acta Paediatrica, 85,* 425–429.

Kopp, P. (2001). The TSH receptor and its role in thyroid disease. *Cellular and Molecular Life Science, 58,* 1301–1322.

LaFranchi, S. (1999). Congenital hypothyroidism: Etiologies, diagnosis, and management. *Thyroid, 9,* 735–740.

Lavado-Autric, R., Auso, E., Garacia-Velasco, J. V., del Carmen Arufe, M., Escobar del Rey, F., Berbel, P., & Morreale de Escobar, G. (2003). Early maternal hypothyroxinemia alters histogenesis and cerebral cotex cytoarchitecture of the progeny. *The Journal of Clinical Investigation, 111,* 1073–1082.

Legler, J., & Brouwer, A. (2003). Are brominated flame retardants endocrine disruptors? *Environment International, 29,* 879–885.

Legrand, J. (1984). Effects of thyroid hormones on central nervous system development. In J. Yanat (Ed.), *Neurobehavioral teratology* (pp. 331–363). Amsterdam.

Leneman, M., Buchanan, L., & Rovet, J. (2001). Where and what visuospatial processing in children with congenital hypothyroidism. *Journal of the International Neuropsychology Society, 7,* 556–562.

Maiorana, R., Carta, A., Floriddia, G., Leonardi, D., Buscema, M., Sava, L., et al. (2003). Thyroid hemiagenesis: Prevalence in normal children and effect on thyroid function. *Journal of Clinical Endocrinology and Metabolism, 88,* 1534–1536.

Mirabella, G., Westall, C. A., Asztalos, E., Perlman, K., Koren, G., & Rovet, J. (2005). The development of contrast sensitivity in infants with prenatal and neonatal thyroid hormone insufficiencies. *Pediatrics Research, 57,* 902–907.

Moreno, J. C., Bikker, H., Kempers, M. J., von Trotsenburg, A. S., Baas, F., de, J. J., et al. (2002). Inactivating mutations in the gene for thyroid oxidase 2 (THOX2) and congenital hypothyroidism. *New England Journal of Medicine, 347,* 95–102.

Moreno, J. C., de Viljder, J. J., Vulsma, T., & Ris-Stalpers, C. (2003). Genetic basis of hypothyroidism: Recent advances, gaps and strategies for future research. *Trends in Endocrinology and Metabolism, 14,* 318–326.

Morreale de Escobar, G., Obregon, M., & Escobar del Rey, F. (2000). Is neuropsychological development related to maternal hypothyroidism or to maternal hypothyroxinemia? *Journal of Clinical Endocrinology and Metabolism, 85,* 3975–3987.

Morreale de Escobar, G., Obregon, M. J., & Escobar del Rey, F. (2004). Role of thyroid hormone during early brain development. *European Journal of Endocrinology, 151,* U25–U37.

Moschini, L., Costa, P., Marinelli, E., Maggioni, G., Sorcini Carta, M., Fazzini, C., et al. (1986). Longitudinal assessment of children with congenital hypothyroidism detected by neonatal screening. *Helvetica Paediatrica Acta, 41,* 415–424.

Muir, T., & Zegarac, M. (2001). Societal costs of exposure to toxic substances: Economic and health costs of four case studies that are candidates for environmental causation. *Environmental Health Perspectives, 109,* 885–903.

Ng, L., Hurley, J. B., Dierks, B., Srinivas, M., Salto, C., Vennstrom, B., et al. (2001). A thyroid hormone receptor that is required for the development of green cone photoreceptors. *Nature Genetics, 27,* 94–98.

Oerbeck, B., Sundet, K., Kase, B. F., & Heyerdahl, S. (2003). Congenital hypothyroidism: Influence of disease severity and L-thyroxine treatment on intellectual, motor, and school-associated outcomes in young adults. *Pediatrics, 112,* 923–930.

Oerbeck, B., Sundet, K., Kase, B. F., & Heyerdahl, S. (2005). Congenital hypothyroidism: No adverse effects of high dose thyroxine treatment on adult memory, attention, and behaviour. *Archives Diseases of Childhood, 90,* 132–137.

Roberts, M. R., Srinivas, M., Forrest, D., Morreale de Escobar, G., & Reh, T. A. (2006). Making the gradient: Thyroid hormone regulates cone opsin expression in the developing mouse retina. *Proceedings of the National Academy of Science, 103,* 6218–6223.

Rosman, N., Malone, M., Helfenstein, M., & Kraft, E. (1972). The effect of thyroid deficiency on myelination of the brain. *Neurology, 22,* 99–106.

Rovet, J. F. (1992). Neurodevelopmental outcome in infants and preschool children following newborn screening for congenital hypothyroidism. *Journal of Pediatric Psychology, 17,* 187–213.

Rovet, J. (1995). Congenital hypothyroidism and nonverbal learning disabilities. In B. Rourke (Ed.), *Syndrome of NLD: Manifestations in neurological disease, disorder, and dysfunction* (pp. 255–281). New York: Guilford Press.

Rovet, J. F. (1999a). Outcome in congenital hypothyroidism. *Thyroid, 9,* 741–748.

Rovet, J. (1999b). Long-term neuropsychological sequelae of early-treated congenital hypothyroidism: Effects in adolescence. *Acta Paediatric, 432,* 88–95.

Rovet, J. F. (2000). Neurobehavioral consequences of congenital hypothyroidism identified by newborn screening. In B. Stabler & B. Bercu (Eds.), *Therapeutic outcome of endocrine disorders: Efficacy, innovation, and quality of life* (pp. 235–254). New York: Springer-Verlag.

Rovet, J. (2003a). Congenital hypothyroidism: Persisting deficits and associated factors. *Child Neuropsychology, 8,* 150–162.

Rovet, J. (2003b). Neurospychological follow-up of early-treated congenital hypothyroidism following newborn screening. In J. de Vildjer, G. Morreale de Escobar, S. Butz, & U. Hostalek (Eds.), *The thyroid and brain* (pp. 242–258). Stuttgart Germany: Schattauer.

Rovet, J. (2005). Congenital hypothyroidism: Treatment and outcome. *Current Opinion in Endocrinology and Metabolism, 12,* 42–52.

Rovet, J., & Alvarez, M. (1996). Thyroid hormone and attention in congenital hypothyroidism. *Journal of Pediatric Endocrinology and Metabolism, 9,* 63–66.

Rovet, J., & Daneman, D. (2003). Congenital hypothyroidism: A review of current diagnostic and treatment practices in relation to neuropsychologic outcome. *Pediatric Drugs, 5,* 141–149.

Rovet, J., Daneman, D., & Huang, C. (2003). Neuropsychological characteristics of children with atypical hypothyroidism suggest a common profile of attention and math deficits. *Thyroid, 13,* 691.

Rovet, J. F., Desrocher, M., Williamson, M., Nash, K., Blaser, S., & Soreni, N. (2006). Abnormal MRS profiles in children with congenital hypothyroidism. In *International Neuropsychological Society 34th Annual Meeting program & abstracts* (p. 253). Boston.

Rovet, J. F., & Ehrlich, R. M. (1995). Long-term effects of L-thyroxine therapy for congenital hypothyroidism. *Journal of Pediatrics, 126,* 380–386.

Rovet, J., & Ehrlich, R. M. (2000). The psychoeducational characteristics of children with early-treated congenital hypothyroidism. *Pediatrics, 105,* 515–522.

Rovet, J., Ehrlich, R., & Sorbara, D. (1989). The effect of thyroid hormone on temperament in infants with congenital hypothyroidism detected by newborn screening. *Journal of Pediatrics, 114,* 63–69.

Rovet, J. F., & Hepworth, S. (2001a). Attention problems in adolescents with congenital hypothyroidism: A multicomponential analysis. *Journal of the International Neuropsychological Society, 7,* 734–744.

Rovet, J., & Hepworth, S. (2001b). Dissociating attention deficits in children with ADHD and congenital hypothyroidism using multiple CPTs. *Journal of Child Psychology & Psychiatry, 42,* 1049–1056.

Rovet, J., Hepworth, S., & Lobaugh, N. (2006). *Visual search for features and conjunctions in children with attention disorders.* Manuscript submitted for publication.

Rovet, J., Walker, W., Bliss, B., Buchanan, L., & Ehrlich, R. (1997). Long-term sequelae of hearing impairment in congenital hypothyroidism. *Journal of Pediatrics, 127*, 776–783.

Ruiz-Marcos, A., & Ipina, S. L. (1986). Hypothyroidism affects preferentially the dendritic densities on the more superficial region of pyramidal neurons of the rat cerebral cortex. *Brain Research, 393*, 259–262.

Rusch, A., Erway, L., Oliver, D., Vennström, B., & Forrest, D. (1998). Thyroid hormone receptor beta-dependent expression of a potassium conductance in inner hair cells at the onset of hearing. *Proceedings of the National Academy of Science, 95*, 15758–15762.

Schapiro, S. (1976). Metabolic and maturational effects of thyroxine in the infant rat. *Endocrinology, 78*, 527–532.

Siragusa, V., Bofelli, S., Weber, G., Triulzim, F., Orezzim, S., Scottim, G., & Chiumello, G. (1997). Brain magnetic resonance imaging in congenital hypothyroid infants at diagnosis. *Thyroid, 7*, 761–764.

Song, S., Daneman, D., & Rovet, J. (2001). The influence of etiology and treatment factors on intellectual outcome in congenital hypothyroidism. *Journal of Developmental and Behavioral Pediatrics, 22*, 376–384.

Surks, M. I., & Sievert, R. (1995). Drugs and thyroid function. *New England Journal of Medicine, 333*, 1688–1694.

Tillotson, S. L., Fuggle, P. W., Smith, I., Ades, A. E., & Grant, D. B. (1994). Relation between biochemical severity and intelligence in early treated congenital hypothyroidism: A threshold effect. *British Medical Journal, 309*, 440–445.

Trueba, S. S., Augé, S., Mattei, G., Etchevers, H., Martinovic, J., Czernichow, P., Vekemans, M., Polak, M., & Attié-Bitach, T. (2005). PAX8, TITF1, and FOXE1 gene expression patterns during human development: New insights into human thyroid development and thyroid dysgenesis associated malformations. *Journal of Clinical Endocrinology and Metabolism, 90*, 455–462.

Van Vliet, G. (2003). Development of the thyroid gland: Lessons from congenitally hypothyroid mice and men. *Clinical Genetics, 63*, 445–455.

Vargha-Khadem, F., Gadian, D. G., Watkins, K. E., Connelly, A., Van Paesschen, W., & Mishkin, M. (1997). Differential effects of early hippocampal pathology on episodic and semantic memory. *Science, 277*, 376–380.

Vermiglio, F., Lo Presti, V. P., Moleti, M., Sidoti, M., Tortorella, G., Scaffidi, G., et al. (2004). Attention deficit and hyperactivity disorders in the offspring of mothers exposed to mild–moderate iodine deficiency: A possible novel iodine deficiency disorder in developed countries. *Journal of Clinical Endocrinology and Metabolism, 89*, 6054–6060.

Virgili, M., Saverino, O., Vaccari, M., Barnabci, O., & Contestabile, A. (1991). Temporal, regional and cellular selectivity of neonatal alteration of the thyroid state on neurochemical maturation in the rat. *Experimental Brain Research, 83*, 556–561.

Zoeller, R. T. (2004). Editorial: Local control of the timing of the thyroid hormone action in the developing human brain. *Journal of Clinical Endocrinology and Metabolism, 89*, 3114–3116.

Zoeller, R. T., & Rovet, J. (2004). Timing of thyroid hormone action in the developing brain: Clinical observations and experimental findings. *Journal of Neuroendocrinology, 16*, 809–818.

9 Inborn Errors of Metabolism

Kevin M. Antshel and Georgianne Arnold

Inborn errors of metabolism (IEM) fall into a number of classifications. They include disorders of intermediary metabolism (protein, carbohydrate, or fatty acid oxidation disorders), mitochondrial disorders, peroxisomal disorders; and disorders of carbohydrate glycosylation, creatine, or neurotransmitters. For more detailed information on these and other metabolic disorders, the reader is referred to *The Molecular and Metabolic Bases of Inherited Disease* (Scriver et al., 2001). IEM have been referred to as unique "experiments of nature" (Roth, 1986, p. 47).

IEM can have widespread systemic effects including neurological and psychological dysfunction. Neurological signs and symptoms of IEM may include mental retardation, abnormal muscle tone, altered mental status, seizures, and other problems. Non-neurological signs and symptoms may include failure to thrive, renal dysfunction, cardiac dysfunction, ketoacidosis, cardiomyopathy, structural birth defects, or dysfunction in virtually any body system.

Most IEMs affect the central nervous system and may lead to mental retardation but also to more subtle signs or symptoms. The neurodevelopmental specialist is frequently called on to evaluate a child who presents with developmental delays and to investigate whether a diagnosis (and potential treatment) or recurrence risk can be determined. This chapter is geared toward developmental specialists who perform these evaluations as well as researchers who may study IEMs. Our goals for this chapter are threefold: (a) to discuss the broad range of metabolic disorders and provide up-to-date information on genotype–phenotype associations, (b) to convey the impressive range of phenotypes that exist within several metabolic disorders, and (c) to articulate how metabolic disorders can inform neurodevelopmental research. We will begin by considering disorders of intermediary metabolism that typically present with some degree of developmental delay with or without other localizing signs.

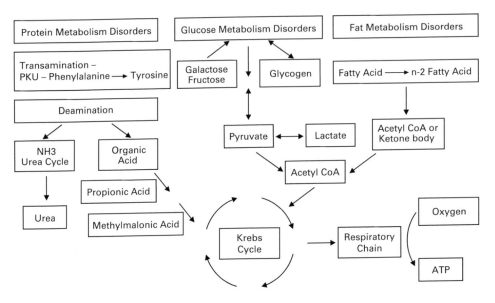

Figure 9.1
Disorders of intermediary metabolism.

Disorders Primarily Presenting with Developmental Delays

Inborn Errors in Protein Metabolism

In typical development, amino acids not needed for protein synthesis or other processes undergo degradation by well-defined pathways. An amino acid can undergo transamination into another amino acid, or the amino acid's nitrogen can be cleaved from the carbon skeleton, forming ammonia (which must be detoxified by the urea cycle) and an organic acid that is eventually metabolized in the Krebs cycle (see figure 9.1). There is a broad range of inborn errors of this protein metabolism. This section will focus on the most common protein metabolism disorder, phenylketonuria (PKU), as well as the most common disorders of the urea cycle and organic acid metabolism.

Phenylketonuria   The most common disorder of amino acid metabolism is PKU (see figure 9.1). PKU is also the best characterized and most researched inborn error of protein metabolism. The amino acid phenylalanine is normally transaminated to tyrosine by the enzyme phenylalanine hydroxylase (with the assistance of a pterin cofactor). This process is disrupted in individuals with PKU. The gene for phenylalanine hydroxylase is located on the distal part of chromosome 12q (Lidsky et al., 1984), and the vast majority of individuals with PKU have a genetic defect in phenylalanine

Table 9.1
Common biochemical tests used in the diagnosis and management of inborn errors of metabolism

Quantitative Plasma Amino Acids: Reports concentrations of essential and nonessential amino acids and urea cycle intermediates. This test is useful for diagnosis of common amino acid disorders.

Quantitative Urine Amino Acids: Reports concentrations of essential and nonessential amino acids and urea cycle intermediates. This test is useful for diagnosis of some transport disorders, homocystinuria, and common amino acid disorders. The results are more sensitive to recent dietary intake than plasma levels and thus are often more easily interpreted in conjunction with plasma amino acids.

Quantitative Cerebral Spinal Fluid (CSF) Amino Acids: Reports concentrations of specific amino acids in CSF. This test is useful for diagnosis of nonketotic hyperglycinemia and serine biosynthesis disorders.

Urine Organic Acids: Reports the presence of common organic acid metabolites. It is useful for diagnosis of common organic acidemias as well as more severe glucose metabolism and fatty acid oxidation disorders.

Plasma Acylcarnitine: Reports concentrations of organic metabolites esterified to carnitine. It is useful for common and more subtle organic acidemias and fatty acid oxidation disorders.

Urine Acylglycine: Reports concentrations of organic metabolites complexed to glycine. It is useful for common and more subtle organic acidemias and fatty acid oxidation disorders.

hydroxylase; therefore phenylalanine accumulates, giving rise to the effects. A small percentage of individuals with PKU have a defect in the pterin cofactor (Scriver et al., 1995). More than 400 mutations have been identified in the phenylalanine hydroxylase gene, which accounts for some of the biochemical phenotypic variability (Ramus et al., 1999).

PKU is inherited in an autosomal recessive manner. The prevalence is approximately 1 in 15,000 in the United States but is higher in Ireland, Scandinavia, and Turkey. Today, most countries with well-developed public health systems provide newborn screening for PKU. Initial screening involves determining free levels of phenylalanine and tyrosine. However, newborn screening programs are not 100% sensitive. Thus, PKU (and other metabolic disorders) should be considered in all children with unexplained developmental delay/mental retardation. In the past, a urine ferric chloride or a qualitative urine amino acid analysis was performed for the diagnosis of PKU. However with today's technology, a quantitative plasma amino acid assay (table 9.1) is the preferred diagnostic test.

Treatment requires restricting dietary phenylalanine, usually to approximately 150–300 mg/day. As phenylalanine is an essential amino acid, some is required in the diet from relatively small amounts of "natural" food, typically fruits and nonstarchy nonlegume vegetables. The diet is highly restrictive; for example a "small" order of fries or a 2 oz. serving of potato chips typically has about 120 mg of phenylalanine. Meat, dairy, soy, legumes, nuts, and other high protein foods are forbidden. Therefore, essential amino acid, caloric, and vitamin needs are all met with "medical foods" consisting of essential amino acids and other nutrients. New treatment modalities are in the development phase, including an injectable enzyme to degrade phenylalanine.

Untreated PKU usually causes profound progressive mental retardation, often with autistic-like features. Up to 1% of adults with idiopathic mental retardation were born before newborn screening, and thus many have undetected and untreated PKU. However, when treated from birth, children with PKU have normal intelligence yet may experience more subtle residual cognitive difficulties. Cognitive vulnerabilities frequently described in children with early and *consistently* treated PKU include executive dysfunction, poor attention, information processing, and visuospatial abilities (Anderson et al., 2004; Antshel & Waisbren, 2003a; Arnold et al., 1998; Gassio et al., 2005; Feldmann et al., 2005; Huijbregts et al., 2002a; Leuzzi et al., 2004; White et al., 2001); and immature academic attainment, especially in math (Azen et al., 1996; Chang, Gray, & O'Brien, 2000). Nearly all of the extant pediatric PKU neuropsychological literature suggests that both lifetime and concurrent history of metabolic control (history of phenylalanine levels) are negatively associated with cognitive performance. In other words, the higher the levels of phenylalanine, both present and past, the worse the performance on cognitive and neuropsychological tests.

Two hypotheses have been posed to describe the neuropsychological profile commonly reported in PKU. First, Diamond (1996) and colleagues (Diamond et al., 1997) proposed the prefrontal cortex dysfunction hypothesis as etiologically relevant. By lacking phenylalanine hydroxylase, children with PKU are unable to break phenylalanine into the dopamine precursor, tyrosine. In addition, phenylalanine competes with tyrosine and tryptophan and other large neutral amino acids for transport across the blood–brain barrier. Thus, as a function of lacking phenylalanine hydroxylase and having elevated levels of phenylalanine, children with PKU are doubly susceptible to having lower levels of dopamine. The prefrontal dysfunction hypothesis posits that these neurotransmitter anomalies are most likely to affect the dorsolateral prefrontal area, a region that is especially sensitive to dopamine depletion (Goldman-Rakic, 1987). Via lower levels of dopamine in the dorsolateral region, Diamond's hypothesis suggests that children with PKU will be at elevated risk of having working memory deficits and being less able to inhibit prepotent responses. Research supports this model (e.g., Antshel & Waisbren, 2003a; Huijbregts et al., 2002a; Weglage et al., 1996; Welsh et al., 1990; White et al., 2002).

Myelin abnormalities, particularly in posterior or periventricular areas (Anderson et al., 2004; Dezortova et al., 2001; Pietz et al., 1996), have been forwarded as a second explanation of the PKU neuropsychological profile (for reviews, see Dyer, 1999; Welsh & Pennington, 2000). These white matter abnormalities have been hypothesized to represent increased water content in the myelin and abnormal myelin production (Pietz, 1998). Associations between phenylalanine levels, again, both past and present, and white matter abnormalities have been empirically demonstrated (Cleary et al., 1994; Pietz et al., 1996). There is some evidence that white matter anomalies are decreased with stricter phenylalanine control (Cleary et al., 1995), lending further support for an association between white matter anomalies and elevated levels of phenylalanine.

Given the dopaminergic system involvement in PKU, it is not surprising that increased prevalence of attention deficit/hyperactivity disorder (ADHD) has been reported in PKU (Antshel & Waisbren, 2003b; Arnold et al., 2004). However, given that most research suggests a positive relationship between phenylalanine levels and inattentive symptoms (Antshel & Waisbren, 2003b; Feldmann et al., 2005; Huijbregts et al., 2002b; Weglage et al., 1996), it remains unclear whether the higher ADHD prevalence rate in PKU represents "true" ADHD or what Pearl, Weiss, and Stein (2001) have termed a "medical mimic." In other words, if a child with PKU demonstrates inattentive symptoms only during periods of poor dietary adherence, does this truly represent ADHD? Children with PKU who are treated with methylphenidate have higher phenylalanine levels than those who are untreated (Arnold et al., 2004); thus, the "validity" of ADHD in PKU might well have public health considerations and be more than just a difficult differential diagnosis.

One method of investigating the validity of ADHD in PKU involves the endophenotype model (Gottesman & Gould, 2003), to examine whether there is a higher rate of familial ADHD in children with PKU and ADHD (PKU+ADHD) than in children with only PKU. A shared predisposing vulnerability should be familial; although not all relatives of children with PKU+ADHD will have ADHD (the vulnerability presumably combines with other factors in only *some* family members to cause the full disorder), we may observe an increased prevalence of ADHD in this population. This basic premise has been relatively well validated in schizophrenia and ADHD, conditions that share neuropsychological vulnerabilities (prefrontal mechanisms; Asarnow et al., 2002).

Much of the previous work in PKU has relied on blood phenylalanine levels as a gauge of brain phenylalanine levels. However, magnetic resonance spectroscopy (MRS) research has demonstrated that despite having similar *blood* phenylalanine levels, individuals with PKU can have very different *brain* phenylalanine levels (Koch et al., 2000; Moats et al., 2000; Moller et al., 2003). Brain:blood ratios in PKU generally range from 0.2–0.7; individual variations in blood–brain barrier phenylalanine transport and brain phenylalanine expenditure rate may account for the variations (Moller et al., 2003). Although tremendous progress has been made on elucidating the pathophysiology of PKU neurological abnormalities, these individual variations observed in brain:blood phenylalanine ratios indicate that much work still remains to be done. These individual variations also help to explain why genotype–phenotype associations in PKU are modest at best.

At one time it was believed that treatment of PKU could be safely stopped at approximately 6 years of age when brain growth was believed to be completed.

However, in light of what is now known about brain development and continued myelination throughout adolescence (Giedd et al., 1999), it is not surprising that findings from the largest longitudinal project, the Phenylketonuria Collaborative Study, have demonstrated earlier termination of the PKU diet (at early to middle childhood) is associated with more significant cognitive difficulties than is dietary compliance through adolescence and adulthood (Koch et al., 2002). In fact, most PKU clinics have now adopted a "diet-for-life" position for optimal management of PKU.

A disorder related to PKU that is relevant to those working in the neurodevelopmental disorders field is maternal PKU (MPKU). Phenylalanine is a teratogen; so women with PKU must carefully control their blood phenylalanine levels during pregnancy to avoid structural and systemic anomalies that are remarkably similar to those reported in fetal alcohol syndrome (Costa et al., 2002). When the mother is not adequately treated during pregnancy, MPKU is associated with mental retardation in 97% of the offspring, and with microcephaly (73%), low birth weight (40%), and congenital heart disease (12%; Lenke & Levy, 1980; Levy & Ghavami, 1996; Rouse et al., 2000). Undetected MPKU should be considered in women who have more than one child with unexplained mental retardation, as a small percentage of individuals with PKU born before newborn screening escaped mental retardation and thus may not be diagnosed.

In untreated or very late treated MPKU pregnancies, corpus callosum hypoplasia is a frequent finding, yet in well-treated MPKU pregnancies, structural brain abnormalities have not been reported (Levy et al., 1996). White matter changes noted in individuals with PKU are not present in MPKU offspring (Levy et al., 1996). Despite normal structural findings in offspring from well-treated MPKU pregnancies, developmental and neuropsychological outcome of MPKU offspring is quite variable and appears strongly related to maternal metabolic control. The MPKU Collaborative Study, a longitudinal prospective study that began in 1984, offers the most extensive findings on the issue of prenatal exposure to elevated levels of phenylalanine (Koch et al., 2000). Overall, the children from mothers with PKU scored significantly lower (<1.0 SD) than children of mothers without PKU on measures of general cognitive ability. Important factors in the children's cognitive development were the timing of maternal metabolic control during pregnancy and the overall average level of phenylalanine exposure (Pearson's $r = -.58$; Waisbren et al., 2000). Those mothers who had less well controlled pregnancies generally had the offspring with the most neurodevelopmental delays. Compared to children with PKU, MPKU offspring also appear to have higher rates of hyperactivity and impulsivity, a finding that is less common in PKU (Antshel & Waisbren, 2003b); thus, in addition to the level of phenylalanine to which the child is exposed, the developmental timing of phenylalanine exposure is an important variable to consider in predicting cognitive phenotypes.

As its name suggests, mild hyperphenylalaninemia (HPA) is less severe than PKU and is diagnosed in untreated children with plasma phenylalanine values between 2–6 mg/dL (normal levels are <2 mg/dL). Children with HPA are generally not treated with a phenylalanine-restricted diet, and most research suggests that cognitive functioning is less affected than is observed in PKU (Gassio et al., 2005; Smith et al., 2000). In addition, phenylalanine restricted diets are not generally prescribed for pregnant women with HPA (Levy et al., 2003). In short, HPA is generally considered to be rather benign.

In conclusion, PKU and MPKU are profound examples of gene–environment interactions. Horst Bickel's 1953 discovery of the PKU diet and Robert Guthrie's 1961 introduction of newborn screening blood assays for PKU both represent impressive environmental modifications of this genetic condition. In the span of 10 years, children with PKU were saved from mental retardation. A similar process occurred in the 1980s once the newborns of the 1960s reached childbearing age and MPKU emerged. Our ability to now prevent mental retardation in both populations provides strong evidence that "genetic" does not mean "predetermined." Likewise, over 400 mutations have been identified in the phenylalanine hydroxylase gene; nonetheless, even within those children with the *same* phenylalanine hydroxylase mutation, phenotypic variability continues to be the rule, not the exception.

Cystathionine Beta-Synthase Deficiency   Classical homocystinuria is an autosomal recessive disorder associated with cystathionine beta-synthase (CBS) deficiency. In reality, there are several disorders that fall under the category "homocystinuria." Thus, this class of disorders is not really a disorder but rather a biochemical finding. In classic homocystinuria, decreased CBS activity leads to increased plasma levels of methionine and homocyst(e)ine, as well as decreased plasma levels of cyst(e)ine (see table 9.1). Plasma homocyst(e)ine levels may be falsely normal unless the sample is specially prepared for this analysis by immediate deproteinization.

Clinical manifestations of classic homocystinuria may include tall stature, a Marfanoid habitus, and lens dislocation (Mudd, Levy, & Skovby, 1995). This disorder is quite rare, and the worldwide prevalence rate is 1:335,000 live births. Prevalence rates are highest in Ireland and Italy. High doses of pyridoxine (Vitamin B_6) and a methionine-restricted diet are typical treatments for classical homocystinuria. Two clinical forms of classical homocystinuria have been identified on the basis of pyridoxine responsiveness (Mudd et al., 1995). As in all conditions with hyperhomocysteinemia, myelinopathy is the most common neuropathology yet thrombotic strokes and small vascular occlusions may also occur (Van der Knaap & Valk, 1995).

Mental retardation is more common in the pyridoxine nonresponsive form of classical homocystinuria (De Franchis et al., 1998); approximately half of the pyridoxine responders have mental retardation, yet nearly 80% of the nonresponders have full scale IQs < 70. In one of the largest homocystinuria studies, Mudd et al. (1985) reported on 268 individuals; the mean IQs were 57 and 79 in the nonresponders and responders, respectively. Less than 5% of the pyridoxine nonresponders had IQs in the average range, while 22% of the pyridoxine responders had IQs > 90. More recently, Yap et al. (2001) investigated IQ in groups of children with classical homocystinuria identified via newborn screening. The groups were dichotomized according to lifetime history of treatment adherence (good/poor). Those children with a good history of treatment (mean age at assessment = 14 years, range = 4–24 years) had IQs in the average range (mean IQ = 105.8, range = 84–120). These children performed significantly better than the poor treatment adherers (mean IQ = 80.8, range = 40–103). Interestingly, in both groups of children with classical homocystinuria, Verbal IQ (VIQ) scores were significantly higher than Performance IQ (PIQ) scores, signifying possible difficulties in nonverbal, perceptual; or fluid reasoning. The Yap et al. (2001) data suggest that, as is the case for PKU, treatment adherence appears to be a salient variable to consider when predicting cognitive outcomes, in addition to treatment responsiveness.

In addition to cognitive differences between pyridoxine responsive and nonresponsive forms of classical homocystinuria, psychiatric functioning also appears to be mediated by pyridoxine responsiveness. For example, 10% of pyridoxine responders vs. 33% of nonresponders have a psychiatric disorder (De Franchis et al., 1998). Although anecdotal reports of schizophrenia in individuals with classical homocystinuria are relatively common (Abbott et al., 1987; Bracken & Coll, 1985; Ryan et al., 2002), few investigations have systematically considered the prevalence rates of schizophrenia in the classical homocystinuria population or vice versa (elevated levels of homocysteine in the schizophrenia population). Nonetheless, a recent review (Picker & Coyle, 2005) nicely outlines the possible connection between low maternal folate levels and neurodevelopmental anomalies that may lead to schizophrenia.

Prenatally, folate deficiencies elevate plasma homocysteine levels by decreasing activity of the folate-sensitive methylenetetrahydrofolate reductase genetic polymorphisms (Kumar et al., 2003). Increased homocysteine levels in the mother are directly passed on to the developing fetus and affect methyl donation and the N-methyl-D-aspartate receptor (NMDAR), both increasing and decreasing NMDAR activity (Lipton et al., 1997). NMDAR activity alterations, in turn, have been empirically demonstrated to produce neurodevelopmental deficits that are similar to those reported in schizophrenia. Clearly, much work remains to be done regarding the association of elevated levels of homocysteine and schizophrenia; nonetheless, Picker and Coyle (2005) have outlined a testable hypothesis.

An alternate form of homocystinuria is found in which affected individuals have a defect in processing of vitamin B_{12} that impairs the remethylation of homocyst(e)ine back to methionine. Some of these defects affect only the form of B_{12} involved in remethylation of homocyst(e)ine (methyl B_{12}), and some affect a precursor to both methyl B_{12} and adenosyl B_{12}, resulting in a combined homocystinuria and methylmalonic acidemia. Clinical and developmental effects can be similar to classical homocystinuria. Treatment typically includes administration of large doses of vitamin B_{12}, typically parenterally.

Tyrosinemia Type II   Tyrosinemia type II is caused by tyrosine aminotransferase deficiency and has a worldwide prevalence rate of 1:250,000 live births (Huhn et al., 1998; Mitchell et al., 2001). Children with tyrosinemia type II frequently have abnormal keratinazataion of the cornea, palms, and soles; photophobia (sensitivity to light); and variable degrees of developmental delay. (A dermatologist or ophthalmologist quite often initially suspects the diagnosis.) Treatment for tyrosinemia type II involves a low-protein diet and medical formula containing essential amino acids minus phenylalanine and tyrosine; treatment also greatly improves optic and dermatological symptoms, generally within days. Much like MPKU, maternal tyrosinemia requires strict dietary management throughout pregnancy (Cerone et al., 2002). Most of the extant neurodevelopmental research in tyrosinemia type II is case reports. For example, Sener (2005) reported globus pallidus white matter anomalies in a preschool girl with tyrosinemia type II. Nonetheless, it is generally accepted that earlier diagnosis and dietary treatment can improve neurological functioning (Mitchell et al., 2001).

Maple Syrup Urine Disease   Maple syrup urine disease (MSUD) is a disorder of the branched chain amino acids valine, leucine, and isoleucine and commonly presents in the neonatal period with ketosis, acidosis, and the odor of maple syrup in urine and cerumen (Chuang & Shih, 2001). MSUD occurs rarely in the general population, possibly as infrequently as 1:290,000 (Levy, 1973). Nonetheless, the disorder is quite common in the Mennonite population, with prevalence rates as high as 1:176 live births (DiGeorge et al., 1982). There are several subtypes of MSUD, yet most research has focused on the "classic" severe form that has a neonatal onset and accounts for 75%–80% of all MSUD cases. Treatment for classical MSUD generally involves leucine-restricted diets and branched-chain amino acid level monitoring.

Despite the relatively low prevalence rate of MSUD, there have been several neurodevelopmental research studies that have assessed relationships between cognitive functioning and physiological variables. For instance, LeRoux et al. (2006) reported that the mean IQ in a group of adults with classic MSUD was in the borderline range (PIQ = 76; VIQ = 81) with a considerable performance range (54–113). A negative association emerged between IQ and age of diagnosis; the earlier the diagnosis, the higher the intellectual functioning. These data are consistent with pediatric data (Hilliges, Awiszus, & Wendel, 1993; Nord, van Doorninck, & Greene, 1991) and suggest that general cognitive abilities are developmentally delayed in MSUD. Nonetheless, others (Kaplan et al., 1991) have reported that children with MSUD can have IQs in the normal range; likewise, Hoffman et al. (2006) reported normal IQs, although these were reported in a sample of five children with MSUD who had chronically low levels of leucine (indicating excellent metabolic control and/or a milder variant of the disorder). In fact, the mean plasma leucine level in these children was 189 ± 82 μmol/L, just out of the normal range of 77–153 μmol/L (Lepage et al., 1997).

Magnetic resonance imaging (MRI) studies of neonatal MSUD are quite consistent; in fact, localized edemas to the cerebellar white matter, posterior brain stem, cerebral peduncles, thalami, and posterior centrum semiovale that co-occur are called a "MSUD edema" (Heindel et al., 1995). Thalamic and globus pallidus myelination delays appear to be the most commonly reported residual effects. These myelin delays persist after diagnosis and treatment have been initiated and continue to persist into adolescence and young adulthood (Ha et al., 2004; Schonberger et al., 2004; Temudo et al., 2004).

Glutaric Acidemia Type I   Glutaric acidemia (GA) type I is an autosomal recessive disorder that results from a defect in the metabolism of tryptophan, lysine, and hydroxylysine and results in glutaric acid accumulation in the blood and brain (Strauss et al., 2003). Over 60 different mutations have been reported on the glutaryl-CoA dehydrogenase gene, located on chromosome 19p13.2 (Goodman et al., 1998). Worldwide, the prevalence rate of GA type I is 1:100,000, although the disorder is more common in French Canadians and old-order Amish (Lindner et al., 2004).

MRI studies shortly after birth have consistently documented macrocephaly; however, despite an enlarged head circumference, children with GA type I often have what has been termed "micrencephalic macrocephaly," due to frontotemporal atrophy, ventricular enlargement, and widening of the Sylvian fissures (Strauss et al., 2003). Metabolic crises are most common between 6 and 18 months of age and are most often triggered by a febrile intercurrent illness. During metabolic stress, children may incur damage to the basal ganglia with loss of developmental milestones (Desai et al., 2003; Neumaier-Probst et al., 2004).

Bjugstad and colleagues (2000) published the largest GA type I developmental outcome study. Archival data were gathered from 42 published reports of children with GA type I. One hundred fifteen children with GA type I were used in the stepwise regression analyses predicting outcome. The strongest predictor of both outcome and motor deficits was age at diagnosis; in both models, having a younger age at diagnosis was associated with more favorable outcomes. Treatment after the onset of symptoms was not associated with outcomes in any of the models; this suggests that in GA type I, early detection is extremely important.

Urea Cycle Disorders   Amino acids are metabolized for energy by removing the nitrogen as ammonia (NH_3) and processing the remaining carbon skeleton as an organic acid and into the Krebs cycle (see Disorders of Organic Acid Metabolism). The ammonia is detoxified via the urea cycle, where it is changed to urine soluble urea and excreted. Caused by defects in the metabolism of the extra nitrogen produced by the breakdown of proteins, urea cycle disorders encompass a range of disorders that are due to deficiencies or absence of any of the urea cycle enzymes (e.g., ornithine transcarbamylase [OTC]). Most urea cycle disorders are inherited in an autosomal recessive manner, with equal numbers of males and females affected. The exception is OTC deficiency, the most prevalent (1:14,000 live births) urea cycle disorder, which is inherited on the X chromosome, although it is commonly penetrant in females as well as males.

Deficiencies of these enzymes lead to progressive accumulation of ammonia during the neonatal period. Hyperammonemic coma, seizures, and distal hypertonia secondary to neurological irritability often emerge acutely in the neonatal period (Brusilow & Horwich, 2001). Having a neonatal onset is associated with significant risk for mortality; an 84% mortality rate for neonatal-onset urea cycle disorders has been reported (Nassogne et al., 2005). Nonetheless, urea cycle disorders can present at any time, often with changes in diet (such as weaning from breast milk to the higher protein content of formula) or during intercurrent illness when protein breakdown from muscle (gluconeogenesis) is enhanced during fasting. Approximately 10% of cases present after the first year of life, documented as late as the seventh decade. Accordingly, age should not be used as a reason to exclude a urea cycle defect from the differential diagnosis of unexplained mental status changes or developmental delays.

Plasma ammonia (free flowing, on ice, analyzed stat) should be measured on any individual with unexplained mental status changes. Plasma amino acid analysis can help to identify which specific urea cycle defect is present, and urine organic acid analysis (table 9.1) should be done to rule out other disorders that also cause elevated ammonia levels. Some urea cycle disorders can be diagnosed by tandem mass spectroscopy on expanded newborn screen, but at this time the most common urea cycle disorder, OTC deficiency, cannot.

The treatment of urea cycle defects generally involves a restricted protein diet, being careful to consume sufficient protein to maintain positive nitrogen balance without excess intake. Hemodialysis or extracorporeal membrane oxygenation may be indicated to lower ammonia levels in a crisis. Drugs that enhance ammonia excretion are useful both chronically and acutely. Liver transplantation is essentially curative for defects "early" in the cycle (OTC deficiency and possibly citrullinemia, a disorder of argininosuccinate synthesase) yet cannot reverse existing cognitive damage.

During periods of metabolic stress, most commonly from intercurrent illnesses, affected individuals can have life-threatening elevations of ammonia. Some degree of mental retardation with or without spasticity is the rule in neonatal onset urea cycle disorders; in fact, nearly two thirds of neonatal onset cases exhibit severe to profound developmental deficits (Gropman & Batshaw, 2004; Bachmann, 2003). However, neurological deficits can occur even without profound hyperammonemia; for example, children with arginase deficiency typically present with severe spasticity and significant mental retardation without having significant ammonia elevations.

The neuropathophysiology of urea cycle disorders is not completely understood. However, one theory posits that high levels of ammonia result in glutamate being converted to glutamine, predominantly in astrocytes. Accumulating glutamine, in turn, leads to astrocyte swelling and intracranial hypertension (Brusilow & Horwich, 2001). Neuroimaging research in OTC deficiency has generally supported this theory (Connelly et al., 1993; Takanishi et al., 2002).

The most consistent neuroimaging findings are generally separated according to age at diagnosis. Neonatal onset is associated with severe and diffuse cerebral edema with accompanying atrophy (Choi & Yoo, 2001). Neuropathologies noted in children with later onset (postneonate) OTC deficiency include infarct-like abnormalities with acute hemiplegia (Bajaj et al., 1996; Connelly et al., 1993; de Grauw et al., 1990) and lesions in the cingulate gyri, temporal lobes, and insular cortex (Takanishi et al., 2002).

Much of the extant urea cycle developmental research has focused on OTC deficiency. Boys with OTC deficiency often do not survive the neonatal period (Nassogne et al., 2005); hence, most developmental research has followed girls with OTC deficiency. Age of diagnosis and plasma level of ammonia at time of diagnosis seem to be the best predictors of cognitive outcome; IQ is positively associated with age of diagnosis, yet ammonia levels at time of diagnosis are negatively associated with cognitive outcomes (Nicolaides et al., 2002). In girls heterozygous for OTC deficiency, phenotypic expression is less variable and the vast majority (85%) are asymptomatic (Maestri et al., 1998). Additional research such as this focusing on the cognitive phenotype of atypical (and less severe) males and females with partial OTC deficiency is needed.

Disorders of Organic Acid Metabolism

Methylmalonic and Propionic Acidemia Before an amino acid is metabolized for energy, the nitrogen is removed (see Urea Cycle Disorders), leaving the remaining carbon skeleton as an organic acid. A series of specific metabolic processes then convert that carbon skeleton to a unique Krebs cycle intermediate. (See figure 9.1.) The most common group of organic acidemia disorders is caused by a defect in an enzymatic step in the degradation pathway common to valine, odd chain fatty acids, methionine, isoleucine, and threonine during the metabolism of propionic acid or methylmalonic acid. Genetic defects in the enzymes propionyl CoA carboxylase or methylmalonyl CoA mutase result in the buildup of propionic acid or methylmalonic acid, respectively.

Methylmalonic acidemia (MMA) and propionic acidemia (PA) are the most prevalent forms of branched-chain organic acidemias and biochemically and clinically present very similarly (Saudubray & Charpentier, 2001). The neurological presentation of MMA or PA is typically part of a neonatal metabolic crisis including altered mental status, irritability, seizures, and non-neurological signs and symptoms such as ketoacidosis, vomiting, bone marrow suppression, and hyperammonemia. Later onset or more chronic presentations are common, often including mental retardation/developmental delay, hypotonia and/or spasticity, failure to thrive, seizures, and other nonspecific findings often in the absence of acidosis or ketosis (Saudubray & Charpentier, 2001). Recurrent metabolic crises can be precipitated by intercurrent illnesses or metabolic stress and can be fatal in the initial or later episodes.

Treatment for neonatal or intermittent crisis may require hemodialysis. In the chronic state, treatment is by supplementation with carnitine and careful control of protein intake such that positive nitrogen balance is maintained without consuming excess protein. Cobalamin (vitamin B_{12}) is also frequently used as a treatment. Cobalamin-responsive children appear to have a more favorable cognitive outcome, although neurological abnormalities increase with age in both cobalamin-responsive and nonresponsive children (Nicolaides, Leonard, & Surtees, 1998). Other useful adjuncts may include treatment with metronidazole or similar antibiotics to reduce intestinal formation of propionate, and supplementation with nonpropiogenic essential amino acids. Given the relatively poor outcomes that have been reported in well-treated children, liver transplant has been forwarded as a potential treatment. Nonetheless, even when occurring very early in life, liver transplant in the organic acidemias does not prevent the basal ganglia deterioration that often ensues from the initial metabolic crises (Chakrapani et al., 2002; Nyhan et al., 2002).

As many as 10% of children with organic acidemias may present with chronic mental retardation, hypotonia, failure to thrive, or other noncritical findings in the absence of ketoacidosis. Therefore, a urine organic acid analysis is indicated in children with unexplained developmental delay/mental retardation even in the absence of ketosis, acidosis, or metabolic crises. Plasma amino acids commonly show elevated plasma glycine. Plasma acylcarnitine and urine acylglycine (table 9.1) can also be helpful diagnostically when a metabolic disorder is suspected based on signs or symptoms of an organic acidemia (e.g., metabolic crises, ketoacidosis, failure to thrive, hypotonia, bone marrow suppression, etc.), particularly in mild cases in which organic acids can appear relatively normal when the patient is not metabolically stressed. This disorder can be diagnosed by tandem mass spectroscopy on expanded newborn screening although with somewhat lesser sensitivity and specificity than for other common metabolic disorders.

The most common neuropathological finding in the organic acidemias is infarct-like episodes with prominent basal ganglia involvement, especially the globus pallidus (Surtees, Matthews, & Leonard, 1992; Nicolaides et al., 1998; Ogier de Baulny et al., 2005). Neurological deficits may show stepwise progression during episodic metabolic crises. Extrapyramidal symptoms often develop in the organic acidemias.

Similar to the urea cycle disorders, mortality is rather high in the neonatal onset organic acidemias. In those with neonatal onset organic acidemias who survive, the neurodevelopmental outcome can be varied. In general, cognitive impairment is less significant in MMA compared to PA; children with MMA can have profound mental retardation, but a recent survey found IQ > 75 in 60% of individuals with MMA and IQ > 90 in 40% (Ogier de Baulny et al., 2005). In fact, a case report of an early adolescent female with late-onset MMA with a history of metabolic crises reported an IQ in the superior range and very strong academic attainment (Varvogli et al., 2000). Notably, she had a less severe form of the disorder that is associated with only partial apoenzyme activity absence.

Disorders of Carbohydrate Metabolism

Carbohydrates are metabolized for energy as glucose and stored as glycogen or processed through the glycolytic process, Krebs cycle, and respiratory chain to produce energy. Relatively few inborn errors of the glycolytic process have been described, but they include glycogen storage disorders, galactosemia, hereditary fructose intolerance, pyruvate dehydrogenase deficiency, and a few rare inborn errors of the Krebs cycle or respiratory chain. Alternate carbohydrates such as fructose and galactose are also subject to inborn errors in the process of conversion to glucose.

Galactosemia   An autosomal recessive disorder, galactosemia is due to a deficiency of the galactose-1-phosphate uridyltransferase (GALT) enzyme. This deficiency results in an accumulation of galactose-1-phosphate. (See figure 9.1.) The GALT gene is located on chromosome 9p13, and many different mutations exist, the most common of which is the Q188R. This mutation is the most prevalent yet is associated with the least enzyme activity (Leslie et al., 1992) and the most affected phenotype. Other variants include S135L, observed commonly in African Americans (Lai et al.,

1996) and associated with a milder phenotype as well as the Duarte variant (Kelly & Segal, 1989), generally associated with very little morbidity or mortality.

Nearly all states test for galactosemia on newborn screening panels. However, infants may already be ill by the time the screening result is available. Infants having a positive newborn screen for galactosemia should be seen by a physician immediately, as serious liver dysfunction or gram-negative sepsis can be present. Galactose should be withheld until the confirmatory testing results are available.

Treatment consists of dietary restriction of galactose. Sources that must be avoided include milk and milk products, legumes, and foods containing casein and whey. Tablet medications frequently contain lactose as a filler and should be avoided unless the absence of lactose can be verified. Affected individuals must seek alternate sources of calcium.

The pathophysiology of the cognitive damage is not known. The buildup of toxic metabolites of galactose, in particular intracellular accumulation of galatose-1-phosphate, has been suggested as a mechanism. Prior studies of extreme dietary galactose deprivation using elemental diets have found that this toxic buildup cannot be fully prevented by diet alone, as endogenous galactose synthesis takes place even in the absence of any galactose intake. An alternate mechanism is end product deficiency of uridyldiphosphate galactose. However studies of uridine supplementation have not shown improved cognitive performance. More recently, abnormal protein galactosylation, particularly of galactosylceramide and sulfatide, has been proposed to cause deficits in myelin and oligodendrocytes (Lebea & Pretorius, 2005). This theory is supported by studies identifying diffuse white matter abnormalities in children with galactosemia (Nelson et al., 1992; Z. I. Wang et al., 2001).

The cognitive outcome in galactosemia is variable, although some relative consistencies have emerged. For example, even with treatment, mean IQ is typically in the low-average range (Antshel, Epstein, & Waisbren, 2004; Kaufman et al., 1995; Waggoner, Buist, & Donnell, 1990). Slowed general processing speed and word retrieval difficulties have also been reported with relative consistency (Antshel et al., 2004; Waisbren et al., 1983; Widhalm et al., 2002). Cognitive problems are more severe in poorly treated or late treated children. However, among children in good metabolic control, there is no clear relationship between markers of metabolic control (e.g., plasma galactose-1-phosphate or urine galactitol) and cognitive outcome (Antshel et al., 2004). Much like PKU, genotype–phenotype correlations in galactosemia seem modest at best; moreover, even in well-treated children (see case 9.1), cognitive outcome can be quite variable, to some degree possibly due to individual differences in endogenous galactose production.

Case 9.1: Paul (Galactosemia) Paul is a 9-year-old boy with the common Q188R variant of galactosemia. He was identified via newborn screening and had been on a lifetime galactose-restricted diet. His mean galactose-1-phosphate milligram percentage level at the time of his neuropsychological assessment was 3.2 (normal value < 1; normal value for galactosemics on galactose-free diet = 2–5), and his galactitol level was 4.5 (normal value < 0.5; normal value for galactosemics on galactose-free diet = 2.5–7.2). According to his hospital chart, these values were a good representation of Paul's lifetime history of metabolic control. Paul was in the fourth grade and was academically retained as a first-grader due to "speech and language difficulties." He was served on a comprehensive individualized education program and had received several years of speech/language therapy as part of his integrated curriculum. His mother reported significant progress in Paul's speech and language. She also reported that Paul "desperately wanted" to have friends yet seemed "too socially inhibited" to engage in conversation with peers.

As shown in table 9.2, Paul's neuropsychological assessment revealed low-average general intellectual abilities and academic attainment. (These results were consistent with a similar protocol administered when he was a first-grader.) Paul's performance on the Rey Osterrieth Complex Figure was particularly interesting, as he recalled the overall gestalt of this abstract design quite well yet struggled to recall virtually any of the internal details. His mother's report on the rating scales reflected her concern about his emotional functioning, his internalizing behavioral symptoms and his difficulties maintaining attention.

Paul had previously been treated with methylphenidate with limited efficacy. He had also participated in a structured social skills training group, but his mother reported, "limited change" in his social functioning after the 8-week treatment program. Compared to Paul's mother's concerns, Paul's teachers were less concerned about his social and academic functioning and reported that Paul was a "great kid" who consistently "tried his best."

Pyruvate Dehydrogenase Deficiency Pyruvate is converted into acetyl-CoA by the pyruvate dehydrogenase complex, a multienzyme complex that consists of five subunits. Most children with this metabolic disorder have deficient pyruvate dehydrogenase activity due to a mutation in the gene encoding the pyruvate dehydrogenase (E1) alpha subunit, located on the X chromosome at position p22 (B. H. Robinson, 2001). Many different mutations have been reported, although females tend to have a more homogeneous and less affected phenotypic expression. Lactic acidosis during the neonatal period is the most common clinical presentation (De Meirleir et al., 1993), although many children, especially females, may present in early childhood with ataxia, hypotonia, and seizures. Elevated pyruvate cerebrospinal levels are diagnostically significant in pyruvate dehydrogenase deficiency (B. H. Robinson, 2001).

Corpus callosum agenesis and neuronal migration anomalies (e.g., abnormal cerebellar Purkinje cells) are the most frequently reported neuropathology in pyruvate dehydrogenase deficiency (Otero et al., 1995; Shevell et al., 1994). An antenatal onset for the neurological symptoms has been hypothesized (Takakubo & Dahl, 1994; J. N. Robinson et al., 2001). Although there have been multiple neuroimaging studies, very few, if any, investigations have assessed cognitive functioning in pyruvate dehydrogenase deficiency.

Table 9.2
Case 9.1—Galactosemia: Cognitive assessment raw data

Wechsler Intelligence Scale for Children (4th ed.)

Verbal	Scaled Score	Performance	Scaled Score
Similarities	6	Block design	8
Vocabulary	8	Picture concepts	8
Comprehension	8	Matrix reasoning	5
Information	(9)	Picture completion	(6)
Working Memory	*Scaled Score*	*Processing Speed*	*Scaled Score*
Digit span	8	Coding	8
Letter–number	7	Symbol search	6
Arithmetic	(8)	Cancellation	(6)

Composite Scores
$M = 100$, $SD = 15$

	Composite Score	95% Confidence Interval
Verbal comprehension	85	79–93
Perceptual reasoning	82	76–91
Working memory	86	79–95
Processing speed	83	76–94
Full scale	79	75–85

Wechsler Individual Achievement Test (2nd ed.)
$M = 100$, $SD = 15$

Subtests	Standard Score
Word reading	85
Reading comprehension	75
Pseudoword decoding	88
Reading composite	81
Numerical operations	71
Math reasoning	77
Math composite	72
Spelling	86
Written expression	81
Written language	82
Listening comprehension	88
Oral expression	92
Oral language	87
Total composite	78

California Verbal Learning Test—Children's edition
Mean T Score = 50, $SD = 10$
Mean Standard Score = 0.0, $SD = 0.5$

	T Score	Standard Score
List A trials 1–5	45	NA
List A trial 1	NA	−1.5
List A trial 5	NA	0.0
List B recall	NA	−1.0
Short delay recall	NA	1.0
Long delay recall	NA	1.0
Perseverations	NA	0.0
Intrusions	NA	0.0

Table 9.2
(continued)

Rey-Osterrieth Complex Figure

	Percentile/T Score
Copy	>16th percentile
Recall	31
Delay	37

Stroop Color and Word Test
Mean T Score = 50, $SD = 10$

	T Score
Word	43
Color score	38
Color/word	30
Interference	39

Continuous Performance Task—Gordon Diagnostic System
Mean Z Score = 0.0, $SD = 1.0$

	Z Score
Total correct	−0.76
Total commissions	0.34
Block 1 latency	−0.50
Block 2 latency	−1.00
Block 3 latency	−0.50
Total latency	−0.70

Behavior Assessment System for Children—Parent Report
Mean T Score = 50, $SD = 10$

Clinical Scales	T Score
Hyperactivity	56
Aggression	65
Conduct problems	50
Externalizing	58
Anxiety	81
Depression	80
Somatization	62
Internalizing	77
Atypicality	69
Withdrawal	61
Attention problems	78
Behavioral symptom index	78
Social skills	35
Leadership	28
Adaptive composite	30

Behavioral Rating Inventory of Executive Functioning
Mean T Score = 50, $SD = 10$

Scale	T Score
Inhibit	51
Shift	53
Emotional control	48
Behavioral regulation	49
Initiate	55
Working memory	77
Plan/organize	65
Organization of materials	52
Monitor	63
Metacognitive	64
General executive composite	61

Respiratory Chain Disorders

Respiratory chain disorders can be primary (from a genetic abnormality in respiratory chain function) or secondary (from shock, hypoxia, exercise, etc., affecting respiratory chain function). In children, it can sometimes be difficult to differentiate primary from secondary mitochondrial dysfunction.

Mitochondrial Disorders   The enzymes of the respiratory chain perform their function in the mitochondria. Thirteen proteins involved in oxidative phosporylation and the transfer RNAs necessary for their translation are coded for within the mitochondrial DNA. The remainder of the enzymes required for oxidative phosphorylation are coded in the nucleus and transported into the mitochondria to do their work. Thus, mitochondrial disease can be acquired (from accumulation of spontaneous mutations in the mitochondria), inherited maternally (as mitochondria are inherited almost exclusively from the mother), or inherited by Mendelian mechanisms.

Some mitochondrial disorders fit a well-defined phenotype, such as, mitochondrial encephalopathy, lactic acidosis, and stroke like episodes (MELAS) and myoclonic epilepsy, ragged red fibers. In addition, there are other some mutations in transfer RNAs or mitochondrial DNA deletion syndromes that also have well-defined phenotypes. In general, adult mitochondrial disease often conforms to a described phenotype. However, pediatric mitochondrial disease can be much more difficult to diagnose and have a wider range of presentation.

Most cases of pediatric mitochondrial disease affect the central nervous system. Typical findings include hypotonia, developmental delay, mental retardation, ataxia, seizures, and other neurological findings. However, these findings are by themselves nonspecific; thus, other diagnostic clues are necessary to prompt the physician to consider mitochondrial disease in the differential diagnosis. Features suggestive (but not diagnostic) of mitochondrial involvement include involvement of other energy-requiring organ systems (such as cardiomyopathy, renal tubular acidosis, liver dysfunction, pigmentary retinopathy, or marked anemia), characteristic changes on MRI (particularly cystic changes in the basal ganglia or periventricular white matter), an abnormally large peak of lactate on cranial MRS scan, or abnormal metabolic studies such as elevated plasma alanine on amino acid analysis, or elevation of lactate, pyruvate, or Krebs cycle intermediates on urine organic acid analysis.

Plasma lactate and pyruvate are highly subject to the conditions of the specimen sample and alone do not differentiate between primary disorders of the mitochondria and secondary lactic acidosis caused by conditions of the actual draw (e.g., tourniquet or excess crying) or poor sample preparation (e.g., failure to ice the sample or process immediately). Plasma lactate levels alone are not reliable markers of mitochondrial disease and, when performed with a tourniquet, can result in a label of "lactic acidosis" inappropriately and subject a child to unnecessary invasive testing.

Evaluation for suspected mitochondrial disease should include plasma amino acids (looking for elevated alanine), urine organic acids (looking for Krebs cycle intermediates or elevated lactate/pyruvate), and consideration of other nonmetabolic causes of neurological or developmental abnormalities (e.g., profound hypotonia secondary to peroxisomal disease or chromosomal abnormalities such as Prader–Willi syndrome, which results from the absence of genes from paternally derived chromosome 15). Blood studies for mitochondrial mutations or muscle biopsy may be indicated. However muscle biopsy findings are often normal in children with obvious mitochondrial disease.

There are few effective treatments for respiratory chain disorders. Some individuals respond to coenzyme Q, an electron carrier that may improve respiratory chain function. Others may show some improvement on vitamin "cocktails" that also have antioxidant or alternative electron carrier properties, such as vitamin E, vitamin K, biotin, lipoic acid and others, carnitine, or creatine.

Mitochondrial Encephalopathy, Lactic Acidosis, and Stroke-like Episodes MELAS was first described by Pavlakis (1984). MELAS is most often diagnosed in elementary-school-age children (5–10 years old), and the vast majority of children with the mitochondrial disorder have an A to G point mutation in the dihydrouridine loop of the tRNA$^{Leu (UUR)}$ gene at position 3243 (A3243G) (Tanji et al., 2001). The most common neuropathological finding in MELAS is multifocal cell death, most often in diffuse cortical regions or basal ganglia white matter, as well as calcification of the basal ganglia (Sparaco et al., 1993). Some have hypothesized that that there is increased blood–brain barrier permeability in children with MELAS due to cortical microvasculature mitochondrial respiratory failure (Tanji et al., 2001). Although much is known about the neuropathology, few, if any, data have considered brain–behavior relationships in MELAS. Moreover, we presently know very little about the cognitive phenotype.

Disorders of Fatty Acid Oxidation

Fatty acids are metabolized for energy through the process of beta-oxidation, in which the two carbons at the carboxyl end of the fat are cleaved in a four-step process, resulting in a molecule of acetyl CoA (which can be converted to a ketone body) and a fatty acid shortened by two carbons. The process is repeated until the fat is fully metabolized. The acetyl CoA molecule can be metabolized in the Krebs cycle for energy or can be converted into a ketone body (acetoacetate or betahydroxybutyrate) and exported to distal tissues. In the interim the fatty acid passes through various lengths (long, medium, or short) with unique enzymes specific to each fatty acid length. Fatty acid oxidation is particularly important for energy production during times of increase demand such as fasting or during an intercurrent illness. The most common disorder of fatty acid oxidation is medium chain acylCoA dehydrogenase (MCAD) deficiency.

Medium Chain acylCoA Dehydrogenase Deficiency   With prevalence rates between 1:6,000 and 1:10,000, MCAD deficiency is one of the most common metabolic disorders (Roe & Ding, 2001). Affected children are normal until they undergo a metabolic fast, usually with an intercurrent illness. Approximately half of affected children do not have access to presymptomatic diagnosis by newborn screening and die or experience permanent cognitive damage and subsequent mental retardation with their first episode of metabolic stress. MCAD deficiency has also been suggested to be associated with an increased risk for sudden infant death syndrome (Brink, 2005; Iafolla, Thompson, & Roe, 1994), although this remains controversial (S. S. Wang et al., 2000).

Children with developmental delays who reportedly had normal acquisition of milestones until a catastrophic intercurrent illness should be suspected of having MCAD (see Case 9.2). The disorder has been added to the expanded newborn screen in many states and countries, yet testing is far from universal. Diagnosis is commonly made by characteristic findings on urine organic acid analysis, but when suspicion is high, more sensitive tests such as plasma acylcarnitine and urine acylglycine (table 9.1) studies are indicated, as urine organic acids can appear normal in the well state.

Case 9.2: Quinn   Quinn, a 26-month-old boy, was referred for a clinical assessment of his moderate global developmental delays. His previous medical history was significant for normal developmental milestones prior to having a hypoglycemic seizure at age 11 months. Routine metabolic testing revealed diagnostic metabolites for MCAD on urine organic acids. Quinn's cognitively unimpaired siblings were subsequently tested for MCAD, and two sisters were also diagnosed with this disorder; they were treated with intravenous glucose during subsequent intercurrent illnesses associated with decreased caloric intake and did not endure any developmental delays.

Prevention of fasting did not reverse developmental delays, yet no further episodes of neurological/cognitive losses occurred.

The pathophysiology of the cognitive damage during a metabolic crisis is not known but could be secondary to hypoglycemia or to accumulation of toxic organic metabolites. Children diagnosed by newborn screening who are treated with intravenous glucose during intercurrent illnesses appear to have normal cognitive and neurological outcome, although large-scale formal cognitive and neuropsychological studies are lacking. Treatment is quite straightforward and consists of prevention of fasting. Children with MCAD deficiency are also at risk for carnitine deficiency, which when extreme can affect strength, tone, and motor functions. The utility of low-fat diets is controversial.

Disorders of both long and short chain fatty acid oxidation have been described and can be associated with developmental disabilities, but few cognitive studies have been performed in these populations.

Disorders Primarily Presenting with Seizures

Seizures frequently accompany disorders associated with developmental delays. However, there are some disorders in which seizures are the central feature, usually with mental retardation or other neurological concerns such as abnormal tone or altered mental status. The value of examination of cerebral spinal fluid (CSF) for amino acids, neurotransmitters, and other metabolites is becoming more apparent as the recognition of this group of metabolic disorders is growing.

Neonatal seizures merit special consideration. Neonatal seizures can be found after sepsis, prenatal or perinatal hypoxia, or other nonmetabolic conditions. However, pervasive, uncontrollable seizures, particularly when accompanied by a burst suppression pattern on EEG, are of particular metabolic concern, as common metabolic testing may fail to detect some underlying metabolic disorders associated with this phenotype. Two uncommon (but likely underdiagnosed) disorders in this differential diagnosis are nonketotic hyperglycinemia and molybdenum cofactor defect (sulfite oxidase deficiency).

Nonketotic Hyperglycinemia   Nonketotic hyperglycinemia (NKH), also known as glycine encephalopathy, is an autosomal recessively inherited disorder of glycine metabolism. The diagnosis is made in the presence of elevated glycine in the CSF and elevated ratio of CSF:plasma glycine on amino acid analysis. Most affected children represent the classical phenotype of neonatal onset profound seizures and neurological abnormalities. Common clinical findings in addition to seizures can include hiccups, hypotonia, and respiratory drive abnormalities (Hamosh & Johnston, 2001).

Mortality rates in classical NKH are quite high, and the majority of infants with classic NKH who survive the newborn period have profound mental retardation. A survey study of surviving children with NKH older than age 3 years noted that only about half could sit independently, 44% could walk, and almost one third could sign or use words (Hoover-Fong et al., 2004). Boys appear more likely to survive the newborn period and were far more likely to be able to walk or sign. While further research is clearly needed, the gender effect favoring boys with NKH is interesting.

However, with increased recognition, a growing number of cases are being diagnosed with an atypical presentation with later onset, including older infants with seizures and milder mental retardation; a sudden onset form during an intercurrent illness with loss of milestones, seizures, and vertical gaze palsy; or a chronic form with developmental regression spastic paraparesis and/or choreathetosis (Applegarth & Toone, 2001; Dinopoulos et al., 2005; Flusser et al., 2005). In the infantile variant of NKH, infants are normal at birth but present later with mild to moderate psycho-motor delay, primarily affecting expressive language. In later onset NKH, a less common variant of the disorder, affected children present with mild cognitive decline and behavioral problems. A transient form has also been described with resolution of hyperglycinemia and relatively normal developmental outcome. Although classical NKH is more prevalent (Hamosh & Johnston, 2001), these variant forms of NKH may also come to the attention of neurodevelopmental specialists.

Children with NKH are treated with benzoate and dextromethorphan (Hoover-Fong et al., 2004). Treatment is aimed at lowering glycine levels by complexing with sodium benzoate, forming hippuric acid that is excreted in the urine, and by sta-bilizing the NMDA receptor with dextromethorphan. In the absence of placebo clin-ical trials and with the natural variability in outcome, it is difficult to determine the clinical effectiveness of treatment in improving cognitive outcome. However, there is evidence that lowering glycine levels can improve seizure control yet does not prevent developmental delays (Hamosh et al., 1998).

In the CNS, gylcine is an inhibitory neurotransmitter in the spinal cord and modulates excitation at the N-methyl-D-aspartate glutamate receptors in cortex, hip-pocampus, and cerebellum. Elevated levels of glycine are hypothesized to lower sei-zure threshold levels, possibly due to decreased levels of gamma aminobutyric acid (GABA; Oh et al., 2002). The most common neuroimaging findings in NKH are myelin abnormalities (e.g., myelin vacuolation), especially obvious in areas like the brainstem, corpus callosum, and cerebellar peduncles that myelinate relatively early (Sener, 2003).

Molybdenum Cofactor Deficiency   Molybdenum cofactor deficiency, also known as sulfite oxidase deficiency, is a deficiency of the enzyme sulfite oxidase and, like NKH, results in a pattern of burst-suppression neonatal seizures. The disorder can be due to isolated deficiency of sulfite oxidase itself, the enzyme that detoxifies sulfite to sulfate, but is commonly associated with a defect in the molybdenum containing cofactor required for the enzymes sulfite oxidase, aldehyde oxidase, and xanthine dehydro-genase (Johnson & Duran, 2001).

The classic neonatal presentation consists of intractable seizures, often with a burst suppression EEG pattern. Some infants have dysmorphic features including bifrontal narrowing and lens dislocation, although these may only become apparent over months to years. Infants often demonstrate opisthotonic posturing and profound axial hypotonia with later development of distal spasticity (Topcu et al., 2001). There are increasingly numerous reports of delayed onset or "atypical" cases, sometimes with developmental regression.

Some children have shown biochemical and limited clinical improvement to dietary restriction of cysteine and methionine (precursors of sulfite), but profound mental retardation is the rule. Attempts to reduce sulfite production using betaine or to chelate excess sulfate have not shown clinical utility.

This disorder also requires clinical suspicion. The characteristic metabolite, s-sulfocysteine, can be overlooked on the amino acid chromatogram in the absence of clinical suspicion. Thus, the laboratory should always be alerted when this disorder is suspected. Bedside diagnostic testing for sulfite using test strips can be helpful, but the urine must be fresh, and both false negative and false positive tests have been reported. Other metabolites can be assayed including urinary urothione, a product of the cofactor that can help to distinguish isolated sulfite oxidase deficiency from absence of the molybdenum cofactor.

The pathophysiology of the disorder appears secondary to sulfite oxidase deficiency. The recent identification of a mouse model suggests cell death associated with elevated sulfite levels may be the cause of CNS abnormalities (Reiss et al., 2005). Structural CNS lesions, spongiosis, and gliosis are commonly found.

Creatine Deficiency Syndromes   Creatine stores energy as creatine phosphate and is required in the brain. Defects have been described in the biosynthesis of creatine from arginine and glycine including arginine:glycine aminotransferase (AGAT) deficiency, guanidinoacetate methyltransferase (GAMT) deficiency, and one disorder of creatine transport, X-linked creatine transporter deficiency; (for a review, see Schulze, 2003). AGAT deficiency is detected by low plasma/urine guanidinoacetate (GAA; Item et al., 2001). In GAMT deficiency, plasma/urine GAA is markedly increased (von Figura et al., 2001). In both disorders, creatine is low. In contrast creatine transporter deficiency is characterized by increased urinary creatine/creatinine ratio in males (Degrauw et al., 2001), but plasma creatine and GAA are normal. Thus, while AGAT and GAMT deficiencies can be identified in both urine and plasma (although plasma is more sensitive), the transporter deficiency can only be identified by analysis of urine (Schulze, 2003).

Still, in all three disorders, low plasma and urine creatinine is not a consistent finding and should not be used as a screen to determine who should have further testing. However, brain creatine, measured by MRS, is decreased or absent in all three disorders (Van der Knapp et al., 2000).

These creatine deficiency syndromes, a relatively new group of disorders, can only be identified by measuring GAA and creatine in blood or urine or by specifically ordering an MRS. Routine metabolic testing such as amino and organic acid analyses will not identify these disorders (Schulze, 2003). Thus, if not specifically tested for, these creatine deficiency syndromes may never be identified.

Creatine disorders present clinically with CNS effects. These include intractable seizures, speech delay, autism, hyperactivity, movement disorders, and hypotonia (Van der Knaap et al., 2000; Wyss & Schulze, 2002). GAMT deficiency results in a buildup of GAA and a depletion of creatine (Schulze et al., 1997). As an agonist of $GABA_A$ receptors and an inhibitor of Na^+–K^+-ATPase activity, GAA can act as a neurotoxin and/or neuromodulator (Schulze, 2003; Torremans et al., 2005).

Furthermore, although the phenotype of GAMT deficiency can be quite severe and, thus, may be tested for on the basis of seizures and a movement disorder, there have been reports of a milder phenotype where the primary findings are delays in development and language, hypotonia, and in some cases autism (Schulze, 2003). The same is true for the relatively few case reports of AGAT deficiency and for the X-linked creatine transporter deficiency (Schulze, 2003).

Thus these disorders include a wide range of cognitive and behavioral effects. Creatine supplementation may be beneficial in the two disorders of creatine synthesis (Item et al., 2001; Leuzzi et al., 2000). Thus, pre/posttreatment studies could be very informative in determining the efficacy of creatine supplementation in reducing the cognitive and behavioral morbidity associated with these disorders.

Supplementation with creatine may help restore brain levels, yet in GAMT deficiency, dietary restriction of arginine may also be required (Schulze, 2003). Clinical trials addressing the effectiveness of creatine therapy are indicated in this family of disorders.

Disorders Primarily Presenting with Hypotonia

Hypotonia is common in children with or without mental retardation. The myriad origins of hypotonia include central causes, spinal cord and anterior horn cell causes, peripheral neuropathies, neuromuscular junction defects, and myopathies. Metabolic disease can cause or contribute to hypotonia in most of these processes.

When hypotonia is central in origin, it often coexists with some degree of distal spasticity. However, the absence of mild spasticity in hypotonic children over 3 months of age implicates that the hypotonia is not central in origin and that it may instead be of a metabolic or myopathic origin. Common genetic causes of CNS dysfunction, such as chromosomal abnormalities, should also be evaluated. In particular, Prader–Willi syndrome should be considered (which may present with nonspecific abnormalities on urine organic acid analysis), as should congenital myotonic dystrophy, a disorder often overlooked in the differential diagnosis of congenital hypotonia. In cases where profound hypotonia is a presenting feature, peroxisomal disease should be considered.

Peroxisomal Disorders   The peroxisome is the site for a number of critical metabolic processes including very long chain fatty acid oxidation and detoxification of free radicals. Peroxisomal disorders commonly presenting with significant hypotonia include neonatal adrenoleukodystrophy, a less severe single-enzyme deficiency, and Zellweger syndrome, a peroxisome biogenesis disorder associated with a more severe phenotype (Gould, Raymond, & Valle, 2001), is typically fatal in infancy. Longer survival is possible in milder forms of peroxisomal disease such as adrenoleukodystrophy.

The etiology of the hypotonia and mental retardation in these disorders is not precisely known, yet neuronal migration abnormalities of the brain are quite common, resulting in a structurally anomalous brain with abnormal myelination (Faust et al., 2005) that typically begins in parieto-occipital regions and progresses asymmetrically in an anterior direction (Powers, Liu, Moser, & Moser, 1992; Powers & Moser, 1998). Gray matter appears less affected in adrenoleukodystrophy. Very few, if any, data have been reported on correlations between neuroimaging findings and cognitive outcomes in children with peroxisomal disorders.

Other Inborn Errors of Metabolism

Barth Syndrome   Barth syndrome is an X-linked recessive disorder of mitochondrial function of cardiolipin (Barth et al., 1983). Affected males manifest multisystem problems including cardiomyopathy, cyclic neutropenia, short stature, and excretion of 3-methylglutaconic acid (a derivative of leucine) in urine, detectable by urine organic acid analysis. With a prevalence rate of 1:250,000, Barth syndrome is associated with mutations in the tafazzin (TAZ) gene, located on chromosome Xq28.12 (Bione et al., 1996). Boys with the syndrome are generally short in stature relative to peers during early childhood yet catch up with and may surpass peers during adolescence (Kelley et al., 1991).

Cognitive and neuropsychological testing of a cohort of boys with Barth syndrome has demonstrated a relatively consistent cognitive phenotype that includes diminished visual–spatial skills yet reading skills comparable to same-age peers (Mazzocco & Kelley, 2001). Math difficulties (Mazzocco, Henry, & Kelley, 2007) also appear to be a salient feature of the cognitive phenotype. At present it is unknown whether this cognitive phenotype is primary or secondary to school absence due to illness or fatigue. The specificity of reported deficits implicates at least partial primary roots (Mazzocco et al., 2007).

Neurotransmitter Disorders   Neurotransmitter disorders are being recognized with increasing frequency as a cause of developmental and neurological abnormalities. These disorders affect the synthesis, metabolism, and catabolism of neurotransmitters.

Clinical features commonly include developmental delay, mental retardation, speech delay, hypotonia, ataxia, movement disorder, oculogyric crises, or sleep disorders. Some neurotransmitter disorders are amenable to treatment; thus, it is important to consider this group of disorders. Diagnosis is made by analysis of CSF collected in specially prepared tubes and analyzed in a limited number of laboratories. The best characterized of the neurotransmitter disorders is pyridoxine-dependent seizure disorder, an autosomal GABA metabolism disorder (Baxter, 2003). Very little, if any, extant data are available regarding cognitive outcomes in children with neurotransmitter disorders who are identified early.

Cholesterol Biosynthesis Disorders   A variety of disorders have been described in the biosynthesis of cholesterol, which is an important component of brain development and steroid hormone biogenesis. These disorders can have a broad range of presentation including skin abnormalities, such as in CHILD syndrome, or congenital hemidysplasia with ichthyosiform erythroderma and limb defects as well as mental retardation, dysmorphic features, and structural birth defects. The most common disorder is Smith–Lemi–Opitz syndrome (SLOS), a defect in the final step of cholesterol synthesis that is caused by loss-of-function mutations on both copies of the 7-dehydrocholesterol reductase (DHCR7) gene (Waterham et al., 1998).

SLOS has a prevalence rate of 1:60,000 live births and is equally represented in males and females (Kelley & Hennekam, 2000). Children with SLOS may manifest mental retardation, 2,3 syndactyly of the toes, ambiguous genitalia or male genital hypoplasia, characteristic facies, and polydactyly (Kelley & Hennekam, 2000). In addition to mental retardation, children with SLOS have also been reported to be at greatly increased risk of having autism (Tierney et al., 2001b). In their study, over half of individuals with SLOS (age range 3–32 years) met formal *Diagnostic and Statistical Manual of Mental Disorders* (4th ed.) diagnostic criteria for autism. Self-injurious behaviors, aggression, sensory hyperreactivity, and irritability were also noted to be phenotypic traits in SLOS (Tierney et al., 2001b). Milder phenotypes of SLOS exist (Languis et al., 2003); some children with SLOS have been reported to have general cognitive abilities in the low-average to average range for age (Mueller et al., 2003). Almost all children with SLOS have frontal lobe hypoplasia; abnormalities of the cerebellum or corpus callosum are also reported, but less frequently (Caruso et al., 2004; Kelley et al., 1996).

Diagnosis of SLOS is by measurement of 7-dehydrocholesterol in plasma, and cholesterol supplementation is the standard of treatment care. Some children with SLOS have improved behavior and cognitive performance after such treatment (Irons et al., 1997). Even autistic behaviors may lessen after cholesterol supplementation, although the evidence for this effect is limited (Tierney et al., 2001a). Some researchers have not reported any developmental improvements after cholesterol supplementation (Sikora et al., 2004).

Summary

Clinically, mental retardation and nonspecific neurological findings like seizures and tone abnormalities are common in metabolic disorders. A minimum standard metabolic evaluation for children with developmental abnormalities should include plasma and urine amino acids and urine organic acids. Plasma acylcarnitine and urine acylglycine should be considered if organic acidemias or fatty acid oxidation disorders are in the differential diagnosis. More specific tests such as CSF amino acids, CSF neurotransmitters, cranial imaging with spectroscopy, and other testing for specific disorders may well be indicated as targeted by presentation. In short, children with unexplained developmental delays may benefit from evaluation of underlying genetic and metabolic causes, particularly in the presence of a positive family history or when developmental regression, or multisystem dysfunction is present. Even though the yield is likely to be rather low (Hunter, 2000), metabolic testing should be considered in unexplained developmental delays as there may be significant implications (e.g., genetic counseling, initiation of effective treatments) that arise from a positive test result (Poplawski et al., 2002; Van Buggenhout et al., 2001).

There has also been significant progress in defining the pathophysiology, neuroanatomy, and neuropsychology of the metabolic disorders in the last 15 years. Despite the genetic, molecular, and biological heterogeneity of the metabolic disorders, the following cross-disorder consistencies have emerged: (a) Metabolic disorders clinically present very early in life, generally during the neonatal period; (b) metabolic disorders appear to affect cerebral white matter more than gray matter; and (c) the degree of neuropsychological impairment in the metabolic disorders seems to parallel the degree of morphologic abnormalities as demonstrated by neuroimaging analysis. Nonetheless, most research suggests that there is a rather weak genotype–phenotype relationship across most metabolic disorders (Dipple & McCabe, 2000; Scriver & Waters, 1999). Thus, the metabolic disorders demonstrate that the etiology and genotype may not be as important as the extent of neural cell loss in determining neurodevelopmental outcome. Environmental parameters are also important to consider when predicting outcomes in metabolic disorders (Chakravarti & Little, 2003; Scriver, 2004).

Relationships between brain and behavior are clearly illustrated in the metabolic disorders. As noted in table 9.3, myelin abnormalities are a very consistent neuroimaging finding in the heterogeneous metabolic disorders. Myelin serves a variety of roles in the CNS, including insulating axons, propagating action potentials, and providing trophic support for axons (for a metabolic-focused review of myelin, see Barkovich, 2005). The process of myelination begins during the second prenatal trimester and proceeds in a rostral fashion. The first 2 postnatal years constitute the most rapid myelination time frame (Yakovlev & Lecours, 1967). Given the neonatal

Table 9.3
Most consistent neurological and psychological findings in metabolic disease

Disease	Neuroimaging Outcomes	Cognitive/Behavioral Outcomes
Phenylketonuria	Myelin anomalies, particularly in posterior areas	Attention, visuospatial, executive functioning deficits, slow general processing speed; outcomes dependent on treatment adherence
Classical homocystinuria	Myelinopathy	B_6 nonresponsive: Mental retardation B_6 responsive: Verbal IQ > Performance IQ
Tyrosinemia type 2	Basal ganglia myelin anomalies	—
Maple syrup urine disease	"Maple syrup urine disease edema": cerebellar brain stem and basal ganglia white matter anomalies	IQ negatively associated with age of diagnosis; generally low-average to borderline IQ levels
Glutaric acidemia type 1	"Microencephalic macroencephaly": Frontotemporal atrophy; ventricular enlargement	IQ negatively associated with age of diagnosis; generally low-average to borderline IQ levels
Ornithine transcarbamylase deficiency	Neonatal onset: Diffuse edema and atrophy Childhood onset: Infarct-like abnormalities, lesions in cingulate gyri, temporal lobe, and insular cortex	Neonatal onset: Mental retardation Childhood onset: IQ positively associated with age of diagnosis
Methylmalonic acidemia/ propionic acidemia	Infarct-like episodes with globus pallidus involvement	Generally low-average to borderline IQ levels; methylmalonic acidemia more affected than propionic acidemia
Galactosemia	Abnormal myelination	Low-average IQ; word retrieval and slow general processing speed; outcomes seem independent of treatment adherence
Pyruvate dehydrongenase deficiency	Corpus callosal agenesis; neuronal migration anomalies	—
Mitochondrial disorders	Periventricular and basal ganglia myelin anomalies	—
Medium chain acylCoA dehydrogenase deficiency	—	Newborn screened without metabolic crises: Normal outcomes
Nonketotic hyperglycinemia	Brainstem, corpus callosum myelin abnormalities	Mental retardation
Molybdenum cofactor deficiency	Diffuse spongiosis, gliosis	Mental retardation
Peroxisomal disorders	Migration abnormalities; anomalous myelination	—
Barth syndrome	—	Visuospatial, math difficulties
Smith–Lemli–Opitz	Frontal lobe hypoplasia; agenesis of corpus callosum	Mental retardation; increased risk for autism; milder variants exist

onset for most metabolic disorders, it is not surprising that the brainstem, cerebellum, and basal ganglia are the most commonly affected regions.

At this point, one of the primary methodological limitations of the metabolic disorder literature is the relative lack of interdisciplinary, longitudinal data. Looking forward, children with metabolic disorders and, more generally, the field of neurogenetic developmental disorders will be served best by interdisciplinary, longitudinal research designs that focus on the developmental progression of cognitive and behavioral functioning. By adopting a longitudinal perspective, we will improve our abilities to not only better understand interindividual differences but also to gain a more complete appreciation of intra-individual changes across time. Within this longitudinal framework, correlating neuropsychological data with physiological data will be important in broadening our knowledge of brain–behavior relationships in this population.

References

Abbott, M. H., Folstein, S. E., Abbey, H., & Pyeritz, R. E. (1987). Psychiatric manifestations of homocystinuria due to cystathionine beta-synthase deficiency: Prevalence, natural history, and relationship to neurologic impairment and vitamin B6-responsiveness. *American Journal of Medical Genetics, 26,* 959–969.

Anderson, P. J., Wood, S. J., Francis, D. E., Coleman, L., Warwick, L., Casneslia, S., et al. (2004). Neuropsychological functioning in children with early-treated phenylketonuria: Impact of white matter abnormalities. *Developmental Medicine & Child Neurology, 46,* 230–238.

Antshel, K. M., Epstein, I. O., & Waisbren, S. E. (2004). Cognitive strengths and weaknesses in children and adolescents homozygous for the galactosemia Q188R mutation: A descriptive study. *Neuropsychology, 18,* 658–664.

Antshel, K. M., & Waisbren, S. E. (2003a). Timing is everything: Executive functions in children exposed to elevated levels of phenylalanine. *Neuropsychology, 17,* 458–468.

Antshel, K. M., & Waisbren, S. E. (2003b). Developmental timing of exposure to elevated levels of phenylalanine is associated with ADHD symptom expression. *Journal of Abnormal Child Psychology, 31,* 565–574.

Applegarth, D. A., & Toone, J. R. (2001). Nonketotic hyperglycinemia (glycine encephalopathy): Laboratory diagnosis. *Molecular Genetics and Metabolism, 74,* 139–146.

Arnold, G. L., Kramer, B. M., Kirby, R. S., Plumeau, P. B., Blakely, E. M., Sanger-Cregan, L. S., & Davidson, P. W. (1998). Factors affecting cognitive, motor, behavioral and executive functioning in children with phenylketonuria. *Acta Paediatrica, 87,* 565–570.

Arnold, G. L., Vladutiu, C. J., Orlowski, C. C., Blakely, E. M., & DeLuca, J. (2004). Prevalence of stimulant use for attentional dysfunction in children with phenylketonuria. *Journal of Inherited Metabolic Disease, 27,* 137–143.

Asarnow, R. F., Nuechterlein, K. H., Subotnik, K. L., Fogelson, D. L., Torquato, R. D., Payne, D. L., et al. (2002). Neurocognitive impairments in nonpsychotic parents of children with schizophrenia and attention-deficit/hyperactivity disorder. *Archives of General Psychiatry, 59,* 1053–1060.

Azen, C., Koch, R., Freedman, E., Wenz, E., & Fishler, K. (1996). Summary of findings from the United States Collaborative Study of children treated for phenylketonuria. *European Journal of Pediatrics, 155*(Suppl. 1), S29–S32.

Bachmann, C. (2003). Outcome and survival of 88 patients with urea cycle disorders: A retrospective evaluation. *European Journal of Pediatrics, 162,* 410–416.

Bajaj, S. K., Kurlemann, G., Schuierer, G., & Peters, P. E. (1996). CT and MRI in a girl with late-onset ornithine transcarbamylase deficiency: Case report. *Neuroradiology, 38,* 796–799.

Barkovich, A. J. (2005). Magnetic resonance techniques in the assessment of myelin and myelination. *Journal of Inherited Metabolic Disease, 28,* 311–343.

Barth, P. G., Scholte, H. R., Berden, J. A., Van der Klei-Van Moorsel, J. M., Luyt-Houwen, I. E., Van't Veer-Korthof, E. T., et al. (1983). An X-linked mitochondrial disease affecting cardiac muscle, skeletal muscle and neutrophil leucocytes. *Journal of Neurological Sciences, 62,* 327–355.

Baxter, P. (2003). Pyridoxine-dependent and pyridoxine-responsive seizures. *Developmental Medicine & Child Neurology, 43,* 416–420.

Bione, S., D'Adamo, P., Maestrini, E., Gedeon, A. K., Bolhuis, P. A., & Toniolo, D. (1996). A novel X-linked gene, G4.5, is responsible for Barth syndrome. *Nature Genetics, 4,* 385–389.

Bjugstad, K. B., Goodman, S. I., & Freed, C. R. (2000). Age at symptom onset predicts severity of motor impairment and clinical outcome of glutaric acidemia type 1. *Journal of Pediatrics, 137,* 681–686.

Bracken, P., & Coll, P. (1985). Homocystinuria and schizophrenia. Literature review and case report. *Journal of Nervous and Mental Disease, 173,* 51–55.

Brink, S. (2005, May 30). Rare but deadly. *U.S. News & World Report, 138,* pp. 44–46.

Brusilow, S. W., & Horwich, A. L. (2001). Urea cycle enzymes. In C. R. Scriver, A. L. Beaudet, W. S. Sly, & D. Valle (Eds.), *The metabolic and molecular bases of inherited disease* (8th ed., pp. 1909–1963). New York: McGraw-Hill.

Caruso, P. A., Poussaint, T. Y., Tzika, A. A., Zurakowski, D., Astrakas, L. G., Elias, E. R., et al. (2004). MRI and 1H MRS findings in Smith–Lemli–Opitz syndrome. *Neuroradiology, 46,* 3–14.

Cerone, R., Fantasia, A. R., Castellano, E., Moresco, L., Schiaffino, M. C., & Gatti, R. (2002). Case report: Pregnancy and tyrosinemia type II. *Journal of Inherited Metabolic Disease, 25,* 317–318.

Chakrapani, A., Sivakumar, P., McKiernan, P. J., & Leonard, J. V. (2002). Metabolic stroke in methylmalonic acidemia five years after liver transplantation. *Journal of Pediatrics, 140,* 261–263.

Chakravarti, A., & Little, P. (2003). Nature, nurture and human disease. *Nature, 421,* 412–414.

Chang, P. N., Gray, R. M., & O'Brien, L. L. (2000). Patterns of academic achievement among patients treated early with phenylketonuria. *European Journal of Pediatrics, 159*(Suppl. 2), S96–S99.

Choi, C. G., & Yoo, H. W. (2001). Localized proton MS spectroscopy in infants with urea cycle defect. *American Journal of Neuroradiology, 22,* 834–837.

Chuang, D. T., & Shih, V. E. (2001). Maple syrup urine disease (branched-chain ketoaciduria). In C. R. Scriver, A. L. Beaudet, W. S. Sly, & D. Valle (Eds.), *The metabolic and molecular bases of inherited disease* (8th ed., pp. 1971–2005). New York: McGraw-Hill.

Cleary, M. A., Walter, J. H., Wraith, J. E., Jenkins, J. P. R., Alani, S. M., Tyler, K., & Whittle, D. (1994). Magnetic resonance imaging of the brain in phenylketonuria. *Lancet, 344,* 87–90.

Cleary, M. A., Walter, J. H., Wraith, J. E., White, F., Tyler, K., & Jenkins, J. (1995). Magnetic resonance imaging in phenylketonuria: Reversal of cerebral white matter change. *Journal of Pediatrics, 127,* 251–255.

Connelly, A., Cross, J. H., Gadian, D. G., Hunter, J. V., Kirkham, F. J., & Leonard, J. V. (1993). Magnetic resonance spectroscopy shows increased brain glutamine in ornithine carbamoyl transferase deficiency. *Pediatric Research, 33,* 73–81.

Costa, L. G., Guizzetti, M., Burry, M., & Oberdoerster, J. (2002). Developmental neurotoxicity: Do similar phenotypes indicate a common mode of action? A comparison of fetal alcohol syndrome, toluene embryopathy and maternal phenylketonuria. *Toxicology Letters, 127,* 197–205.

De Franchis, R., Sperandeo, M. P., Sebastio, G., Andria, G., & the Italian Collaborative Study Group on Homocystinuria. (1998). Clinical aspects of cystathionine ß-synthase deficiency: How wide is the spectrum? *European Journal of Pediatrics, 157*(Suppl. 2), S67–S70.

Degrauw, T. J., Cecil, K. M., Ball, W. S., Wong, B., Jakobs, C., & Verhoeven, N. M. (2001). A new disorder of creatine metabolism: A patient with possible creatine transport defect. *Journal of Inherited Metabolic Disease, 23,* 211.

de Grauw, T. J., Smit, L. M. E., Brockstedt, M., Meijer, Y., Moorsel, J. V. D. K., & Jakobe, C. (1990). Acute hemiparesis as the presenting sign in a heterozygote for ornithine transcarbamylase deficiency. *Neuropediatrics, 21,* 133–135.

De Meirleir, L., Lissens, W., Denis, R., Wayenberg, J. L., Michotte, A., Brucher, J. M., et al. (1993). Pyruvate dehydrogenase deficiency: Clinical and biochemical diagnosis. *Pediatric Neurology, 9,* 216–220.

Desai, N. K., Runge, V. M., Crisp, D. E., Crisp, M. B., & Naul, L. G. (2003). Magnetic resonance imaging of the brain in glutaric acidemia type I: A review of the literature and a report of four new cases with attention to the basal ganglia and imaging technique. *Investigative Radiology, 38,* 489–496.

Dezortova, M., Hajek, M., Tintera, J., Hejcmanova, L., & Sykova, E. (2001). MR in phenylketonuria-related brain lesions. *Acta Radiology, 42,* 459–466.

Diamond, A. (1996). Evidence for the importance of dopamine for prefrontal cortex functions early in life. *Philosophical Transactions of the Royal Society of London, Series B: Biological Sciences, 351,* 1483–1493.

Diamond, A., Prevor, M. B., Callender, G., & Druin, D. P. (1997). Prefrontal cortex cognitive deficits in children treated early and continuously for PKU. *Monographs of the Society for Research in Child Development, 62* (4, Serial No. 252).

DiGeorge, A. M., Rezvani, I., Garibaldi, L. R., & Schwartz, M. (1982). Prospective study of maple-syrup-urine disease for the first four days of life. *New England Journal of Medicine, 307,* 1492–1495.

Dipple, D. M., & McCabe, E. R. (2000). Phenotypes of patients with "simple" Mendelian disorders are complex traits: Thresholds, modifiers, and systems dynamics. *American Journal of Human Genetics, 66,* 1729–1735.

Dinopoulos, A., Kure, S., Chuck, G., Sato, K., Gilbert, D. L., Matsubara, Y., & Degrauw, T. (2005). Glycine decarboxylase mutations: A distinctive phenotype of nonketotic hyperglycinemia in adults. *Neurology, 64,* 1255–1257.

Dyer, C. A. (1999). Pathophysiology of phenylketonuria. *Mental Retardation and Developmental Disabilities Research Reviews, 5,* 104–112.

Faust, P. L., Banka, D., Siriratsivawong, R., Ng, V. G., & Wikander, T. M. (2005). Peroxisome biogenesis disorders: The role of peroxisomes and metabolic dysfunction in developing brain. *Journal of Inherited Metabolic Disease, 28,* 369–383.

Feldmann, R., Denecke, J., Grenzebach, M., & Weglage, J. (2005). Frontal lobe-dependent functions in treated phenylketonuria: Blood phenylalanine concentrations and long-term deficits in adolescents and young adults. *Journal of Inherited Metabolic Disease, 28,* 445–455.

Flusser, H., Korman, S. H., Sato, K., Matsubara, Y., Galil, A., & Kure, S. (2005). Mild glycine encephalopathy (NKH) in a large kindred due to a silent exonic GLDC splice mutation. *Neurology, 64,* 1426–1430.

Gassio, R., Artuch, R., Vilaseca, M. A., Fuste, E., Boix, C., Sans, A., & Campistol, J. (2005). Cognitive functions in classic phenylketonuria and mild hyperphenylalaninemia: Experience in a pediatric population. *Developmental Medicine & Child Neurology, 47,* 443–448.

Giedd, J. N., Blumenthal, J., Jeffries, N. O., Castellanos, F. X., Liu, H., Zijdenbos, A., Paus, T., Evans, A. C., & Rapoport, J. L. (1999). Brain development during childhood and adolescence: A longitudinal MRI study. *Nature Neuroscience, 2,* 861–863.

Goldman-Rakic, P. S. (1987). Circuitry of the primate prefrontal cortex and the regulation of behavior by representational memory. In F. Plum (Ed.), *Handbook of physiology: The nervous system: Vol. 5. Higher functions of the brain* (pp. 373–417). Baltimore: American Physiological Society.

Goodman, S. I., Stein, D. E., Schlesinger, S., Christensen, E., Schwartz, M., Greenberg, C. R., & Elpeleg, O. N. (1998). Glutaryl-CoA dehydrogenase mutations in glutaric acidemia (type I): Review and report of thirty novel mutations. *Human Mutations, 12,* 141–144.

Gottesman, I. I., & Gould, T. D. (2003). The endophenotype concept in psychiatry: Etymology and strategic intentions. *American Journal of Psychiatry, 160,* 1–10.

Gropman, A. L., & Batshaw, M. L. (2004). Cognitive outcome in urea cycle disorders. *Molecular Genetics and Metabolism, 81*(Suppl. 1), S58–S62.

Gould, S. J., Raymond, D. V., & Valle, D. (2001). The peroxisome biogenesis disorders. In C. R. Scriver, A. L. Beaudet, W. S. Sly, & D. Valle (Eds.), *The metabolic and molecular bases of inherited disease* (8th ed., pp. 3181–3217). New York: McGraw-Hill.

Ha, J. S., Kim, T. K., Eun, B. L., Lee, H. S., Lee, K. Y., Seol, H. Y., & Cha, S. H. (2004). Maple syrup urine disease encephalopathy: A follow-up study in the acute stage using diffusion weighted MRI. *Pediatric Radiology, 34,* 163–166.

Hamosh, A., & Johnston, M. V. (2001). Nonketotic hyperglycinemia. In C. R. Scriver, A. L. Beaudet, W. S. Sly, & D. Valle (Eds.), *The metabolic and molecular bases of inherited disease* (8th ed., pp. 2065–2078). New York: McGraw-Hill.

Hamosh, A., Maher, J. F., Bellus, G. A., Rasmussen, S. A., & Johnston, M. V. (1998). Long-term use of high-dose benzoate and dextromethorphan for the treatment of nonketotic hyperglycinemia. *Journal of Pediatrics, 132,* 709–713.

Heindel, W., Kugel, H., Wendel, U., Roth, B., & Benz-Bohm, G. (1995). Proton magnetic resonance spectroscopy reflects metabolic decompensation in maple syrup urine disease. *Pediatric Radiology, 25,* 296–299.

Hilliges, C., Awiszus, D., & Wendel, U. (1993). Intellectual performance of children with maple syrup urine disease. *European Journal of Pediatrics, 152,* 144–147.

Hoffmann, B., Helbling, C., Schadewaldt, P., & Wendel, U. (2006). Impact of longitudinal plasma leucine levels on the intellectual outcome in patients with classic MSUD. *Pediatric Research, 59,* 17–20.

Hoover-Fong, J. E., Shah, S., Van Hove, J. L., Applegarth, D., Toone, J., & Hamosh, A. (2004). Natural history of nonketotic hyperglycinemia in 65 patients. *Neurology, 63,* 1847–1853.

Huhn, R., Stoermer, H., Klingele, B., Bausch, E., Fois, A., Farnetani, M., et al. (1998). Novel and recurrent tyrosine aminotransferase gene mutations in tyrosinemia type II. *Human Genetics, 102,* 305–313.

Huijbregts, S. C., deSonneville, L. M., Licht, R., van Spronsen, F. J., Verkerk, P. H., & Sergeant, J. A. (2002b). Sustained attention and inhibition of cognitive interference in treated phenylketonuria: Associations with concurrent and lifetime phenylalanine concentrations. *Neuropsychologia, 40,* 7–15.

Huijbregts, S. C., deSonneville, L. M., van Spronsen, F. J., Licht, R., & Sergeant, J. A. (2002a). The neuropsychological profile of early and continuously treated phenylketonuria: Orienting, vigilance, and maintenance versus manipulation-functions of working memory. *Neuroscience & Biobehavioral Review, 26,* 697–712.

Hunter, A. G. (2000). Outcome of the routine assessment of patients with mental retardation in a genetics clinic. *American Journal of Medical Genetics, 90,* 60–68.

Iafolla, A. K., Thompson, R. J., & Roe, C. R. (1994). Medium-chain acyl-coenzyme A dehydrogenase deficiency: Clinical course in 120 affected children. *Journal of Pediatrics, 124,* 409–415.

Irons, M., Elias, E. R., Abuelo, D., Bull, M. J., Greene, C. L., Johnson, V. P., et al. (1997). Treatment of Smith–Lemli–Opitz syndrome: Results of a multicenter trial. *American Journal of Medical Genetics, 68,* 311–314.

Item, C. B., Stockler-Ipsiroglu, S., Stromberger, C., Muhl, A., Alessandri, M. G., Bianchi, M. C., et al. (2001). Arginine:glycine amidinotransferase deficiency: The third inborn error of creatine metabolism in humans. *American Journal of Human Genetics, 69,* 1127–1133.

Johnson, J. L., & Duran, M. (2001). Molybdenum cofactor deficiency and isolated sulfite oxidase deficiency. In C. R. Scriver, A. L. Beaudet, W. S. Sly, & D. Valle (Eds.), *The metabolic and molecular bases of inherited disease* (8th ed., pp. 3163–3177). New York: McGraw-Hill.

Kaplan, P., Mazur, A., Field, M., Berlin, J. A., Berry, G. T., Heidenreich, R., et al. (1991). Intellectual outcome in children with maple syrup urine disease. *Journal of Pediatrics, 119,* 46–50.

Kaufman, F. R., McBride-Chang, C., Manis, F. R., Wolff, J. A., & Nelson, M. (1995). Cognitive functioning, neurologic status, and brain imaging in classical galactosemia. *European Journal of Pediatrics, 154*(Suppl. 2), S2–S5.

Kelley, R. I., Cheatham, J. P., Clark, B. J., Nigro, M. A., Powell, B. R., Sherwood, G. W., et al. (1991). X-linked dilated cardiomyopathy with neutropenia, growth retardation, and 3-methylglutaconic aciduria. *Journal of Pediatrics, 119,* 738–747.

Kelley, R., & Segal, S. (1989). Evaluation of reduced activity galactose-1-phosphate uridyl transferase by combined radioisotopic assay and high-resolution isoelectric focusing. *Journal of Laboratory & Clinical Medicine, 114,* 152–156.

Kelley, R. I., & Hennekam, R. C. (2000). The Smith–Lemli–Opitz syndrome. *Journal of Medical Genetics, 37,* 321–335.

Kelley, R. L., Roessler, E., Hennekam, R. C., Feldman, G. L., Kosaki, K., Jones, M. C., et al. (1996). Holoprosencephaly in RSH/Smith–Lemli–Opitz syndrome: Does abnormal cholesterol metabolism affect the function of sonic hedgehog? *American Journal of Medical Genetics, 66,* 478–484.

Koch, R., Burton, B., Hoganson, G., Peterson, R., Rhead, W., Rouse, B., et al. (2002). Phenylketonuria in adulthood: A collaborative study. *Journal of Inherited Metabolic Disease, 25,* 333–346.

Koch, R., Moats, R., Guttler, F., Guldberg, P., & Nelson, M. (2000). Blood–brain phenylalanine relationships in persons with phenylketonuria. *Pediatrics, 58,* 46–54.

Kumar, K. S., Govindaiah, V., Naushad, S. E., Devi, R. R., & Jyothy, A. (2003). Plasma homocysteine levels correlated to interactions between folate status and methylene tetrahydrofolate reductase gene mutation in women with unexplained recurrent pregnancy loss. *Journal of Obstetrics and Gynecology, 23,* 55–58.

Lai, K., Langley, S. D., Singh, R. H., Dembure, P. P., Hjelm, L. N., & Elsas, L. J. (1996). A prevalent mutation for galactosemia among Black Americans, *Journal of Pediatrics, 128,* 89–95.

Languis, F. A., Waterham, H. R., Romeijn, G. J., Oostheim, W., de Barse, M. M., Dorland, L., et al. (2003). Identification of three patients with a very mild form of Smith–Lemli–Opitz syndrome. *American Journal of Medical Genetics, 122,* 24–29.

Lebea, P. J., & Pretorius, P. J. (2005). The molecular relationship between deficient UDP-galactose uridyl transferase (GALT) and ceramide galactosyltransferase (CGT) enzyme function: A possible cause for poor long-term prognosis in classic galactosemia. *Medical Hypotheses, 65,* 1051–1057.

Lenke, R. R., & Levy, H. L. (1980). Maternal phenylketonuria and hyperphenylalaninemia: An international survey of the outcome of untreated and treated pregnancies. *New England Journal of Medicine, 303,* 1202–1208.

Lepage, N., McDonald, N., Dallaire, L., & Lambert, M. (1997) Age-specific distribution of plasma amino acid concentrations in a healthy pediatric population. *Clinical Chemistry, 43,* 2397–2402.

LeRoux, C., Murphy, E., Hallam, P., Librum, M., Orlowska, D., & Lee, P. (2006). Neuropsychometric outcome predictors for adults with maple syrup urine disease. *Journal of Inherited Metabolic Disease, 29,* 201–202.

Leslie, N. D., Immerman, E. B., Flach, J. E., Florez, M., Fridovich-Keil, J. L., & Elsas, L. J. (1992). The human galactose-1-phosphate uridyltransferase gene. *Genomics, 14,* 474–480.

Leuzzi, V., Bianchi, M. C., Tosetti, M., Carducci, C., Cerquiglini, C. A., Cioni, G., & Antonozzi, I. (2000). Brain creatine depletion: Guanidinoacetate methyltransferase deficiency (improving with creatine supplementation). *Neurology, 55,* 1407–1409.

Leuzzi, V., Pansini, M., Sechi, E., Chiarotti, F., Carducci, C., Levi, G., & Antonozzi, I. (2004). Executive function impairment in early-treated PKU subjects with normal mental development. *Journal of Inherited Metabolic Disease, 27,* 115–125.

Levy, H. L. (1973). To genetic screening. *Advances in Human Genetics, 4,* 389–394.

Levy, H. L., & Ghavami, M. (1996). Maternal phenylketonuria: A metabolic teratogen. *Teratology, 53,* 176–184.

Levy, H. L., Lobbregt, D., Barnes, P. D., & Poussaint, T. Y. (1996). Maternal phenylketonuria: Magnetic resonance imaging of the brain in offspring. *Journal of Pediatrics, 128,* 770–775.

Levy, H. L., Waisbren, S. E., Guttler, F., Hanley, W. B., Matalon, R., Rouse, B., et al. (2003). Pregnancy experiences in the woman with mild hyperphenylalaninemia. *Pediatrics, 112,* 1548–1552.

Leuzzi, V., Pansini, M., Sechi, E., Chiatotti, F., Carducci, C., Levi, G., & Antonozzi, I. (2004). Executive function impairment in early-treated PKU subjects with normal mental development. *Journal of Inherited Metabolic Disease, 27,* 115–125.

Lidsky, A. S., Robson, K. J. H., Thirumalachary, C., Barker, P. E., Ruddle, F. H., & Woo, S. L. C. (1984). The PKU locus in man is on chromosome 12. *American Journal of Human Genetics, 36,* 527–533.

Lindner, M., Kolker, S., Schulze, A., Christensen, E., Greenberg, C. R., & Hoffmann, G. F. (2004). Neonatal screening for glutaryl-CoA dehydrogenase deficiency. *Journal of Inherited Metabolic Disease, 27,* 851–859.

Lipton, S. A., Kim, W. K., Choi, Y. B., Kumar, S., D'Emilia, D. M., Rayudu, P. V., et al. (1997). Neurotoxicity associated with dual actions of homocysteine at the N-methyl-D-aspartate receptor. *Proceedings of the National Academy of Sciences, 94,* 5923–5928.

Maestri, N. E., Lord, C., Glynn, M., Bale, A., & Brusilow, W. (1998). The phenotype of ostensibly healthy women who are carriers for ornithine transcarbamylase deficiency. *Medicine, 77,* 389–397.

Mazzocco, M. M. M., Henry, A. E., & Kelley, R. I. (2007). Barth syndrome is associated with a cognitive phenotype. *Journal of Developmental & Behavioral Pediatrics.*

Mazzocco, M. M. M., & Kelley, R. I. (2001). Preliminary evidence for a cognitive phenotype in Barth syndrome. *American Journal of Medical Genetics, 102,* 372–378.

Mitchell, G. A., Grompe, M., Lambert, M., & Tanguay, R. (2001). Hypertyrosinemia. In C. R. Scriver, A. L. Beaudet, W. S. Sly, & D. Valle (Eds.), *The metabolic and molecular bases of inherited disease* (8th ed., pp. 1777–1805). New York: McGraw-Hill.

Moats, R. A., Koch, R., Moseley, K., Guldberg, P., Guttler, F., Boles, R. G., & Nelson, M. D. (2000). Brain phenylalanine concentration in the management of adults with phenylketonuria. *Journal of Inherited Metabolic Disease, 23,* 7–14.

Moller, H. E., Weglage, J., Bick, U., Widermann, D., Feldmann, R., & Ullrich, K. (2003). Brain imaging and proton magnetic resonance spectroscopy in patients with phenylketonuria. *Pediatrics, 112,* 1580–1583.

Mudd, S. H., Levy, H. L., & Skovby, F. (1995). Disorders of transsulfuration. In C. R. Scriver, A. L. Beaudet, W. S. Sly & D. Valle (Eds.), *The metabolic and molecular bases of inherited disease* (pp. 1279–1327). New York: McGraw-Hill.

Mudd, S. H., Skovby, F., Levy, H. L., Pettigrew, K. D., Wilcken, B., Pyeritz, R. E., et al. (1985). The natural history of homocystinuria due to cystathionine beta-synthase deficiency. *American Journal of Human Genetics, 37,* 1–31.

Mueller, C., Patel, S., Irons, M., Antshel, K., Salen, G., Tint, G. S., & Bay, C. (2003). Normal cognition and behavior in a Smith–Lemli–Opitz syndrome patient who presented with Hirschsprung disease. *American Journal of Medical Genetics, 123,* 100–106.

Nassogne, M. C., Heron, B., Touati, G., Rabier, D., & Saudubray, J. M. (2005). Urea cycle defects: Management and outcome. *Journal of Inherited Metabolic Disease, 28,* 407–414.

Nelson, M., Wolff, J., Cross, C., Donnell, G., & Kaufman, F. (1992). Galactosemia: Evaluation with MR imaging, *Radiology, 184,* 255–261.

Neumaier-Probst, E., Harting, I., Seitz, A., Ding, C., & Kolker, S. (2004). Neuroradiological findings in glutaric aciduria type I (glutaryl-CoA dehydrogenase deficiency). *Journal of Inherited Metabolic Disease, 27,* 869–876.

Nicolaides, P., Leonard, J., & Surtees, R. (1998). Neurological outcome of methylmalonic acidaemia. *Archives of Disease in Childhood, 78,* 508–512.

Nicolaides, P., Liebsch, D., Dale, N., Leonard, J., & Surtees, R. (2002). Neurological outcome of patients with ornithine carbamoyltransferase deficiency. *Archives of Disease in Childhood, 86,* 54–56.

Nord, A., van Doorninck, W. J., & Greene, C. (1991). Developmental profile of patients with maple syrup urine disease. *Journal of Inherited Metabolic Disease, 14,* 881–889.

Nyhan, W. L., Gargus, J. J., Boyle, K., Selby, R., & Koch, R. (2002). Progressive neurologic disability in methylmalonic acidemia despite transplantation of the liver. *European Journal of Pediatrics, 161,* 377–379.

Ogier de Baulny, H., Benoist, J. F., Rigal, O., Touati, G., Rabier, D., & Saudubray, J. M. (2005). Methylmalonic and propionic acidaemias: Management and outcome. *Journal of Inherited Metabolic Disease, 28,* 415–423.

Oh, S. H., Lee, K. Y., Im, J. H., & Lee, M. S. (2002). Chorea associated with non-ketotic hyperglycemia and hyperintensity basal ganglia lesion on T1-weighted brain MRI study: A meta-analysis of 53 cases including four present cases. *Journal of Neurological Science, 200*, 57–62.

Otero, L. J., Brown, G. K., Silver, K., Arnold, D. L., & Matthews, P. M. (1995). Association of cerebral dysgenesis and lactic acidemia with X-linked PDH E1 alpha subunit mutations in females. *Pediatric Neurology, 13*, 327–332.

Pavlakis, S. G. (1984). Mitochondrial myopathy, encephalomyopathy, lactic acidosis and stroke-like episodes: A distinctive clinical syndrome. *Annals of Neurology, 16*, 481–488.

Pearl, P. L., Weiss, R. E., & Stein, M. A. (2001). Medical mimics: Medical and neurological conditions simulating ADHD. *Annals of the New York Academy of Sciences, 931*, 97–112.

Picker, J. D., & Coyle, J. T. (2005). Do maternal folate and homocysteine levels play a role in neurodevelopmental processes that increase risk for schizophrenia? *Harvard Review of Psychiatry, 13*, 197–205.

Pietz, J. (1998). Neurological aspects of adult phenylketonuria. *Current Opinion in Neurology, 11*, 679–688.

Pietz, J., Kreis, R., Schmidt, H., Meyding-Lamadé, U. K., Rupp, A., & Boesch, C. (1996). Phenylketonuria: Findings at MR imaging and localized in vivo H-1 MR spectroscopy of the brain in patients with early treatment. *Radiology, 201*, 413–420.

Poplawski, N. K., Harrison, J. R., Norton, W., Wiltshire, E., & Fletcher, J. M. (2002). Urine amino and organic acids analysis in developmental delay or intellectual disability. *Journal of Pediatric & Child Health, 38*, 475–480.

Powers, J. M., Liu, Y., Moser, A. B., & Moser, H. W. (1992). The inflammatory myelinopathy of adrenoleukodystrophy: Cells, effector molecules, and pathogenetic implications. *Journal of Neuropathology & Experimental Neurology, 51*, 630–643.

Powers, J. M., & Moser, H. W. (1998). Peroxisomal disorders: Genotype, phenotype, major neuropathologic lesions, and pathogenesis. *Brain Pathology, 8*, 101–120.

Ramus, S. J., Forrest, S. M., Pitt, D. D., & Cotton, R. G. (1999). Genotype and intellectual phenotype in untreated phenylketonuria patients. *Pediatric Research, 45*, 474–481.

Reiss, J., Bonin, M., Schwegler, H., Sass, J. O., Garattini, E., Wagner, S., et al. (2005). The pathogenesis of molybdenum cofactor deficiency, its delay by maternal clearance, and its expression pattern in microarray analysis. *Molecular Genetics & Metabolism, 85*, 12–20.

Robinson, B. H. (2001). Lactic acidemia (disorders of pyruvate carboxylase, pyruvate dehydrogenase). In C. R. Scriver, A. L. Beaudet, W. S. Sly, & D. Valle (Eds.), *The metabolic and molecular bases of inherited disease* (8th ed., pp. 2275–2295). New York: McGraw-Hill.

Robinson, J. N., Norwitz, E. R., Mulkern, R., Brown, S. A., Rybicki, F., & Tempany, C. M. (2001). Prenatal diagnosis of pyruvate dehydrogenase deficiency using magnetic resonance imaging. *Prenatal Diagnosis, 21*, 1053–1056.

Roe, C. R., & Ding, J. H. (2001). Mitochondrial fatty acid oxidation disorders. In C. R. Scriver, A. L. Beaudet, W. S. Sly, & D. Valle (Eds.), *The metabolic and molecular bases of inherited disease* (8th ed., pp. 2297–2326). New York: McGraw-Hill.

Roth, K. S. (1986). Newborn metabolic screening: A search for "nature's experiments." *Southern Medical Journal, 79*, 47–54.

Rouse, B., Matalon, R., Koch, R., Azen, C., Levy, H., Hanley, W., et al. (2000). Maternal phenylketonuria syndrome: Congenital heart defects, microcephaly, and developmental outcomes. *Journal of Pediatrics, 136*, 57–61.

Ryan, M. M., Sidhu, R. K., Alexander, J., & Megerian, J. T. (2002). Homocystinuria presenting as psychosis in an adolescent. *Journal of Child Neurology, 17*, 859–860.

Saudubray, J. M., & Charpentier, C. (2001). Clinical phenotypes: Diagnosis/algorithms. In C. R. Scriver, A. L. Beaudet, W. S. Sly, & D. Valle (Eds.), *The metabolic and molecular bases of inherited disease* (8th ed., pp. 1327–1403). New York: McGraw-Hill.

Schonberger, S., Schweiger, B., Schwahn, B., Schwarz, M., & Wendel, U. (2004). Dysmyelination in the brain of adolescents and young adults with maple syrup urine disease. *Molecular Genetics & Metabolism, 82*, 69–75.

Schulze, A. (2003). Creatine deficiency syndromes. *Molecular & Cellular Biochemistry, 244,* 143–150.

Schulze, A., Hess, T., Wevers, R., Mayatepek, E., Bachert, P., Marescau, B., et al. (1997). Creatine deficiency syndrome caused by guanidinoacetate methyltransferase deficiency: Diagnostic tools for a new inborn error of metabolism. *Journal of Pediatrics, 131,* 626–631.

Scriver, C. R., Beaudet, A. L., Sly, W. S., Valle, D., Childs, B., Kinzler, K. W., & Vogelstein, B. (2001). *The metabolic and molecular bases of inherited disease* (Vols. 1–4). New York: McGraw-Hill.

Scriver, C. R., Kaufman, S., Eisensmith, R. C., & Woo, S. L. C. (1995). The hyperphenylalaninemias. In C. R. Scriver, A. L. Beaudet, W. S. Sly, & D. Valle (Eds.), *The metabolic and molecular bases of inherited disease* (7th ed., pp. 1015–1075). New York: McGraw-Hill.

Scriver, C. R., & Waters, P. J. (1999). Monogenic traits are not simple: Lessons from phenylketonuria. *Trends in Genetics, 15,* 267–272.

Scriver, C. R. (2004). After the genome—the phenome? *Journal of Inherited Metabolic Disease, 27,* 305–317.

Sener, R. N. (2003). Nonketotic hyperglycinemia: Diffusion magnetic resonance imaging findings. *Journal of Computerized Assisted Tomography, 27,* 538–540.

Sener, R. N. (2005). Brain magnetic resonance imaging in tyrosinemia. *Acta Radiologica, 46,* 618–620.

Shevell, M. I., Matthews, P. M., Scriver, C. R., Brown, R. M., Otero, L. J., Legris, M., et al. (1994). Cerebral dysgenesis and lactic acidemia: An MRI/MRS phenotype associated with pyruvate dehydrogenase deficiency. *Pediatric Neurology, 11,* 224–229.

Sikora, D. M., Ruggiero, M., Petit-Kekel, K., Merkens, L. S., Connor, W. E., & Steiner, R. D. (2004). Cholesterol supplementation does not improve developmental progress in Smith–Lemli–Opitz syndrome. *Journal of Pediatrics, 144,* 783–791.

Smith, M. L., Saltzman, J., Klim, P., Hanley, W. B., Feigenbaum, A., & Clarke, J. T. (2000). Neuropsychological function in mild hyperphenylalaninemia. *American Journal of Mental Retardation, 105,* 69–80.

Sparaco, M., Bonilla, E., DiMauro, S., & Powers, J. M. (1993). Neuropathology of mitochondrial encephalomyopathies due to mitochondrial DNA defects. *Journal of Neuropathology and Experimental Neurology, 52,* 1–10.

Strauss, K. A., Puffenberger, E. G., Robinson, D. L., & Morton, D. H. (2003). Type I glutaric aciduria: I. Natural history of 77 patients. *American Journal of Medical Genetics, Part C: Seminars in Medical Genetics, 121C,* 38–52.

Surtees, R. A., Matthews, E. E., & Leonard, J. V. (1992). Neurologic outcome of propionic acidemia. *Pediatric Neurology, 8,* 333–337.

Takakubo, F., & Dahl, H. M. (1994). Analysis of pyruvate dehydrogenase expression in embryonic mouse brain: Localization and developmental regulation. *Developmental Brain Research, 77,* 63–76.

Tanji, K., Kunimatsu, T., Vu, T. H., & Bonilla, E. (2001). Neuropathological features of mitochondrial disorders. *Seminars in Cell & Developmental Biology, 12,* 429–439.

Temudo, T., Martins, E., Pocas, F., Cruz, R., & Vilarinho, L. (2004). Maple syrup disease presenting as paroxysmal dystonia. *Annals of Neurology, 56,* 749–750.

Tierney, E., Nwokoro, N. A., Porter, F. D., Bukelis, I., Garrett, E. S., & Kelley, R. I. (2001a). *Smith–Lemli–Opitz syndrome: Changes in ADI-R scores with cholesterol supplementation.* Paper presented at the 9th Annual Scientific Meeting of the Society for the Study of Behavioral Phenotypes, Oxford, England.

Tierney, E., Nwokoro, N. A., Porter, F. D., Freund, L. S., Ghuman, J. K., & Kelley, R. I. (2001b). Behavior phenotype in the RSH/Smith–Lemli–Opitz syndrome. *American Journal of Medical Genetics, 98,* 191–200.

Topcu, M., Coskun, T., Haliloglu, G., & Saatci, I. (2001). Molybdenum cofactor deficiency: Report of three cases presenting as hypoxic–ischemic encephalopathy. *Journal of Child Neurology, 16,* 264–270.

Torremans, A., Marescau, B., Possemiers, I., Van Dam, D., D'Hooge, R., Isbrandt, D., & De Devyn, P. P. (2005). Biochemical and behavioural phenotyping of a mouse model for GAMT deficiency. *Journal of Neurological Sciences, 231,* 49–55.

Van Buggenhout, G. J., Trijbels, J. M., Wevers, R., Trommelen, J. C., Hamel, B. C., Brunner, H. G., & Fryns, J. P. (2001). Metabolic studies in older mentally retarded patients: Significance of metabolic testing and correlation with the clinical phenotype. *Genetic Counseling, 12,* 1–21.

Van der Knaap, M. S., & Valk, J. (1995). *Magnetic resonance of myelin, myelination, and myelin disorders* (2nd ed.). Berlin, Germany: Springer.

Van der Knaap, M. S., Verhoeven, N. M., Maaswinkel-Mooij, P., Pouwels, P. J., Onkenhout, W., Peeters, E. A., et al. (2000). Mental retardation and behavioral problems as presenting signs of a creatine synthesis defect. *Annals of Neurology, 47,* 540–543.

Varvogli, L., Repetto, G. M., Waisbren, S. E., & Levy, H. L. (2000). High cognitive outcome in an adolescent with mut-methylmalonic acidemia. *American Journal of Medical Genetics, 96,* 192–195.

von Figura, K., Hanefeld, F., Isbrandt, D., & Stöckler-Ipsirogly, S. (2001). Guanidinoacetate methyltransferase deficiency. In C. R. Scriver, A. L. Beaudet, W. S. Sly, & D. Valle (Eds.), *The metabolic and molecular bases of inherited disease* (8th ed., pp. 1897–1908). New York: McGraw-Hill.

Waggoner, D. D., Buist, N. M. R., & Donnell, G. N. (1990). Long-term prognosis in galactosemia: Results of a survey of 350 cases. *Journal of Inherited Metabolic Disorders, 13,* 802–818.

Waisbren, S. E., Hanley, W., Levy, H. L., Shifrin, H., Allred, E., Azen, C., et al. (2000). Outcome at age 4 years in offspring of women with maternal phenylketonuria: The Maternal PKU Collaborative Study. *Journal of the American Medical Association, 283,* 756–762.

Waisbren, S. E., Norman, T. R., Schnell, R. R., & Levy, H. L. (1983). Speech and language deficits in early-treated children with galactosemia. *Journal of Pediatrics, 102,* 75–77.

Wang, S. S., Fernhoff, P. M., & Khoury, M. J. (2000). Is the G985A allelic variant of medium-chain acyl-CoA dehydrogenase a risk factor for sudden infant death syndrome? A pooled analysis. *Pediatrics, 105,* 1175–1176.

Wang, Z. I., Berry, G. T., Dreha, S. F., Zhao, H., Segal, S., & Zimmerman, R. A. (2001). Proton magnetic resonance spectroscopy of brain metabolites in galactosemia. *Annals of Neurology, 50,* 266–269.

Waterham, H. R., Wijburg, F. A., Hennekam, R. C., Vreken, P., Poll-The, B. T., Dorland, L., et al. (1998). Smith–Lemli–Opitz syndrome is caused by mutations in the 7-dehydrocholesterol reductase gene. *American Journal of Human Genetics, 63,* 329–338.

Weglage, J., Pietsch, M., Fuenders, B., Koch, H. G., & Ullrich, K. (1996). Deficits in selective and sustained attention processes in early treated children with phenylketonuria—Result of impaired frontal lobe functions? *European Journal of Pediatrics, 155,* 200–204.

Welsh, M. C., & Pennington, B. F. (2000). Phenylketonuria. In K. O. Yeates, M. D. Ris, & H. G. Taylor (Eds.), *Pediatric neuropsychology: Research, theory and practice* (pp. 275–299). New York: Guilford Press.

Welsh, M. C., Pennington, B. F., Ozonoff, S., Rouse, B., & McCabe, E. R. B. (1990). Neuropsychology of early-treated phenylketonuria: Specific executive functions deficits. *Child Development, 61,* 1697–1713.

White, D. A., Nortz, M. J., Mandernach, T., Huntington, K., & Steiner, R. D. (2001). Deficits in memory strategy use related to prefrontal dysfunction during early development: Evidence from children with phenylketonuria. *Neuropsychology, 15,* 221–229.

White, D. A., Nortz, M. J., Mandernach, T., Huntington, K., & Steiner, R. (2002). Age-related working memory impairments in children with prefrontal dysfunction associated with phenylketonuria. *Journal of the International Neuropsychological Society, 8,* 1–11.

Widhalm, K., Miranda-da-Cruz, B., & de Sonneville, L. M. (2002). Information processing characteristics and uridine treatment in children with classical galactosemia. *Nutrition Research, 22,* 257–270.

Wyss, M., & Schulze, A. (2002). Health implications of creatine: Can oral creatine supplementation protect against neurological and atherosclerotic disease? *Neuroscience, 112,* 243–260.

Yakovlev, P. I., & Lecours, A. R. (1967). The myelogenetic cycles of regional maturation of the brain. In A. Minkowski (Ed.), *Regional development of the brain in early life* (pp. 3–70). Oxford, England: Blackwell.

Yap, S., Rushe, H., Howard, P. M., & Naughten, E. R. (2001). The intellectual abilities of early-treated individuals with pyridoxine-nonresponsive homocystinuria due to cystathionine beta-synthase deficiency. *Journal of Inherited Metabolic Disease, 24,* 437–447.

10 Neurodevelopmental Effects of Childhood Exposure to Heavy Metals: Lessons from Pediatric Lead Poisoning

Theodore I. Lidsky, Agnes T. Heaney, Jay S. Schneider, and John F. Rosen

An unfortunate result of industrialization has been the increasing exposure of the population to chemicals with neurotoxic potential. Children, due to a variety of physiological and behavioral factors, represent a particularly vulnerable target for some of these toxins with the developing brain the most significant casualty.[1] Heavy metals, metals with high atomic weight, pose one of the most prominent neurodevelopmental threats. However, despite growing awareness of the dangers of heavy metals, regulation by government agencies charged with protecting public health has been slow to keep up with the information provided by science and even slower to react. Due to shortcomings of regulatory bodies, children continue to be adversely affected by neurotoxins long after research has clearly demonstrated their pernicious effects.

By far the most heavily studied of these heavy metals is lead, a neurotoxin that is particularly dangerous to the developing nervous system of children. Awareness that lead poisoning poses a special risk for children dates back over 100 years, and there has been increasing research on the developmental effects of this poison over the past 60 years. Despite this research and growing public awareness of the dangers of lead to children, government regulation has lagged behind scientific knowledge; legislation has been ineffectual in critical areas, and many new cases of poisoning occur each year.

Lead, however, is not the only neurotoxic metal that presents a danger to children. Several other heavy metals, such as mercury and manganese, are also neurotoxic, have adverse effects on the developing brain, and can be encountered by children. Although these other neurotoxic metals have not been as widely studied as lead, there has been important research describing their effects on the brain. The purpose of the present chapter is to review the neurotoxicology of lead poisoning as well as what is known concerning the neurtoxicology of mercury and manganese. The purpose of this review is to provide information that might be of some help in avoiding repetition of the mistakes that were made in attempting to protect children from the dangers of lead poisoning.

Lead: A Child's Poison

The archetypical neurotoxic heavy metal is lead. Known for millennia to be generally poisonous and for more than a century to be especially poisonous to children, this metal continues to claim hundreds of thousands of young victims in the United States and millions internationally. Recognized by scientists long before public health officials as a danger to development, the effects of lead on the brain and behavior have been the subject of intensive study. Despite its disappointing history in public health, there are a number of insights that can be gained from a review of the research on lead poisoning that are generalizable to other neurotoxins and that might be of some help in avoiding repetition of the mistakes that were made in attempting to protect children from the dangers of lead poisoning.

Unique Vulnerability

Although the earliest reports of lead poisoning date back at least to the Roman empire, the singular vulnerability of young children to this metal was first noted in 1897 (Pueschel et al., 1996). In the first half of the 20th century, public health policy was primarily concerned with occupational exposures and as a result focused on adults. However, accumulating scientific information about children's exquisite sensitivity to this neurotoxin, especially (though certainly not exclusively) during the latter part of the 20th century, eventually resulted in public health regulation addressed to the specific protection of children.[2]

Children are more susceptible to the neurotoxic effects of lead for several physiological reasons (Leggett, 1993; Hartman, 1995). With similar degrees of exposure, children, in comparison to adults, (a) absorb more lead, (b) retain more lead (i.e., excrete proportionally less of the absorbed lead), and (c) deposit relatively more of the retained lead in the brain.

In addition, the developing brain is more damaged by lead than is the mature brain. Human brain development continues well past birth into the teenage years and, for certain systems, into the 20s (Giedd, 2004).

There are several possible mechanisms for the increased vulnerability of the developing brain to lead; these are not mutually exclusive.[3] Lead, at very low concentrations, affects the activity of second messengers. For example, both protein kinase C (PKC) and calmodulin are activated by lead at concentrations that are well below the equivalent of the toxic threshold in children. Both second messengers participate in many important cellular functions including proliferation and differentiation. In addition, PKC is also involved in long-term potentiation, a form of neuronal plasticity that may be involved in memory and learning. Lead also disrupts synaptic release of the excitatory neurotransmitter glutamate and also alters glutamate receptors. Normal transmission involving glutamate is critical during development for cell migration, differentiation, and cell survival. Acute lead exposure has been shown to decrease activity of CNPase, an enzyme preferentially located in myelin and shown to be an integral protein for myelin synthesis during development. Lead also can produce anemia, both by interfering with heme synthesis and by decreasing iron absorption from the gut. Severe iron deficiency and iron deficiency anemia are associated with impaired cognitive and neuropsychological development. Lead also disrupts thyroid hormone transport into the brain. Thyroid hormones are critical to the normal development of the brain with severe deficiencies causing mental retardation.

In addition to the biological determinants of a child's vulnerability, there are also behavioral factors that increase risk. The primary source of lead is in dust, either from deteriorating lead-based paint or from soil contaminated by leaded gasoline. Crawling infants are closer to surfaces on which lead dust is likely to be located, a proximity that results in increased exposure both from breathing in the dust and also from ingestion due to hand to mouth activities (Weiss, 2000).

The greater sensitivity of children to lead's effects on the brain is reflected in a lower threshold for poisoning. Exposure levels are typically measured in micrograms of lead per deciliter of blood. In the early 1960s the upper acceptable limit for children was 60 µg/dl, the level at which lead poisoning could cause such physical symptoms as vomiting, clumsiness and hyperirritability. However, as research led to the recognition that lower blood lead levels that may lack clear physical symptoms were also neurotoxic, the threshold was lowered to 40 µg/dl in 1970. With further research demonstrating adverse effects at ever lower levels of exposure, what was considered to be an "acceptable" blood lead level has been successively decreased; in 1975 it was dropped to 30 µg/dl, in 1985 to 25 µg/dl, and finally, in 1991, to 10 µg/dl (Pueschel et al., 1996). Most recently, the Centers for Disease Control and Prevention (CDC; 2005) reported that they no longer consider *any* blood lead level to be safe for children. In contrast, 40 µg/dl is the action threshold established by the Occupational Safety and Health Administration for adults.

Another factor that influences vulnerability is socioeconomic status (SES). Traditionally, SES has been treated simply as a confounding factor because lower SES is associated with increased risk of exposure and also because of SES's effect on certain components of standard intelligence tests, the typical endpoint in the seminal epidemiological studies of lead's effects on neurodevelopment. However, to assume that SES is simply a confound might be incorrect. Rutter (1983) theorized that the neurodevelopmental status of economically disadvantaged children, rendered fragile by environmental influences, might be more susceptible to the neurotoxic effects of lead. Findings in accord with this idea were reported by Winneke and Kraemer (1984). SES *interacted* with lead's effects on visual–motor integration and reaction time; performance deficits were greater in poorer lead exposed children than their more economically fortunate counterparts. Similar results and conclusions were reported by Bellinger (2000) for prenatal lead exposure.

Although the mechanisms of the effect of SES on lead's neurotoxicity are not known, there are several possible alternatives. Lead absorption from the gut is increased by several dietary conditions (i.e., deficiencies in calcium, iron, zinc, or protein) that are more frequently encountered in economically disadvantaged people (Chisolm, 1996; Cheng et al., 1998). Calcium deficiency also increases lead uptake in an in vitro model of the blood–brain barrier (Kerper & Hinkle 1997); it has been hypothesized that increased uptake of lead kills capillary endothelial cells and thereby disrupts the blood–brain barrier (Anderson et al., 1996). However, dietary differences do not completely explain the moderating effects of SES since analogous effects can be observed in laboratory rats. Rat pups were put in either impoverished or enriched environments. Half of the animals in each environment were exposed to lead via drinking water. Although similar levels of lead were observed in the blood and in the brain, only lead-exposed rats reared in impoverished environments showed learning deficits. Dietary considerations do not explain the differential sensitivity of the groups of rats since, apart from lead exposure, diet was identical (Schneider et al., 2001).

Neurodevelopmental Effects of Lead

In laboratory research, lead has been demonstrated to have a variety of adverse effects on brain development and functioning that include disruption of synaptic transmission, disruption of intracellular neurochemical processes, and impaired cellular metabolism that results in abnormal neuronal development, reduced neuronal plasticity, and, in some cases, death of neuronal elements (Lidsky & Schneider, 2003).

Lead's neurotoxic effects are manifest in children in a dose-dependent fashion. At higher blood levels (typically ≥ 70 μg/dl but, in some children, at levels of 50 μg/dl), encephalopathy can result. The symptoms include vomiting, clumsiness, and ataxia, ultimately progressing to alternating periods of hyperirritability and stupor and then finally coma and seizures. Children who survive have severe cognitive impairments including mental retardation (Byers & Lord, 1943).

Lower blood lead levels, which can be asymptomatic or associated with nonspecific complaints (e.g., stomachaches, constipation, or loss of appetite), can also be neurotoxic, although the consequences of such poisoning are different in degree and perhaps in type. Except in a developmentally fragile child, lower blood-lead levels do not result in retardation but have adverse consequences for neurocognitive development. Although scanning techniques, only recently used with lead poisoned patients (Trope et al., 2001; Meng et al., 2005), demonstrate a variety of brain abnormalities associated with neuronal loss, behavioral assessments are currently most useful for identifying lead's effects in children.

The pioneering research on the neurocognitive effects of nonencephalopathic lead poisoning on neurocognitive development was performed by Needleman and associates (e.g., 1979). These investigations demonstrated that overall level of cognitive functioning as represented by IQ[4] decreased as blood lead level increased. Needleman's findings have been replicated and extended by more than 30 studies by different groups of investigators studying children in various parts of the world. Lead's adverse effects on cognition are observed with blood levels below 10 µg/dl; no safe level has been identified (Canfield et al., 2003; Lanphear et al., 2005).

Lead's effects on IQ have been further investigated by the use of neuropsychological tests, assessment instruments that are designed to target specific cognitive functions that could be affected by brain injury. These studies have shown that lead poisoning can have deleterious effects on a child's fine motor functioning, memory, language functioning, ability to pay attention, and executive functioning (Bellinger et al., 1994; Faust & Brown, 1987; Dietrich et al., 1992; Stiles & Bellinger, 1993; Stokes et al., 1998; Walkowiak et al., 1998; T. F. Campbell et al., 2000; Wasserman et al., 2000; White et al., 1993a; Winneke & Kramer, 1997, Ris et al., 2004; Canfield et al., 2004). As with lead's influences on IQ, many of these functions are affected at blood levels below 10 µg/dl.

When any source of brain injury produces symptoms of great similarity in each patient, it is said to have a behavioral signature: Lead lacks a behavioral signature. Lead poisoning, like the majority of causes of brain injury, affects different neuropsychological processes in different children. For example, while one child might evidence problems in verbal memory, a second child could have deficiencies in executive functioning.

In addition to lead's adverse effects on cognition, children who have had elevated lead levels as infants will subsequently have reduced proficiency in basic academic skills (e.g., reading, arithmetic) and lessened achievement at school (e.g., Needleman et al., 1990; Lanphear et al., 2000; Wang et al., 2002). For every 1 µg/dl increase in blood lead, there was about a 0.7 point decrease in average math scores and about a 1 point decrease in average reading scores (Lanphear et al., 2000). Lead-poisoned children are also at increased risk for antisocial behavior and delinquency (e.g., Dietrich et al., 2001).

The effects of lead poisoning, even at lower blood lead levels, persist through the teenage years into early adulthood and appear to be permanent (e.g., Needleman et al., 1990; Fergusson et al., 1997; Ris et al., 2004). In a recent dose-response study, functional imaging was used evaluate cortical activation patterns during a verb generation task in individuals between the ages of 20 and 23 years who had been poisoned with low lead levels in infancy (Cecil et al., 2005). Activation of the left frontal inferior gyrus (Broca's area) showed an inverse relationship with blood lead level while the right temporal region, the *contralateral* area to the traditional Wernicke's area, showed a strong positive association. These effects were seen in a dose-dependent fashion with blood lead levels ranging from about 5 to about 30 µg/dl.

Diagnostic Considerations

In the majority of cases, lead poisoning is diagnosed by blood test. With severe poisoning, the presence of overt signs of encephalopathy can alert a physician to the possibility of severe lead poisoning, a diagnosis that would be confirmed with a blood test. Lower blood lead levels can also be neurotoxic, but the particulars of the condition present diagnostic problems for the clinician. At lower blood lead levels, poisoning does not produce clinical symptoms on physical examination that are informative with respect to etiology. Although some children experience stomachaches, constipation, or loss of appetite during periods of elevated blood lead levels, other children have no such complaints. Similarly, anemia is seen in some but not all children with lower blood lead levels. Even when children do exhibit some of these symptoms, any of a myriad of etiologies are possible; lead poisoning is not the only or most obvious candidate.

Diagnosis of lead poisoning at nonencephalopathic levels is often due to routine screening or surveillance of at-risk populations (see below). Lead has a fairly short half-life in the blood, 35 days with a simple exposure. Therefore, if not performed close in time to the actual exposure, blood tests can result in false negatives or underestimation of the degree of poisoning (Erkkila et al., 1992).

Estimates of total body burden of lead have been attempted by use of chelation with CaEDTA (ethylenediaminetetraacetic acid). Excretion of lead, mobilized from tissue storage, is measured in urine. Body burden is also estimated by examination of bone, wherein more than 90% of lead is stored, via x-ray flourescence techniques. However, it is unclear which pools of lead (e.g., cortical, trabecular) are being assessed, as well as what the threshold of detection is (Cory-Schlecta & Schaumberg, 2000).

Nonencephalopathic lead levels, because they are neurotoxic, clearly do produce brain injury and, as a consequence, neurocognitive symptoms. However, there are two reasons that the behavioral effects of lead poisoning are not useful in diagnosis. First, lead poisoning, like the majority of causes of brain injury, lacks a behavioral signature. Thus, there is no set of impairments that would identify lead poisoning as the culprit rather than, for example, traumatic brain injury or perinatal asphyxia. Second, lead-poisoning-induced neurocognitive impairments demonstrate a "lag" effect; symptoms are often not evident for a considerable time after the initial intoxication, well after blood lead levels have declined to normal (Bellinger & Rappaport, 2002). Three transition points have been identified at which a child could show the aftereffects of early lead poisoning. The first is at 5 to 7 years of age when a child is learning to read; the second is beginning at 8 to 10 years (and thereafter) when the child begins to use reading as a tool for learning; the third is when a child enters adolescence and is required to make use of mature executive functions (e.g., planning, concept formation, self-monitoring). Some children show problems immediately as infants, while others seem normal until the first transition point, the second, or even the third (Bellinger & Rappaport, 2002).

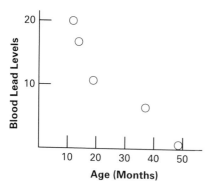

Figure 10.1
Blood lead levels (in micrograms per deciliter) in case 10.1 (Albert) as a function of age.

Case 10.1: Albert   Albert was delivered by normal spontaneous vaginal delivery following a full-term pregnancy. Although there were variable heart rate decelerations during delivery, resuscitation was not needed and Apgar scores were 9 at 1 minute and at 5 minutes. The pregnancy was significant for group B hemolytic streptococcus infection and also chlamydia, both treated during the intrapartum period.

Developmental milestones in all areas were reached in an age-appropriate fashion through at least 20 months. However, at about 13 months of age, Albert was found to be lead poisoned. His history of blood lead test results is summarized in figure 10.1. At about 5 years of age, Albert was diagnosed with severe expressive and receptive language delays and attention deficit/hyperactivity disorder (ADHD) Combined Type, and, due to persisting acting out behavior, he was also diagnosed with oppositional defiant disorder. His ADHD is being treated with Ritalin.

Albert experienced considerable academic difficulty since he first started formal education. Evaluated for an individualized education program while in kindergarten, it was noted that "Reading, Writing and Math were all areas of concern..." as were language delays. The Evaluation Report stated: "The language deficit is not caused by: visual or auditory acuity deficits, emotional disturbance, mental retardation, dialectal differences or second language influence, environmental or economic disadvantage, or cultural difference." On administration of the Stanford–Binet Intelligence Scale (4th ed.), a composite score of 81 (4th percentile) was attained. To address his deficiencies, Albert is now receiving special educational services that include preferential seating, modified assignments, seating next to a "study buddy," small group instruction in a separate setting, and extra time to complete schoolwork.

A comprehensive neuropsychological evaluation was conducted when Albert was about $8\frac{1}{2}$ years old. Results showed normal performance in tests of verbal fluency, attention, and aspects of executive functioning (e.g., planning). However, in association with these areas of normalcy, Albert showed impairments of naming, fine motor functioning, verbal memory, visuospatial memory, auditory working memory, verbal concept formation, and cognitive flexibility. These deficiencies observed in association with normal functioning in other neurocognitive domains and interpreted in the context of Albert's history are indicative of brain injury (Lezak, Howieson, & Loring, 2004; Lidsky & Schneider, 2006). Lead was determined to be the causative factor by the process of differential diagnosis. Thus, in addition to lead poisoning, review of Albert's available medical history indicated no factors or events capable of producing brain injury. Impairments similar to those seen in Albert have been described as sequelae of early childhood exposure to lead (Lidsky & Schneider, 2006).

Treatment

Encephalopathic lead levels are treated with chelation, a procedure that rapidly lowers blood lead level and removes some lead stored in soft tissues. Rebound increases in blood lead levels are common as stored lead leaches out from various tissue compartments; repeat chelation is often necessary (Chisolm, 1996). Chelation, by rapidly reducing blood lead albeit sometimes only temporarily, decreases the acute toxic effects of lead on the brain and other organ systems and has dramatically reduced mortality (Dietrich et al., 2004). Chelation, however, does not appreciably reduce lead stored in the brain (Cremin et al., 1999) and does not prevent the well-documented effects of severe poisoning on neurocognitive development. As previously discussed, lead exposures that are well below those that can cause encephalopathy are also neurotoxic and also result in neurocognitive damage. Attempts have been made to treat these lower lead levels ($\leq$ 44 μg/dl) with chelation. Unfortunately chelation also does not mitigate the detrimental effects of lower lead levels on a child's cognitive development (Dietrich et al., 2004; Rogan et al. 2001).

As of yet, no treatment modalities have been identified that can prevent the neurotoxic effects of lead, once a child has been exposed, as evidenced in an elevated blood lead level. The use of calcium supplementation has been advocated as a way to reduce lead absorption and thereby reduce the toxic dose. However, while there is a clear rationale for this procedure based on research using laboratory animals, there is no strong clinical evidence for the efficacy of this treatment in children (Ballew & Bowman, 2001). There appears to be more support for the use of iron supplementation in reducing lead absorption (Hammad et al., 1996).

Since the effects of lead poisoning on a child's brain are permanent and there is no effective treatment to prevent the adverse effects of lead exposure on neurocognitive development once a child has been poisoned, prevention of lead exposure is the only *cure* for this disease; once a child has been poisoned, the most effective actions may mitigate but will not prevent damage. In the United States, government regulations led to the banning of lead in paint in 1978 (*several* decades after Australia and some parts of Europe) and the removal of lead from gasoline in 1985. Unfortunately these regulations have not been effective at prevention; although they reduced the addition of more lead into the child's environment, they did nothing to remove lead that was already present in a child's surroundings. For example, the U.S. Environmental Protection Agency (EPA, 1996a) estimates that about three quarters of housing built in the United States before 1978 still contains lead paint (approximately 64 million houses). As a result, new cases of childhood lead poisoning from old paint continue to occur with an alarming frequency.

Another example of the inadequacy of government regulation is seen in the ineffectiveness of special legislative efforts that have been made in public housing. Because much public housing was built before 1978 and has lead paint, there are regulations specifically targeted toward preventing lead poisoning of children in these dwellings. However, a recent comparison of children in public housing in New Orleans with other high-risk children in private residences showed no differences in the incidence of lead poisoning. Thus, children living in public housing were no safer from lead poisoning despite the existence of special legislation. The authors concluded "... public housing does not appear to protect children from elevated lead levels, calling into question the efficacy of existing regulations" (Rabito, Shorter, & White, 2003).

There are also other sources of lead exposure that can result in poisoning. Leaded solder used in older plumbing can contaminate drinking water, a hazard that affects not only homes but also day care facilities, schools, and restaurants. A variety of other commodities, particularly those imported from outside the United States, are also sources of lead poisoning; certain alternative medicines, confections, glazed pottery and dishes, inexpensive children's jewelry, some candlewicks, and certain cosmetics have all been implicated in lead poisoning (Jones et al., 1999; CDC, 2003). The CDC Web site (http://www.cdc.gov/nceh/lead/lead.htm) provides current information about product recalls and other recently identified sources of lead poisoning.

For those cases of childhood lead poisoning that have already occurred, and those that inevitably will occur absent a tightening of public health regulations, modalities of treatment are those that are applied to mitigate the effects of brain injury from virtually any etiology. Thus, cognitive remediation, with the goal of teaching an injured patient to use remaining functioning to attempt to compensate for deficits, pharmacotherapy when appropriate (e.g., for some attentional disorders), and counseling are all possible approaches to try to lessen the aftereffects of childhood lead poisoning.

Summary

Lead poisoning causes brain damage that can impair a child's fine motor functioning, memory, language functioning, ability to pay attention, and executive functioning, as well as social and behavioral development. These effects are irreversible and permanent (Lidsky & Schneider, 2003). Often there is a lag in the emergence of symptoms; cognitive impairments may not be observable until a child, poisoned during early infancy, is an adolescent.

Since the negative effects of lead on child development are mediated by brain damage, evaluations must employ techniques suited to assessing this type of injury. Thus, neuropsychological testing, rather than administration of IQ test batteries, is the methodology of choice. Although IQ will often decrease with brain injury, this is not always the case (e.g., Dlugos et al., 1999). Further, even when IQ does decrease with brain injury, the magnitude of the decrease underestimates the severity of the injury (Lezak et al., 2004, Lidsky & Schneider, 2006).

Given the ubiquity of sources of lead exposure and the ineffectual nature of governmental regulation, new cases of lead poisoning will continue to occur. For this reason, efforts at early detection are crucial to minimize exposure as much as possible. Unfortunately, there are two formidable obstacles to early detection. First, blood lead testing, the most accurate way to determine exposure, if not performed close in time to the actual exposure, can result in false negatives. Second, since nonencephalopathic levels of lead exposure lack overt clinical findings on physical examination that would suggest the possibility that a child has been poisoned, one must depend on serendipity for a child to be brought to a physician at a time that would be optimal to detect an elevated blood lead level. For these reasons, the only sure treatment for childhood lead poisoning is prevention, a goal that can only be reached by removal of existing leaded paint and contaminated soils and strict regulation of other sources of lead exposure (*vide supra*).

Mercury

The use and misuse of mercury, like that of lead, dates back to antiquity. As reviewed by Hartman (1995),

In the second and third centuries A.D. the Chinese philosopher Pao Pu Tzu recommended mixing pills of three parts cinnabar (red mercuric sulfide) and one part honey to induce immortality.... Hippocrates was said to have employed mercuric compounds in his pharmacopeia around 400 B.C....and Indian physicians of the Braham period (800 B.C.–A.D. 1000) employed mercury to treat smallpox and syphilis...

Mercury has also been used to "treat" children for worms and sore throat (Hartman, 1995).

Because mercury is not curative for any of the diseases for which it was used as a treatment and is, in fact, toxic, a fact that has been recognized for centuries, this metal is no longer employed in conventional medicine. In contrast, its use lingers on in folk medicine:

For example, various Chinese patent medicines have been found to be the source of several cases of severe mercury poisoning, including in a New York City four year old whose mother systematically fed him a Chinese medicine called Tse Koo Choy, which contains mercurous chloride. The child developed progressive neurological deterioration, with drooling, dysphagia, and irregular movements... recovery was incomplete (Hartman, 1995),

with evidence of both neurological and neurocognitive damage (Hartman, 1995).

There are three principal forms of mercury—elemental mercury, inorganic mercury salts, and organic forms (methylmercury and ethylmercury). Although each compound is toxic, they differ in potency and bioavailablity (Verity & Sarafian, 2000).

Elemental Mercury and Inorganic Salts

Toxicology The primary sources of elemental mercury are emissions from coal-burning electric power generators. Much of this mercury, however, eventually is converted to organic forms via biotransformation (see below; Trasande, Landrigan, & Schechter, 2005). The primary sources of elemental mercury and its inorganic salts that are involved cases of in human exposure are occupational (e.g., miners, photo engravers, and dental technicians) and from home accidents (broken thermometer), alternative/ethnic medicines, and some cultural/religious practices. In addition, dental fillings are also a source of elemental mercury and also organic mercury compounds. Fillings made of amalgam, an alloy that is up to 54% mercury, give rise to levels that "continue to be detectable for 1 year after amalgam implant" (Hartman, 1995) although at low levels. Whether or not these levels are neurotoxic or have adverse neuropsychological effects is not known (Hartman, 1995).

Because elemental mercury is liquid at room temperature and, because it is easily aerosolized or vaporized, one of the principal routes of exposure is via respiration. Mercury then enters the circulation, wherein it is transported to the brain and other organs; elemental mercury readily crosses the blood–brain barrier (e.g., Warfvinge et al., 1992; Pamphlett & Waley, 1996). Although inorganic mercury apparently does not easily cross the blood–brain barrier, it does enter the brain in adults in regions lacking the barrier (e.g., area postrema; Verity & Sarafian, 2000) and in infants due to an incompletely developed barrier (Trasande et al., 2005).

There is also efficient placental to fetal transfer of mercury (Yoshida, 2002), and the fetal brain accumulates more mercury than does the brain of the mother (Feng et al., 2004). Respired mercury, in addition to entering the brain via the circulation, also may do so by a more direct route; mercury is absorbed through the olfactory mucosa, taken up by olfactory nerves and transported to the olfactory bulbs (Henriksson & Tjalve, 1998). Mercury is also absorbed transdermally (Verity & Sarafian, 2000) and can enter the brain either via the circulation or, potentially, by uptake at the neuromuscular junction, and perhaps other nerve endings, followed by axonal transport (Arvidson, 1992).

Once in the brain, inorganic mercury disrupts the normal functioning of a variety of neurotransmitters including aminergic, cholinergic, and glutamatergic systems (Oudar, Caillard, & Fillion, 1989; Hare et al., 1990; Castoldi et al., 1996; Allen, Mutkus, & Aschner, 2001; Moretto et al., 2004). Cellular activity is impaired by disruption of calcium currents (Szucs et al., 1997) and by generation of reactive oxygen species with resulting oxidative stress (Hussain et al., 1997). Inorganic mercury also has an indirect effect on brain development by affecting thyroid status of the mother during pregnancy (Takser et al., 2005).

Clinical Effects   In the adult brain, elemental mercury is deposited both cortically and subcortically as well as in the brainstem and cerebellum (Pamphlett & Waley, 1996). There was a preferential deposition in motor cortical neurons, though glial cells were affected throughout the brain (Pamphlett & Waley, 1996). In animal studies, the hippocampus and cerebellum were particularly vulnerable to mercury deposition (Feng et al., 2004).

Case 10.2: The B. Family   The consequences of elemental mercury exposure to the brain were demonstrated in a case of exposure involving a family of seven (Cherry et al., 2002). The B. family was exposed via elemental mercury that had been spilled on a carpet prior to their moving into the home. The mercury had been absorbed and was not visually detectable; poisoning occurred via fumes. Symptoms were observed only in the youngest member of the family, Claudia, a 3-year-old girl. Prior to hospital admission and detection of elevated blood mercury levels, Claudia exhibited "progressive weight loss, limping, ataxia, irritability, 'screaming,' and regression in speech capability." When admitted to the hospital, she was drooling, hypotonic, ataxic, and mute with a tremor that disappeared during sleep. The toxic threshold in adults, measured in micrograms of mercury per liter of blood, is 50, while less than 10 is expected in unexposed individuals. Such exposure guidelines for infants and young children have not been developed. The young child in this case had a blood mercury level of 295 μg/l. The child underwent 3 rounds of chelation therapy with dimercaptosuccinic acid (DMSA), and her symptoms gradually resolved over a 4-month period. Unfortunately, this child has not undergone neuropsychological testing, and review of the literature indicates no case reports of the cognitive aftereffects of elemental mercury poisoning in young children. In adults, persisting neurocognitive deficits have been reported including "specific problems with cognitive flexibility, cognitive tracking, inhibiting perseveration, fine manual motor coordination, visuospatial analysis and organization, memory for visuospatial information, affect and personality." (White et al., 1993b). [all names are pseudonyms]

The nature of the symptoms of poisoning from elemental and inorganic mercury results in diagnostic difficulties: "The non-specific psychosomatic symptoms of mercury poisoning would likely be misdiagnosed as psychiatric illness unless special inquiry and blood screen were conducted on symptomatic patients from high risk populations" (Hartman, 1995).

Organic Compounds—Methylmercury

Mercury is generated primarily from the combustion of coal but also from volcanic sources, burning of waste, manufacturing processes that use mercury (e.g., fabrication of paper), and chemical production (EPA, 1996; Verity & Sarafian, 2000; Trasande et al., 2005). This mercury, typically in elemental form, travels some distance in the atmosphere and is eventually deposited in water and soil, where it is converted to methylmercury by bacteria, a process that takes place particularly in water. It thereby enters and bioaccumulates up the food chain, reaching very high concentrations in some fish. Consumption of fish is the primary route by which humans are exposed to methylmercury (California Office of Health Hazard Assessment, 2001).

Toxicology   Because it is more easily and efficiently absorbed (EPA, 1996) and also because it readily crosses the blood–brain barrier (Aschner & Clarkson, 1989; Verity & Sarafian, 2000), methylmercury is far more toxic than elemental or inorganic mercury. Once deposited in the brain, methylmercury is slowly demethylated to form inorganic mercury (Friberg & Mottet, 1989).

Methylmercury disrupts normal neuronal electrophysiological activity by affecting both Ca^{2+} and K^+ channels. Methylmercury's neurotoxic effects include influences on a variety of neurotransmitter systems (Oudar et al., 1989; Castoldi et al., 1996). Notable is its influence on astroglia that results in reduced uptake of extracellular glutamate (Fitsanakis & Aschner, 2005). Increasing concentrations of glutamate resulting from decreased clearance are excitotoxic and cause neuronal cell death (Olney, 1994). Methylmercury also causes damage by generation of reactive oxygen species (Shanker et al., 2005).

Clinical Effects: High Mercury Levels   At high concentrations methylmercury causes severe toxic encephalopathy. The symptoms of severe poisoning were illustrated by the victims of large outbreaks of mercury poisoning in Iraq, Pakistan, and Guatemala from ingestion of flour and wheat seeds contaminated with organic mercury agents (Bakir et al., 1973) and in Japan (Minimata Bay and Niigata) from the consumption of mercury-laden fish (D. Campbell et al., 1992). Each of these exposures resulted in widespread poisoning. It is estimated that about 50,000 people consumed bread made with the contaminated flour; 459 died, and 6,530 were hospitalized. It is not known how many suffered adverse effects due to lower doses. In the Japanese exposures, the government officially recognizes 2,265 victims, including 1,435 who have died. Another 15,000 people have registered with the government as poisoning victims (Grimel, 2001). D. Campbell et al. describe several types of symptoms:

(a) psychologic—difficult concentrating, short- and long-term memory loss, emotional volatility, depression, decreased intellectual abilities, and ultimately coma; (b) cerebellar-generalized ataxia with stumbling gait, dysdiadochokinesia, and uncoordination; (c) sensory numbness and stocking-glove paresthesias of distal extremities and mouth, deafness, tunnel vision, visual field constriction, scanning speech with slurring, dysphagia; (d) motor-spasticity, tremors of hands, face, or legs, and weakness proceeding to paralysis. The initial symptoms are fatigue and perioral/extremity paresthesias, followed by difficulty with hand movements. Sensation and visual disturbances occur next. Electrocardiographic abnormalities (changes in S–T segment waves) were noted in about one third of cases from the last Iraqi poisoning. Important aspects of methylmercury toxicity include its predisposition for the CNS, its insidious onset, and its poor prognosis for improvement.

When mercury poisoning occurs during pregnancy, the congenital effects in the neonate are particularly severe. In some cases infants are born with CNS mercury toxicity to mothers whose symptoms were so mild that they were unaware of their own poisoning. Signs and symptoms in the neonate include severe mental retardation, cerebral palsy-like movement problems, both cerebellar and basal ganglia associated dyskinesias, and seizure disorders (D. Campbell et al., 1992). The more severe outcome associated with the congenital form of organic mercury poisoning is probably due to a variety of factors including the undeveloped nature of the fetal blood–brain barrier, the increased susceptibility of the developing nervous system to neurotoxins, and the greater affinity of fetal hemoglobin for mercury that results in higher fetal brain concentrations of mercury (D. Campbell et al., 1992; Trasande et al., 2005).

The National Research Council of the National Academy of Sciences, reviewed the extensive literature on the mass poisoning in Minimata Bay. It concluded that there was evidence for both delayed emergence of symptoms, sometimes decades after the initial exposure, and symptom progression. While acknowledging that continued exposure to mercury cannot be ruled out in these cases, the National Research Council pointed out that delayed emergence and progression of effects was also observed in laboratory research employing animals.

Two biomarkers have been used to quantify mercury dose—mercury concentrations in hair and in blood. Many of the studies of encephalopathy have relied on hair measurements, which reflect average exposure over time. Severe symptoms are seen in children whose mother's hair had 165–320 parts per million (ppm) of mercury, while more mild effects were observed when maternal hair mercury content was in the range of 68–180 ppm (California Office of Health Hazard Assessment, 2001). Although hair and blood mercury concentrations are correlated, there are some suggestions that the former is more imprecise than the latter and blood measurements may be preferred (Budtz-Jørgensen et al., 2004).

Case 10.3: The Doe Family   Over a 3-month period, a family consumed pork from a hog that had been fed seed grain that was treated with a methylmercury-containing fungicide. Following this period, 3 children in the family became ill and exhibited signs of a central nervous system disorder. Following are the details of the case of Eli, a boy who was 13 years old at the time of the poisoning. During the acute phase of intoxication, Eli was somnolent or agitated and showed choreoathetosis. He also exhibited cortical blindness, right hemiparesis, and loss of proprioception, as well as hyperactive reflexes and Babinski signs. Eli's mercury levels were 0.21 ppm in urine, 2.91 ppm in serum and 3.33 ppm in cerebral spinal fluid. Although he was treated with chelation, his neurological signs were not reversed. Upon reevaluation 22 years after the initial poisoning, Eli was found to have a Verbal IQ of 99. However, he remained cortically blind with mild ataxia and hyperactive reflexes; there were no Babinski signs. His speech was dysarthric and dysfluent, and he exhibited a mild attentional deficit, a moderate learning deficit, and problems with word retrieval and response inhibition. Magnetic resonance imaging (MRI) of the brain showed tissue loss in visual cortex, parietal cortex, and cerebellar folia. Notably, although both of Eli's parents were also exposed to methylmercury, neither developed symptoms, though his mother had showed cerebellar atrophy on MRI examination. The mother was pregnant at the time of the poisoning, and the congenitally exposed child, Fiama, was most severely affected, being both blind and mute and showing severe mental retardation, quadriparesis, choreoathetosis, and seizures (Davis et al., 1994).

Another child from this family, Gustav, was poisoned at the age of 8 years. He developed severe mental retardation, quadriplegia, and blindness. Gustav died at the age of 30 years and on postmortem showed cortical atrophy, particularly in paracentral and parieto-occipital areas, loss of neurons, and gliosis. Notably, although the mercury content of his internal organs did not differ from that of an adult without know mercury exposure, Gustav's brain mercury levels were about 51 times control levels (Davis et al., 1994). Thus, after severe poisoning, mercury appears to remain in the brain indefinitely.

Clinical Effects: Moderate to Low Mercury Levels There have been several prospective studies of the effects of low to moderate levels of methylmercury on adults. The participants for several of these studies were drawn from populations with a large daily consumption of fish caught in waters polluted with mercury (Amazon Basin, and St. John's Bay, Quebec); mercury dose was typically based on hair samples. In reviewing these studies, the National Research Council (2000) concluded that hair mercury concentrations less than "50 ppm are significantly associated with disturbances of the visual system (chromatic discrimination, contrast sensitivity, and peripheral fields) and with neuromotor deficits (tremor, dexterity, grip strength, complex movement sequences, hand–eye coordination, and rapid alternating movement)." A recent study also reported neuropsychological sequelae: problems of attention, verbal learning, and memory (Yokoo et al., 2003). In an older adult population (50–70 years of age) with median blood mercury levels of 2.1 µg/l (range = 0–16 µg/l), no adverse effects on neurocognitive performance were identified (Weil et al., 2005). Unlike those studies reporting sensory, motor, and cognitive aftereffects of mercury poisoning, the adults in this latter study were drawn from the United States and were exposed to mercury through a diet with fish consumption typical of the U.S. population; their exposure levels were low.

In view of the greater sensitivity to methylmercury's adverse effects shown by the fetuses of exposed mothers in the Minimata and Iraqi mass poisonings, a number of investigations have assessed the influences of lower levels of exposure during pregnancy on infant development. As in the research on low to moderate methylmercury exposure in adults, the infants for several of the investigations of fetal effects were drawn from populations with a large daily consumption of fish caught in waters polluted with mercury. The National Research Council reviewed the findings of those studies published up to the year 2000 and concluded that there was an increased occurrence of abnormal findings on neurological examinations in congenitally exposed children.

Several large prospective studies have evaluated effects of prenatal methylmercury on neurocognitive development. Mother–infant pairs from the Faroe Islands were studied longitudinally for more than a decade (Grandjean et al., 1997; Grandjean et al., 1999). The Faroe Islands are in the North Atlantic northwest of Scotland and halfway between Iceland and Norway. Mercury exposure in this cohort is from dietary consumption of whale meat and blubber. Prenatal exposure resulted in decreased functioning in several neuropsychological domains (language, attention, memory, visuospatial, and fine motor functioning). The associations of decreased neuropsychological functioning with organic mercury exposure remained after adjustment for covariates and were seen with hair concentrations of less than 10 ppm. Mean maternal hair mercury levels were 4.3 ppm (Grandjean et al., 1997).

A second large cohort came from the Republic of Seychelles in the middle of the Indian Ocean (Myers et al., 2003; Huang et al., 2005). Unlike the diet from the Faroe Islands, wherein exposure was primarily from whale meat and blubber, the mercury exposure of the pregnant mothers from Seychelles was from ocean fish. The mothers' consumption of fish (12 meals per week that included fish) far exceeded that of a typical diet in the United States. Average maternal hair mercury concentrations were 6.8 ppm. Extensive analysis of the effects of prenatal exposure on IQ, academic skills, executive functioning, learning and memory, attention, language, and fine motor functioning failed to show any adverse effect.

There are several important differences between the studies of the Faroes cohort and the Seychilles cohort. First, although the average exposure of the Seychilles group was higher than in the Faroes studies (average maternal mercury hair concentration 6.8 vs. 4.3 ppm), the average concentration of organic mercury in whale meat (1.6 μg/g) is much greater than in ocean fish (0.3 μg/g). Thus, the Faroes Islands cohort received a much bigger bolus of mercury than the mothers in the Seychilles group.

A second difference is that whale meat and blubber, in addition to being contaminated with organic mercury, also have a high content of a number of organic pollutants including PCBs, known neurotoxins. Although attempts were made to control for possible confounding due to PCBs (Grandjean et al., 1997), there were effects on language that were difficult to attribute solely to mercury exposure. In addition, possible interactions between mercury and PCB neurotoxicities could not be ruled out (Grandjean et al., 2001).

A third difference between the two studies is that fish, unlike whale blubber, also contains a number of compounds that are important for brain development and may also be neuroprotective. Long chain polyunsaturated fatty acids, iron, iodine, and choline are each found in fish and are each important for brain development. There is also some evidence that choline mitigates excitotoxicity. It is plausible that the negative influences of lower levels of mercury are offset by the positive effects of these nutrients (Clarkson & Strain, 2003).

In view of the controversy about the effects of exposure of the developing fetus to lower levels of mercury, concerns have been raised about whether or not fish should be consumed during pregnancy. A recent study (Oken et al., 2005) addressed this issue, weighing the risk of mercury's possible toxicity at low doses against the benefits of a fish diet, rich in nutrients that facilitate brain development. Associations between maternal fish intake during pregnancy and maternal hair mercury at delivery with infant cognition at 6 months of age were evaluated in 135 mother–infant pairs. Infant cognition was assessed via a test of visual recognition memory, a measure that is weakly correlated with Full Scale IQ at 6 years of age. The findings were that as fish consumption increased, hair mercury concentrations increased and cognitive scores decreased. However, fish consumption per se was associated with *higher* cognitive scores. The most beneficial effects were observed in infants whose mothers consumed more fish but had lower mercury levels. The authors recommended that "women should continue to eat fish during pregnancy but choose varieties with lower mercury contamination."

Clinical Effects: Mercury and Autism In 2001, Bernard et al. proposed that thimerosal, a preservative containing organic mercury that is used in many vaccines given to infants, induced "many cases of idiopathic autism." Thimerosal is about 49% ethylmercury; Bernard et al. attributed the hypothesized thimerosal-induced autism to mercury exposure. This hypothesis was based in part on the increasing use of thimerosal, the increasing incidence of autism, the known neurtoxicity of ethylmercury, and that mercury exposure "can cause immune, sensory, neurological, motor and behavioral dysfunctions similar to traits defining or associated with autism" (Bernard et al., 2001). In infants who receive several vaccinations, as a function of body weight and vaccination type, certain patients receive substantial exposure to organic mercury that may exceed governmental guidelines.

As Bernard et al. (2001) suggest, the reported incidence of autism has increased from about 2 to 4 cases per 10,000 when Kanner first described the disorder in 1943 to the present rate of 30 to 60 cases per 10,000. However, it is unclear to what extent the increased incidence reflects an actual increment in cases as opposed to broadening of diagnostic criteria and greater public awareness, resulting in enhanced identification (Rutter, 2005).

In evaluating thimerosal's possible role in autism, attention has been directed to the Danish childhood vaccination program. Since 1970, only pertussis vaccine contained thimerosal and, in March of 1992, that inoculation was replaced with a thimerosal-free vaccine. Although the incidence of autism has increased in Denmark as in other countries, the incidence continued to rise after thimerosal was eliminated and there was no increased risk of autism for children innoculated with or without thimerosal-containing vaccine (Hviid et al., 2003; Madsen et al., 2003). In contrast, Geier and Geier (2005) reported increased risk of autism as well as other developmental disorders (e.g., mental retardation) based on reporting to the U.S.'s Vaccine

Adverse Event Reporting System comparing diphtheria–tetanus–acellular pertussis vaccine with and without thimerisol.

Review of the epidemiological literature offers little support for the thimerosal–autism link. In 2000, the Institute of Medicine (IOM) of the National Academies of Science, at the request of the CDC and the National Institutes of Health, evaluated the evidence that use of thimerosal-containing vaccines was associated with increased risk of autism. The first report was issued in 2001 and then was updated in 2004 due to the publication of several new studies. According to both IOM evaluations, there was no evidence of an association between thimerosal use and autism (IOM, 2004).

Parker et al. (2004) reviewed the original data from 10 epidemiological studies and concluded that "the preponderance of epidemiological evidence does not support an association between thimerosal-containing vaccines and ASD [autistic spectrum disorders]," further noting that those "studies that support an association are of poor quality and cannot be interpreted." In addition, while ethylmercury and methylmercury are assumed to have similar neurotoxic mechanisms, there are toxicokinetic differences between the two compounds that render ethylmercury less damaging to the brain. Ethylmercury does not pass through the blood–brain barrier as easily as methylmercury and has a shorter half-life (Parker et al., 2004).

Manganese

Unlike lead and mercury, manganese is an essential metal that is found in all tissues and is required for normal amino acid, lipid, protein, and carbohydrate metabolism (Erikson et al., 2005). Manganese plays an essential role in a variety of physiological functions and systems, including but not limited to immune system functioning, regulation of cellular energy, bone growth, and blood clotting (Erikson et al., 2005). In the brain, manganese functions as a cofactor for important enzymes including superoxide dismutase (a critical antioxidant enzyme) and glutamine synthetase (important for brain ammonia metabolism; Hurley & Keen, 1987). Manganese also has effects on metabolism of the neurotransmitters dopamine and serotonin by playing a role in the activities of monoamine oxidase and catechol-o-methyltransferase enzymes (Golub et al., 2005).

Even though manganese is viewed as an essential element, there is no consensus regarding optimal intake of manganese. The National Academy of Sciences (NAS) has recommended an adequate intake (AI) for adult men at 2.3 mg/day and for adult women at 1.8 mg/day (NAS, 2001), taking into account decreased gastrointestinal absorption in men versus women (Finley et al., 1994). AIs for infants (0.003 to 0.6 mg/day) and children (1.2 to 1.5 mg/day) have also been recommended (NAS, 2001).

Manganese deficiency in a variety of animal species can lead to multiple problems including stunted growth, skeletal defects, abnormal glucose tolerance, and altered lipid and carbohydrate metabolism (Erikson et al., 2005). However, "frank manganese deficiency has not been clinically recognized in humans" (Erikson et al., 2005). In contrast, manganese toxicity from exposure to elevated levels of manganese has serious negative implications for human health and has particularly damaging effects on the central nervous system.

Toxicology

Sources of excess intake of manganese are excess dietary intake, occupational exposures, and environmental exposures. Excess dietary intake of manganese is most typical in infants fed soy-based formulas, which contain higher levels of manganese than breast milk or cow's-milk-based formulas (Lonnerdal, 1994). Occupational exposures occur in workers in certain industries such as alloy production, mining, battery manufacturing, and welding. Recently, the possible relationship between manganese, welding, and Parkinson's disease has received considerable attention (Racette et al., 2001; Racette et al., 2005), although a causal relationship between these factors is still considered by some to be speculative and tentative (Jankovic, 2005). Environmental exposures can occur via drinking contaminated water, from environmental deposition of methylcyclopentadienyl manganese tricarbonyl (MMT) used as an antiknock additive to gasoline, and from organo-manganese agricultural fungicides (Vezar, 2005). Even though the environmental level of manganese from MMT may be quite low, the neurotoxic effects of chronic low-level manganese exposure are unknown.

The main routes of exposure are inhalation and ingestion. Following ingestion, inorganic manganese, in trivalent form, is absorbed in the intestine (Cotzias et al., 1971). Once absorbed, manganese is bound to plasma proteins and is readily taken up in the brain as a free ion or in a transferrin-bound form (Aschner & Gannon, 1994). Manganese is deposited preferentially in mitochondria-rich tissues such as liver, pancreas, and brain. The brain is a primary target in chronic manganese exposure (Roels et al., 1987), and the turnover of manganese in the brain is slower than in other parts of the body (Feldman, 1992). Among cell types in the brain, manganese has been shown to accumulate in astrocytes and neurons. Respiratory symptoms of cough, bronchitis, and impaired pulmonary function are associated with inhaled manganese particulate and may reflect direct pulmonary toxicity induced by manganese (Erikson et al., 2005). Although respiratory effects are important, again, the most sensitive organ for manganese toxicity is the brain (Erikson et al., 2005). The basal ganglia are a particular target for manganese deposition (Josephs et al., 2005).

The transport of manganese into the brain may be aided by iron deficiency. Both manganese and iron are transported into the brain via transferrin-mediated endocytosis (Crowe & Morgan, 1992). Iron deficiency causes increased brain regional tranferrin and transferrin receptor levels, particularly in basal ganglia regions (Erikson et al., 1997). Iron deficiency may also cause an increase in divalent metal transporter-1 levels, which may also foster manganese accumulation in brain (Erikson et al., 2004).

Clinical Effects

A number of reports in the literature describe outbreaks of manganism (a syndrome characterized by a movement disorder including tremor, dystonia, and/or rigidity and psychiatric disorders) following ingestion of contaminated well water (Erikson et al., 2005). However, many of these studies are difficult to intrepret due to the suspected presence of other metals and toxins in the water. Thus, an indisputable link between chronic manganese consumption in drinking water and heightened risk of neurological disorders has not yet been established.

Manganism is typically associated with elevated brain levels of manganese, particularly in basal ganglia regions. A biologic marker for manganese accumulation in the brain is an increased T1 MRI signal, particularly within the globus pallidus but also in the striatum (Josephs et al., 2005). Patients (career welders) with manganese evidenced on MRI had a variety of neurological symptoms (many of which are Parkinson-like in nature) including tremor, ataxia, rigidity, bradykinesia, headaches, memory loss, reduced learning capacity, decreased flexibility, and cognitive slowing. Symptoms persisted even after removal from exposure (Josephs et al., 2005). Manganese accumulation in specific basal ganglia structures appears to be related to diverse neurological outcomes and may be causative, but currently this remains speculative.

The developing nervous system appears to be a target for manganese neurotoxicity, as it is for mercury and lead neurotoxicity. Most of the studies relating brain manganese accumulation to brain damage or dysfunction have been performed in animals. The increased susceptibility of young animals to manganese neurotoxicity is likely related to several factors including increased absorption from the gastrointestinal tract, an incompletely formed blood–brain barrier, and immature biliary excretory mechanisms (Erikson et al., 2005).

In contrast to an extensive literature describing manganese effects on brain and behavior in developing animals, there are scant reports concerning the effects of developmental manganese toxicity in children. Excess manganese has been suggested to cause hyperactivity (Barlow, 1983), psychosis and motor dysfunction (above 7.5 µg/l blood; Mergler et al., 1999). Impaired psychomotor development and a variety of cognitive deficits (e.g., in verbal learning, visual recognition, and digit span) have been noted (Takser et al., 2003). Takser et al. prospectively investigated developmental effects of low-level manganese exposures in humans in 247 pregnant Canadian women and their babies to determine effects of in utero manganese exposure on psychomotor development. After controlling for several potentially confounding factors such as maternal educational level and child's gender, negative relationships were observed between cord blood manganese levels and several factors including attention, nonverbal memory, and manual dexterity measured at 3 years of age.

Other reports demonstrate the ill effects of higher level manganese exposures on children. A child developed severe epilepsy after exposure to welding fumes that resulted in blood manganese levels of 15–20 µg/l (Herraro Hernandez et al., 2003). Chelating treatment reduced blood manganese levels, and seizures abated. Tremor and seizures have been reported in a child receiving parenteral nutrition (Komaki et al., 1999). Blood manganese levels were elevated, and T1-weighted MRI images showed hyperintensities in basal ganglia, brainstem, and cerebellum. Symptoms and MRI abnormalities disappeared after withdrawal of manganese-containing formula. Neurobehavioral deficits have been described in Chinese children who drank water containing high levels of manganese (from an area with high-level manganese sewage irrigation). Children with elevated manganese levels scored lower on tests of digit span, manual dexterity, digit symbol, and visual memory than did children from a control area (He, Liu, & Zhang, 1994).

Case 10.4: Helen Helen is an 8-year-old girl with end-stage cholestatic liver disease due to Aligille's syndrome. She presented with episodes of dystonia and cramping of her hands and arms (Devenyi, Barron, & Mamourian, 1994). These episodes had been occurring over a period of 2 months. Each instance lasted several minutes with a gradual return to normal motor functioning; consciousness was not altered. Helen's history was also significant for vitamin E deficiency and a stable peripheral neuropathy. On neurological examination cognitive screening was within normal limits as was speech. Helen exhibited a low-amplitude resting tremor that intensified with intention; strength was normal. There was decreased muscle bulk, but tone was normal. "sensory testing revealed decreased thermal, vibratory, and pinprick sensation in a fiber-length distribution. Romberg's sign was markedly positive. Tests of coordination revealed mild dysmetria bilaterally. No truncal titubation was noted. Helen had marked propulsion, retropulsion, and a poor check response bilaterally. Reflexes were 1+ in the upper extremities and absent in the lower; plantar responses were flexor. Her gait was narrow based, but she was unable to tandem-gait."

Helen's whole blood manganese levels were elevated at 27 µg/L (normal range = 1–14 µg/L). Her head MRI showed symmetrical hyperintense globus pallidi and subthalamic nucleus with T1 weighting but not with T2 weighting. The morphology of her basal ganglia as well as the rest of her brain was otherwise normal. Helen had a liver transplant 1 year after the onset of her symptoms and 2 months later her whole blood manganese level had dropped to 8.6 µg/L, all symptoms except peripheral neuropathy had disappeared, and the abnormalities noted previously on the brain MRI were gone.

The case of Helen illustrates several features common to manganese poisoning. Individuals with liver problems are at increased risk for manganese intoxication.

Extrapyramidal motor abnormalities are typically observed, and reversibility of neurological signs and symptoms (e.g., motor symptoms, seizures; Herraro Hernandez et al., 2003, *vide supra*) often occurs with reduction of manganese levels. However, irreversibility of symptoms can occur, particularly with prolonged exposure. In addition, cognitive impairments are also frequently observed in manganese neurotoxicity (Devenyi et al., 1994).

Summary

Manganese is essential for the normal functioning of a variety of physiological processes. Excess levels of manganese can be dangerous to children as well as adults and can result in a variety of motor and cognitive/psychiatric disturbances. In some instances, the effects of acute manganese toxicity may be reversible. It is unclear at this time whether the effects of chronic manganese poisoning can be reversed. Additionally, while much is known about the manifestations of chronic occupational exposures, virtually nothing is known about the effects of chronic low-level environmental exposures on neurodevelopment and behavior.

Summary—Lessons to be Learned from Lead Poisoning

Lead, known to be a potent developmental neurotoxin for more than a century, continues to cause brain damage in large numbers of children. Extensive research on the diagnosis, treatment, and prognosis of pediatric lead poisoning has indicated that the detrimental effects of lead poisoning are permanent, irreversible, and largely untreatable. Ongoing research is addressed toward determining the toxic threshold as well as genetic and other factors that influence vulnerability.

Prevention of exposure is the only "cure" for this disease, while early detection is critical to limiting exposure in those children who have already been poisoned. Unfortunately, there are a number of unique features of childhood lead poisoning that pose serious obstacles to early detection. These include the short half-life of lead in blood and the lack of specific symptoms of neurotoxic levels of exposure that could alert a clinician to elevated blood lead levels. Another problem is that the neurocognitive effects of lead poisoning may not be observable until years after the poisoning, when the patient's blood lead levels have dropped below regulatory agencies' threshold of concern.

Mercury and manganese, heavy metals that are developmentally neurotoxic, have only recently been the subject of increasing investigation. Inasmuch as the neurotoxic effects of mercury on the child's brain also appear to be permanent, early detection is crucial to minimizing harm. Research directed toward this goal should be guided by knowledge of the factors identified in studies of lead poisoning to be important for diagnosis.

Notes

1. Lead also has toxic effects on other organ systems including the kidneys, lungs, heart, hematopoetic system, and reproductive system. The present chapter only addresses effects of lead on the brain.

2. For a comprehensive history of lead and public health, the reader is referred to *Brush with Death: A Social History of Lead Poisoning*, by C. Warren, The Johns Hopkins University Press, Baltimore, 2000.

3. These are reviewed in Lidsky and Schneider (2003), wherein detailed references are provided.

4. General Cognitive Index from the McCarthy Scales of Children's Abilities; Full Scale IQ from the Wechsler intelligence batteries and Test Composite from the Stanford Binet Test of Intelligence.

References

Allen, J. W., Mutkus, L. A., & Aschner, M. (2001). Mercuric chloride, but not methylmercury, inhibits glutamine synthetase activity in primary cultures of cortical astrocytes. *Brain Research, 891,* 148–157.

Anderson, A. C., Pueschel, S. M., & Linakis, J. G. (1996). Pathophysiology of lead poisoning. In S. M. Pueschel, J. G. Linakis, & A. C. Anderson (Eds.), *Lead poisoning in children* (pp. 75–96). Baltimore: Brookes.

Arvidson, B. (1992). Inorganic mercury is transported from muscular nerve terminals to spinal and brainstem motoneurons. *Muscle and Nerve, 15,* 1089–1094.

Aschner, M., & Clarkson, T. W. (1989). Methylmercury uptake across bovine brain capillary endothelial cells in vitro: The role of amino acids. *Pharmacology & Toxicology, 64,* 293–297.

Aschner, M., & Gannon, M. (1994). Manganese (mn) transport across the rat blood–brain barrier: Saturable and transferrin-dependent transport mechanisms. *Brain Research Bulletin, 33,* 345–349.

Bakir, F., Damluji, S. F., Amin-Zaki, L., Murtadha, M., Khalidi, A., al-Rawi, N. Y., et al. (1973). Methylmercury poisoning in Iraq. *Science, 181,* 230–241.

Ballew, C., & Bowman, B. (2001). Recommending calcium to reduce lead toxicity in children: A critical review. *Nutrition Reviews, 59,* 307–308.

Barlow, P. J. (1983). A pilot study on the metal levels in the hair of hyperactive children. *Medical Hypotheses, 11,* 309–318.

Bellinger, D., Hu, H., Titlebaum, L., & Needleman, H. L. (1994). Attentional correlates of dentin and bone levels in adolescents. *Archives of Environmental Health, 49,* 98–105.

Bellinger, D. C. (2000). Effect modification in epidemiological studies of low-level neurotoxicant exposures and health outcomes. *Neurotoxicology & Teratology, 22,* 133–140.

Bellinger, D., & Rappaport, L. (2002). Developmental assessment and interventions. In B. Harvey (Ed.), *Managing elevated blood lead levels among young children: Recommendations from the advisory Committee on Childhood Lead Poisoning Prevention* (pp. 77–95). U.S. Department of Health and Human Services.

Bernard, S., Enayati, A., Redwood, L., Roger, H., & Binstock, T. (2001). Autism: A novel form of mercury poisoning. *Medical Hypotheses, 56,* 462–471.

Budtz-Jørgensen, E., Grandjean, P., Jørgensen, P. J., Weihe, P., & Keiding, N. (2004). Association between mercury concentrations in blood and hair in methylmercury-exposed subjects at different ages. *Environmental Research, 95,* 385–393.

Byers, R. K., & Lord, E. E. (1943). Late effects of lead poisoning on mental development. *Journal of Diseases of Childhood, 66,* 471–494.

California Office of Health Hazard Assessment. (2001, October). Mercury. Prioritization of Toxic Air Contaminants. Children's Environmental Health Protection Act.

Campbell, D., Gonzales, M. S., & Sullivan, J. B. (1992). Mercury. In J. B. Sullivan & G. R. Krieger (Eds.), *Hazardous materials toxicology: Clinical principles of environmental health* (pp. 824–833). Baltimore: Williams & Wilkins.

Campbell, T. F., Needleman, H. L., Riess, J. A., & Tobin, M. J. (2000). Bone lead levels and language processing performance. *Developmental Neuropsychology, 18,* 171–186.

Canfield, R. L., Gendle, M. H., & Cory-Schlechta, D. A. (2004). Impaired neuropsychologial functioning in lead-exposed children. *Developmental Neuropsychology, 26,* 513–540.

Canfield, R. L., Henderson, C. R., Jr., Cory-Slechta, D. A., Cox, C., Jusko, T. A., & Lanphear, B. P. (2003). Intellectual impairment in children with blood lead concentrations below 10 microg per deciliter. *New England Journal of Medicine, 348,* 1517–1526.

Castoldi, A. F., Candura, S. M., Costa, P., Manzo, L., & Costa, L. G. (1996). Interaction of mercury compounds with muscarinic receptor subtypes in the rat brain. *Neurotoxicology, 17,* 735–741.

Cecil, K., Yuan, W., Holland, S., Wessel, S., Dietrich, K., Ris, D., & Lanphear, B. (2005). The influence of childhood lead exposure on language function in young adults: An fMRI study. *Int Soc Magnetic Resonance Imaging, 12 Scientific Meeting and Exhibition,* A1443.

Centers for Disease Control. (2004). Childhood lead poisoning from French ceramic dinnerware—New York City, 2003. *Morbidity and Mortality Weekly Report, 53,* 584–586.

Centers for Disease Control. (2005, August). Preventing lead poisoning in children. *A statement by the Centers for Disease Control and Prevention.* Washington, DC: U.S. Department of Health and Human Services, Public Health Service.

Cheng, Y., Willett, W. C., Schwartz, J., Sparrow, D., Weiss, S., & Hu, H. (1998). Relation of nutrition to bone lead and blood lead levels in middle-aged to elderly men: The Normative Aging Study. *American Journal of Epidemiology, 147,* 1162–1174.

Cherry, D., Lowry, L., Velez, L., Cotrell, C., & Keyes, D. C. (2002, January). Elemental mercury poisoning in a family of seven. *Family & Community Health, 24,* 1–8.

Chisolm, J. J., Jr. (1996). Medical management. In S. M. Pueschel, J. G. Linakis, & A. C. Anderson (Eds.), *Lead poisoning in children* (pp. 141–162). Baltimore: Brookes.

Clarkson, T. W., & Strain, J. J. (2003). Nutritional factors may modify the toxic actions of methyl mercury in fish-eating populations. *Journal of Nutrition, 133* (5 Suppl. 1), 1539S–1543S.

Cory-Slechta, D. A., & Schaumburg, H. H. (2000). Lead, inorganic. In P. S. Spencer, H. H. Schaumberg, & A. C. Ludolph (Eds.), *Experimental and Clinical Neurotoxicology* (2nd ed., pp. 708–720). New York: Oxford University Press.

Cotzias, G. C., Papavasiliou, P. S., Ginos, J., Steck, A., & Duby, S. (1971). Metabolic modification of Parkinson's disease and of chronic manganese poisoning. *Annual Review of Medicine, 22,* 305–326.

Cremin, J. D., Jr., Luck, M. L., Laughlin, N. K., & Smith, D. R. (1999). Efficacy of succimer chelation for reducing brain lead in a primate model of human lead exposure. *Toxicology & Applied Pharmacology, 161,* 283–293.

Crowe, A., & Morgan, E. H. (1992). Iron and transferrin uptake in brain and cerebrospinal fluid in rat. *Brain Research, 592,* 8–16.

Davis, L. E., Kornfeld, M., Mooney, H. S., Fiedler, K. J., Haaland, K. Y., Orrison, W. W., et al. (1994). Methylmercury poisoning: Long-term clinical, radiological, toxicological, and pathological studies of an affected family. *Annals of Neurology, 35,* 680–688.

Devenyi, A. G., Barron, T. F., & Mamourian, A. C. (1994). Dystonia, hyperintense basal ganglia, and high whole blood manganese in Alagille's syndrome. *Gastroenterology, 106,* 1068–1071.

Dietrich, K. M., Succop, P. A., Berger, O. G., & Keith, R. W. (1992). Lead exposure and the central auditory processing abilities and cognitive development of urban children: The cincinnati lead study cohort at age 5 years. *Neurotoxicology and Teratology, 14,* 51–56.

Dietrich, K. N., Ris, M. D., Succop, P. A., Beger, O. G., & Bornschein, R. L. (2001). Early exposure to lead and juvenile delinquency. *Neurotoxicology Teratology, 23,* 511–518.

Dietrich, K. N., Ware, J. H., Salganik, M., Radcliffe, J., Rogan, W. J., Rhoads, G. G., et al. (2004). Treatment of lead-exposed children clinical trial group: Effect of chelation therapy on the neuropsychological and behavioral development of lead-exposed children after school entry. *Pediatrics, 114,* 19–26.

Dlugos, D. J., Moss, E. M., Duhaime, A.-C., & Brooks-Kayal, A. R. (1999). Language-related cognitive declines after left temporal lobectomy in children. *Pediatric Neurology, 21,* 444–449.

Erikson, K. M., Pinero, D. J., Connor, J. R., & Beard, J. L. (1997). Regional brain iron, ferritin and transferrin concentrations during iron deficiency and iron repletion in developing rats. *Journal of Nutrition, 127,* 2020–2038.

Erikson, K. M., Syversen, T., Aschner, J. L., & Aschner, M. (2005). Interactions between excessive manganese exposures and dietary iron-deficiency in neurodegeneration. *Environmental Toxicology and Pharmacology, 19,* 415–421.

Erikson, K. M., Syversen, T., Steinnes, E., & Aschner, M. (2004). Globus pallidus: A target brain region for divalent metal accumulation associated with dietary iron deficiency. *Journal of Nutritional Biochemistry, 15,* 335–341.

Erkkila, J., Armstrong, R., Riihimaki, V., Chettle, D. R., Paakkari, A., Scott, M., et al. (1992). In vivo measurements of lead in bone at four anatomical sites: Long-term occupational and consequent endogenous exposure. *British Journal of Industrial Medicine, 49,* 631–644.

Faust, D., & Brown, J. (1987). Moderately elevated blood lead levels: Effects on neuropsychologic functioning in children. *Pediatrics, 80,* 623–629.

Feldman, R. G. (1992). Manganese. In F. A. de Wolff (Ed.), *Handbook of clinical neurology: Intoxications of the nervous system* (Part I, Vol. 20, pp. 303–322). Amsterdam: Elsevier.

Feng, W., Wang, M., Li, B., Liu, J., Chai, Z., Zhao, J., & Deng, G. (2004). Mercury and trace element distribution in organic tissues and regional brain of fetal rat after in utero and weaning exposure to low dose of inorganic mercury. *Toxicology Letters, 25,* 223–234.

Fergusson, D. M., Horwood, L. J., & Lynskey, M. T. (1994). Early dentine lead levels and educational outcomes at 18 years. *Journal of Child Psychology Psychiatry, 38,* 471–478.

Finley, J. W., Johnson, P. E., & Johnson, L. K. (1994). Sex affects manganese absorption and retention by humans from diet adequate in manganese. *American Journal of Clinical Nutrition, 60,* 949–955.

Fitsanakis, V. A., & Aschner, M. (2005). The importance of glutamate, glycine, and gamma-aminobutyric acid transport and regulation in manganese, mercury and lead neurotoxicity. *Toxicology & Applied Pharmacology, 204,* 343–354.

Friberg, L., & Mottet, N. K. (1989). Accumulation of methylmercury and inorganic mercury in the brain. *Biological Trace Element Research, 21,* 201–206.

Geier, D. A., & Geier, M. R. (2005). A two-phased population epidemiological study of the safety of thimerosal-containing vaccines: A follow-up analysis. *Medical Science Moniter, 11,* CR160–170.

Giedd, J. N. (2004). Structural magnetic resonance imaging of the adolescent brain. *Annals of the New York Academy of Science, 1021,* 77–85.

Golub, M. S., Hogrefe, C. E., Germann, S. L., Tran, T. T., Beard, J. L., Crinella, F. M., & Lonnerdal, B. (2005). Neurobehavioral evaluation of rhesus monkey infants fed cow's milk formula, sow formula or soy formula with added manganese. *Neurotoxicology and Teratology, 27,* 615–627.

Grandjean, P., Budtz-Jorgensen, E., White, R. F., Jorgensen, P. J., Weihe, P., & Debes, F., Keiding, N. (1999). Methylmercury exposure biomarkers as indicators of neurotoxicity in children aged 7 years. *American Journal of Epidemiology, 150,* 301–305.

Grandjean, P., Weihe, P., Burse, V. W., Needham, L. L., Storr-Hansen, E., Heinzow, B., et al. (2001). Neurobehavioral deficits associated with PCB in 7-year-old children prenatally exposed to seafood neurotoxicants. *Neurotoxicology and Teratology, 23,* 305–317.

Grandjean, P., Weihe, P., White, R. F., Debes, F., Araki, S., Yokoyama, K., et al. (1997). Cognitive deficit in 7-year-old children with prenatal exposure to methylmercury. *Neurotoxicology and Teratology, 19,* 417–428.

Grimel, H. (2001, October 10). Minimata Bay mercury victims could double. *Associated Press.* Retrieved from http://www.mindfully.org/Pesticide/Minimata-Mercury-Victims.htm October 8, 2006.

Hammad, T. A., Sexton, M., & Langenberg, P. (1996). Relationship between blood lead and dietary iron intake in preschool children: A cross-sectional study. *Annals of Epidemiology, 6,* 30–33.

Hare, M. F., Rezazadeh, S. M., Cooper, G. P., Minnema, D. J., & Michaelson, I. A. (1990). Effects of inorganic mercury on [^{3}H] dopamine release and calcium homeostasis in rat striatal synaptosomes. *Toxicology Applied Pharmacology, 102,* 316–330.

Hartman, D. E. (1995). *Neuropsychological toxicology* (2nd ed.). New York: Plenum Press.

He, P., Liu, D. H., & Zhang, G. Q. (1994). Effects of high level manganese sewage irrigation on children's neurobehavior. *Zhonghua Yu Fang Yi Xue Za Zhi, 28,* 216–218.

Henriksson, J., & Tjalve, H. (1998). Uptake of inorganic mercury in the olfactory bulbs via olfactory pathways in rats. *Environmental Research, 77,* 130–140.

Herrero Hernandez, E., Discalzi, G., Dassi, P., Jarre, L., & Pira, E. (2003). Manganese intoxication: The cause of an inexplicable epileptic syndrome in a 3 year old child. *Neurotoxicology, 24,* 633–639.

Huang, L. S., Cox, C., Myers, G. J., Davidson, P. W., Cernichiari, E., Shamlaye, C. F., et al. (2005). Exploring nonlinear association between prenatal methylmercury exposure from fish consumption and child development: Evaluation of the Seychelles Child Development Study nine-year data using semiparametric additive models. *Environmental Research, 97,* 100–108.

Hurley, L. S., & Keen, C. L. (1987). Manganese. In E. Underwood, & W. Mertz (Eds.), *Trace Elements in Human Health and Animal Nutrition* (pp. 185–225). New York: Academic Press.

Hussain, S., Rodgers, D. A., Duhart, H. M., & Ali, S. F. (1997). Mercuric chloride-induced reactive oxygen species and its effect on antioxidant enzymes in different regions of rat brain. *Journal of Environment Science & Health Part B, 32,* 395–409.

Hviid, A., Stellfeld, M., Wohlfahrt, J., & Melbye, M. (2003). Association between thimerosal-containing vaccine and autism. *Journal of the American Medical Association, 290,* 1763–1766.

Institute of Medicine. (2004). *Vaccines and autism: An Institute of Medicine (IOM) report.* Washington, DC: The National Academies Press.

Jankovic, J. (2005). Searching for a relationship between manganese and welding and Parkinson's disease. *Neurology, 64,* 2021–2028.

Jones, T. F., Moore, W. L., Craig, A. S., Reasons, R. L., & Schaffner, W. (1999). Hidden threats: Lead poisoning from unusual sources. *Pediatrics, 104,* 1223–1225.

Josephs, K. A., Ahlskog, J. E., Klos, K. J., Kumar, N., Fealey, R. D., Trenerry, M. R., & Cowl, C. T. (2005). Neurologic manifestations in welders with pallidal MRI T1 hyperintensity. *Neurology, 64,* 2033–2039.

Kanner, L. (1943). Autistic disturbances of affective contact. *Nervous Child, 2,* 217–250.

Kerper, L. E., & Hinkle, P. M. (1997). Lead uptake in brain capillary endothelial cells: Activation by calcium store depletion. *Toxicology & Applied Pharmacology, 146,* 127–133.

Komaki, H., Maisawa, S., Sugai, K., Kobayashi, Y., & Hashimoto, T. (1999). Tremor and seizures associated with chronic manganese intoxication. *Brain Development, 21,* 122–124.

Lanphear, B. P., Dietrich, K., Auinger, P., & Cox, C. (2000). Cognitive deficits associated with blood lead concentrations < 10 microg/dL in U.S. children and adolescents. *Public Health, 115,* 521–529.

Lanphear, B. P., Hornung, R., Khoury, J., Yolton, K., Baghurst, P., Bellinger, D. C., et al. (2005). Low-level environmental lead exposure and children's intellectual function: An international pooled analysis. *Environmental Health Perspectives, 113,* 894–899.

Leggett, R. W. (1993). An age-specific kinetic model of lead metabolism in humans. *Environmental Health Perspectives, 101,* 598–616.

Lezak, M., Howieson, D. B., & Loring, D. W. (2004). *Neuropsychological Assessment* (4th ed.). New York: Oxford University Press.

Lidsky, T. I., & Schneider, J. S. (2003). Lead neurotoxicity in children: Basic mechanisms and clinical correlates. *Brain, 126,* 5–19.

Lidsky, T. I., & Schneider, J. S. (2006). Adverse effects of childhood lead poisoning: The clinical neuropsychological perspective. *Environmental Research, 100,* 284–293.

Lonnerdal, B. (1994). Manganese nutrition in infants. In D. Klimis-Ravantzis (Ed.), *Manganese in health and disease* (pp. 175–191). Boca Raton, FL: CRC Press.

Madsen, K. M., Lauritsen, M. B., Pedersen, C. B., Thorsen, P., Plesner, A. M., Andersen, P. H., & Mortensen, P. B. (2003). Thimerosal and the occurrence of autism: Negative ecological evidence from Danish registry data. *Pediatrics, 112*(Pt 1), 604–606.

Meng, X.-M., Zhu, D.-M., Ruan, D.-Y., She, J.-Q., & Luo, L. (2005). Effects of chronic lead exposure on ^{1}H MRS of hippocampus and frontal lobes in children. *Neurology, 64,* 1644–1647.

Mergler, D., Baldwin, M., Belanger, S., Larribe, F., Beuter, A., Bowler, R., et al. (1999). Manganese neurotoxicity, a continuum of dysfunction: Results from a community-based study. *Neurotoxicology, 20,* 327–342.

Moretto, M. B., Lermen, C. L., Morsch, V. M., Bohrer, D., Ineu, R. P., da Silva, A. C., et al. (2004). Effect of subchronic treatment with mercury chloride on NTPDase, 5'-nucleotidase and acetylcholinesterase from cerebral cortex of rats. *Journal of Trace Elements in Medicine & Biology, 7,* 255–260.

Myers, G. J., Davidson, P. W., Cox, C., Shamlaye, C. F., Palumbo, D., Cernichiari, E., et al. (2003). Prenatal methylmercury exposure from ocean fish consumption in the Seychelles child development study. *Lancet, 361,* 1686–1692.

National Academy of Sciences. (2001). Dietary reference intakes for vitamin a, vitamin k, arsenic, boron, chromium, copper, iodine, iron, manganese, molybdenum, nickel, silicon, vanadium and zinc. Panel on Micronutrients, Subcommittee on Upper Reference Levels of Nutrients and of Interpretation and Use of Dietary Reference Intakes, and the Standing Committee on the Scientific Evaluation of Dietary Reference Intakes. Retrieved from www.nap.edu/books/0309072794/html/ October 8, 2006.

National Research Council. (2000). *Toxicological effects of methylmercury.* Committee of the Toxicological Effects of Methylmercury, Board on Environmental Studies and Toxicology. Washington, DC: National Academy Press.

Needleman, H. L., Gunnoe, C., Leviton, A., Reed, R., Peresie, H., Maher, C., & Barrett, P. (1979). Deficits in psychologic and classroom performance of children with elevated dentine lead levels. *New England Journal of Medicine, 300,* 689–695.

Needleman, H. L., Schell, A., Bellinger, D., Leviton, A., & Allred, E. N. (1990). The long-term effects of exposure to low doses of lead in childhood. An 11-year follow-up report. *New England Journal of Medicine, 322,* 83–88.

Oken, E., Wright, R. O., Kleinman, K. P., Bellinger, D., Amarasiriwardena, C. J., Hu, H., et al. (2005). Maternal fish consumption, hair mercury, and infant cognition in a U.S. cohort. *Environmental Health Perspectives, 113,* 1376–1380.

Olney, J. W. (1994). New mechanisms of excitatory transmitter neurotoxicity. *Journal of Neural Transmission Supplement, 43,* 47–51.

Oudar, P., Caillard, I., & Fillion, G. (1989). In vitro effect of organic and inorganic mercury on the serotonergic system. *Pharmacology & Toxicology, 65,* 245–248.

Pamphlett, R., & Waley, P. (1996). Uptake of inorganic mercury by the human brain. *Acta Neuropathologica (Berlin), 92,* 525–527.

Parker, S. K., Schwartz, B., Todd, J., & Pickering, L. K. (2004). Thimerosal-containing vaccines and autistic spectrum disorder: A critical review of published original data. *Pediatrics, 114,* 793–804.

Pueschel, S. M., Linakis, J. G., & Anderson, A. C. (1996). Lead poisoning: A historical perspective. In S. M. Pueschel, J. G. Linakis, A. C. Anderson (Eds.), *Lead poisoning in childhood* (pp. 1–13). Baltimore: Brookes.

Rabito, F. A., Shorter, C., & White, L. E. (2003). Lead levels among children who live in public housing. *Epidemiology, 14,* 257–258.

Racette, B. A., McGee-Minnich, L., Moerlein, S. M., Mink, J. W., Videen, T. O., & Perlmutter, J. S. (2001). Welding-related parkinsonism: Clinical features, treatment, and pathophysiology. *Neurology, 56,* 8–13.

Racette, B. A., Tabbal, S. D., Jennings, D., Good, L., Perlmutter, J. S., & Evanoff, B. (2005). Prevalence of parkinsonism and relationship to exposure in a large sample of Alabama welders. *Neurology, 64,* 230–235.

Ris, M. D., Dietrich, K. N., Succop, P. A., Berger, O. G., & Bornstein, R. L. (2004). Early exposure to lead and neuropsychological outcome in adolescence. *Journal of the International Neuropsychological Society, 10,* 261–270.

Roels, H., Lauwerys, R., Buchet, J. P., Genet, P., Sarhan, M. J., Hanotiau, I., et al. (1987). Epidemiological survey among workers exposed to manganese: Effects on lung, central nervous system and some biological indices. *American Journal of Industrial Medicine, 11,* 307–327.

Rogan, W. J., Dietrich, K. N., Ware, J. H., Dockery, D. W., Salganik, M., Radcliffe, J., et al. (2001). The effect of chelation therapy with succimer on neuropsychological development in children exposed to lead. *New England Journal of Medicine, 344,* 1421–1426.

Rutter, M. (1983). Low level lead exposure: Sources, effects and implications. In M. Rutter, & Russell-Jones (Eds.), *Lead versus health* (pp. 333–370). Chichester, England: John Wiley.

Rutter, M. (2005). Aetiology of autism: Findings and questions. *Journal of Intellectual Disability Research, 49*(Pt 4), 231–238.

Schneider, J. S., Lee, M. H., Anderson, D. W., Zuck, L., & Lidsky, T. I. (2001). Enriched environment is protective against lead-induced neurotoxicity. *Brain Research, 896,* 48–55.

Shanker, G., Syversen, T., Aschner, J. L., & Aschner, M. (2005). Modulatory effect of glutathione status and antioxidants on methylmercury-induced free radical formation in primary cultures of cerebral astrocytes. *Brain Research. Molecular Brain Research, 137,* 11–22.

Stiles, K. M., & Bellinger, D. C. (1993). Neuropsychological correlates of low-level lead exposure in school-age children: A prospective study. *Neurotoxicology & Teratology, 15,* 27–35.

Stokes, L., Letz, R., Gerr, F., Kolczak, M., McNeil, F. E., Chettle, D. R., & Kaye, W. E. (1998). Neurotoxicity in young adults 20 years after childhood exposure to lead: The Bunker Hill experience. *Occupational & Environmental Medicine, 55,* 507–516.

Szucs, A., Angiello, C., Salanki, J., & Carpenter, D. O. (1997). Effects of inorganic mercury and methylmercury on the ionic currents of cultured rat hippocampal neurons. *Cellular & Molecular Neurobiology, 17,* 273–288.

Takser, L., Mergler, D., Baldwin, M., de Grosbois, S., Smargiassi, A., & Lafond, J. (2005). Thyroid hormones in pregnancy in relation to environmental exposure to organochlorine compounds and mercury. *Environmental Health Perspectives, 113,* 1039–1045.

Takser, L., Mergler, D., Hellier, G., Sahuquillo, J., & Huel, G. (2003). Manganese, monoamine metabolite levels at birth, and child psychomotor development. *Neurotoxicology, 24,* 667–674.

Trasande, L., Landrigan, P. J., & Schechter, C. (2005). Public health and economic consequences of methylmercury toxicity to the developing brain. *Environmental Health Perspectives, 113,* 590–596.

Trope, I., Lopez-Villegas, D., Cecil, C. M., & Lenkinski, R. E. (2001). Exposure to lead appears to selectively alter metabolism of cortical gray matter. *Pediatrics, 107,* 1437–1442.

U.S. Environmental Protection Agency. (1996a, March). *Fact sheet* (Report No. EPA-747-F-96-002).

U.S. Environmental Protection Agency. (1996b). *Mercury Study Report to Congress Volumes I to VII* (Report No. EPA-452-R-96-001b). Washington, DC: Office of Air Quality Planning and Standards.

Verity, M. A., & Sarafian, T. A. (2000). Mercury and mercury compounds. In *Experimental and Clinical Neurotoxicology* (pp. 763–770). Edited by P. S. Spencon, H. H. Schaumburg, A. C. Ludolph. New York: Oxford University Press.

Vezer, T., Papp, A., Hoyk, Z., Varga, C., Naray, M., & Nagymajtenyi, L. (2005). Behavioral and neurotoxicological effects of subchronic manganese exposure in rats. *Environmental Toxicology and Pharmacology, 19,* 797–810.

Walkowiak, J., Altmann, L., Krämer, U., Sveinsson, K., Turfeld, M., Weishoff-Houben, M., & Winneke, G. (1998). Cognitive and sensorimotor functions in 6 year old children in relation to lead and mercury levels: Adjustment for intelligence and contrast sensitivity in computerized testing. *Neurotoxicology & Teratology, 20,* 511–521.

Wang, C. L., Chuang, H. Y., Ho, C. K., Yang, C. Y., Tsai, J. L., Wu, T. S., & Wu, T. N. (2002). Relationship between blood lead concentrations and learning achievement among primary school children in Taiwan. *Environmental Research, 89,* 12–18.

Warfvinge, K., Hua, J., & Berlin, M. (1992). Mercury distribution in the rat brain after mercury vapor exposure. *Toxicology and Applied Pharmacology, 117,* 46–52.

Wasserman, G. A., Musabegovic, A., Liu, X., Kline, J., Factor-Litvak, P., & Graziano, J. H. (2000). Lead exposure and motor functioning in $4\frac{1}{2}$-year-old children: The Yugoslavia prospective study. *Journal of Pediatrics, 137,* 555–561.

Weil, M., Bressler, J., Parsons, P., Bolla, K., Glass, T., & Schwartz, B. (2005). Blood mercury levels and neurobehavioral function. *Journal of the American Medical Association, 293,* 1875–1882.

Weiss, B. (2000). Vulnerability of children and the developing brain to neurotoxic hazards. *Environmental Health Perspectives, 108*(Suppl. 3), 375–381.

White, R. F., Diamond, R., Proctor, S., Morey, C., & Hu, H. (1993a). Residual cognitive deficits 50 years after lead poisoning during childhood. *British Journal of Industrial Medicine, 50,* 613–622.

White, R. F., Feldman, R. G., Moss, M. B., & Proctor, S. P. (1993b). Magnetic resonance imaging (MRI), neurobehavioral testing, and toxic encephalopathy: Two cases. *Environmental Research, 61,* 117–123.

Winneke, G., & Krämer, U. (1984). Neuropsychological effects of lead in children: Interactions with social background variables. *Biological Psychology & Pharmacopsychology, 11,* 195–202.

Winneke, G., & Krämer, U. (1997). Neurobehavioral aspects of lead neurotoxicity in children. *Central European Journal of Public Health, 2,* 65–69.

Yokoo, E. M., Valente, J. G., Grattan, L., Schmidt, S. L., Platt, I., & Silbergeld, E. K. (2003). Low level methylmercury exposure affects neuropsychological function in adults. *Environmental Health.* Retrieved from http://www.ehjournal.net/content/2/1/8

Yoshida, M. (2002). Placental to fetal transfer of mercury and fetotoxicity. *Tohoku J Experimental Medicine, 196,* 79–88.

III REACTIONS AND RESPONSES: BEYOND THE DIAGNOSIS

11 Beyond the Diagnosis: The Process of Genetic Counseling

Allyn McConkie-Rosell and Julianne O'Daniel

The diagnosis of a genetic disorder may be perceived by family members as a threatening, stressful life event because of the lack of either prior experience or the knowledge to adequately cope with this new situation (McConkie-Rosell & Sullivan, 1999). This reaction may lead to feelings of loss of control or powerlessness. Thus, one of the major objectives of genetic counseling is to facilitate adaptive coping through interventions designed to provide families with the knowledge, skills, and resilient self-beliefs required to cope, adjust, and affect control over their lives (McConkie-Rosell & Sullivan, 1999). These objectives are reflected in the recent definition of genetic counseling, which is the process of helping people understand and adapt to the medical, psychological, and familial implications of genetic contributions to disease (Resta et al., 2006). This process integrates the following steps:

- Interpretation of family and medical histories to assess the chance of disease occurrence or recurrence
- Education about inheritance, testing, management, prevention, resources, and research
- Counseling to promote informed choices and adaptation to the risk or condition

In this chapter we will briefly describe the process of genetic counseling both during and after the diagnosis of a genetic disorder. Shiloh noted that the very "nature of genetic conditions limits their generalizability" (Shiloh, 1996, p. 476). That is, the variability of each disorder exemplified by the number and type of symptoms, their onset, and their severity, is equally matched by the variability in the emotional and coping response of each patient and family.[1] Human development and relationships are not static, so the meaning and need for genetic counseling will evolve as the family develops. For example, although adults are often the focus of initial genetic counseling sessions, children—both affected and unaffected—may and will have questions of their own as they mature. In addition, the heritability of genetic disorders creates the potential for genetic risk to extended relatives. This evolution of needs and perspectives can greatly benefit from a similarly dynamic genetic counseling approach. Thus, we utilized a developmental family life cycle approach to frame the pediatric genetic counseling process described in this chapter.

Genetic Counseling and the Diagnostic Process

Although most individual genetic disorders are rare, collectively they are common. Approximately 3%–4% of children are born with a birth defect (Wilcox & Marks, 1999) such as cleft lip, club foot, congenital heart defects, or spina bifida. In addition, genetic and genetically influenced disorders have been reported to account for approximately 71% of pediatric in-patient hospital admissions (McCandless, Brunger, & Cassidy, 2004). Online Mendelian Inheritance in Man (OMIN, 2000) is a continuously updated catalogue of human genes and genetic diseases, which, as of February 2006, contained more than 5,560 different entries for disorders with a known or suspected genetic basis.

Referral to the Medical Genetics Clinic

The referral to the medical genetics clinic may arise from many different sources. Parents may seek an evaluation based on personal concerns about their child's development. In other situations, the developmental concerns may be brought to the parents' attention by the pediatrician. For others, a teacher may be the first to notice a school or learning difficulty and alert the parents to the possibility of a problem that should be discussed with their child's physician. Regardless of the initial source of the referral, parents who learn that their child may have a genetic disorder are frequently faced with learning about not only numerous possible disorders in the differential diagnosis for their child but also the plethora of testing options and strategies that can be used throughout the diagnostic evaluation process.

Medical Genetics Evaluation

The objective of a diagnostic medical genetics evaluation is the elucidation of the presence or suspicion of an underlying genetic etiology that explains a child's symptomatology. The diagnostic tools used in a medical genetics evaluation are structurally similar to those used as part of any medical evaluation. The process is usually led by a medical geneticist, a physician who has specialty training in the area of clinical medical genetics. The evaluation involves obtaining relevant medical and family history, performing a physical examination, discussing the different diagnostic possibilities, and recommending laboratory or other diagnostic studies.

There are now genetic tests clinically available for over 930 different genetic conditions (www.genetests.org, 1993–2006). Significant technological advances in molecular (Mitterer et al., 2005), chromosomal (Speicher & Carter, 2005), and biochemical (Chace & Kalas, 2005) analyses continue to lead to improved diagnostic tools. Despite the multitude of testing options and continuous advances in genetics and genomic science, many inherited disorders are not associated with a testable marker, and for some there is a paucity of significant research on which to establish a definitive test. Due to the intricate complexity of many available genetic tests, some tests can be performed at only a few specialized laboratories. Among these tests, analysis may take several months. Further, the detection rates (the ability of the test to actually find the causative gene change in the clinically affected individual) vary widely depending upon the condition, the test method, and sometimes even the ethnic background of the patient (O'Daniel & McConkie-Rosell, 2005). Knowledge of patient-specific factors such as clinical symptoms, ethnic background, and testing methodologies are all essential to the accurate interpretation of a test result, especially when determining what a negative (normal) result has actually ruled out. Thus, even with the tremendous advances in genetic testing technology, a test that confirms the diagnosis is not always available or even possible. In these situations, the patient(s) must rely on the clinical expertise of the medical geneticist.

To aid medical geneticists and other physicians in developing a strategy for evaluating a child with developmental delay, two algorithmic approaches have been published (Shevell et al., 2003; Battaglia & Carey, 2003). Both algorithms address prioritizing genetic testing while considering other sources of information such as neuroimaging, ophthalmologic, or audiologic assessments. When utilizing these algorithms, medical geneticists are trained to attend to the continual evolution in genetic science and testing technologies.

Genetic testing is not limited to children and their families. It can also be performed on a fetus during pregnancy. Prenatal genetic testing usually involves a tissue or cell sample that must be cultured (grown) in a laboratory for several days before testing can be performed. Diagnostic prenatal genetic testing is most often performed on cells collected from the amniotic fluid surrounding the fetus via amniocentesis, which can typically be performed after the 15th week of gestation. During amniocentesis, the cells collected from the amniotic fluid are derived from the fetus's skin cells (fibroblasts). In contrast, during chorionic villus sampling (CVS), cells are collected from the tissues that surround the fetal sac (the chorionic villi); this can be performed between the 10th and 13th weeks of pregnancy. Through a more rarely used procedure, percutaneous umbilical blood sampling (PUBS), fetal blood is obtained via the umbilical cord. PUBS may be performed after 16 weeks of pregnancy.

Although diagnostic prenatal genetic testing is highly accurate in over 99% of cases, an inconclusive result is possible and thus requires additional testing. In CVS testing, an inconclusive result occurs in up to 1% of cases. In addition, prenatal testing procedures are invasive to different extents and thus carry a risk for miscarriage or pregnancy complication, with PUBS having the highest risk (approximately 2%–3%). Lastly, the different tissues collected during pregnancy can affect the total amount of time required to analyze the sample. Couples considering diagnostic genetic testing during a pregnancy are strongly encouraged to meet with a genetic counselor or specialist obstetrician prior to or very early in pregnancy to discuss which prenatal procedures are best for them.

In addition to diagnostic testing, women may be offered routine screening tests such as a multiple marker screening or first-trimester screening. It is important to understand that screening modalities such as these assist the clinician in identifying pregnancies that are at an increased risk for certain birth defects such as open neural tube defects (spina bifida), Down syndrome, trisomy 18 and/or trisomy 13. These screening tests involve obtaining a blood sample from the pregnant mother and may also involve ultrasonographic measurements. Women whose pregnancies are identified as being at an increased risk for these disorders will be offered additional diagnostic tests (such as amniocentesis or CVS) to further investigate the specific risk.

The accuracy and wide availability of diagnostic prenatal genetic testing may create additional stress during the medical genetics evaluation process as families anxiously await diagnostic testing in their child. In some cases, the wait may be several weeks for the genetic analysis. If a genetic diagnosis can be confirmed with testing of a child, then (in most cases) the family can utilize that specific genetic test for prenatal diagnosis in future pregnancies. Individuals and their family members may struggle with decisions regarding how to best use this information in current and future family planning. Emotional conflicts may arise as family members (including parents, adult siblings, and extended family members) strive to resolve their feelings for the affected child with their own desire to have an unaffected child.

Components of Pediatric Genetic Counseling

Genetic counselors often work with a medical geneticist, as part of a team, obtaining family and medical history and helping to alleviate the confusion that may surround the diagnostic process. In the early stage of the genetic evaluation, an important role of the genetic counselor is that of "guide," explaining the individual steps and limitations in the genetic diagnostic process such as collection of medical, family, and pregnancy history; the types of testing available (e.g., biochemical, molecular, chromosomal); the limitations of that testing; and the differential diagnoses. Both the information exchanged and the manner in which it occurs sets the framework for the relationship with the patient(s). Typical components of an initial genetic counseling session(s) include the following:

- Contracting
- Collection/review of family medical history

• Discussion of clinical suspicion and findings
• Discussion and formulation of the diagnostic plan

Contracting is the process of identifying mutually agreed upon goals and the steps necessary to reach those goals. It is one of numerous interviewing techniques utilized by genetic counselors to "elicit, comprehend, evaluate, clarify, and confirm information about the family" (Baker, 1998, p. 55). Through contracting, the genetic counseling goals are presented and the expectations of the patient(s) are sought. Perceptions of the reason for referral to the genetics clinic are discussed, and areas of dissonance addressed. The candid discussion of these perceptions and expectations is essential to the foundation of an open, mutually trusting relationship between the genetic counselor and patient. The establishment of this manner of open rapport where information is not withheld from or by the patient results in greater satisfaction with the genetics clinic experience (Michie, Marteau, & Bobrow, 1997).

Collection/review of family medical history is often one of the strongest relationship-building tools in the genetic counseling process (Bennett, 2004). Family medical histories may be emotionally charged, often containing intimate information about illness, death, and relationships within the family (Bennett, 2004; Schuette & Bennet, 1998). Reviewing these histories of medical concerns present in the family affords the genetic counselor a chance to explore the family's experience with, and perception of, the concerns being addressed, including the severity and perceived burden of the disease and beliefs about the transmission of disease within the family. This review includes discussions of who is or is not at risk (Bennett, Hampel, Mandell, & Marks, 2003). Genetic counseling aims to incorporate this knowledge into the language and approach used in future discussions.

The family history information is routinely recorded in the format of a pedigree utilizing standard symbols (Bennett et al., 1995). This graphical depiction (figure 11.1) of family members can also be a useful educational tool, serving as a visual aid when discussing genetic risk assessment and inheritance patterns for disease within the family.

Discussion of clinical suspicion and findings can occur at numerous points throughout the diagnostic process. This discussion frequently incorporates complex genetic risk assessments based upon the family and medical histories or findings from a physical examination (Ogino & Wilson, 2004). The language used to describe these findings can be exclusionary of the patient, leading to mistrust of and frustration with the health care provider (Chapple, Campion, & May, 1997). Many patients have had little, if any, formal training in genetics, and much of their understanding of genetic terms and concepts has been influenced by the media (Lanie et al., 2004). Therefore, genetic terminology can present a unique challenge, as familiarity does not necessarily correlate with understanding (Lanie et al., 2004). The manner in which genetics is

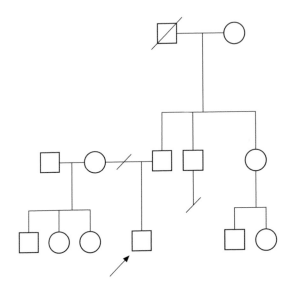

Common Pedigree Symbols

☐ Male	│	Vertical line = Generation; Descent from parents
○ Female	──	Horizontal line = Relationship
◇ Unknown sex	☐─○	Relationship (marriage)
↗ Indicates primary patient	☐─╱○	Relationship has ceased
⊠⊘ Deceased male, female	☐○	Sibling relationship

Figure 11.1
Sample pedigree.

portrayed in the popular media is often in accurate or in complete (Caulfield, 2004; Holtzman et al., 2005). Further, some words, like "syndrome" or "mutation," may frighten or alarm the patient and family based on the imagery associated with these terms (Chapple et al., 1997). Identifying areas of misconception may help alleviate some of the anxiety that patients and families may feel when referred for a genetics evaluation (Chapple et al., 1997; McGowan, 1999).

Careful attention is thus allotted to the descriptions and explanations given to the family. Genetics concepts, as they relate to the differential diagnosis, are introduced and explained in an appropriate manner; medical descriptions of physical character-istics such hypertelerism (wide set eyes) or fifth-finger clinodactyly (crooked pinky fingers) are explained. Maintaining the open rapport established through contracting, the genetic counselor and clinical genetics team discuss findings with the family. This inclusionary discussion can aid in the reduction of negative feelings such as parents becoming uncomfortable with or offended by the process (McGowan, 1999).

Discussion and formulation of the diagnostic plan are the natural conclusions to the clinical genetic evaluation. A summary of the differential diagnosis is presented. The diagnostic suspicion may be targeted to one specific disorder or encompass several related disorders. The suggested testing scenario(s) is discussed with the patient and family including the possible ramifications of positive (abnormal) or negative (normal) results. Some but not all genetic tests of children require the informed consent of the patient or guardian. During this stage, it is not unusual for the patient and family to seek advice on choosing a course of action (Karp, 1983). Building from the developing relationship with the patient and family, the genetic counseling can help the family make decisions that are consistent with their personal goals and values (O'Daniel & Wells, 2002).

For some families, the diagnostic process may be very straightforward. This is more commonly the case when the genetic condition is associated with easily recognizable physical features such as in Down syndrome or neurofibromatosis type 1 (NF-1). However, for many others, the diagnostic process requires patience and perseverance, frequently requiring multiple evaluations and medical tests. For some families, the investigative process may take several years before a definitive diagnosis is reached, and for others, an underlying genetic diagnosis may never be confirmed.

For example, a common reason for a medical genetics or other evaluation is to determine whether there is a genetic cause of a child's autism and developmental delay. Although autism describes a specific pattern of social, communicative, and cognitive delays, there are multiple genetic disorders associated with autism as a clinical feature. These disorders include Rett syndrome, Down syndrome, fragile X syndrome, tuberous sclerosis, untreated phenylketonuria, and small chromosome deletions or duplications (Veenstra-VanderWeele, Christain, & Cook, 2004). However, these specific genetic causes of autism account for only a small percentage of idiopathic autism. Therefore, for some children, even after extensive testing utilizing the most recent applicable technologies, the underlying cause of autism remains unknown. Although numerous variables are involved, such as patient population studied, extent of testing, and the year data were collected, different studies have suggested estimates of 20%–80% of patients remained undiagnosed following diagnostic evaluations (Battaglia, Bianchini, & Carey, 1999; Curry et al., 1997; Hunter, 2000).

Genetic counseling for families for whom a diagnosis remains elusive often includes a discussion of genetic testing results and the disorders that have been ruled out. The genetic counseling also includes a frank discussion of the level of suspicion regarding the possibility of an underlying genetic cause of the clinical symptoms. For some families the suspicion may be low, based on the outcome of the medical genetic evaluation. In this situation the family may be reassured that a genetic disorder is unlikely and thus should not reoccur in the family. For other families, the possibility of a genetic disorder based on the medical genetic evaluation remains high, and an empirical risk for recurrence of the suspected condition is given. In these families, follow-up assessment(s) is often essential as the child, medical knowledge, and diagnostic testing continually evolve.

The Diagnosis

Learning that your child has a genetic diagnosis is a life-changing, potentially life-shattering event (McGowan, 1999). Although the answers made possible by a definitive diagnosis may bring a sense of relief to a parent, this information can also lead to a feeling of isolation from others experiencing "normal parenting" (Barlow-Stewart & Gaff, 2003; Skirton, 2004). The experience has been likened to the bereavement process, where the child and the newly altered expectations of parenting that child are far removed from what was anticipated prior to the genetic concern. Furthermore, the altered expectations and perceptions associated with the diagnosis of a genetic disorder may also lead to a diminished sense of personal control. This sense of diminished perceived personal control was found to be strongest when the genetic diagnosis was associated with a cognitive disability (Berkenstadt et al., 1999).

One of the greatest benefits to knowing the genetic diagnosis is the possibility of anticipatory guidance. Although each patient is unique, the ability to learn from the health, developmental, and behavioral concerns faced by other individuals with the same diagnosis affords preventative measures through focused evaluations. Preventative health guidelines exist for several genetic conditions including Down syndrome (American Academy of Pediatrics Committee on Genetics, 2001), Turner syndrome (Frias, Davenport, & Endocrinology, Committee on Genetics and Section on Endocrinology, 2003), and NF-1 (American Academy of Pediatrics Committee on Genetics, 1995). In other less common genetic conditions, review of the scientific literature can provide guidance regarding possible concerns.

In addition to the health benefits of screening and early detection, anticipatory follow-up may also result in the child's receiving a greater benefit from timely developmental interventions. Parents may focus on one major feature of a genetic disorder to the exclusion of another, just as concerning clinical complication. For example, mild learning disabilities may go unnoticed until a child is behind in school and struggling to keep up. Knowing about an increased risk for learning difficulties can significantly aid early detection and initiate school intervention.

This anticipatory guidance can be exemplified by considering the case of a young patient with NF-1 from early childhood to adolescence. NF-1 is a relatively common condition, affecting approximately 1 person in 5,000 in the general population. It has a wide range of clinical symptoms that may affect both physical appearance and neurodevelopment and may result in significantly increased morbidity (see Slopis & Moore, chapter 5, this volume).

Case 11.1: Jamie Jamie first presented to the genetics clinic at 3 years of age. At birth she was found to have several faint birthmarks, which now seemed to be darkening. In addition, her parents thought there were two new very faint spots on her right foot. More out of curiosity than concern, they showed them to Jamie's pediatrician. The pediatrician told them that the spots could mean nothing at all but could also be associated with a genetic disorder called neurofibromatosis and referred them to the genetics clinic.

On physical examination by the medical geneticist, Jamie was found to have eight small birthmarks: two on her chest, one beside her belly button, one on her shoulder, one on her lower back, one on her left thigh, and two on her right foot. The genetics team (the medical geneticist and genetic counselor) explained that the birthmarks were consistent with café-au-lait spots seen in neurofibromatosis. In addition, Jamie had three tiny freckles in her right armpit that were consistent with axillary freckling also seen in neurofibromatosis. The genetics team talked with the parents and explained that these two different symptoms were enough to fulfill the clinical diagnostic criteria for NF-1. The diagnosis and clinical features of NF-1 were discussed with Jamie's parents. The availability of direct molecular testing for NF-1 was also discussed as were the possible benefits and limitations of the testing. Jamie was the only person in the family with any symptoms; this is consistent with reports that approximately 50% of NF-1 cases are sporadic rather than familial. Jamie's parents understood that they could still have very mild presentations of NF-1 but did not plan on having any more children. They decided to not pursue genetic testing at this time and allow that to be Jamie's decision later in life when she wanted that information for her own family. Instead, they chose to have eye examinations for the presence of Lisch nodules, which are found in greater than 95% of adults with NF-1. Normal eye examinations on the parents would be further evidence that Jamie was the first person in her family with NF-1.

At this visit, preventative screening guidelines for NF-1 were reviewed with Jamie's parents, and appointments were made for an ophthalmology evaluation and a 1-year follow-up visit in the genetics clinic for Jamie.

The ophthalmology evaluation revealed Jamie had several Lisch nodules, benign symptoms of NF-1, but did not have any evidence of optic glioma, a serious tumor of the optic nerve. Neither of Jamie's parents showed any evidence of NF-1 (figure 11.2).

At their 1-year follow-up visit, Jamie's parents were well adjusted to her diagnosis. They had attended a support group educational conference and were able to recognize that Jamie's case was mild. They became more knowledgeable about the various symptoms associated with NF-1 and eagerly discussed the latest research findings they had learned at the educational conference. At this time, Jamie is 3 years old and is developing normally. Her mother takes care of her in the home and reports no concerns.

At 5 years of age, Jamie and her family return to the genetics clinic. When discussing the interval history, Jamie's mother reports that Jamie is now in kindergarten. The teacher has mentioned that Jamie has some trouble with sitting still during circle time. The possibility of learning and behavior problems in children with the diagnosis of NF-1 was reviewed with the family. The parents state that they are not overly concerned, as they had expected Jamie would have an adjustment period since she did not attend preschool and that many 5-year-olds exhibit the same behaviors her teacher reports.

At 7 years of age, Jamie and her family return to the genetics clinic. When asked about school, Jamie's parents report they are becoming frustrated. In first grade, Jamie was a little behind in her

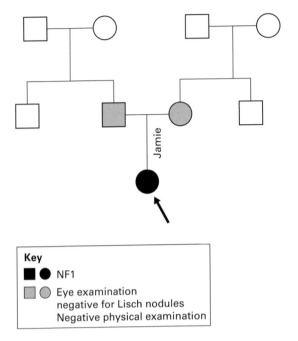

Figure 11.2
Family history of sporadic case of neurofibromatosis type 1 (NF-1). Although the parents elected to not have molecular testing of the NF-1 gene, the parental eye examination that is negative for Lisch nodules and a negative physical examination suggests that Jamie's neurofibromatosis is a new mutation. Jamie faces a 50% risk for having children with NF-1. Her parents' risk of having another affected child is greatly reduced.

reading abilities and was assigned to a small group for reading support. At first they were not concerned with her lack of progress, as Jamie is quite shy in groups, especially since she is smaller than most children her age (short stature is a clinical feature of NF-1). When spring came and she was still not progressing like the other children in her group, the parents asked if she could receive one-on-one tutoring. They were told this was not available but that they could seek private tutoring outside of school (but see chapter 15, this volume). Because of the cost of private tutoring, Jamie's parents tried to work with her each night and throughout the summer. Now, in the first month of second grade, Jamie was still not up to grade level and had again been assigned to the small group.

The medical genetics team reviewed that greater than 50% of children with NF-1 have learning difficulties, the most common of which is reading difficulties (Hyman, Shores, & North, 2005). Jamie's parents were surprised that this could be the NF-1. They thought that the learning problems would have shown up as a more significant developmental concern. They had not planned on telling the school about the NF-1 because they were fearful it could bias some educators to seek out learning and behavior problems in Jamie. The genetics team talked with Jamie's parents about the importance of informing the school about the diagnosis and discussed some of the services Jamie might qualify for because of her medical diagnosis. Although they had originally decided to keep Jamie's diagnosis from her teachers, they now sought information specific to the learning disabilities in NF-1 to share with her teachers and school.

> At 11 years of age Jamie and her parents return to the genetics clinic. School is improving for Jamie; however, her parents think that Jamie is becoming self-conscious about her spots. They state that she refused to take her t-shirt off when swimming and have seen her pull at her clothes, possibly to cover the spots on her legs and shoulder. They know that it is normal for any girl to become more self-conscious as she enters puberty but now wonder how the NF-1 could also be affecting Jamie's body image.
>
> The genetics team reviews that some symptoms of NF-1 may worsen during periods of hormonal changes like puberty and pregnancy. Although Jamie only has two small neurofibromas, she could develop more throughout her life because NF-1 is a progressive disorder. Even though Jamie would not be expected to develop severe cutaneous symptoms given her mild presentation thus far, she may continue to develop several café-au-lait spots and/or neurofibromas and is at risk for other symptoms as well.
>
> The genetics team, along with Jamie's parents, begin discussions with Jamie regarding her "spots" and "bumps" and how she feels about them. They work with Jamie and her parents to come up with honest answers to questions about her skin changes. The genetic counselor suggests Jamie could benefit from a pen pal her age with NF-1 and provides the family with contact information to set it up. The medical genetics team continues to maintain a relationship with Jamie and her parents as she matures into adulthood to help them address potential issues including genetic testing and recurrence risk for Jamie's future offspring.

Immediately following the diagnosis of a genetic disorder, genetic counseling sessions tend to focus on the parents and their informational needs, often including the provision of concrete resource materials that can be reviewed and shared with others. These may include the following:

· Patient letters to review the diagnosis and summarize the genetics clinic discussions

· Family letters to be shared with nonpresent family members that review the medical and genetic implications of the diagnosis

· Support group contact information

· Additional educational materials to help review the concepts

· Periodic follow-up

Return visits remain important following a confirmed diagnosis, allowing the complex, highly technical information to be spread out over several visits, thus providing time for review and assimilation (Barr, 1999). This approach also takes into account the potentially high emotional state of the patient and family when learning of a genetic diagnosis, which may interfere with retention and comprehension (McCarthy Veach, Truesdell, LeRoy, & Bartels, 1999). Because of the complexity of much of the genetic information combined with the emotional response to the diagnosis, follow-up visits may be used by genetic counselors to guide the discussions to include information on the social, medical, and educational concerns related to their child's disorder. Over time, the children will be included in the genetic counseling in an age-appropriate manner.

The potential for developmental disabilities may be dismissed in some disorders in which there is an apparently normal physical appearance and early development. Although there is significant variability with regard to the presence or severity of developmental disabilities in each of the conditions discussed in this book, it is important to be aware of the associations and to seek evaluation and assessment so that appropriate developmental, educational, behavioral, and social interventions can be put into place.

Genetic Counseling Beyond the Diagnosis

The educational process of understanding inheritance and clinical implications of a disorder is often only the beginning of the genetic counseling relationship. Parents of children with genetic disorders are also concerned about their child's social and emotional adjustment. Acknowledging and discussing the potential difficulties faced when attempting to adjust to a genetic diagnosis in the family can help provide tools to be used when and if those problems are encountered (McCarthy Veach et al., 1999; Bernhardt, Biesecker, & Mastromarino, 2000). For example, the reproductive risk of a newly diagnosed 2-year-old with NF-1 may be of little concern to the parents. However, these same parents, 13 years later, will often have significant concerns about how NF-1 affects their child's ability to integrate with peers and to someday have children.

Continued follow-up, with genetic counseling beyond the diagnosis, enables consideration of the family life stage, the developmental age of the child(ren) in the family, and the implications of the diagnosis itself. It also allows the counselor to focus on the family's current educational and psychosocial needs and to provide anticipatory guidance. Just as families change and develop over time, the genetic counseling role can be flexible and tailored to the current as well as future needs of the family. The presence of a genetic disorder in the family may affect normal family life stages and the achievement of developmental tasks and the transitions between them. Genetic counseling can help the family identify aspects of their family life in which developmental tasks may be affected by the genetic disorder, thus helping to identify major developmental tasks that will become important in the next year and anticipate future tasks for the affected child(ren), parents, and siblings. Once developmental tasks are identified, the discussion can focus on how the genetic disorder may influence the successful completion of those tasks. The genetic counselor can also help to resolve concerns by providing information about community resources. Proactively addressing these types of questions helps the family plan for successful transitions (Rolland, 1994).

Families have strengths and resilience (Boss, 1988), and genetic counseling can help tap into those strengths. Exploration of how parents perceive the diagnosis, adjust, and cope is an important ongoing aspect of the genetic counseling. The exploration of parental coping often informs how children in the family are also responding. The genetic disorder itself, and the morbidity and mortality associated with it, as well as whether or not there is medical treatment for the disorder, will directly influence how the family perceives the diagnosis. Parents' interactions with their child related to the genetic diagnosis and their responses to the disorder set the stage for the child's long-term adjustment (Weil, 2000).

Learning to Talk about the Diagnosis and Use New Information

An important part of adjusting to having a genetic condition in the family is learning how to talk about it. Helping parents answer questions about their child's diagnosis can be an important step. Initially, parents report wanting to know the facts about their child's diagnosis (Starke & Moller, 2002); however, these informational needs change over time. Parents may be the individuals informing educational, developmental, and other health professionals about the diagnosis. They may also be the persons primarily responsible for talking with their child(ren) about the diagnosis and possible prognosis (Hodgkinson & Lester, 2002). Genetic counseling can aid in the process as family members transition from the role of learner to advocate.

In addition to becoming an advocate for their child outside the family, parents may need to take on the role of advocate within their own families. Genetic disorders differ from other conditions as the diagnosis of one child may have significant implications beyond the parents and siblings. For some disorders, there can be significant risks to more distantly related family members. Therefore, families must learn to talk with each other about the diagnosis. As exemplified by Jed and his family in the following case, the diagnosis of fragile X syndrome has direct implications for Jed as well as for multiple relatives. In order to help meet the needs of the family, multiple clinic visits are required.

Case 11.2: Jed Jed is a 3-year-old with mild global developmental delay. Jed's parents said that they first became worried about his development when he was 2 years old because he did not have any clear words and communicated through crying and pointing. He now has only two to three words. Jed's mother reported that his medical history was significant only for multiple ear infections. His pediatrician has recommended pressure-equalizing tubes and initially felt that Jed would start talking when his hearing improved. When that didn't happen, his pediatrician referred Jed for a developmental evaluation. Jed was referred by his local Developmental Evaluation program to the Medical Genetics Clinic for additional evaluation of his developmental delay.

The physical examination by the medical geneticist found no dysmorphic features. Jed is a well-grown little boy whose height, weight, and head circumference are all in the 75th percentile. The family history was nonspecific. Jed has one older sister, Janet. Jed's parents reported that Janet was in kindergarten and is doing well. However, her teachers have commented that she is a little shy and has some difficulty making friends. There is a first cousin, a boy, who was also a little

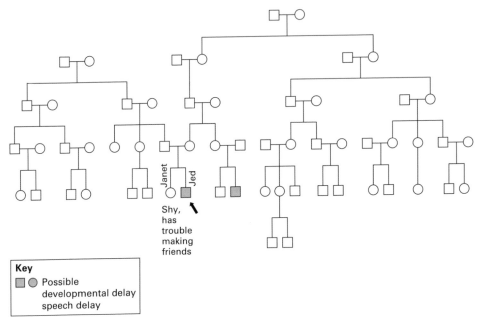

Key
Possible
  developmental delay
  speech delay

Figure 11.3
Jed's family history obtained at the initial appointment in the medical genetics clinic. The family history is dynamic and changes over time as relatives learn about the disorder and are tested.

slow to talk and may have some mild motor delays but is now felt by the family to be "coming around" (figure 11.3). As part of his evaluation, fragile X DNA analysis and a chromosome study were carried out.

The chromosome study was normal, 46, XY. The fragile X study was positive, demonstrating that Jed had both size and methylation mosaicism, confirming a diagnosis of fragile X syndrome (see Cornish, Levitas, & Sudhalter, this volume).

Jed, his sister, and his parents came back to the medical genetics clinic to discuss the diagnosis and implications for their family. Throughout the diagnostic process, Jed's parents have been focused solely on his developmental delay. All they wanted to know was when he was going to start talking. Now that the diagnosis of fragile X syndrome has been made, Jed's parents realize that this is not just speech delay but also has long-term implications for Jed as well as other family members. The focus of the initial counseling session with Jed's parents is on the clinical features and inheritance of fragile X syndrome and the need for comprehensive developmental interventions.

The genetic counselor reviews the family history with specific attention paid to who in the family could carry an unstable fragile X gene and for the mild clinical features of this disorder. With the diagnosis of fragile X syndrome, additional problems and concerns for other family members become apparent. During their previous clinic visit, Jed's parents had expressed no concerns about Jed's sister or other family members. The risk that his sister also has fragile X syndrome is 50%. The genetic counselor explained that sometime a child can seem fine, when compared to their more affected sibling, so that the developmental and educational concerns for the more mildly affected sibling can be overlooked. As part of the genetic counseling, parents have to be prepared that their "normal" child may also be affected. The parents decide to have Janet tested and schedule a return appointment to discuss the results of Janet's fragile X test.

Janet does, in fact, have a fragile X full mutation. At this visit, the focus is now on Janet. The parents were confused about how Jed could be so much more affected than his sister. The genetic counselor explains the process of X inactivation and the variability in the clinical presentation of fragile X syndrome in girls. Because of random X inactivation, some girls present with developmental concerns as significant as their affected brother while others have little to no clinical symptoms. The genetic counselor recommends that Janet be evaluated by the local developmental/ school program to assess for mild features of fragile X syndrome. If developmental concerns are present, then Janet's parents can work with her teacher and the school programs to develop an appropriate individualized educational program (see Sudhalter, this volume). Additionally, because of the expanding triplet repeat, there is new concern for the cousin who was previously thought to be a "slow talker like Jed." The genetic counselor discusses with Jed's parents different approaches to informing family members about the diagnosis of fragile X syndrome and the risk that relatives may also have an unstable FMR1 gene. The genetic counselor also provides Jed's parents with a family letter to be given to relatives, explaining the diagnosis. The family letter contains information on not only fragile X syndrome but also whom to contact if a relative is interested in learning more. The genetic counselor also works with the family to develop a follow-up plan for Jed, his sister, and his parents. Jed's parents would like to come back to the clinic in 3–6 months after they have had some time to digest all the information.

Six months later, Jed, Janet, and their parents return to the medical genetics clinic. They have made some progress in getting developmental services for both children. Jed's cousin has also been diagnosed with fragile X syndrome, and Jed's maternal grandfather has been found to be a carrier. However, no one else in the family has been tested, and the parents are very frustrated because no one seems to be interested or to believe them about how fragile X is inherited. The genetic counselor again reviews the family history, now knowing that the unstable repeat originated on the maternal grandfather's side of the family. Based on this information, the risk to other relatives can be more specifically determined. Additionally, the genetic counselor questions the parents, looking for a reliable relative who can help inform the family about fragile X. The parents identify Aunt May as the one everyone turns to when there is a problem. A follow-up plan is made with the parents to ask Aunt May to come to clinic with them at their next appointment.

Three months later, Aunt May, along with Jed's grandparents, attends the clinic appointment to learn more about fragile X syndrome. With Jed's parents' permission, the genetic counselor discusses the triplet repeat inheritance of fragile X syndrome. As Aunt May and Jed's grandparents learn more about fragile X syndrome and the implications for the extended family, Aunt May decides that she needs to start telling "her people" about fragile X. Over the next several years, various relatives contact the genetic counselor to find out about fragile X, and some decide to be tested (figure 11.4). The genetic counselor continues to work with the original proband family as well as the newly identified relatives.

Informing relatives about the diagnosis can be difficult when there are genetic risk implications for those family members (McConkie-Rosell et al., 1995). Relatives may not believe the genetic risk is real, especially when the disorder exhibits a complex inheritance pattern such as that seen in fragile X syndrome (McConkie-Rosell et al., 1995). Genetic counseling can facilitate the communication of genetic risk information to relatives by helping the patient's family first to identify "at-risk" relatives and then to develop informational strategies for successful communication. Genetic counselors often provide the patient's family with a general informational letter that

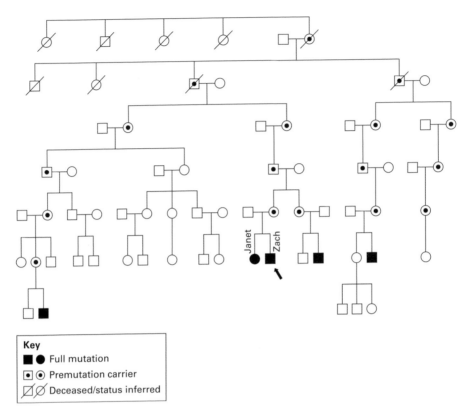

Figure 11.4
Zach's family history at a follow-up visit several years after the diagnosis of fragile X syndrome.

can be distributed among other family members. Such a letter includes a description of the disorder recently diagnosed in the family, how it is inherited, and the risk to relatives. Included with this letter is contact information for a medical genetics program, for relatives interested in obtaining more information (Baker, Eash, Schuette, & Uhlmann, 2002; McConkie-Rosell et al., 1995).

Family Talk: What a Child Hears and Understands

While a 2-year-old may have no memory of the diagnostic process, over time the child may incorporate the family "stories" about the diagnosis into that "memory." In describing how young children recall traumatic events, Fivush (1998) found that children not only are affected by the event as it is occurring but are even more affected by how it is discussed afterwards. Children may learn more from their parents' reaction and how they themselves experience that reaction than from what is simply said (Koopman, Baars, Chaplin, & Zwinderman, 2004). Thus, children may not understand the implications of the diagnosis but will often focus on the emotion with which it is presented.

Children overhear conversations being held by adults both at home and in the clinical setting with professionals. From these conversations, children may begin drawing their own conclusions. They may overhear conversations among family members going through testing themselves, including discussions of who is and who is not a carrier in the family. Tercyak et al. (2001) found that the greatest exposure of children to genetic information was indirectly through contact with family members who were affected or who were undergoing testing themselves. Simple statements that are easily comprehended by an adult may be misunderstood by a child such as a comment about terminating a pregnancy. It is critically important that possible misunderstandings are anticipated and addressed. For example, children have expressed concerns about "catching" a genetic disorder (Fanos, 1999; Fanos, Davis, & Puck, 2001). Therefore, even in families with very young children, the genetic counseling includes discussion of how parents and close family members describe the disorder to others, including children.

Talking with children about either their own or their sibling's diagnosis of a genetic disorder is not simply a matter of using different words; the children's developmental age and ability to understand must also be taken into account. Children often have questions about the disorder. Genetic counseling can also enhance a child's understanding about the disorder as well as provide an "opportunity for expressing, validating, and addressing their emotions" (Weil, 2000, p. 181). Repeated sessions, occurring over many years, allow the opportunity to address misinformation and provide new information regarding the diagnosis, including medical or educational interventions, as well as an opportunity to manage the maturing emotional responses to the diagnosis.

Children affected by genetic disorders have to adapt to the physical, cognitive, and social effects of their disorder (Weil, 2000). When the diagnosis of a progressive disorder such as NF-1 is made in a young child, there is uncertainty. It is impossible to predict how much disfigurement and physical impairment will result or how the NF-1 will affect educational and social issues. A child may have more or fewer clinical features than an affected parent. Just as parents learn to manage the uncertainty, with time, so does the child.

Talking to a child who has cognitive disabilities as a result of a genetic disorder can be especially challenging. The child's cognitive level of understanding and emotional maturity have to be considered in determining how information is discussed. For example, although children with Williams syndrome may only be able to understand their diagnosis at a very basic level, it can be helpful to practice the words to respond to specific questions about the diagnosis.

Talking about Recurrence Risks

Besides the physical and emotional effects on the child and family, a genetic diagnosis may also carry significant implications for current and future family members. The move from diagnosis to recurrence risk is often very difficult, as is talking to children about genetic risk. Parents often worry about the potential harm genetic risk knowledge may have on their child's developing self-concept and at the same time search for ways to help their child positively adapt to this information (McConkie-Rosell, Spiridigliozzi, Dawson, Sullivan, & Lachiewicz, 2002; McConkie-Rosell, Spiridigliozzi, Iafolla, Tarleton, & Lachiewicz, 1997; McConkie-Rosell et al., 1999). Parents are also faced with difficult questions regarding when and how to provide genetic risk information to a child who faces a risk for having affected offspring in the future. A child with NF-1 faces a 50% chance of passing on this autosomal dominant disorder. A girl with the fragile X full mutation also faces a 50% chance of passing the altered X to her offspring. Conversely, instead of a risk for having an affected child, disorders such as Turner syndrome or Klinefelter syndrome carry a loss of reproductive potential. Genetic counseling for these disorders includes a discussion of infertility in the context of life decisions and timing for reproduction (Sybert, 2001).

Parents of children with genetic disorders that cause significant developmental disabilities face a combination of concerns related to their child's sexuality and reproduction. These concerns include the possibility of their affected child having affected offspring, protecting the child who may be vulnerable to predators (Levy & Packman, 2004), and helping the child make realistic decisions about having a baby of their own (Finucane, 1998). Genetic counseling can help parents start thinking through the process of talking with their children about genetic information.

Discussions also need to be sensitive to the emotional development and concerns for the maturing child. When counseling a young woman with cognitive disabilities, Finucane (1998) has emphasized the importance of shifting the focus of the genetic counseling from educational facts about the disorder and genetic risk to exploration of the emotions related to wanting to become a mother. Others have also emphasized the importance of focusing on the social and emotional development of a young person with cognitive disabilities, not just the developmental level of that individual (Thomasgard & Metz, 2004).

There may also be concerns regarding the reproductive risks for the clinically unaffected child(ren) in the family. Parents report that they have a parental right to decide when to inform children of the genetic risk and when to seek carrier testing (McConkie-Rosell et al., 1999). Although some families actively address this concern, others do not know where to begin. Additionally, the child(ren) may view the information quite differently from their parents (either as more positive and less threatening or as more negative). Genetic counseling aims to help families formulate an approach to this information (McConkie-Rosell & Spiridigliozzi, 2004) by considering the following:

· What is the age of the child(ren) in the family?

· What are the implications of genetic information at different ages and developmental stages?

· What are the implications of learning the information now versus a staged approach in the future?

When appropriate, a genetic counselor seeks to engage the child directly or indirectly through the parents or caretakers in order to explore the following:

· What is their personal experience with the disorder?

· What have they been told about the specific disorder?

· What do they know/understand about the specific disorder?

· What is their perception of the family's emotional response?

· What do they do to manage negative emotions?

· What do they know/understand about their risk for being a carrier or to be affected and what this might mean for them individually?

· Do they have a motivating factor for wanting genetic testing?

· Do they understand what the test results might mean?

These questions can be framed for inclusion of either the affected child or the unaffected sibling.

What about Me? Other Children in the Family

Siblings frequently do not understand why their brother or sister is the focus of family attention and the adjustments to daily life required to accommodate the child (Weil, 2000). If the parent(s) is overwhelmed by the needs of the affected child, the parent may become emotionally less available to the unaffected child(ren) (Fanos, 1997). Resentment of the affected child, including parental attention and necessary accommodations, can be a source of difficulty for the family and negatively affect the sibling's relationships with family members. These feelings of anger and jealousy toward an affected brother or sister can also lead to feelings of guilt, which may be exacerbated by the genetics of the disorder (Weil, 2000).

Opperman and Alant (2003) found that adolescent siblings (12–16 years of age) of children with severe disabilities did not have detailed knowledge about their own brother or sister's disability. They concluded that in order to help the unaffected sibling develop effective coping strategies, it is important that the sibling be well informed about the disorder and its consequences. Siblings need to have an opportunity to practice responses to questions like "What is wrong with your brother—why does he act that way?" In addition, adult siblings have been found to carry misunderstanding about genetic information learned as a child into their adulthood (Fanos et al., 2001; Fanos & Gatti, 1999). The needs of the unaffected siblings will change over time. These siblings may express conflict between loving their affected sibling and not wanting to be the parent of a child with the same disorder. Additionally, they may have to identify when in a romantic relationship they feel they should inform someone about their personal reproductive genetic risk as well as the probability of a life-long responsibility to their affected sibling.

Unaffected siblings' attitudes about themselves, their family, and their affected sibling are influenced by the quality of the sibling relationship, family interactions, personality characteristics and communication style, and the parent–child relationships (McConkie-Rosell & Spiridigliozzi, 2004; Opperman & Alant, 2003). Inclusion of the clinically unaffected siblings is an important component of genetic counseling and encourages the message that their opinions matter, too. The focus of the counseling is the exploration of how the sibling views his or her affected brother or sister and to identify and discuss their specific concerns.

Conclusion

Families are constantly changing, growing, and developing. In a pediatric setting, genetic counseling includes discussions aimed at helping the family identify the many ways in which their family is responding to the diagnosis. By partnering with the family to provide accurate, appropriate, and timely information, genetic counseling can help empower families to take control of the genetic information and to apply it in a meaningful way.

Note

1. Throughout this chapter reference to the patient includes cases of individual adults, couples, a child, or a family.

References

American Academy of Pediatrics Committee on Genetics. (1995). Health supervision for children with neurofibromatosis. *Pediatrics, 96*(2, Pt 1), 368–372.

American Academy of Pediatrics: Committee on Genetics. (2001). *American Academy of Pediatrics: Health supervision for children with Down syndrome. Pediatrics, 107,* 442–449.

Baker, D. L. (1998). Interviewing techniques. In D. L. Baker, J. L. Schuette, & W. R. Uhlmann (Eds.), *A guide to genetic counseling* (pp. 55–98). New York: Wiley-Liss.

Baker, D. L., Eash, T., Schuette, J. L., & Uhlmann, W. R. (2002). *Guidelines for writing letters to patients. Journal of Genetic Counseling, 11,* 399–418.

Barlow-Stewart, K., & Gaff, C. (2003). Working in partnership with support services in the era of the "new genetics." *Medical Journal of Australia, 178,* 515–519.

Barr, O. (1999). Genetic counselling: A consideration of the potential and key obstacles to assisting parents adapt to a child with learning disabilities. *British Journal of Learning Disabilities, 27,* 30–36.

Battaglia, A., Bianchini, E., & Carey, J. (1999). Diagnostic yield of the comprehensive assessment of developmental delay/mental retardation in an institute of child neuropsychiatry. *American Journal of Medical Genetics, 82,* 60–66.

Battaglia, A., & Carey, J. (2003). Diagnostic evaluation of developmental delay/mental retardation: An overview. *American Journal of Medical Genetics (Semin. Med. Genet.), 117C,* 3–14.

Bennett, R. (2004). The family medical history. *Primary care: Clinics in office practice, 31,* 479–495.

Bennett, R., Hampel, H., Mandell, J., & Marks, J. (2003). Genetic counselors: Translating genomic science into clinical practice. *Journal of Clinical Investigation, 112,* 1274–1279.

Bennett, R., Steinhaus, K., Ulrich, S., O'Sullivan, C., Resta, R., Lochner-Doyle, D., et al. (1995). Recommendations for standardized pedigree nomenclature. *American Journal of Human Genetics, 56,* 745–752.

Berkenstadt, M., Shiloh, S., Barkai, G., Katznelson, M.-M., & Goldman, B. (1999). Perceived personal control (ppc): A new concept in measuring outcome of genetic counseling. *American Journal of Medical Genetics, 82,* 53–59.

Bernhardt, B., Biesecker, B., & Mastromarino, C. (2000). Goals, benefits and outcomes of genetic counseling: Client and genetic counselor assessment. *American Journal of Medical Genetics, 94,* 189–197.

Boss, P. (1988). *Family stress management* (Vol. 8). Newbury Park, London: Sage.

Caulfield, T. (2004). Biotechnology and the popular press: Hype and the selling of science. *Trends in Biotechnology, 22,* 337–339.

Chace, D. H., & Kalas, T. A. (2005). A biochemical perspective on the use of tandem mass spectrometry for newborn screening and clinical testing. *Clinical Biochemistry, 38,* 296–309.

Chapple, A., Campion, P., & May, C. (1997). Clinical terminology: Anxiety and confusion amongst families undergoing genetic counseling. *Patient Education and Counseling, 32,* 81–91.

Cheung, S., Shaw, C., Yu, W., Li, J., Ou, Z., Patel, A., et al. (2005). Development and validation of a CGH microarray for clinical cytogenetic diagnosis. *Genetics in Medicine, 7,* 422–432.

Curry, C., Stevenson, R., Aughton, D., Byrne, J., Carey, J., Cassidy, S., et al. (1997). Evaluation of mental retardation: Recommendations of a consensus conference. *American Journal of Medical Genetics, 72,* 468–477.

Fanos, J. (1999). The missing link in linkage analysis: The well sibling revisited. *Genetic Testing, 3,* 273–278.

Fanos, J. H. (1997). Developmental tasks of childhood and adolescence: Implications for genetic testing. *American Journal of Medical Genetics, 71,* 22–28.

Fanos, J. H., Davis, J., & Puck, J. M. (2001). Sib understanding of genetics and attitudes toward carrier testing for x-linked severe combined immunodeficiency. *American Journal of Medical Genetics, 98,* 46–56.

Fanos, J. H., & Gatti, R. A. (1999). A mark on the arm: Myths of carrier status in sibs of indivdiuals with ataxia-telangiectasia. *American Journal of Medical Genetics, 86,* 338–346.

Finucane, B. (1998). Acculturation in women with mental retardation and its impact on genetic counseling. *Journal of Genetic Counseling, 7,* 31–47.

Fivush, R. (1998). Children's recollections of traumatic and nontraumatic events. *Development and Psychopathology, 10,* 699–717.

Frias, J., Davenport, M., & Endocrinology, Committee on Genetics and Section on Endocrinology. (2003). Health supervision for children with Turner syndrome. *Pediatrics, 111,* 692–702.

Genetests: Medical genetics information resource [Database online]. Copyright University of Washington, Seattle. 1993–2006. Updated weekly. Retrieved February 6, 2006 from http://www.geneclinics.org.

Hodgkinson, R., & Lester, H. (2002). Stresses and coping strategies of mothers living with a child with cystic fibrosis: Implications for nursing professionals. *Journal of Advanced Nursing, 39*(4), 377–383.

Holtzman, N., Berhardt, B., Mountcastle-Shah, E., Rodgers, J., Tambor, E., & Geller, G. (2005). The quality of media reports on discoveries related to human genetic diseases. *Community Genetics, 8,* 133–144.

Hunter, A. (2000). Outcome of the routine assessment of patients with mental retardation in a genetic clinic. *American Journal of Medical Genetics, 90,* 60–68.

Hyman, S., Shores, A., & North, K. (2005). The nature and frequency of cognitive deficits in children with neurofibromatosis type 1. *Neurology, 65,* 1037–1044.

Karp, L. (1983). The terrible question. *American Journal of Medical Genetics, 14,* 1–4.

Koopman, H. M., Baars, R. M., Chaplin, J., & Zwinderman, K. H. (2004). Illness through the eyes of the child: The development of children's understanding of the causes of illness. *Patient Education and Counseling, 55,* 363–370.

Lanie, A., Jayaratne, T., Sheldon, J., Kardia, S., Anderson, E., Feldbaum, M., et al. (2004). Exploring the public understanding of basic genetic concepts. *Journal of Genetic Counseling, 13,* 305–320.

Levy, H., & Packman, W. (2004). Sex abuse prevention for individuals with mental retardation: Considerations for genetic counselors. *Journal of Genetic Counseling, 13,* 189–205.

McCandless, S., Brunger, J., & Cassidy, S. (2004). The burden of genetic disease on inpatient care in a children's hospital. *American Journal of Human Genetics, 74,* 121–127.

McCarthy Veach, P., Truesdell, S., LeRoy, B., & Bartels, D. (1999). Client perceptions of the impact of genetic counseling: An exploratory study. *Journal of Genetic Counseling, 8,* 191–216.

McConkie-Rosell, A., Robinson, H., Wake, S., Staley, L., Heller, K., & Cronister, A. (1995). The dissemination of genetic risk information to relatives in the fragile X syndrome: Guidelines for genetic counselors. *American Journal of Medical Genetics, 59,* 426–430.

McConkie-Rosell, A., & Spiridigliozzi, G. A. (2004). "Family matters": A conceptual framework for genetic testing in children. *Journal of Genetic Counseling, 13,* 9–29.

McConkie-Rosell, A., Spiridigliozzi, G., Dawson, D., Sullivan, J., & Lachiewicz, A. (2002). Carrier testing in fragile x syndrome: When to tell and test. *American Journal of Medical Genetics, 110,* 36–44.

McConkie-Rosell, A., Spiridigliozzi, G. A., Iafolla, T., Tarleton, J., & Lachiewicz, A. M. (1997). Carrier testing in the fragile x syndrome. *American Journal of Medical Genetics, 68,* 62–69.

McConkie-Rosell, A., Spiridigliozzi, G. A., Rounds, K., Dawson, D., Sullivan, J. A., Burgess, D., et al. (1999). Parental attitudes regarding carrier testing in children at-risk for fragile x syndrome. *American Journal of Medical Genetics, 82,* 206–211.

McConkie-Rosell, A., & Sullivan, J. (1999). Genetic counseling—Stress, coping, and the empowerment perspective. *Journal of Genetic Counseling, 8,* 345–358.

McGowan, R. (1999). Beyond the disorder: One parent's reflection on genetic counselling. *Journal of Medical Ethics, 25,* 195–199.

Michie, S., Marteau, T., & Bobrow, M. (1997). Genetic counselling: The psychological impact of meeting patients' expectations. *Journal of Medical Genetics, 34,* 237–241.

Mitterer, G., Bodamer, O., Harwanegg, C., Maurer, W., Mueller, M., & Schmidt, W. (2005). Microarray-based detection of mannose-binding lectin 2 (mbl2) polymorphisms in a routine clinical setting. *Genetic Testing, 9,* 6–13.

O'Daniel, J., & McConkie-Rosell, A. (2005). Test results: Communication and counseling. In N. F. Sharpe & R. F. Carter (Eds.), *Genetic testing: Care, consent, and liability* (pp. 355–397). New York: Wiley.

O'Daniel, J., & Wells, D. (2002). Approaching complex cases with a crisis intervention model and teamwork. *Journal of Genetic Counseling, 11,* 369–376.

Ogino, S., & Wilson, R. (2004). Bayesian analysis and risk assessment in genetic counseling and testing. *Journal of Molecular Diagnostics, 6,* 1–9.

OMIN. (2000). Online Mendelian inheritance in man, OMIN™. Retrieved June 29, 2005, from http://www.ncbi.nlm.nih.gov/omim/

Opperman, S., & Alant, E. (2003). The coping response of the adolescent siblings of children with severe disabilities. *Disability and Rehabilitation, 25,* 441–454.

Resta, R., Bowles Biesecker, B., Bennett, R. L., Blum, S., Estabrooks-Hahn, S., Strecker, M. N., et al. (2006). A new definition of genetic counseling: National Society of Genetic Counselors' Task Force Report. *Journal of Genetic Counseling, 15,* 77–83.

Rolland, J. S. (1994). *Families, illness, and disability.* New York: Basic Books.

Schuette, J., & Bennet, R. (1998). Lessons in history: Obtaining the family history and constructing a pedigree. In D. Baker, J. Schuette, & W. Uhlmann (Eds.), *A guide to genetic counseling* (pp. 27–51). New York: Wiley-Liss.

Shevell, M., Ashwal, S., Donley, D., Flint, J., Gingold, M., Hirtz, D., et al. (2003). Practice parameter: Evaluation of the child with global developmental delay: Report of the Quality Standards Subcommittee of the American Academy of Neurology and the Practice Committee of the Child Neurology Society. *Neurology, 60,* 367–380.

Shiloh, S. (1996). Genetic counseling: A developing area of interest for psychologists. *Professional Psychology: Research and Practice, 27,* 475–486.

Skirton, H. (2004). More than just science: One family's story of a chromosome translocation diagnosis. *Paediatric Nursing, 16*(10), 18–21.

Speicher, M. R., & Carter, N. P. (2005). The new cytogenetics: Blurring the boundaries with molecular biology. *Nature, 6,* 782–792.

Starke, M., & Moller, A. (2002). Parents' needs for knowledge concerning the medical diagnosis of their children. *Journal of Child Health Care, 6,* 245–257.

Sybert, V. P. (2001). Turners syndrome. In S. B. Cassidy & J. E. Allanson (Eds.), *Management of genetic syndromes* (pp. 459–484). New York: Wiley-Liss.

Tercyak, K., Hughes, C., Main, D., Snyder, C., Lynch, J., Lynch, H., et al. (2001). Parental communication of BRCA1/2 genetic test results to children. *Patient Education and Counseling, 42,* 213–224.

Thomasgard, M., & Metz, W. P. (2004). Promoting child social–emotional growth in primary care settings: Using a developmental approach. *Clinical Pediatrics, 43,* 119–127.

Veenstra-VanderWeele, J., Christain, S. L., & Cook, E. H. (2004). Autism as a paradigmatic complex genetic disorder. *Annual Review of Genomics and Human Genetics, 5,* 379–405.

Weil, J. (2000). *Psychosocial genetic counseling.* New York: Oxford University Press.

Wilcox, L., & Marks, J. (1999). *From data to action. Center for Disease Control's public health surveillance for women, infants and children.* Atlanta, GA: U.S. Department of Health and Human Services, Public Health Service, Centers for Disease Control and Prevention.

From Diagnosis to Adaptation: Optimizing Family and Child Functioning When a Genetic Diagnosis Is Associated with Mental Retardation

Laraine Masters Glidden and Sarah A. Schoolcraft

Mental retardation is a condition characterized by "significantly subaverage intellectual functioning (an IQ of approximately 70 or below) with onset before age 18 years and concurrent deficits or impairments in adaptive functioning" (American Psychiatric Association, 2000, p. 39). Of the three definitional components—IQ, adaptive behavior, and age—the most straightforward is the age of onset, although not all definitions of mental retardation specify age 18; some pinpoint age 22 as a cutoff (Jacobson & Mulick, 1996). The older age criterion may reflect a belief in a longer developmental trajectory as well as concern for eligibility for educational services to which children with disabilities are entitled only until their 22nd birthday.

In this chapter, in addition to defining and describing mental retardation, we review important societal and family issues associated with raising children with mental retardation. We highlight national and international movements that have resulted in massive changes in the way individuals with mental retardation and their families live their lives. We also emphasize the roles that medical and health professionals can play to help families adapt to the rearing of a child with mental retardation. Positive adaptation leads to a more optimal environment for the child and other family members, both parents and siblings. Because adaptation is a dynamic process that takes place over extended periods of time, we have organized that section chronologically, focusing first on the diagnosis and factors that influence family reaction to it, and then on adaptation during childhood and the variables that are important to it. In each period, we highlight the critical challenges that must be met for adaptation to be successful, specifically those challenges that may vary depending on the level of severity of the mental retardation.

Heterogeneity of Functioning

Although the dual criteria of intelligence and adaptive behavior are formally part of most definitions of mental retardation, levels of mental retardation are frequently specified only by IQ ranges. For example, the *Diagnostic and Statistical Manual of Mental Disorders* (4th ed., text revision; American Psychiatric Association, 2000, p. 42) specifies four degrees of severity—mild, moderate, severe, and profound—with IQ levels of 50–55 to approximately 70, 35–40 to 50–55, 20–25 to 35–40, and below 20–25, respectively. These ranges generally correspond to IQ scores that are 2–3, 3–4, 4–5, and below 5 *SD*s from the mean. Ranges rather than absolute IQ scores are used because different IQ tests have standard deviations of different sizes, and because measurement error puts some reliance on the clinical judgment of the diagnostician. Although precise figures are unknown, it is generally agreed that at least 60% of school-age children with mental retardation have IQ scores in the mild range, with some estimates as high as 75% (McLaren & Bryson, 1987).

The definition and assessment of adaptive behavior is rooted in the kinds of daily tasks that an individual of a given age and culture is expected to perform successfully. The American Psychiatric Association (2000) uses a criterion of significant limitations in at least two of the following domains: communication, self-care, self-direction, social and interpersonal skills, home living, academic tasks, health, safety, leisure, use of community resources, and work, as did the 1992 definition of the American Association on Mental Retardation (AAMR). However, in its latest edition of a definition and classification manual (AAMR, 2002), the AAMR[1] described adaptive behavior in terms of three skill dimensions: conceptual, social, and practical. Conceptual skills are those mostly closely linked with the lay concept of intelligence, such as the language-based activities of listening, speaking, reading, and writing. Social skills include mostly those activities that involve others. Examples would be interpersonal interaction and compliance with formal and informal rules. Practical skills are those that include activities of daily living such as eating, toileting, hygiene, and using mass transportation.

Recently developed or revised standardized tests assess adaptive behaviors. They are usually completed by someone who knows the person with mental retardation quite well and has had an opportunity to observe and interact with him or her in a variety of settings over time. Family members, other caretakers, and teachers are frequently the informants. Examples of well-regarded instruments for adaptive behavior measurement are the AAMR Adaptive Behavior Scale (Lambert, Nihira, & Leland, 1993), the Adaptive Behavior Assessment System II (Harrison & Oakland, 2002), and the Vineland Adaptive Behavior Scale (Sparrow, Cicchetti, & Balla, 2005).

Clearly, adaptive behavior skills are linked to developmental level. During the infancy period, adaptive behaviors consist mostly of gross and fine motor skills with communication such as joint attention, pointing, receptive expression, and single-word utterances becoming relevant as the infant approaches toddlerhood. By adulthood, all three dimensions of conceptual, social, and practical skills are important, and deficits in any of them can lead to significantly reduced quality of life and the need for greater intensity of supports to successfully engage in the society, whether it be for vocational, family, or recreational pursuits.

Diagnostic and Etiological Challenges

Lags in both cognitive and adaptive behavior skills are important in identifying children with mental retardation. Those with moderate, severe, and profound mental retardation are typically identified in infancy because they fail to meet motor milestones such as sitting up, crawling, and walking. Moreover, early language acquisition such as single words at 12–18 months and two-word utterances at 24 months are almost always delayed. Most disagreement with regard to diagnosis occurs with individuals at the mild level of mental retardation. Because mental retardation may not have a known medical etiology, its diagnosis is, in part, based on the expectation for behavior in the society. In a simple society where demands for abstract thinking or advanced literacy or numeracy are minimal, many individuals with mild mental retardation may not be identified. Indeed, in our own society, many children with mild mental retardation are diagnosed not by medical practitioners but rather by psychologists in the educational setting, where their academic failures may be the first formal indication of intellectual and adaptive behavior deficits. However, even children with mild mental retardation may display delays that are noticeable in the preschool period, particularly with regard to academic readiness skills such as visual identification of letters and numbers, as well as memory problems for sequences such as counting and days of the week. Their vocabulary is likely to be much smaller than that of other children their age, and they are likely to have difficulty with abstractions, such as recognizing that apples and oranges are both fruits.

Diverse Etiology

The etiology of mental retardation is diverse, with genetic or other biological characteristics often interacting with psychosocial environmental contexts to produce deficits in both IQ and adaptive behavior. Effects are often complex and interactive with pre-, peri- and postnatal factors all combining to elevate and cumulate risk. Consider the following case: A poor, uneducated, young, single pregnant woman receives little or no prenatal care. During her pregnancy, she drinks, smokes, and uses other drugs suspected of being harmful to prenatal development. She has a difficult labor and birth and her child is low birth weight. Following the birth, she receives little or no support from her family of origin or from the father of her child. She lives in inadequate housing and has little money available even for the basic necessities of food, clothing, shelter, and health. Many factors contribute to the risk that her child will have lowered IQ and adaptive behavior. They include prenatal toxins such as alcohol; poor prenatal care; anoxia during birth, and respiratory or brain damage associated with other birth difficulties and low birth weight; poor sanitation and nutrition after birth coupled with lack of good health care; and lack of educational stimulation of the sort that would likely be provided by a parent whose access to resources afforded easy access to basic survival needs. Because of this complexity and cumulative risk, often a specific underlying etiology of mental retardation is difficult to identify. Although estimates vary, there is some consensus that in at least 50% of all cases of mental retardation, no single cause can be determined (Beirne-Smith, Patton, & Kim, 2006), with even higher percentages of unkown etiology associated with milder mental retardation (Durkin & Stein, 1996). This may seem surprising in light of the known genetic etiologies of mental retardation such as Down syndrome or fragile X syndrome, but not in light of the complex range of genetic and environmental influences on development as exemplified in chapters 8 and 9, and chapter 10, respectively.

Regardless of the etiology, intensive early intervention is generally regarded as an effective form of primary, secondary, and tertiary prevention (Ramey & Ramey, 1992; Ramey, Ramey, Lanzi, & Cotton, 2002; Guralnick, 1997), although effects may be small, and not all children are equally benefited (Farran, 2000). For example, in the multisite Infant Health and Development Program, intensive intervention was provided to low-birth-weight infants who weighed less than 2,500 g. Results at 36 months indicated general improvement in intellectual functioning in comparison to those for whom intensive intervention was not provided, but the heavier children with birth weight between 2,001 and 2,500 g improved relatively more than did the children weighing 2,000 g or less (Hill, Brooks-Gunn, & Waldfogel, 2003; Ramey, 1998; Ramey et al., 1992).

Even children functioning at profound levels of mental retardation, where measured IQ is below 25, can benefit from education and training. They can show improvements in many areas of adaptive functioning such as personal care and hygiene and communication skills (Breslau, 2001; Ramey et al., 2002). And for children with mild to moderate levels of retardation, far more is possible with appropriate education. As an example, the life course for individuals with Down syndrome born in the early 21st century is remarkably different from what it was for cohorts born in the early 20th century. Life expectancy has increased dramatically, and there is general agreement that both intellectual functioning and adaptive behavior have improved, primarily because of better education (Jancar & Jancar, 1996; Merrick, 2000; Breslau, 2001; Ramey et al., 2002). Hatton and Sudhalter each have chapters in this volume that describe early intervention and educational plans that may enhance the functioning of both children and parents.

Stigmatization

Despite the improved prognosis for children with mental retardation and the increased opportunities available for them, it is among the most feared and stigmatized of all disabilities diagnosed in childhood (Gottlieb & Gottlieb, 1977). In fact, for conditions such as Down syndrome, associated with visible physical characteristics, families may choose cosmetic surgery to reduce or eliminate the noticeable and syndrome-identifying features (Katz & Kravetz, 1989a, 1989b; May, 1988; Katz, Kravetz, & Marks, 1997; Goeke, 2003). Furthermore, this stigma may be responsible for an actual decline in the number of individuals who are diagnosed with mental retardation. In the United States, currently, many children with IQ scores in the 55–70 range who could be classified as having mild mental retardation are instead being labeled as learning disabled. In just 25 years, from 1976 to 2001, school-age children with the mental retardation classification dropped from 26% to just 10.8% of all school-age children with a disability diagnosis (U.S. Department of Education, 2003). Experts have written about the reluctance of parents, educators, and other professionals to use the mental retardation label, and the resulting disappearance of mild mental retardation (MacMillan, Siperstein, & Leffert, 2003; Spitz, 2003).

Uncertainty of Prognosis   This fear and stigma is compounded by the wide range of functioning found within the population of individuals with mental retardation, including those with the same diagnosed condition, making prognoses unreliable (Constable, 2004). Consider the following two children, each of whom has mental retardation:

Case 12.1: Leona   Leona was born with Trisomy-9q, indicating that one of the chromosome 9 homologs has a duplicate copy of the long arm (q). Leona's grandmother was the first to note her "unusual" look (Leona had a large head), and the pediatrician tested for and confirmed the Trisomy-9q. Initially, her physicians provided a very poor prognosis and did not expect Leona to live through her first year. However, instead of placing her in an institution, as advised by the professionals who delivered the diagnosis, her biological parents placed her for adoption, and she joined her new family when she was 12 weeks old.

Leona was quite delayed in early infancy—she had low muscle tone, was generally unresponsive, and seemed frightened of most stimuli in her environment. Within a few weeks of placement with her adoptive parents, however, her doctors remarked upon her rapid improvement. Leona continued on an upward trajectory, and by the time she was 8 years old, she was functioning only 2 years behind her chronological age, a level that would be in the mild to borderline range of mental retardation. Leona's adoptive parents were quite pleased with her development and reported that she was especially caring in her attitudes toward others and that she seemed to be a positive addition not only to their lives but also to the lives of friends and neighbors. Leona continued to achieve far beyond the original prognosis, and as a young adult has graduated from high school, works part-time, and has a full social life, including dating. Her vocational goal is to work as a veterinarian's assistant.

Leona is an example of an inaccurate prognosis in which eventual functioning was far better than expected. Melvin, described next, is also an example of heterogeneity of outcomes, but in his case, functioning was more limited than most individuals with his diagnosis of Williams syndrome. Williams syndrome, caused by a micro-deletion on chromosome 7, generally results in functioning at the upper levels of the mental retardation range. For example, Mervis, Robinson, Row, Becerra, & Klein-Tasman, 2003) report a mean Kaufman composite IQ of 67 (with a range of 40–108) for 250 individuals with Williams syndrome. Melvin was outside this range.

Case 12.2: Melvin   As Melvin reached the ages where he should have achieved developmental milestones but did not, it became clear to his parents that something was wrong. By 12 months of age, he was far enough behind that the family was referred to a team at a specialty hospital, and he was diagnosed with Williams syndrome. Melvin's parents were provided with a prognosis for him, based on the "typical" Williams syndrome profile. His doctors informed his parents of possible out-comes such as mild mental retardation or anxiety and suggested the possibility of remarkable music ability or the ability to live on his own when he grew up. Melvin, however, did not follow this tra-jectory (see also Mervis & Moore, chapter 7, this volume). He is severely to profoundly retarded, and at age 18 years he was functioning at less than a 3-year-old level. Melvin currently lives at home, but his mother is hoping to move him into a group home setting one day.

Melvin, like Leona, did not develop according to the prognosis that was originally provided. Follow-up care in a genetics clinic is especially important given the diffi-culty in predicting a specific outcome for each individual. Indeed, there is much vari-ability in phenotypic expression for even some of the most well-understood genetic disorders, as demonstrated in the first seven chapters of this volume. There are also varying degrees of accuracy in the "common knowledge" available for many dis-orders, adding to the potential challenges of long term predictions.

Dimensions of Classification   In spite of this variability and unpredictability, genetic and other organic conditions that may result in mental retardation can be catego-rized along known dimensions, and the understanding of those dimensions is useful for prevention and treatment. Prognosis for level of functioning mentioned earlier is one of them. Risk of recurrence is another of these dimensions. Some conditions have implications for substantial risk of recurrence in future pregnancies, whereas recurrence risk for other conditions is only slightly elevated, if at all. For example, because of its pattern of inheritance and relatively high risk of recurrence, a child's diagnosis of fragile X syndrome has implications for all immediate nuclear family members as well as those in the extended family. Diagnostic DNA testing becomes relevant for adults, other children, and fetuses in current or future pregnancies. (For more detail, see chapters on fragile X syndrome and genetic counseling in this volume.)

Another important dimension is when the diagnosis is likely to occur. In the case of fragile X, diagnosis is not typically before or at birth if there is no known family history. Indeed, many children are not diagnosed until the preschool or school-age years, even though parents and professionals had recognized earlier that the child's functioning was delayed or atypical (Bailey, Skinner, & Sparkman, 2003). This pattern is in marked contrast to Down syndrome or phenylketonuria (PKU) in which diagnosis is almost always at birth or even during the prenatal period. This dimension of timing of diagnosis has implications for the beginning of treatment—as in the case of PKU—that can prevent mental retardation or ameliorate its severity. It has implications also for family reaction and adjustment, which will be discussed at greater length in a later section.

Despite the stigma associated with mental retardation, the prognosis for life quality for children and adults with this condition improved dramatically during the last half of the 20th century. Social movements, catalyzed in large measure by parent advocacy groups such as The Arc (originally Association for Retarded Children), led to the acceptance of the principle that persons with mental retardation were entitled to "normal" lives. This principle of normalization (Nirjie, 1969; Wolfensberger, 1972) spurred other changes such as where persons with mental retardation lived, what kind of medical treatment they received, where and how they were educated, and what other entitlements they deserved.

Deinstitutionalization

Although most children with mental retardation have lived with their families of origin throughout history, during the latter half of the 20th century, residential options for individuals with mental retardation changed and increased dramatically. For example, in 1977, 35.8% of residents in institutions for persons with mental retardation or other developmental disabilities were 21 years old or younger. In 2000, only 4.5% were in that age group (Smith, Prouty, Polister, Kwak, & Lakin, 2001). Moreover, in a 30-year period, the overall institutional population declined from 169,214 residents in 1974 to only 41,792 in 2004 (Prouty, Coucouvanis, & Lakin, 2005), despite an increase in the U.S. population from approximately 210 million to 290 million (U.S. Bureau of the Census, 2005). Thus, when a family receives a diagnosis that includes mental retardation, the reality is that the child will almost certainly live with them. An exception to this trend is the increased number of children with mental retardation and other developmental disabilities who are adopted (Dumaret et al., 1998; Glidden, 1989, 1994, 2005; Glidden, Valliere, & Herbert, 1988).

Medical Treatment

During this same time period of the latter half of the 20th century, recognition developed that persons with mental retardation had the right to life and to medical treatment that would extend that life (Rogers & Roizen, 1991; Wolraich, Siperstein, & Reed, 1991; Cooley & Olson, 1996; Woodhouse, 1998; Chase, Osinowo, & Pary, 2002). A series of Baby Doe cases in the 1970s and 1980s established this right as superseding the guardianship rights of parents (Dybwad, 1973; Mitchell, 1985; "Baby Doe," 1996). This same battle was later refought with regard to sterilization (Dickin & Ryan, 1983; Melton & Scott, 1984; Ashman, 1990; Beyer, 1991; Elkins, 1992). Although this right to medical treatment is now generally recognized, the devaluation of persons with mental retardation may still influence medical decision making, especially when scarce resources need to be allocated, as in the case of some transplants (Hardie, 2000, as cited in Beirne-Smith et al., 2006).

Mainstreaming and Inclusion

Although the right to education is regarded as constitutionally given in the United States, it was not until 1975 that federal legislation was passed that guaranteed a free and appropriate education to children with disabilities (P.L. 94–142). During various amendments to this public law, and challenges to its provisions, it has generally been regarded that children should be placed in an educational environment that is the least restrictive possible. For many, but not all, children with mental retardation this placement will entail at least some inclusion in classrooms with children without disabilities.

Other Civil Rights

In addition to rights to treatment and education, persons with mental retardation are entitled to other rights for which they qualify as citizens of the United States. Particular instances of these rights have included the right to marry, to bear children, and to vote, as well as the right to equal protection and due process. Of interest, recently, is the dilemma that is posed for advocates of these rights in light of the Supreme Court ruling that persons with mental retardation should not be subject to the death penalty because their cognitive limitations rendered them "categorically less culpable than the average criminal" (Atkins v. Virginia; Legal Information Institute, 2002; Weeks, 2003).

In sum, the outlook for children and adults with mental retardation is quite different from what it was 50 or 100 years ago. Many individuals, even those with severe and profound mental retardation, can expect to live longer lives and lives of higher quality than used to be possible. These widespread social changes are both a reflection of attitude change and a stimulus for that change. In 1989, Chris Burke, a 24-year-old man with Down syndrome, played a feature part in the television serial, *Life Goes On* (McMurran, 1989; "Life goes on," 1990). Enduring for 5 years, the program helped to educate the public about the potential accomplishments of young adults with Down syndrome and possibly dispel some of the stigma associated with it. However, that this television show aired and was popular was, to some extent, a reflection of changes that had already occurred. For example, decades earlier, families on the leading edge of this societal change had begun to welcome children with mental retardation into their families by knowingly and willingly adopting them (Glidden, 1989).

The Diagnosis and Reacting to It

The Timing of the Diagnosis

The timing of the diagnosis may have an impact in determining how parents adapt and adjust to their child's disability. In general, parents want to know of any potential disability or developmental delay as soon as possible (Cunningham, Morgan, & McGucken, 1984; Skotko, 2005). Diagnoses of many syndromes and disabilities, such as Down syndrome, can be detected as early as the first trimester prenatally (see, e.g., Skotko, 2005), but other diagnoses, especially those concerning a nonspecific disability, may not be known and communicated until 2 or even 3 years after the birth of the child (Quine & Pahl, 1987; Bailey et al., 2003). Indeed, infants and young children with mild mental retardation may not have observable physical or social characteristics linked to their intellectual deficits. For many of these children, diagnosis will be made not by medical practitioners, but by educators. It is only when these children begin to fail academic tasks that they are referred for psychoeducational testing and they obtain "significantly subaverage" IQ scores.

Prenatal Screening

Prenatal screening has become an increasingly utilized tool to assess the risk of giving birth to a child with a disability. Although prenatal testing is clearly valuable for a variety of reasons, it is not universally accepted. Skotko (2005) reports that some parents who receive a positive result from prenatal screening may feel rushed into making a decision as to whether or not to continue the pregnancy. Some parents have reported being told little, if anything at all, of the quality of life they might expect for their child, nor were they provided with much information concerning the actual disability assessed prenatally (Roberts, Stough, & Parrish, 2002). When such information is provided, one advantage of prenatal screening is that parents receive early information on their child's disability. Prenatal and newborn screening are discussed further elsewhere in this volume (McConkie-Rosell & O'Daniel, this volume chapter 11).

Neonatal Screening

Screening newborns for a variety of disorders that have not been diagnosed prenatally has become more common in the United States. According to the Web site of

the National Newborn Screening and Genetics Resource Center (2005) (http://genes-
r-us.uthscsa.edu/nbsdisorders.pdf), all states require at least *some* neonatal screening. Although there are some disorders that are screened in all or almost all of the
50 states, such as PKU and sickle cell, there is little uniformity with regard to most
disorders. Bailey (2004) reviewed the guidelines for how decisions regarding newborn
screening were made. He found that, despite the lack of a standardized system, most
task forces agree that screening should be done for a disorder if the disorder can be
screened quickly, accurately, and effectively; if the disorder can somehow be eradi-
cated from the individual (or at least if its trajectory can be significantly altered); or
if the disorder severely impacts affected individuals.

For some disorders, such as fragile X syndrome, in some individuals there may be
few if any clinical features, particularly in childhood. In these cases, diagnosis can be
very difficult without utilizing specialized testing such as direct DNA testing of the
fragile X mental retardation gene—1. Thus, families are often frustrated by the lack
of explanation for their child's aberrant behavior and development. Indeed, Bailey
(2004) argues that fragile X may often be diagnosed months or years after birth despite the fact that it could be easily detected at birth if newborn DNA screening were
in place. More importantly, early identification of the disorder increases the likelihood of obtaining early access to intervention programs. Furthermore, parents may
be unaware of their carrier status and, thus, without a diagnosis, may bear additional
children at risk for fragile X before the first child is diagnosed.

In contrast to fragile X, Down syndrome is easily detectable at birth, and many
argue that the certainty of an early diagnosis, although potentially shocking, may facilitate parental adjustment. Lenhard et al. (2005), for example, found that mothers
of children with Down syndrome fared as well on a variety of outcomes as mothers
of children without disabilities, whereas mothers of children with undiagnosed disabilities fared worse. An early diagnosis gives parents more time to adjust to and
cope with the needs of their newborn child; it also gives them more opportunities to
identify and make use of available supports.

As biotechnological innovations and improvements continue, it will become easier
and more cost-efficient for a variety of disorders to be detectable at birth. To reiter-
ate a common theme among parents and researchers, it is evident that diagnoses are
received best when they come early. A specific diagnosis may ease parental feelings
of anxiety or guilt, which, in turn, will enable the parents to utilize resources more
effectively to enhance their child's development, as well as increase family functioning as a whole.

Nature of the Disability

As described earlier in this chapter, "mental retardation" is a term that encompasses
a wide range of functioning, manifested even within the same diagnostic condition. It

includes children who are nonambulatory, are nonverbal, and have multiple disabilities that might include physical and sensory impairments, as well as other health problems. It also refers to individuals who will graduate from high school, win medals in Special Olympics, live independently as adults, marry, and bear and raise children. Therefore, it is essential that parents and other family members, as well as professionals who provide services to the individual with mental retardation and his or her family members, recognize the heterogeneity that is possible. Many conditions have their own behavioral phenotypes that include relative strengths as well as deficits. For example, there is now good evidence that language functioning is a relative strength for children and adults with Williams syndrome, whereas it is a relative weakness for individuals with Down syndrome (Chapman, 2003; Mervis et al., 2003).

Preparation that will remediate the weaknesses and capitalize on the strengths is an ongoing strategy to optimize the functioning of individuals with mental retardation. Thus, speech and language therapy for children with Down syndrome can start very early given the likelihood that it is an area of functioning that will need extensive and intensive remediation (Chapman, 2003). With regard to capitalizing on strengths, music camps for children and adults with Williams syndrome have been established on a national scale, and some of the attendees have become known for the high quality of their performances (Williams Syndrome Foundation, 2005).

Ideal Practice for Delivering the Diagnosis

Despite the sensitive nature of receiving a diagnosis associated with disability, an established protocol outlining the best way to deliver a diagnosis to parents and family members does not exist (Skotko, 2005; Cunningham et al., 1984; Svarstad & Lipton, 1977). Although some health professionals are curt when delivering the diagnosis, others take their time; some professionals accentuate the negative, and others accentuate the positive. Some parents are provided with up-to-date information, whereas others are provided with out-of-date information, or no information at all (see, e.g., Abramsky, Hall, Levitan, & Marteau, 2001).

Throughout the years, however, parents and researchers representing a variety of cultures have specifically described methods they believe are best when delivering a diagnosis. These methods are mostly in agreement with each other, as they propose similar recommendations (Hatton, Akram, & Robertson, 2003; Svarstad & Lipton, 1977; Skotko, 2005). One such model attempting to standardize the diagnostic procedure and increase parental satisfaction was provided by Cunningham and colleagues (1984), based on previous research and extensive interviews with parents. Parents, they concluded, should be told together and in a private place, if possible, as soon as the doctor knows or suspects any abnormality. For neonatal or postnatal diagnoses, the infant should be in the same room as the parents and doctor, preferably being held by the doctor, and parents should be provided ample time to air any questions and concerns they may have. Furthermore, parents should be allowed a private setting afterwards to discuss with one another what they have heard and its implications. Recognizing that the initial diagnosis can be a shock and parents may not have time to think of all questions they could possibly have, a follow-up interview should be arranged to address any additional questions or concerns.

The Cunningham analysis and protocol for best practice was published in 1984 but appears to have had minimal impact in the ensuing 2 decades. Many parents still report dissatisfaction with the diagnostic process and, when asked how this process could be improved, parents make suggestions akin to those made by Cunningham and earlier researchers.

Attention to the diagnostic process is especially important because the delivery of prenatal diagnoses may influence family adaptation. Consider the case study reported by two parents whose child was diagnosed prenatally with Down syndrome (Beach Center on Disability, 2005). The diagnosis was given in the late 1990s, but none of the aforementioned Cunningham's recommendations was followed. In this case, the mother received the diagnosis by phone, and was given the responsibility of conveying the diagnosis to her husband. Their obstetrician informed the parents that a decision regarding termination of the pregnancy was needed within 1 week. When the parents decided against termination, their obstetrician suggested the possibility of institutionalization. This is in contrast to cases where the Cunningham recommendations are followed as described above or when a genetic counselor is involved (McConkie-Rosell & O'Daniel, this volume).

The initial diagnosis is the beginning of a lengthy journey along a landscape with many peaks and valleys. Parents and other family members encounter a variety of rewards and challenges as they learn to adapt to their child with disabilities. The next section outlines the crucial components of this adaptation process.

Adaptation During Childhood

Regardless of when the diagnosis is initially suggested or confirmed, it will activate many responses in parents. If the diagnosis is unexpected, as it frequently is when it comes during the prenatal period or at birth, parents are almost always in a negative emotional state and they will typically experience depression and an array of existential reactions including a questioning of life's meaning and of religious beliefs. However, regardless of the intensity and duration of these reactions, parents also crave information that provides them with reduction of ambiguity about the future. They want a prognosis, both for the near term and the long term. Sometimes this prognosis is difficult, almost impossible to provide, either because little is known about the etiology of the mental retardation or because there is substantial variability in the functioning of individuals with the diagnosis. However, there are general guidelines that are influenced by the level of mental retardation and the specific condition.

Level and Type of Functioning

Mild Mental Retardation   Although most children with mild mental retardation will not be identified until they are school-age, some have conditions that will ensure earlier identification. For example, some children with Down syndrome function in the mild mental retardation range, as do many children with Williams syndrome and fragile X syndrome. In general, although these children will be somewhat late in attaining developmental milestones such as walking, running, bowel and urinary control, receptive and expressive language, the practical dimensions of their adaptive behavior may be less impaired. Individuals with Down syndrome, for example, frequently exhibit adaptive behavior strengths in daily living and socialization skills (Dykens, Hodapp, & Evans, 1994).

Moderate/Severe/Profound Mental Retardation   Children with intellectual functioning at these levels will almost always be identified during the infancy period or earlier. With more severe mental retardation, there is also an increased likelihood of other disabilities such as physical impairments, sensory impairments, and a variety of complicating health conditions. For families, a difficult challenge, in addition to the psychological one of adjusting to the diagnosis and prognosis, is the management of a daily routine that may involve complicated regimens, as in the following case:

Case 12.3: Naomi   Naomi was born at 26 weeks' gestation, weighing less than 1,000 g. Her cerebral palsy was diagnosed in infancy, and by the time she was 30 months old, she had been hospitalized more than 80 times, was subject to four kinds of seizures, and had endured 22 episodes of pneumonia.

Naomi is nonambulatory and nonvocal. Even her crying is mute, requiring someone to be with her constantly in case of difficulties that arise quite frequently because she requires tube feeding and ventilator support for breathing. Leaving the house requires extensive preparation. Naomi's mother described it matter-of-factly after adapting to the regimen:

"She's got the tray, and all the GTs (gastrointestinal tubes). When she's got wires hanging from her, she can be, to someone that's not used to her, kind of frightening. Anyplace you go, you've got to take this entourage of stuff…you have to keep it on her all the time, you have that kind of monitor, the tray, the suctioner, and the wheelchair, it can get kind of difficult."

Behavioral Phenotypes   Genetic conditions are associated with an increased likelihood not only of identifiable physical manifestations but also behavioral characteristics. Collectively, these behavioral tendencies are called "behavioral phenotypes," and recent research has identified strengths and weaknesses associated with several neurogenetic conditions, including Down syndrome, Williams syndrome, fragile X syndrome, Prader–Willi syndrome, and others (Dykens & Rosner, 1999; Dykens, Rosner, Ly, & Sagun, 2005; Finucane, Dirrigl, & Simon, 2001). Although these phenotypes should be interpreted probabilistically rather than as "biology is destiny," they do provide some guidance for parents and for professionals as to what to expect and what services and enrichments are advisable. They also can link parents into a variety of sources of support in the form of professional groups, parent networks, targeted Internet mailing and discussion lists, and even national and regional meetings.

Family Characteristics and Resources

Families differ on many dimensions such as size; number of parents; number of children; psychological and material resources that are available to the family; values, including even the concept of the role of the family; and so forth. These family characteristics and resources can exert substantial influence on the process of adaptation to the rearing of a child with mental retardation. The next several sections summarize what we know about some of these influences.

Family Composition   One element of family composition is whether the child with mental retardation has siblings. In the October 2005 issue of the journal *Mental Retardation*, a special section was devoted to sibling perspectives. Emphases included a need to focus on positive outcomes (Dykens, 2005; Hodapp, Glidden, & Kaiser, 2005; McMillan, 2005; Swenson, 2005), a need that was described by both family members and researchers. There is general agreement that typically developing siblings, especially girls, offer a variety of help to their brothers and sisters with mental retardation (Cuskelly & Gunn, 2003; Hannah & Midlarsky, 2005). This help begins quite early in childhood, and there is good evidence that it is lifelong (Orsmond & Seltzer, 2000; Seltzer, Greenberg, Orsmond, & Lounds, 2005). Whereas some interpretations of these data have focused on the burden of helping and other psychological negative effects, others have been positive, emphasizing the development of qualities such as empathy, patience, tolerance, altruism, and nurturance (Cuskelly & Gunn, 2003; Hannah & Midlarsky, 2005; Stoneman, 2005). McMillan (2005), the mother of a son, Will, who has Down syndrome, and two other children who are typically developing, cites the response of her 18-year-old son when asked about who has had the biggest impact on his life: "The answer is my brother, Will. From him, I have learned patience, and also what is really important."

The presence or absence of siblings is only one facet of family composition. Another aspect that has drawn considerable research attention is marital status. Early on in the study of family reaction to the diagnosis of disability, it was assumed that single parents would be more vulnerable to negative outcomes because of the greater burden of caring and the potentially lower level of social support. The research evidence is mixed, however (Shapiro, Blacher, & Lopez, 1998). In addition, some research has indicated that marital discord and disruption are the result of the mental retardation diagnosis and subsequent challenges, but the evidence for this finding is also mixed (Glidden & Schoolcraft, 2007). Finally, when the mental retardation is the result of a genetic disorder, single parenting presents a difficulty in addition to those of burden of care and lack of social support. The need for genetic counseling for the absent parent and related family members may go unfulfilled. This can happen when a parent abandons the family. However, every effort is made to include the whole family when possible (McConkie-Rosell & O'Daniel, this volume).

Finally, the extended family can also be important in adaptation to the child with mental retardation. Grandparents, for example, can offer considerable help and are sometimes even the primary caretakers when, for various reasons, the parent(s) of the child with mental retardation are unable or unwilling to assume that role (Kinney, McGrew, & Nelson, 2003).

Parental Personality   Adaptation is influenced by stable and consistent traits, namely, the personality, of the individuals who must adapt. Glidden and Schoolcraft (2003), using the NEO Five Factor Inventory (Costa & McCrae, 1992), measured five factors of personality in parents rearing children with developmental disabilities, many of whom had mental retardation as a result of genetic conditions. We found that Neuroticism, or a general mental health/stability trait, was related to the report of depression when the children were, on average, 11 years old. Follow-ups to this research have extended this finding to other variables, to fathers as well as mothers, and to the adolescent years of the children with mental retardation (Glidden & Jobe, 2005, 2006).

Religiousness   Religious beliefs and participation in religious activities play a role in the adaptation to many life challenges, including the diagnosis of a child's disability and the subsequent adjustment to it (Pargament, 2003; Glidden, Rogers-Dulan, & Hill, 1999). Religious beliefs can help parents find a meaning and understanding of the disability and its role in their lives, and religious practices and a religious community can offer support both in a tangible form, such as babysitting help or donations of needed clothing or equipment, and in enhancement of psychological well-being. Professionals providing services to families should be aware that religiousness might be an important factor that influences the immediate and long-term adaptation of the family to the child with mental retardation.

Economic Resources   As long as the economic circumstances of families are not dire, they appear to have little effect on psychological adaptation (Shapiro et al., 1998). An exception is the relation of financial resources to variables that specifically measure financial burden (Glidden, 1993). Families of poverty, however, are frequently not included in samples (Stoneman, 1997), so it is likely that economic resources could influence family adaptation if they dropped below a certain threshold. Certainly, models of adaptation and coping frequently include economic resources as a component (e.g., McCubbin & Patterson, 1982). Practically, families who do not have to worry about their financial status will be able to afford a quality and quantity of care that will protect them from some of the burdens of rearing a child with disabilities. For example, access to best medical care is linked to economic circumstances with lack of health insurance remaining an obstacle for some children with mental retardation.

Social Support

The existence or lack of social supports is another factor influencing how a family will adapt to a mental retardation diagnosis, and health professionals can make this adaptation easier by informing parents and families of available supports. Broadly speaking, there are two types of support that a family may receive: informal or formal (Glidden & Schoolcraft, 2007). Informal support networks are most often composed of family and friends who typically provide emotional support (i.e., offering motivation or encouragement to the parent) or instrumental support (offering to babysit, etc.). Formal support networks are often composed of professionals, including doctors, teachers, social workers, and others. These professionals typically provide informational, medical, or psychological support.

A multitude of research has pointed to the importance of social support and its relation to more positive outcomes. In a review of the literature, for example, Glidden and Schoolcraft (2007) found that researchers have linked greater levels of social support with better family functioning, lower maternal depression, lower maternal anxiety, and lower maternal distress. Higher levels of social support have also been found to keep children with mental retardation in their natural homes longer (Bruns, 2000).

Of course, rarely is the influence of any variable uniformly positive, and social support is no exception. Not every source of support is positive; for example, a persistent friend or neighbor may be perceived as intrusive, and an abundance of well-intentioned advice may make a mother feel incapable of caring for her child on her own. Various researchers, such as Lunsky and colleagues, have found that unwanted supports are associated with negative maternal outcomes, such as maternal depression (Lunsky & Benson, 2001). For the most part, however, higher levels of perceived social support have been shown to help protect families of children with mental retardation, and good relationships with health care professionals may enable parents to more quickly adapt to their child.

Multicultural Issues

Increasingly, we are a multicultural society, and therefore it is essential that cultural characteristics be considered when providing a diagnosis or offering support to families. Many parents who speak English as a second language, for example, would prefer that the initial diagnosis and subsequent information pertaining to the type of disability and possible outcomes be provided in their primary language (Hatton, Akram, Robertson, Shah, & Emerson, 2003). Difficulty with the language may delay acceptance of the diagnosis, and parents may have a hard time asking questions, and receiving the answers, if they do not comprehend English as well as their native language.

Additionally, Blacher, Lopez, Shapiro, and Fusco (1997) found that their sample of 148 Latina mothers rearing children with developmental disabilities exhibited greater depressive symptoms than would be expected based on normative samples. They also noted that Latino/a parents are often overlooked and, therefore, are underrepresented in research samples. Thus, primary care physicians and other health care providers may need to more closely monitor these parents to ensure optimal adjustment to their severely altered lifestyle.

Furthermore, culture-specific stigmas associated with mental retardation may make the acceptance of a diagnosis particularly difficult. To provide one example, Chinese societies often label parents of children with mental retardation as immoral, as such a child is believed to be a punishment for some past sin or wrongdoing (Chen & Tang, 1997). Therefore, these parents may have a greater sense of guilt and may react more negatively to the diagnosis. Furthermore, Chen and Tang note the possibility that parents may be reluctant to look to others for support (either formal or informal), as they feel this child is *their* punishment, and a cross they must bear alone. Health care workers, then, should be aware of such stigmas so they can more appropriately help the parents obtain the information and help they need.

Some cultures may offer ways of coping with the rearing of a child with mental retardation that reduce the stress on the family. For example, Glidden et al. (1999) described the ways in which religion is embedded in the cultural framework of African American and Latino families. As examples of religiousness as a source of strength, they described two African American families. In both families, the parents' interpretation of the meaning of their child's mental retardation was embedded in their understanding of God. In addition, their strong ties to their church provided both tangible and intangible coping resources. Tangible resources included clothing and respite care. However, the intangible resources such as acceptance of their child into the community may be just as important in enhancement of the family's well-being.

Conclusions, Recommendations, and Limitations

In this chapter, we have defined "mental retardation," emphasized its heterogeneity, and examined some of the factors that influence families' adaptation to and coping with the rearing of children with mental retardation. These factors include preexisting family and parental characteristics as well as the nature of the neurogenetic condition and its developmental trajectory of child functioning. Also influencing adaptation are context features such as the way the diagnosis is conveyed and the availability of formal and informal supports.

Although substantial research attention has been given to this adaptation process, evidence-based practice is nonetheless in its own infancy. We are still mostly ignorant when it comes to refining clinical intervention to accommodate the myriad of individual differences in the child with mental retardation as well as other nuclear and extended family members. This ignorance remains in part because of the complexity of the research context and the difficulty of doing research with samples that are representative of the full range of families and children with mental retardation. As with much behavioral research, samples are ones of convenience rather than randomly selected.

Nonetheless, we have made progress. We know that best practice with families involves early diagnosis and conveying of that diagnosis by a practitioner or team that is aware of both the challenges that will be associated with adapting to the child and the rewards to be gained from it. The emphasis on rewards and satisfaction is pronounced in recent research utilizing a framework of positive psychology (Flaherty & Glidden, 2000; Glidden & Schoolcraft, 2003). It has overturned the early view that a family with a child with a disability is a disabled family. Although each family is different and some will adapt more quickly and more successfully than others, all do adapt. Professionals who provide services to them will be more effective if they understand how family, child, and context variables influence that adaptation.

Acknowledgments

The writing of this chapter was supported, in part, by Grant No. 21993 from the National Institute of Child Health and Human Development awarded to Laraine Masters Glidden and to faculty development grants from St. Mary's College of Maryland. Thanks go to Colleen Fisher and Caitlin Ward for their assistance.

Note

1. The AAMR is now the AAIDD.

References

Abramsky, L., Hall, S., Levitan, J., & Marteau, T. M. (2001). What parents are told after prenatal diagnosis of a sex chromosome abnormality: Interview and questionnaire study. *British Medical Journal, 322,* 463–466.

American Association on Mental Retardation. (2002). *Mental retardation: Definition, classification, and systems of support* (10th ed.). Washington, DC: Author.

American Psychiatric Association. (2000). Mental retardation. *Diagnostic and statistical manual of mental disorders* (4th ed., text rev.). Washington, DC: Author.

Ashman, A. F. (1990). Sterilization and training for normal sexual development: Human rights and obligations. *Journal of Developmental Disabilities, 16,* 359–368.

(1986). "Baby Doe" records not disclosable. *Mental & Physical Disability Law Reporter, 10,* 364–365.

Bailey, D. B., Jr. (2004). Newborn screening for fragile X syndrome. *Mental Retardation and Developmental Disabilities Research Reviews, 10,* 3–10.

Bailey, D. B., Skinner, D., & Sparkman, K. L. (2003). Discovering fragile X syndrome: Family experiences and perceptions. *Pediatrics, 111,* 407–417.

Beach Center on Disability. (2005, November 4). Expecting a baby with Down syndrome: One couple's story of coping…and carrying on. *Real Stories & Tips.* Retrieved November 11, 2005, from http://www.beachcenter.org/stories/default. asp?intResourceID=1812&act=detail&story=true&type=&id=0

Beirne-Smith, M., Patton, J. R., & Kim, S. H. (2006). *Mental retardation: An introduction to intellectual disabilities* (7th ed.). Upper Saddle River, NJ: Pearson Prentice Hall.

Beyer, H. A. (1991). Litigation involving people with mental retardation. In J. L. Matson & J. A. Mulick (Eds.). *Handbook of mental retardation* (2nd ed., pp. 74–93). Elmsford, NY: Pergamon.

Blacher, J., Lopez, S., Shapiro, J., & Fusco, J. (1997). Contributions to depression in Latina mothers with and without children with retardation: Implications for caregiving. *Family Relations: Interdisciplinary Journal of Applied Family Studies, 46,* 325–334.

Breslau, N. (2001). Academic achievement of low birthweight children at age 11: The role of cognitive abilities at school entry. *Journal of Abnormal Child Psychology, 29,* 273–279.

Bruns, D. A. (2000). Leaving home at an early age: Parents' decisions about out-of-home placement for young children with complex medical needs. *Mental Retardation, 38,* 55–60.

Chapman, R. S. (2003). Language and communication in individuals with Down syndrome. In L. M. Glidden (Series Ed.) & L. Abbeduto (Vol. Ed.), *International review of research in mental retardation: Vol. 27. Language and communication in mental retardation* (pp. 1–34). New York: Academic Press/Elsevier.

Chase, C. D., Osinowo, T., & Pary, R. J. (2002). Medical issues in patients with Down syndrome. *Mental Health Aspects of Developmental Disabilities, 5,* 34–45.

Chen, T. Y., & Tang, C. S. (1997). Stress appraisal and social support of Chinese mothers of adult children with mental retardation. *American Journal on Mental Retardation, 101,* 473–482.

Constable, B. (2004, June 3). Devoted teen with Down syndrome graduates with honors. *Chicago Daily Herald.* Retrieved November 11, 2005, from http://nl.newsbank.com/nl-search/we/Archives?p_product=ADHB&p_

Cooley, W. C., & Olson, A. L. (1996). Developing family-centered care for families of children with special health care needs. In G. H. S. Singer & L. E. Powers (Eds.), *Redefining family support: Innovations in public–private partnerships* (pp. 239–257). Baltimore: Brookes.

Costa, P. T., & McCrae, R. R. (1992). *Revised Personality Inventory (NEO PI-R) and NEO Five-Factor Inventory (NEO-FFI): Professional Manual.* Odessa, FL: Psychological Assessment Resources.

Cunningham, C. C., Morgan, P. A., & McGucken, R. B. (1984). Down's syndrome: Is dissatisfaction with disclosure inevitable? *Developmental Medicine & Child Neurology, 26,* 33–39.

Cuskelly, M., & Gunn, P. (2003). Sibling relationships of children with Down syndrome: Perspectives of mothers, fathers, and siblings. *American Journal on Mental Retardation, 108,* 234–244.

Dickin, K. L., & Ryan, B. A. (1983). Sterilization and the mentally retarded. *Canada's Mental Health, 31,* 4–8.

Dumaret, A. C., De Vigan, C. Julian-Reynier, Goujard, C. J., Rosset, D., & Aymé, S. (1998). Adoption and fostering of babies with Down cyndrome: A cohort of 593 cases. *Prenatal Diagnosis, 18,* 437–445.

Durkin, M. S., & Stein, Z. A. (1996). Classification of mental retardation. In J. W. Jacobson & J. A. Mulick (Eds.), *Manual of diagnosis and professional practice in mental retardation* (pp. 67–73). Washington, DC: American Psychological Association.

Dybwad, G. (1973). Basic legal aspects in providing medical, educational, social, and vocational help to the mentally retarded. *Journal of Special Education, 7,* 39–50.

Dykens, E. M. (2005). Happiness, well-being, and character strengths: Outcomes for families and siblings of persons with mental retardation. *Mental Retardation, 43,* 360–364.

Dykens, E. M., Hodapp, R. M., & Evans, D. W. (1994). Profiles and development of adaptive behavior in children with Down syndrome. *American Journal on Mental Retardation, 98,* 580–587.

Dykens, E. M., & Rosner, B. A. (1999). Refining behavioral phenotypes: Personality–motivation in Williams and Prader–Willi syndromes. *American Journal on Mental Retardation, 104,* 158–169.

Dykens, E. M., Rosner, B. A., Ly, T., & Sagun, J. (2005). Music and anxiety in Williams syndrome: A harmonious or discordant relationship? *American Journal on Mental Retardation, 110,* 346–358.

Elkins, T. E. (1992). Sterilization of persons with mental retardation. *Journal of the Association for Persons with Severe Handicaps, 17,* 19–26.

Farran, D. C. (2000). Another decade of intervention for children who are low income or disabled: What do we know now? In J. P. Shonkoff & S. J. Meisels (Eds.), *Handbook of early childhood intervention* (2nd ed., pp. 510–548). New York: Cambridge University Press.

Finucane, B., Dirrigl, K. H., & Simon, E. W. (2001). Characterization of self-injurious behaviors in children and adults with Smith–Magenis syndrome. *American Journal on Mental Retardation, 106,* 52–58.

Flaherty, E. M., & Glidden, L. M. (2000). Positive adjustment in parents rearing children with Down syndrome. *Early Education & Development, 11,* 407–422.

Glidden, L. M. (1989). *Parents for children, children for parents: The adoption alternative.* (American Association on Mental Retardation Monograph #11). Washington, DC: American Association on Mental Retardation.

Glidden, L. M. (1993). What we do *not* know about families with children who have developmental disabilities: Questionnaire on Resources and Stress as a case study. *American Journal on Mental Retardation, 97,* 481–495.

Glidden, L. M. (1994). Not under my heart, but in it: Families by adoption. In J. Blacher (Ed.), *When there's no place like home: Options for children living apart from their natural families* (pp. 181–209). Baltimore: Brookes.

Glidden, L. M. (2005, June). Families who adopt children with developmental disabilities. *National Council on Family Relations Report, 50*(2), F13–14.

Glidden, L. M., & Jobe, B. M. (2005). *Measuring parental daily rewards and worries in the transition to adulthood.* Manuscript submitted for publication.

Glidden, L. M., & Jobe, B. M. (2006). The longitudinal course of depression in adoptive and birth mothers of children with intellectual disabilities. *Journal of Policy and Practice in Intellectual Disabilities, 3,* 139–142.

Glidden, L. M., Rogers-Dulan, J. R., & Hill, A. E. (1999). "The child that was meant?" or "punishment for sin?": Religion, ethnicity, and families with children with disabilities. In L. M. Glidden (Ed.), *International review of research in mental retardation* (Vol. 22, pp. 267–288). San Diego, CA: Academic Press.

Glidden, L. M., & Schoolcraft, S. A. (2003). Depression: Its trajectory and correlates in mothers rearing children with intellectual disability. *Journal of Intellectual Disability Research, 47,* 250–263.

Glidden, L. M., & Schoolcraft, S. A. (2007). Family assessment and social support. In J. W. Jacobson & J. A. Mulick & J. Rojahn (Eds.), *Handbook of intellectual and developmental disabilities* (pp. 391–422). New York: Kluwer Academic/Plenum.

Glidden, L. M., Valliere, V. N., & Herbert, S. L. (1988). Adopted children with mental retardation: Positive family impact. *Mental Retardation, 26,* 119–125.

Goeke, J. (2003). Parents speak out: Facial plastic surgery for children with Down syndrome. *Education & Training in Developmental Disabilities, 38,* 323–333.

Gottlieb, J., & Gottlieb, B. W. (1977). Stereotypic attitudes and behavioral intentions toward handicapped children. *American Journal on Mental Deficiency, 82,* 65–71.

Guralnick, M. J. (1997). Second-generation research in the field of early intervention. In M. J. Guralnick (Ed.), *The effectiveness of early intervention* (pp. 366–378). Baltimore: Brookes.

Hannah, M. E., & Midlarsky, E. (2005). Helping by siblings of children with mental retardation. *American Journal on Mental Retardation, 110,* 87–99.

Harrison, P., & Oakland, T. (2002). *The Adaptive Behavior Assessment System II.* San Antonio, TX: Harcourt Assessment.

Hatton, C., Akram, Y., Robertson, J., Shah, R., & Emerson, E. (2003). The disclosure process and its impact on South Asian families with a child with severe intellectual disabilities. *Journal of Applied Research in Intellectual Disabilities, 16,* 177–188.

Hill, J. L., Brooks-Gunn, J., & Waldfogel, J. (2003). Sustained effects of high participation in an early intervention for low-birth-weight premature infants. *Developmental Psychology, 39,* 730–744.

Hodapp, R. M., Glidden, L. M., & Kaiser, A. P. (2005). Siblings of persons with disabilities: Toward a research agenda. *Mental Retardation, 43,* 334–338.

Jacobson, J. W., & Mulick, J. A. (1996). Definition of mental retardation. In J. W. Jacobson & J. A. Mulick (Eds.), *Manual of diagnosis and professional practice in mental retardation* (pp. 39–44). Washington, DC: American Psychological Association.

Jancar, J., & Jancar, P. J. (1996). Longevity in Down syndrome: A twelve year study (1984–1995). *Italian Journal of Intellective Impairment, 9,* 27–30.

Katz, S., & Kravetz, S. (1989a). Facial plastic surgery for persons with Down syndrome: Research findings and their professional and social implications. *American Journal on Mental Retardation, 94,* 101–110.

Katz, S., & Kravetz, S. (1989b). Plastic surgery for persons with Down syndrome: From evaluations to recommendations. *American Journal on Mental Retardation, 94,* 119–120.

Katz, S., Kravetz, S., & Marks, Y. (1997). Parents' and doctors' attitudes toward plastic facial surgery for persons with Down syndrome. *Journal of Intellectual & Developmental Disability, 22,* 265–273.

Kinney, J. M., McGrew, K. B., & Nelson, I. M. (2003). Grandparent caregivers to children with developmental disabilities: Added challenges. In B. Hayslip Jr. & J. H. Patrick (Eds.), *Working with custodial grandparents* (pp. 93–109). New York: Springer.

Lambert, N., Nihira, K., & Leland, H. (1993). *AAMR Adaptive Behavior Scale—School* (2nd ed.). Austin, TX: Pro-Ed.

Legal Information Institute. (2002). Supreme Court of the United States: Atkins v. Virginia, Certiorari to the Supreme Court of Virginia. *Supreme Court Collection.* Retrieved September 13, 2005, from http://straylight.law.cornell.edu/supct/html/00-8452.ZS.html

Lenhard, W., Breitenbach, E., Ebert, H., Schindelhauer-Deutscher, H. J., & Henn, W. (2005). Psychological benefit of diagnostic certainty for mothers of children with disabilities: Lessons from Down syndrome. *American Journal of Medical Genetics, 133A,* 170–175.

(1990). Life goes on for disabled TV star. *Current Science, 75*(10), 9.

Lunsky, Y., & Benson, B. A. (2001). Association between perceived social support and strain, and positive and negative outcome for adults with mild intellectual disability. *Journal of Intellectual Disability Research, 45,* 106–114.

MacMillan, D. L., Siperstein, G. N., & Leffert, J. S. (2003). A challenge for classification practices. In H. Switzky & S. Greenspan (Eds.), *What is mental retardation?* (pp. 242–262). Washington, DC: American Association on Mental Retardation.

May, D. C. (1988). Plastic surgery for children with Down syndrome: Normalization or extremism? *Mental Retardation, 26,* 17–19.

McCubbin, H. I., & Patterson, J. M. (1982). Family adaptation to crises. In H. I. McCubbin, A. E. Cauble, & J. M. Patterson (Eds.), *Family stress, coping, and social support* (pp. 26–47). New York: Haworth.

McLaren, J., & Bryson, S. E. (1987). Review of recent epidemiological studies of mental retardation: Prevalence, associated disorders, and etiology. *American Journal of Mental Retardation, 92,* 243–254.

McMillan, E. (2005). A parent's perspective. *Mental Retardation, 43,* 351–353.

McMurran, K. (1989). For Chris Burke, the first actor with Down syndrome to star on TV, "Life Goes On" in a big way. *People, 32*(16), 61–64.

Melton, G. B., & Scott, E. S. (1984). Evaluation of mentally retarded persons for sterilization: Contributions and limits of psychological consultation. *Professional Psychology: Research & Practice, 15,* 34–48.

Merrick, J. (2000). Aspects of Down syndrome. *International Journal of Adolescent Medicine & Health, 12,* 5–17.

Mervis, C. B., Robinson, B. F., Rowe, M. L., Becerra, A. M., & Klein-Tasman, B. P. (2003). Language abilities of individuals with Williams syndrome. In L. M. Glidden (Series Ed.) & L. Abbeduto (Vol. Ed.), *International review of research in mental retardation: Language and communication in mental retardation* (Vol. 27, pp. 35–81). San Diego, CA: Academic Press/Elsevier.

Mitchell, D. R. (1985). Ethical and legal issues in providing medical treatment for seriously ill handicapped persons. *Australia & New Zealand Journal of Developmental Disabilities, 11,* 245–256.

National Newborn Screening and Genetics Resource Center. (2005, November 1). National newborn screening status report. *United States National Screening Status Report.* Retrieved November 11, 2005, from http://genes-r-us.uthscsa.edu/nbsdisorders.pdf

Nirjie, B. (1969). The normalization principle and its human management implications. In R. B. Kugel & W. W. Wolfensberger (Eds.), *Changing patterns in residential services for the mentally retarded* (pp. 179–188). Washington, DC: U.S. Government Printing Office.

Orsmond, G. K., & Seltzer, M. M. (2000). Brothers and sisters of adults with mental retardation: Gendered nature of the sibling relationship. *American Journal on Mental Retardation, 105,* 486–508.

Pargament, K. I. (2003). Religious/spiritual coping. In *Multidimensional measurement of religiousness/spirituality for use in health research* (pp. 43–56). Kalamazoo, MI: John E. Fetzer Institute.

Prouty, R., Coucouvanis, K., & Lakin, K. C. (2005). Fiscal year 2005 institution populations, movement, and expenditures by state with national comparisons to earlier years. *Mental Retardation, 43,* 149–151.

Quine, L., & Pahl, J. (1987). First diagnosis of severe handicap: A study of parental reactions. *Developmental Medicine & Child Neurology, 29,* 232–242.

Ramey, C. T. (1998). Prevention of intellectual disabilities: Early interventions to improve cognitive development. *Preventative Medicine: An International Journal Devoted to Practice & Theory, 27,* 224–232.

Ramey, C. T., Bryant, D. M., Wasik, B. H., Sparling, J. J., Fendt, K. H., & LaVange, L. M. (1992). Infant health and development program for low birth weight, premature infants: Program elements, family participation, and child intelligence. *Pediatrics, 89,* 454–466.

Ramey, C. T., & Ramey, S. L. (1992). Effective early intervention. *Mental Retardation, 30,* 337–345.

Ramey, C. T., Ramey, S. L., Lanzi, R. G., & Cotton, J. N. (2002). Early education interventions for high-risk children: How center based treatment can augment and improve parenting effectiveness. In J. G. Borkowski & S. L. Ramey (Eds.), *Parenting and the child's world: Influences on academic, intellectual, and social–emotional development* (pp. 125–140). Mahwah, NJ: Erlbaum.

Roberts, C. D., Stough, L. M., & Parrish, L. H. (2002). The role of genetic counseling in the elective termination of pregnancies involving fetuses with disabilities. *Journal of Special Education, 36,* 48–55.

Rogers, P. T., & Roizen, N. J. (1991). A life-cycle approach to management of Down syndrome. In A. J. Capute & P. J. Accardo (Eds.), *Developmental disabilities in infancy and childhood* (pp. 441–454). Baltimore: Brookes.

Seltzer, M. M., Greenberg, J. S., Orsmond, G. I., & Lounds, J. (2005). Life course studies of siblings of individuals with developmental disabilities. *Mental Retardation, 43,* 354–359.

Shapiro, J., Blacher, J., & Lopez, S. R. (1998). Maternal reactions to children with mental retardation. In J. A. Burack, R. M. Hodapp, & E. Zigler (Eds.), *Handbook of mental retardation and development* (pp. 606–636). New York: Cambridge University Press.

Skotko, B. G. (2005). Prenatally diagnosed Down syndrome: Mothers who continued their pregnancies evaluate their health care providers. *American Journal of Obstetrics and Gynecology, 192,* 670–675.

Smith, J., Prouty, B., Polister, B., Kwak, N., & Lakin, C. (2001). Large state residential facilities: Status and trends in population characteristics as of June 30, 2000. *Mental Retardation, 39,* 334–337.

Sparrow, S. S., Cicchetti, D. V., & Balla, D. A. (2005). *Vineland Adaptive Behavior Scale* (2nd ed.). Circle Pines, MN: AGS.

Spitz, H. H. (2003). The ideological position of the 1992 classification system. In H. Switzky & S. Greenspan (Eds.), *What is mental retardation?* (pp. 117–124). Washington, DC: American Association on Mental Retardation.

Stoneman, Z. (1997). Mental retardation and family adaptation. In W. E. MacLean Jr. (Ed.), *Ellis' handbook of mental deficiency, psychological theory and research* (pp. 405–437). Mahwah, NJ: Erlbaum.

Stoneman, Z. (2005). Siblings of children with disabilities: Research themes. *Mental Retardation, 43,* 351–353.

Svarstad, B. L., & Lipton, H. L. (1977). Informing parents about mental retardation: A study of professional communication and parent acceptance. *Social Science & Medicine, 11,* 645–651.

Swenson, S. (2005). Families, research, and systems change. *Mental Retardation, 43,* 356–368.

U.S. Bureau of the Census. (2005, September 30). People QuickFacts: Population, 2004 estimate. *U.S. Census Bureau: State & Country QuickFacts.* Retrieved November 11, 2005, from http://quickfacts.census.gov/qfd/states/00000.html

U.S. Department of Education. (2003). *Twenty-fourth annual report to congress on the implementation of the Individuals with Disabilities Education Act.* Office of Special Education Programs, Data Analysis system. Available at http://www.ed.gov.

Weeks, R. M. A. (2003). Comparing children to the mentally retarded: How the decision in Atkins v. Virginia will affect the execution of juvenile offenders. *BYU Journal of Public Law, 17,* 451–485.

Williams Syndrome Foundation. (2005, April 27). Williams syndrome musicians. Retrieved November 11, 2005, from http://www.wsf.org/music/musician/musician.htm

Wolfensberger, W. (1972). *The principle of normalization in human services.* Toronto, Ontario, Canada: National Institute on Mental Retardation.

Wolraich, M. L., Siperstein, G. N., & Reed, D. (1991). Doctors' decisions and prognostications for infants with Down syndrome. *Developmental Medicine & Child Neurology, 33,* 336–342.

Woodhouse, J. M. (1998). Investigating and managing the child with special needs. *Ophthalmic & Physiological Optics, 18,* 147–152.

13 When a Genetic Disorder Is Associated with Learning Disabilities

Michèle M. M. Mazzocco

Approximately 2.8 million children in the United States have a specific learning disability (LD).[1] An important distinction between LD and well-understood genetic disorders is that the latter are each linked to a known biological etiology and are thus medically defined, whereas LD is a behaviorally defined disorder (as are other disorders such as autism and attention deficit hyperactivity disorder; ADHD) despite evidence of genetic underpinnings (Plomin & Kovas, 2005). Since this distinction may not be evident to lay audiences, it may be helpful to clarify the distinction when discussing genetic-syndrome-associated LD. Moreover, the LD diagnosis is often far broader in scope than a disease with a single etiology, even for subclassifications of LD such as "nonverbal learning disability" (NLD). It is possible to lose sight of the descriptive rather than explanatory nature of LD terminology. For instance, after giving a detailed presentation on cognitive and academic skills in girls with Turner syndrome to a parent support group, I was approached by a parent who asked me whether the cognitive features that I had described were present "because of 'their' nonverbal learning disability." This parent's question parallels the proverbial one: "What came first: The chicken or the egg?" Do girls with Turner syndrome (or any children with LD) who have difficulty with math and spatial skills have this difficulty *because* of an NLD, or do we report that girls with Turner syndrome have NLD because of apparent difficulties in math and spatial skills? Although we will revisit this specific question later in this chapter, it is worth pointing out that—unlike the chicken-or-egg dilemma, for which we can clearly identify and describe both the chicken *and* the egg—certain categories of LD are not easy to describe, much less define. This complexity extends to the relationships between defining, classifying, and identifying LD (as discussed by Fletcher, Morris, & Lyon, 2003; and Keogh, 2005).

Defining Learning Disability

In view of the fact that definitions of LD vary—both within and across disciplines—a thorough historical review of these definitions is beyond the scope of this chapter.

The term "learning disability" and its variants have evolved during a relatively brief history (Hallahan & Mock, 2003) from legal terminology used in both the previous and current versions of the Individuals with Disabilities Education Act (IDEA; see Sudhalter, this issue; also see Herr & Bateman, 2003, for a history of the litigation and legislation leading to IDEA) to the commonly used phrase that it is today. A March 2006 Web-based search for a definition of "learning disability" yielded 5 to 13 million hits when using common search engines. Even when compared with 0.8 million hits for the common genetic disorder fragile X syndrome, or fewer than 200,000 hits for the even more common Klinefelter syndrome, the larger number of hits for LD is not surprising, because the term reflects a broader category of "disabilities" than the examples of genetic disorders. The vast amount of readily available information about LD pertains to specific, well-understood LDs including dyslexia (i.e., reading disability; RD) as reviewed by the National Reading Panel (2000), but also other LDs such as writing disorders (e.g., Berninger, Abbott, Thomson, & Raskind, 2001), and mathematical disability (MD; Geary, 1993, 2004) and the extremely broad category of NLD (Rourke, 1995). Three commonly used LD categories are shown in table 13.1. Classification of LDs includes proposed subtypes of RD (e.g., Morris et al., 1998) and MD (e.g., Geary, 1993), including MD with versus without

Table 13.1
Three commonly used learning disability categories

Characteristic	Reading Disability	Math Disability	Nonverbal Learning Disability
Are core deficits known?	Few, specified, well-replicated over decades of research	Proposed	Many, across several domains
Core deficit skills	Specific to phonological awareness and decoding	Proposed in areas of "number sense," working memory, attentional, spatial, and linguistic domains	Most academic skills other than reading; a subset overlaps with math disability
Nature of definition	Empirically based	Theoretically guided, with some empirical support gained in recent decade	Theoretically based
Research basis	30 years of research, as summarized by the National Reading Panel in the United States established in 1997	Relatively young field, National Math Panel established in the United States in 2006	Across many etiologies
Definitions	Relative consensus, specific to core deficit areas	Lack of consensus regarding severity and domains of difficulty that meet criteria for math learning disability	Multilevel (see chapter 1, table 1.3)

RD (Hanich, Jordan, Kaplin, & Dick, 2001), and varying levels of NLD (Tsatsanis & Rourke, 1995). What may be unclear to parents and teachers is how variable the degree of empirical support is across the different major LD classifications and the recent changes in how LD is identified. Until recently, it was customary to define or identify LD on the basis of a discrepancy between aptitude and academic achievement scores. This method has been challenged at both theoretical and empirical levels (Fletcher, Francis, Morris, & Lyon, 2005; Francis, Fletcher, Shaywitz, Shaywitz, & Rourke, 1996; Francis et al., 2005) as inferior to the use of low achievement and "response to intervention" (RTI) methods (Fletcher et al., 2005). More recent challenges to the RTI methodology reflect that the difficulty in defining and identifying LD is ongoing (e.g., Kavale, Holdnack, & Mostert, 2005), despite a large research base. Thus, although the term "learning disability" is useful and informative, the issues surrounding definition and identification of LD may affect the confidence with which we can characterize the LD we attribute to an individual child.

Although there is no single definition of a learning disability, most definitions share several basic components: Specific reference to manifestation of a learning difficulty in *academic domains* such as reading, writing, or mathematics; the notion that this difficulty is a *biologically based* disorder that interferes with understanding or processing information; and recognition that the learning difficulty does not result from mental retardation or environmental influences such as poor or limited instruction. For example, the National Institute of Neurological Disorders and Stroke (2007) defines "learning disabilities" as follows:

disorders that affect the ability to understand or use spoken or written language, do mathematical calculations, coordinate movements, or direct attention. Although learning disabilities occur in very young children, the disorders are usually not recognized until the child reaches school age.

The emphasis on the school-age years reflects how the deficiencies that warrant an LD label are in skills that are deemed, by our society, to be of sufficient importance because they underlie basic academic competence. It is no coincidence that common forms of LD include disorders of reading, mathematics, or writing—skills needed for successful completion of schooling and for the vast majority of adult occupations. Note the lack of other terms such as "musically disabled" or "racquet-sport disabled" in our clinical or research lexicon, despite the range of differences in how well individuals pursue or perform such skills. Were it essential to sing on key in order to complete schooling or pursue most avenues of employment, the term "musically disabled" would likely be included in the IDEA. Since this is not the case, individuals whose genotype contributes to a lack of musical or athletic ability may pursue schooling and an occupation without difficulty and with no diagnostic label reflecting their inability to sing or play tennis. The focus on academic skills should not be misinterpreted as evidence that LD affects children only in school. LD has an impact on home and peer relationships throughout the life span, particularly for LD related to executive dysfunction (e.g., Powell & Voeller, 2004), which is a component of many of the cognitive phenotypes described in part I of this volume. Parents of children with LD may benefit from understanding that their child has a difficulty in an area considered of sufficient importance by our society that intervention and instructional support are warranted.

The biological basis of LD is supported by neuroimaging (e.g., Eden & Zeffiro, 2004) and heritability studies (e.g., Petrill & Plomin, 2007; Plomin & Kovas, 2005), both of which carry implications for the importance of early identification, prompt and sustained intervention, and issues of comorbidity (such as LD and ADHD; Semrud-Clikeman et al., 1992). That is, if biological influences affect reading (or mathematics or writing), these influences are also likely to affect more than these academic skills, depending on the brain circuitry underlying the specific disability. There are also the issues of primary and secondary effects, and interactions via factors that influence LD outcome, such as classroom environment.

The notion of biological basis does not refute the possibility that, for some children, poor achievement is due only (or primarily) to inadequate or absent instruction. In the strictest sense of the term "learning disability," poor instruction does not lead to a learning *disability*, even in the presence of learning *difficulties*. However, this "disability–difficulty" distinction is controversial, and the criteria that differentiate the two constructs can be arbitrary (e.g., at the 10th percentile or 25th percentile, etc.). Also, the distinction is not definitively qualitative, because in some cases LD is viewed as a quantitative difference at the extreme end of a normal continuum, such as in studies of RD (Shaywitz, Escobar, Shaywitz, Fletcher, & Makuch, 1992).

The notion of biologically mediated LDs does not mean that cognitive phenotypes are unaffected by environmental factors. There is much evidence of the contrary: Effectiveness of reading interventions have been documented by behavioral and neuroimaging studies of children with dyslexia (Eden & Zeffiro, 2004); studies of genetic disorders include the well-established and dramatic effects of dietary modification for children with phenylketonuria (PKU) who escape mental retardation through phenylalinine-restricted diets, and the preliminary support for behavioral improvement due to cholesterol supplementation reported in children with Smith–Lemli–Opitz syndrome, both summarized by Antshel and Arnold (chapter 9, this volume). As such, genetic disorders provide a mechanism by which to better understand the influences of both environmental and genetic contributions to learning ability and disability.

Genetic Disorders as "Models" of LD

Because of their biological bases, genetic disorders with associated cognitive phenotypes can serve as models of neurodevelopmental pathways to LD (proposed in chapters 1 through 9 of this volume), regardless of the specificity of a phenotype or of the extent to which biological causal links for a phenotype are understood. When biological changes in brain development or function have demonstrated links to known agents such as environmental neurotoxins (Lidsky, Heaney, Schneider, & Rosen, this volume) or metabolic abnormalities (Antshel & Arnold, this volume), it may be plausible to establish specific biological pathways leading to LD; still, the LD itself may be heterogeneous, because the same biological insult may damage different brain regions or alter different neuroanatomic pathways. Even in the absence of clearly implicated causal links, neuropsychological constructs provide theoretical models for pathways to LD of varying specificity. At one extreme, neurofibromatosis type 1 (NF-1) may affect one or several distinct neuroanotomical regions, which in turn are associated with distinct cognitive effects (Slopis & Moore, this volume). This intradis-order variation results in NF-1 serving as a proposed model of both RD (Denckla, 1996; Mazzocco et al., 1995) and of NLD (Tsatsanis & Rourke, 1995, p. 486). Despite having perhaps the most highly variable cognitive phenotype of any disorder presented in part I of this volume (in terms of the possible number and range of domains affected), NF-1 remains a model of specific LD outcomes. The same is true for other highly variable disorders not included in this volume, such as spina bifida (e.g., Dennis, Landry, Barnes, & Fletcher, 2006).

In addition to serving as models of LD, if specific mechanisms underlying a disorder can be tested, it is possible that the disorder may explain normal variation in the expression of select skills in the general population. From studies of the genetic disorders presented in parts I and II of this volume, we learn about the role of several factors on cognitive development, including CNS anomalies (e.g., NF-1), sex hormones (e.g., Turner syndrome and Klinefelter syndrome), thyroid hormones (e.g., congenital hypothyroidism), specific genes as implicated by studies of gene mapping (e.g., Turner syndrome) or gene dosing (e.g., fragile X and Barth syndromes), or gene regions as assessed for deletion syndromes (such as 22q deletion, Williams syndrome, and Duchenne muscular dystrophy mutations).

Despite the phenotypic variability described in each of the earlier chapters, it is the relative within-group *homogeneity* that gives rise to specific models of LD or of LD subtypes. However, a disorder serving as a "model" of LD does not implicate conformity in learning profiles among individuals from the population in question. This distinction is subject to misinterpretation as illustrated in the case of Olga (p. 420). This is one of the reasons why it may be helpful to address the following points when informing parents or teachers of a child's LD diagnosis or risk for LD:

• the limited knowledge regarding specific causes or correlates of LD within the population in question,

• the degree to which deficits appear to be domain specific (such as in Turner syndrome) or of specific severity levels across domains (such as in NF-1 or spina bifida), and

• sources of interactions associated with variable outcome levels.

Case 13.1: Olga   Olga is a 9-year-old with 45X, classic Turner syndrome. She has many of the physical features described in chapter 1, including short stature and a webbed neck. In school, Olga consistently receives poor grades in both reading and math. Her parents bring her to be evaluated by a psychologist, citing frustration that "girls with Turner syndrome aren't supposed to have problems with reading." The parents cite no behavioral difficulties and believe that Olga has higher intelligence than indicated by her failing grades in reading and math.

During the psychological assessment, Olga scores well below average on tests of academic achievement: Based on a mean score of 100 (SD = 15), Olga's Math Calculations standard score is 64, and her Letter Word Identification score is 84. This is in contrast to her Verbal IQ score of 122, although her Performance IQ score is 78. More telling is her nonword reading score of 67 and the qualitative observations made during that task. Olga's errors include many whole-word guesses, sound substitutions, and other errors that barely approximate the nonwords she is asked to sound out. Her oral reading is slow, inaccurate, and laborious. Assessment of phonological processing skills reveals performance levels below the minimum recommended levels for the typical beginning kindergartner. During the feedback session with Olga's parents, the psychologist explains that Olga's performance meets the criteria for dyslexia and that this may well be independent of her having Turner syndrome. Both parents express frustration over their having been "misled" to believe that "all girls with Turner syndrome have nonverbal learning disability," which they adamantly point out does not include dyslexia. Olga's father adds that he always struggled with reading during school and that as an adult he still does not enjoy reading. He does not wish the same for his daughter. These comments open the door for two related discussions: (a) that the implications of Turner syndrome as a "model" of NLD is not equivalent to expectations that each child with Turner syndrome will have a "classic," or model, NLD profile and (b) the notion that multiple genes and environmental factors contribute to Olga's phenotype as an individual, not just the absent X indicated by her 45X karyotype.

Olga's parents misinterpreted the notion of Turner syndrome as a model of LD as evidence that their daughter would have the model case of that LD, in this case NLD. Plomin and Walker (2003) describe another common misconception of the relation between genetics and cognitive outcome: that genetic causes are "hard wired" (p. 11) and thus unlikely to respond to intervention effects (Sternberg & Grigorenko, 1999). An emphasis on the notion of genes as an influence on, rather than determinant of, behavior, may affect parent's reactions to an LD diagnosis regardless of the extent to which the diagnosis is evident in their child. At the same time, parents need to recognize that additional factors—including the genes not associated with the disorder in question—have some influence on an individual's cognitive phenotype. In addition to the case of Olga, the cases of Pedro and Quillan illustrate two opposing outcomes of failing to recognize this basic information.

Case 13.2: Pedro   Pedro is a 16-year-old with sporadic NF-1, diagnosed at age 3 years when a pediatrician noted multiple café au lait spots during a routine examination. Pedro is now in 11th grade, where he continues to earn mostly A's and occasional B's. He excels in mathematics and is in an accelerated program through which he studies calculus I. Although less successful at reading than mathematics, Pedro is nevertheless performing well within grade-appropriate levels at reading and often reads for pleasure, preferring science fiction. He does not read large quantities of sci-fi novels, but he reports reading every day. Pedro comes to clinical attention via a self-referral to a school psychologist, because he is frustrated by his low college entrance exam scores despite repeated attempts (he has now taken the SAT three times). At the initial visit he is accompanied by his mother (a radiologist) and father (a physicist). Both Pedro and his mother believe that his SAT scores are not an accurate reflection of his ability, which they believe is more accurately indicated by his cumulative high school GPA (3.87). During the intake interview, there is no mention of NF-1 or LD.

Pedro's performance on the psycho-educational assessment is unremarkable, except for significantly lower scores on timed versus untimed testing. Whereas on most math and spatial tasks he scores above the 80th percentile, on all timed tasks such as the Wechsler Block Design he scores below the 40th percentile. The psychologist engages in limit testing, allowing Pedro to complete all block design items untimed; under these conditions, Pedro completely and accurately solves all items from the test. This pattern is repeated on timed tests of mathematics, spatial reasoning, and reading fluency.

During the feedback session, the psychologist asks whether Pedro was ever diagnosed with a learning disability. Mother then reveals the diagnosis of NF-1. (The psychologist is surprised, because of the absence of apparent physical features.) Mother adds that, when given the diagnosis, she had been informed that LD was a likely outcome. But she cites the doctors at having been "wrong, because Pedro clearly does not have a learning disability, he is actually rather intelligent." This comment gives rise to several points of discussion: an accurate definition of LD, its variability in children with NF-1, that gifted students can have LD, and the influences on Pedro's development in addition to NF-1 that may have contributed favorably to his academic skills. Such influences are implicated by parental interview and are associated with the parents' successful education and careers in math-oriented sciences and with the academically oriented environment in which Pedro was raised. A neuropsychological assessment is scheduled to address possible LD and to determine whether Pedro is eligible for untimed testing during the college entrance exams.

Case 13.3: Brothers Quentin and Quillan   Quentin is a 13-year-old boy with moderate mental retardation and Williams syndrome. Quentin's mother and father expressed concern about Quentin's 11-year-old brother, Quillan, who has been acting out at school in the midst of declining grades. Although Quillan had steadily maintained a B average in school through 5th grade, he is now achieving C's and D's and at times fails a class altogether. He seems more active than he has been in the past. Quillan's parents acknowledged that Quillan does not have the significant cognitive impairments most often associated with Williams syndrome, a difference readily apparent to them because Quentin has moderate mental retardation. Yet, being aware of the full range of possible phenotypes associated with Williams syndrome, the parents requested that Quillan receive fluorescence in situ hybridization testing for the syndrome. On the basis of a pedigree analysis, it was determined that it was possible for Quillan to have inherited genes related to Williams syndrome, and genetic testing is carried out.

Two weeks later, the results of Quillan's testing were presented to his parents by a psychologist and pediatrician, both experienced with patients who have Williams syndrome. The test results are negative. Quillan's parents express surprise at this result, and insisted that Quillan "must have Williams syndrome because his behavior and school performance are so poor." During the next 20 minutes, the pediatrician and psychologist explained that not all "negative" or "undesired" behaviors manifested in family members of a child with a syndrome are linked to that syndrome. Additional efforts are made to also address that not all aspects of the Williams syndrome phenotype are negative behaviors.

For Olga (case 13.1), there were probable heritable contributions to her co-occurring (but not necessarily comorbid) dyslexia that did not conform with a "classic" Turner syndrome profile. She had difficulties not expected on the basis of Turner syndrome but that were not surprising given her positive family history for dyslexia. For Pedro (case 13.2), additional influences may have ameliorated the effects leading to an LD profile, but he also may have had a relatively mild case of NF-1, as implicated by the lack of observable physical features. The case reports of Olga and Pedro illustrate how, despite the sheer wealth and range of information available about LD, there is a risk of losing the sense of this breadth when applying the term to an individual. LDs in children with a genetic disorder may not be associated with the disorder in question, and, as in the case of Quentin and his brother, less desirable characteristics of one's phenotype need not all be linked to the genetic disorder as a "scapegoat" for all problem behaviors—including in other family members.

Sharing Information about LD as a Risk, Not a Diagnosis

In cases 13.1 through 13.3 above, each individual demonstrated potential features of LD and came to clinical attention because of those features, at different points during development. This is in contrast to discussions of LD that occur during the information-sharing phase of informing parents of a child's diagnosis. When information about LD is delivered as one component of a syndrome-associated risk for LD, the information may not be directed toward the individual child so much as to the increased risk for a potential LD outcome. In these cases, information about LD may not even be anticipated by parents or teachers of a child with a new diagnosis, as observed in the following cases of Robert and Sasha. This is an issue specific to parents of children whose LD is associated with a genetic disorder or predisposing condition.

Case 13.4: Robert   Robert is a 2½-year-old boy with Klinefelter syndrome. His parents attended a support group meeting within months of learning of Robert's diagnosis. One presentation at that meeting pertained to LD profiles observed in children with Klinefelter syndrome. Robert's parents' surprise was reflected by their facial expressions and by the father's question, "Is there reason for me to believe that my son will have a learning disability?"

When the diagnosis of an LD is the consequence of clinical evaluations of a child's presenting symptoms, the diagnosis is an explanation for concerns or questions already raised by a parent or teacher. This sequence of events differs from the scenario of informing family members of LD associated with a given cognitive phenotype.

The same information that may direct parents to *explanations* for their child's difficulty has the potential to lead parents toward *expectations*, and these expectations may be neither necessary nor accurate. It is possible to provoke expectations—inappropriate or helpful—in parents of any child, and thus presenting information about LD should be done with caution and clarification. It is important to clarify the nature of how LD is defined (and how this differs from defining a known genetic disorder), limitations of applying a definition to an individual child, and the developmental differences in the manifestation of LD. Naturally, it is also important to emphasize when LD characterizations are empirically based versus anecdotal, as well as the degree of risk implied by having a genetic disorder. Any recommendations for intervention should include preventative measures that are believed to be helpful for all children, such as changes to the language arts curriculum that enhance reading skills for children at all reading levels (National Reading Panel, 2000).

> **Case 13.5: Sasha** Sasha is the mother of a 3-year-old boy who has the fragile X full mutation. Like many other parents attending a regional fragile X conference for parents and teachers, Sasha had recently been diagnosed as a carrier of the fragile X premutation. She described the supportive nature of the professionals whose clinical expertise ultimately led her to her son's diagnosis and reported some of the reactions she had to learning that she herself was a carrier. When describing the conversation about her own diagnosis, she noted having been told about "the characteristics of female carriers (of the premutation)" by a genetic counselor, who had followed up the feedback session with a telephone call, during which the counselor proceeded to list the psychological strengths and difficulties associated with the premutation. She told Sasha that women with the premutation had depression and poor mathematics ability. Sasha laughed while recalling this conversation, commenting that at least she now has an excuse for hating math.

Sasha's story is hardly amusing, because both the nature of the information she received and how that information was shared with her were inappropriate. She received clinical information about her psychological functioning without benefit of a psychological assessment. She received information about associated phenotype characteristics that are controversial at best, as some studies have called into question the validity of cognitive or behaviorial effects of the fragile X premutation (Myers et al., 2001; Reiss, Freund, Abrams, Boehm, & Karazian, 1993). In Sasha's case, she may have come to expect behaviors in herself that she would now readily dismiss as resulting from her genetic "disorder."

Knowledge of a cognitive phenotype may affect one's self-expectation. Thus, it stands to reason that it could also affect a parent or teacher's expectation for a child. Indeed, Walker and Plomin (2005) found that most teachers (82%) feel that their method of teaching or following a student would be influenced by knowledge that the child had a genetically influenced LD. There are clear benefits of this effect, in terms of the number of students with genetically influenced LD who would receive appropriate instructional modification when a diagnosis is made available to a teacher. A possible drawback is in changes to instruction that are unwarranted if the genetically influenced LD is not a particularly accurate portrayal of the child in question. (In cases where the instructional modification is one that would benefit all children, such as the language arts curriculum addressed earlier, this is not problematic.) Walker and Plomin found that most teachers participating in their survey had knowledge of the influence of genetics on learning difficulties, intelligence, and mental illness, despite no formal training in genetics. Despite a general increase in attention devoted to genetics within the field of education, formal training is very limited. For instance, in their review of textbook contents, Plomin and Walker (2003) found that educational psychology textbook coverage of genetics is limited to three or fewer pages. Although it is encouraging that teachers are recognizing the contributions of genetics to intellectual function and development, this informally acquired (or limited) knowledge base may be especially prone to misperceptions and inaccuracies. Indeed, in another study of parents' and teachers' beliefs regarding mathematics achievement specifically, Uttal (1997) reported that "Americans hold an unjustified belief that achievement ... is determined largely by innate ability" (i.e., hardwired and not subject to environmental influence, p. 171) and that this belief may "contribute to the poor mathematics performance of American children." Whereas Uttal draws implications from his review for how parents are informed of findings regarding genetic influences on intelligence and achievement, I argue that the same implications can be applied to the manner in which we convey information to parents regarding cognitive phenotypes with associated LD. We must avoid implying that LD is hardwired to the extent that it is not subject to effects of intervention, unless empirical evidence unequivocally supports this notion at some point in the future. Although this is an unlikely situation, we are currently faced with the unfortunate situation of a paucity of empirical research on effective instruction for children with genetically associated LD. Clearly, there will be limits to the contribution of intervention, but such limits do not negate that benefits may occur.

Generalizing Group Findings to Individuals

Whereas phenotype descriptions reported by researchers apply to *groups* of individuals with a disorder, these descriptions rarely if ever describe all (or any) single individual with the disorder. Even the most severely affected child with fragile X syndrome will likely fail to manifest all of the associated features of the fragile X behavior and cognitive phenotypes. Indeed, in many cases, seemingly opposing features characterize the group-based phenotype of the syndrome. For instance, children with fragile X are described as having "relatively intact language skills" (relative to other domains), yet a hallmark of this disorder is delayed language. Language in children with fragile X is often described as perseverative (Belser & Sudhalter, 2001), yet there are cases of reported elective mutism (Hagerman et al., 1999). Social shyness and anxiety are features of fragile X (Sobesky et al., 1994), as is poor inhibition (Bennetto et al., 2001). These descriptions may appear contradictory to the lay person who is attempting to synthesize information about a disability in order to apply that information to an individual child. Such confusion is likely to emerge from descriptions of highly variable disorders, such as LD, particularly broad classifications of LD, such as NLD.

NLD: Multiple Etiologies, Discrepant Profiles

Many of the disorders described in part I have been proposed as an etiology of NLD (Davenport, Hooper, & Zeger, this volume; Cornish, Levitas, & Sudhalter, this volume; Simon, Burg-Malki, & Gothelf, this volume; Slopis & Moore, this volume; Mervis & Morris, this volume). Yet each is quite distinct from the others. Even in cases where global descriptions appear similar, important differences emerge and thereby offer alternative models of brain–behavior relationships underlying cognitive processes. Differences are noted in patterns of reading, math, attention, and social disability such that more recent models of neurodevelopmental disorders are moving away from all-encompassing terms that unify rather than specify diverse conditions. Researchers of these conditions seek to generate testable models based on an analysis of the assets and deficits in each condition (e.g., Dennis et al., 2006; Mazzocco & McCloskey, 2005; Murphy, Mazzocco, & McCloskey, in press; and chapters 1, 3, 6, and 7 in this volume). In my own research laboratory, we carry out studies of cognitive phenotypes for fragile X, Turner, and Barth syndromes. Below I report on a subset of descriptive findings from this ongoing research as a complement to the phenotype descriptions provided elsewhere in this volume (Cornish et al., this volume; Davenport et al., this volume; Antshel & Arnold, this volume, respectively). Although the findings suggest that there is some wisdom in describing the associated LD as *nonverbal*, the findings further illustrate the lack of specificity inherent in the NLD label.

Our comparison is based on IQ test scores of children with fragile X, Turner, or Barth syndrome, including Full Scale, Verbal, and Performance scores. (Note that our studies of children with fragile X include only females, who are high functioning relative to males with the disorder, as a group.) A higher Verbal versus Performance IQ score would conform to a "classic NLD" profile. In order to assess both qualitative and quantitative performance strengths and deficits, we compared IQ scores of each individual child with IQ scores of each child's mother. (There was an insufficient number of scores available from fathers to justify a comparison either with fathers only or with mid-parental IQ.) Although mother–child comparisons do not control for all genetic influences in addition to the disorder in question, such comparisons are a more direct measure of the specific effects of the disorder than are comparisons with other, unrelated children. Our evaluation of the discrepancies in IQ scores for the mother–child pairs reveals differences across the three groups, despite the fact that each is reported to be at risk for NLDs.

For girls with fragile X syndrome, the global deficits are immediately apparent in figure 13.1, despite the restriction of this group to relatively high-functioning individuals with fragile X. Nearly all of the girls with fragile X, in our studies, have lower full scale, Verbal, and Performance IQ scores than do their own mothers (figure 13.1). The mother–child discrepancy ranges from minimal to significant, with a mean full scale IQ discrepancy of 1.5 SDs ($M = 22.88$, $SD = 11.82$). The mother–child discrepancy is more remarkable (and less variable) for Performance IQ scores ($M = 32.62$, $SD = 11.41$) relative to Verbal IQ scores ($M = 9.85$, $SD = 16.96$), but together, these three discrepancies reflect broader ranging deficits in the fragile X group.

The pattern of findings observed for the fragile X group differs from those observed for the two remaining groups. Relative to girls with fragile X, girls with Turner syndrome have more specific but less remarkable deficits, as indicated by the mother–child discrepancy scores. That is, there is no significant tendency for girls to have lower (or higher) full scale IQ scores than their mothers, as seen in figure 13.2. The mother–child discrepancies in verbal IQ scores (or the lack thereof) also fail to support that global cognitive deficits characterize this group. Neither the full scale nor verbal score discrepancy is significant, $ps > .10$. Yet nearly all girls with Turner syndrome have lower Performance IQ scores than do their mothers (to different degrees). The mean mother–child Performance IQ score discrepancy is significant, at nearly 1 SD ($M = 14.20$, $SD = 11.45$), although less than that reported for girls with fragile X. Boys with Barth syndrome fall somewhere between what is observed for the first two groups (figure 13.3): Cognitive effects are more global than seen for the Turner syndrome group (as is also the case for the fragile X group), because boys with Barth syndrome have significantly lower scores than their mothers for full scale IQ, Verbal IQ, and Performance IQ scores, $ps < .018$; but the Performance IQ discrepancy scores ($M = 21.56$, $SD = 16.68$) are smaller and more variable than those observed in the fragile X group and larger (and more variable) than those observed for the Turner syndrome group. The group differences in discrepancy score profiles are not likely to result from characteristics of the mothers. In terms of overall performance levels, figures 13.1 to 13.3 illustrate that mothers' scores are well within the average range for all three groups.

Although we can conclude that primary-school-age children with any of these three disorders have lower Performance IQ scores than their own mothers, the nonverbal difficulties are *more specific* for Turner syndrome, of *greater magnitude* for the group with fragile X, and *more variable* for the group with Barth syndrome. This profile variability is not necessarily inconsistent with descriptions of NLD, which in-

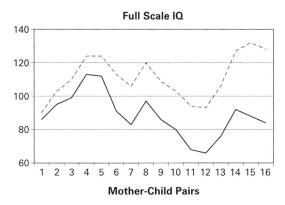

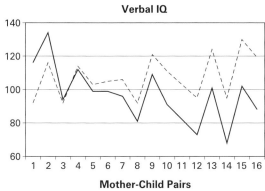

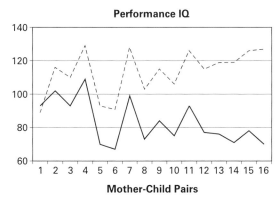

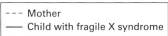

Figure 13.1
Full scale IQ (FSIQ), Verbal IQ (VIQ), and Performance IQ (PIQ) scores for 16 girls with fragile X syndrome and their own mothers. The paired set of data points appears in order of smallest to largest discrepancy between mothers and their own daughters. The girls whose scores are represented in this data set range in age from 7 to 11 years at the time of their IQ assessment.

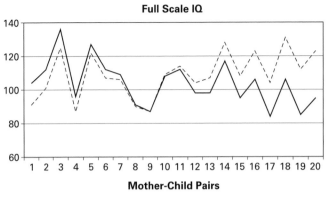

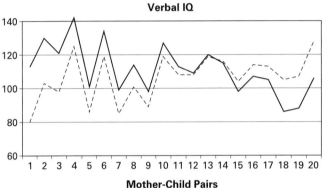

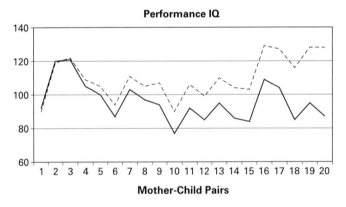

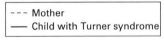

Figure 13.2
Full scale IQ (FSIQ), Verbal IQ (VIQ), and Performance IQ (PIQ) scores for 20 girls with Turner syndrome and their own mothers. The paired set of data points appears in order of smallest to largest discrepancy between mothers and their own daughters. The girls whose scores are represented in this data set range in age from 7 to 10 years at the time of their IQ assessment. Reprinted from International Congress Series, 1298, M. M. M. Mazzocco, The cognitive phenotype of Turner syndrome: Specific learning disabilities, pp. 83–92, with permission from Elsevier.

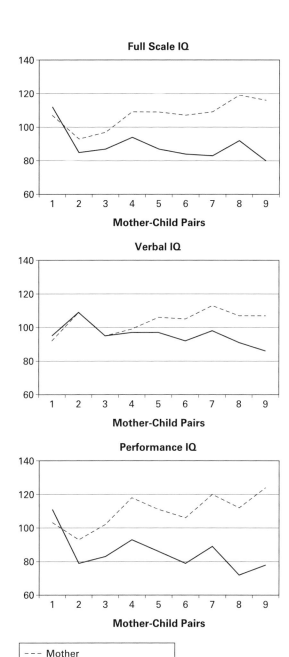

Full Scale IQ

Verbal IQ

Performance IQ

--- Mother
— Child with Barth syndrome

Figure 13.3
Full scale IQ (FSIQ), Verbal IQ (VIQ), and Performance IQ (PIQ) scores for 9 boys with Barth syndrome and their own mothers. The paired set of data points appears in order of smallest to largest discrepancy between mothers and their own sons. The boys whose scores are represented in this data set range in age from 6 to 10 years at the time of their IQ assessment.

clude many primary, secondary, and/or tertiary difficulties (e.g., in tactile perception, psychomotor coordination, visual–spatial skills, nonverbal problem solving, concept formation, and hypothesis testing; distorted sense of time, poor reading comprehension despite strong rote reading skills, weak performance in mathematics, deficits in social perception, and internalized behaviors such as depression and social withdrawal, as reviewed by Davenport et al., this volume, chapter 1). This variability is captured by the classification of NLD at "Levels" 1 to 3, based on whether the phenotype meets all, or a subset, of the "syndrome" criteria (Tsatsanis & Rourke, 1995). Note that Turner syndrome, classified by Rourke as a Level 1 NLD, is in fact associated with more specific nonverbal deficits *than the other syndromes* examined above, but it cannot be said that the cognitive phenotype is homogeneous with respect to the number of features summarized above. It is on this basis that Davenport and colleagues (chapter 1, p. 28) caution us that, "making an NLD 'diagnosis' probably is not warranted, nor even evidence-based, [but] conceptualizing children with Turner syndrome within an NLD framework can help to provide a heuristic for better understanding the problems experienced by many individuals with Turner syndrome and it should help to frame this disorder for health care providers and educators." This caution may be even more applicable to other syndromes associated with NLD, in view of the fact that the Turner syndrome phenotype meets more criteria of NLD than most other syndromes.

If NLD is only the starting point of describing a cognitive phenotype (for a group or an individual), what subsequent steps must follow? Initial phenotyping studies necessarily focus on behaviors that can be measured by general or standardized testing, to assess more broadly defined skills, such as the IQ score profiles summarized above. For each disorder, this type of descriptive approach is needed for initially establishing the general areas of deficits in persons with known disorders, in much the same way that early investigations for candidate genes focus on larger rather then gene-specific locations. This broader (and incomplete) level of knowledge is all that is available for understudied phenotypes, such as those associated with errors of metabolism (Antshel & Arnold, this volume). In cases where the initial groundwork has been summarized, such as for Turner syndrome (Ross & Zinn, 1999), Klinefelter syndrome (Geschwind, Boone, Miller, & Swerdloff, 2000), 22q deletion (Shprintzen, 2000), NF-1 (Kayl & Moore, 2000), Williams syndrome, and fragile X (Hagerman & Hagerman, 2002; Mazzocco, 2000), subsequent studies have examined more specific cognitive mechanisms by testing theories of cognition. Unlike the initial descriptive studies, this approach is informative for teasing apart different pathways to the misleadingly "similar" phenotypes as is evident in chapters 1 through 7 in part I (this volume).

Moreover, comparisons across "similar" syndromes are an effective means by which to identify different neuropathways to comparable (or identical) LD-related outcome behaviors. For example, my own research on mathematics LD in genetic syndromes is based on the hypothesis that the poor mathematics achievement reported for girls with fragile X or Turner syndrome do not conform to the same profile of arithmetic strengths and weaknesses. These hypotheses are supported from our ongoing research: Although girls with either disorder show increased risk for mathematics disability by kindergarten (Mazzocco, 2001), group differences emerged for (a) the age at which specific arithmetic weaknesses emerge (earlier for fragile X; see Murphy, Mazzocco, Gerner, & Henry, 2006), (b) the types of arithmetic errors made (more alignment errors among girls with fragile X; Mazzocco, 1998), (c) the cognitive correlates of math performance (Mazzocco, Singh-Bhatia, & Lesniak-Karpiak, 2006), and (d) the areas of relative strengths and weaknesses such as in math fact retrieval (vs. conceptual understanding of arithmetic) for which the former is a strength for girls with fragile X, and a weakness for girls with Turner syndrome (Murphy & Mazzocco, in press). Just as it is inappropriate to equate the two phenotypes on the basis of their shared poor math achievement, it is even more inappropriate to consider an NLD label to sufficiently and thoroughly reflect the profile characteristics and educational needs of an individual.

Implications for Intervention and Identification

Cognitive profile studies of different syndrome groups may reveal different neurodevelopmental pathways to the same or a similar manifestation. Therefore, despite similar outcomes, different underlying causes suggest that the success of specific interventions may vary across groups. Nevertheless, a logical starting point for intervention is implementation of empirically based and tested instruction for children with a specific LD classification. However, whereas there is a solid evidence-based practice for RDs (e.g., as reviewed by Schatschneider & Torgesen, 2004; National Reading Panel, 2000), there is far less research to guide intervention for mathematics- or "NLD"-related deficits. The same dilemma applies to identification: If we understand the construct and the underlying difficulties of LD, we can test and determine risk prior to manifestation in school. For RD, early rhyming and other phonological awareness indices are associated with later successful reading (Braddley & Bryant, 1983), giving rise to empirically based tools (such as the Comprehensive Test of Phonological Processing; Wagner, Torgesen, & Rachotte, 1999) that can be used with children as young as 5 years of age. Early predictors of mathematics LD have not been definitively established, but the research to date suggests that both concepts of number (e.g., Mazzocco & Thompson, 2005; Jordan, Hanich, & Kaplan, 2003) and executive function skills (Espy et al., 2004, Mazzocco & Kover, 2007) are predictive of risk for later poor math achievement.

Implications for Child Development

In this volume, heightened risk for LD was a component of the cognitive phenotype for all disorders presented. The study of each disorder makes contributions at several levels, specifically by enhancing our understanding of the nature of the learning difficulties in persons with the specific phenotypes in question, the variation of learning difficulties within phenotypes, and models of variation in LDs as observed in the general population. In considering the extent to which this type of research informs the broader field of child development, it is helpful to consider models used to describe how phenotypes develop in children with developmental disorders. Among existing models are the "three-level frameworks" proposed by Frith (2001). At the first level is the contribution and driving force of *biology*; so for the framework to be relevant, it is essential to accurately define the biological condition. With known genetic disorders, the presence or absence of the disorder itself is most often unequivocal, as is the case for all disorders described in part I and many others described in part II. In contrast, the presence or absence of LD is more equivocal for some (but not all) individuals from these groups. This is one advantage of studying conditions with known genetic etiologies. Level 2, *cognition*, is subject to influences from biology (genes, brain function) and environment. Both cognition and the environment influence the third level proposed by Frith, *behavior*. The distinction between cognition (e.g., deficits in phonological decoding or number sense difficulties that may interfere with automatic processing of small quantities) and behavior (slow reading or inaccurate mental addition calculation, respectively) drives the current efforts to delineate the cognitive deficits that underlie genetic-syndrome-associated LD. This distinction may also guide our effort to identify and describe LD in an individual with a given syndrome, rather than forcing the phenotype onto the individual in question. Finally, a focus on specific behaviors as indices of cognitive ability and disability will serve to guide the research on the effectiveness of intervention, and of the additional influences on outcome of the phenotype.

Conclusion

Whether focusing on identification of LD, classification of an LD profile, or intervention for the child with LD, describing LDs as a phenotype-associated outcome is an important preventative measure for parents of children with genetic disorders. We must exercise caution in how such descriptions are presented, to prevent misinterpretation and overgeneralization of group-based findings. We should consider whether the parent anticipates any information about LD, which may affect the degree to which the parent is receptive to discussions at various levels. We must clarify the limitations of the LD label, just as we may address the benefits it affords in terms of special education services and classroom modifications (see Hatton, this volume; Sudhalter, this volume). Group-based risk does not equal individual outcomes, and individual outcomes often will not conform to the group-based models of LD that we develop via research. Just as an LD definition may be a starting point from which a family is to seek appropriate guidance and intervention, for the clinician, the syndrome model is the starting point for making recommendations for a given individual, and for going beyond the syndrome to understand the individual and the contexts in which that child functions. By attending to these cautions, we may maximize the effectiveness of information we share with parents when LD is associated with the genetic disorder present in their child.

Note

1. The term "learning disability," while not clearly defined, is used in this chapter to refer to children whose learning difficulties are not due to mental retardation. This use of the term is consistent with most variations of the definition used in the United States. Elsewhere, such as in the United Kingdom, the term "learning disability" includes mental retardation.

References

Belser, R. C., & Sudhalter, V. (2001). Conversational characteristics of children with fragile X syndrome: Repetitive speech. *American Journal of Mental Retardation, 106,* 28–38.

Bennetto, L., Pennington, B. F., Porter, D., Taylor, A. K., & Hagerman, R. J. (2001). Profile of cognitive functioning in women with the fragile X mutation. *Neuropsychology, 15,* 290–299.

Berninger, V. W., Abbott, R. D., Thomson, J. B., & Raskind, W. H. (2001). Language phenotype for reading and writing disability: A family approach. *Scientific Studies of Reading, 5,* 59–106.

Bradley, L., & Bryant, P. E. (1983). Categorizing sounds and learning to read—A causal connection. *Nature, 301,* 419–421.

Denckla, M. (1996). Neurofibromatosis type 1: A model for the pathogenesis of reading disability. *Mental Retardation and Developmental Disabilities Research Reviews, 2,* 48–53.

Dennis, M., Landry, S. H., Barnes, M., & Fletcher, J. M. (2006). A model of neurocognitive function in spina bifida across the life span. *Journal of the International Neuropsychological Society, 12,* 285–296.

Eden, G. F., & Zeffiro, T. (2004). Neural systems affected in developmental dyslexia revealed by functional neuroimaging. *Neuron, 21,* 279–282.

Epsy, K. A., McDiarmid, M. M., Cwik, M. F., Stalets, M. M., Hamby, A., & Senn, T. E. (2004). The contribution of executive function to emergent mathematic skills in preschool children. *Developmental Neuropsychology, 26,* 465–486.

Fletcher, J. M., Francis, D. J., Morris, R., & Lyon, G. R. (2005). Evidenced-based assessment of learning disabilities in children and adolescents. *Journal of Clinical Child and Adolescent Psychology, 34,* 506–522.

Fletcher, J. M., Morris, R., & Lyon, G. R. (2003). Classification and definition of learning disabilities: An integrated perspective. In H. L. Swanson, K. R. Harris, & S. Graham (Eds.), *Handbook of learning disabilities* (pp. 30–56). New York: Guilford Press.

Francis, D. J., Fletcher, J. M., Shaywitz, B. A., Shaywitz, S. E., & Rourke, B. P. (1996). Defining learning and language disabilities: Conceptual and psychometric issues with the use of IQ tests. *Language, Speech, and Hearing Services in the Schools, 27,* 132–143.

Francis, D. J., Fletcher, J. M., Stuebing, K. K., Lyon, G. R., Shaywitz, B. A., & Shaywitz, S. E. (2005). Psychometric approaches to the identification of LD: IQ and achievement scores are not sufficient. *Journal of Learning Disabilities, 38,* 98–108.

Frith, U. (2001). What framework should we use for understanding developmental disorders? *Developmental Neuropsychology, 20,* 555–563.

Geary, D. C. (1993). Mathematical disabilities: Cognitive, neuropsychological, and genetic components. *Psychological Bulletin, 114,* 345–362.

Geary, D. C. (2004). Mathematics and learning disabilities. *Journal of Learning Disabilities, 37,* 4–15.

Geary, D. C. (2005). Role of cognitive theory in the study of learning disability in mathematics. *Journal of Learning Disabilities, 38,* 305–307.

Geschwind, D. H., Boone, K. B., Miller, B. L., & Swerdloff, R. S. (2000). Neurobehavioral phenotype of Klinefelter syndrome. *Mental Retardation and Developmental Disabilities Research Reviews, 6,* 107–116.

Hagerman, R., & Hagerman, P. (2002). (Eds.). *Fragile X syndrome: Diagnosis, treatment, and research.* Baltimore: Johns Hopkins University Press.

Hagerman, R. J., Hills, J., Scharfenaker, S., & Lewis, H. (1999). Fragile X syndrome and selective mutism. *American Journal of Medical Genetics, 83,* 313–317.

Hallahan, D. P., & Mock, D. R. (2003). A brief history of the field of learning disabilities. In H. L. Swanson, K. R Harris, & S. Graham (Eds.), *Handbook of learning disabilities* (pp. 16–29). New York: Guilford Press.

Hanich, L. B., Jordan, N. C., Kaplan, D., & Dick, J. (2001). Performance across different areas of mathematical cognition in children with learning difficulties. *Journal of Educational Psychology, 92,* 615–626.

Herr, C. M., & Bateman, B. D. (2003). Learning disabilities and the law. In H. L. Swanson, K. R Harris, & S. Graham (Eds.), *Handbook of learning disabilities* (pp. 57–73). New York: Guilford Press.

Jordan, N. C., Hanich, L. B., & Kaplan, D. (2003). A longitudinal study of mathematical compentencies in children with specific mathematics difficulties versus children with comorbid mathematics and reading difficulties. *Child Development, 74,* 834–850.

Kavale, K. A., Holdnack, J. A., & Mostert, M. P. (2005). Responsiveness to intervention and the identification of specific learning disability: A critique and alternative proposal. *Learning Disabilities Quarterly, 28,* 2–16.

Kayl, A. E., & Moore, B. D. (2000). Behavioral phenotype of neurofibromatosis type 1. *Mental Retardation and Developmental Disabilities Research Reviews, 6,* 117–124.

Keogh, B. K. (2005). Revisiting classification and identification. *Learning Disability Quarterly, 28,* 100–102.

Mazzocco, M. M. M. (1998). A process approach to describing mathematics difficulties in girls with Turner syndrome. *Pediatrics, 102,* 492–496.

Mazzocco, M. M. M. (2000). Advances in research on the fragile X syndrome. *Mental Retardation and Developmental Disabilities Research Reviews, 6,* 96–106.

Mazzocco, M. M. M. (2005). Challenges in identifying target skills for math disability screening and intervention. *Journal of Learning Disabilities, 38,* 318–323.

Mazzocco, M. M. M. (2001). Math learning disability and math LD subtypes: Evidence from studies of Turner syndrome, fragile X syndrome, and neurofibromatosis type 1. *Journal of Learning Disabilities, 34,* 520–533.

Mazzocco, M. M. M., & Kover, S. T. (2007). A longitudinal assessment of the development of executive function and their association with math performance. *Child Neuropsychology, 13,* 18–45.

Mazzocco, M. M. M., & McCloskey, M. (2005). Math performance in girls with Turner or Fragile X syndrome. In J. Campbell (Ed.), *Handbook of mathematical cognition.* Hove, UK and New York: Psychology Press, pp. 269–297.

Mazzocco, M. M. M., Singh Bhatia, N. S., & Lesniak-Karpiak, K. (2006). Visuospatial skills and their association with math performance in girls with fragile X or Turner syndrome. *Child Neuropsychology, 12,* 87–110.

Mazzocco, M. M. M., & Thompson, R. E. (2005). Kindergarten predictors of math learning disability. *Learning Disabilities Research and Practice, 20,* 142–155.

Mazzocco, M. M. M., Turner, J. E., Denckla, M. B., Hofman, K. J., Scanlon, D. C., & Vellutino, F. R. (1995). Language and reading deficits associated with neurofibromatosis type 1: Evidence for a not-so-nonverbal learning disability. *Developmental Neuropsychology, 11,* 503–522.

Morris, R. D., Stuebing, S. E., Fletcher, J. M., Shaywitz, S. E., Lyon, G. R., Shankweiler, D. P., et al. (1998). Subtypes of reading disability: Variability around a phonological core. *Journal of Educational Psychology, 3,* 347–373.

Murphy, M. M., Mazzocco, M. M. M., Gerner, G., & Henry, A. E. (2006). Mathematics learning disability in girls with Turner syndrome or fragile X Syndrome. *Brain and Cognition, 6,* 195–210.

Murphy, M. M., & Mazzocco, M. M. M. (in press). Mathematics learning disability in girls with fragile X or Turner syndrome during late elementary school. *Journal of Learning Disabilities.*

Murphy, M. M., Mazzocco, M. M. M., & McCloskey, M. (in press). Mathematics disabilities in fragile X and Turner syndromes. To appear in M. Barnes (Ed.), *Genes, brain, and development: The neurocognition of genetic disorders.* Cambridge University Press.

Myers, G. F., Mazzocco, M. M. M., Madalena, A., & Reiss, A. L. (2001). No widespread.psychological effect of the fragile X premutation in childhood: Evidence from a preliminary controlled study. *Journal of Developmental and Behavioral Pediatrics, 22,* 353–359.

National Institute of Neurological Disorders and Stroke. (2007) NINDS learning disabilities information page. Retrieved January 7, 2006 from http://www.ninds.nih.gov/disorders/learningdisabilities/learningdisabilities.htm

National Reading Panel. (2000). *Teaching children to read: An evidence-based assessment of the scientific research literature on reading and its implications for reading instruction* (NIH Publication No. 00-4754). Washington, DC: National Institute of Child Health and Human Development.

Petrill, S. A., & Plomin, R. (2007). Quantitative genetics and mathematical abilities/disabilities. In D. Berch & M. M. M. Mazzocco (Eds.), *Why is math so hard for some children? The nature and origins of mathematical learning difficulties and disabilities.* Baltimore: Brookes.

Plomin, R., & Kovas, Y. (2005). Generalist genes and learning disabilities. *Psychological Bulletin, 131,* 592–617.

Plomin, R., & Walker, S. O. (2003). Genetics and educational psychology. *British Journal of Educational Psychology, 73,* 3–14.

Powell, K. B., & Voeller, K. K. (2004). Prefrontal executive function syndromes in children. *Journal of Child Neurology, 19,* 785–797.

Reiss, A. L., Freund, L. S., Abrams, M. T., Boehm, C., & Kazazian, H. (1993). Neurobehavioral effects of the fragile X premutation in adult women: A controlled study. *American Journal of Human Genetics, 52,* 884–894.

Ross, J. R., & Zinn, A. (1999). Turner syndrome: Potential hormonal and genetic influences on the neurocognitive profile. In H. Tager-Flusberg (Ed.), *Neurodevelopmental disorders* (pp. 251–268). Cambridge, MA: MIT Press.

Rourke, B. P. (1995). (Ed.). *Syndrome of nonverbal learning disabilities: Neurodevelomental manifestations.* New York: Guilford Press.

Schatschneider, C., & Torgesen, J. K. (2004). Using our current understanding of dyslexia to support early identification and intervention. *Journal of Child Neurology, 19,* 759–765.

Semrud-Clikeman, M., Biederman, J., Sprich-Buckminster, S., Lehman, B. K., Faraone, S. V., Norman, D. (1992). Comorbidity between ADDH and learning disability: A review and report in a clinically referred sample. *Journal of the American Academy of Child and Adolescent Psychiatry, 31,* 439–448.

Shaywitz, S. E., Escobar, M. D., Shaywitz, B. A., Fletcher, J. M., & Makuch, R. (1992). Evidence that dyslexia may represent the lower tail of a normal distribution of reading ability. *The New England Journal of Medicine, 326,* 145–150.

Shprintzen, R. J. (2000). Velo–cardio–facial syndrome: A distinctive behavioral phenotype. *Mental Retardation and Developmental Disabilities Research Reviews, 6,* 142–147.

Simon, T. J., Bearden, C. E., McDonald-McGinn, D., & Zackai, E. (2005). Visuospatial and numerical cognitive deficits in children with chromosome 22q11.2 deletion syndrome. *Cortex, 41,* 145–155.

Sobesky, W. E., Pennington, B. F., Porter, D., Hull, C. E., & Hagerman, R. J. (1994). Emotional and neurocognitive deficits in fragile X. *American Journal of Medical Genetics, 51,* 378–385.

Sternberg, R. J., & Grigorenko, E. L. (1999). Myths in psychology and education regarding the gene–environment debate. *Teachers College Record, 100,* 536.

Tsatsanis, K. D., & Rourke, B. P. (1995). Conclusions and future directions. In B. Rourke (Ed.), *Syndrome of nonverbal learning disabilities: Neurodevelomental manifestations* (pp. 476–496). New York: Guilford Press.

Uttal, D. H. (1997). Beliefs about genetic influences on mathematics achievement: A cross-cultural comparison. *Genetica, 99,* 165–172.

Wagner, R., Torgesen, J., & Rasshotte, C. (1999). Comprehensive Test of Phonological Processing (CTOPP). Austin, TX: Pro-Ed.

Walker, S. O., & Plomin, R. (2005). The nature–nurture question: Teachers' perceptions of how genes and the environment influence educationally relevant behaviour. *Educational Psychology, 25,* 509–516.

14 Early Intervention and Early Childhood Special Education for Young Children with Neurogenetic Disorders

Deborah D. Hatton

Children with disabilities from birth to 5 years of age have been entitled to special supports and special education since 1986 when Public Law 99-457 was passed. Later, this law was reauthorized as part of the Individuals With Disabilities Education Act (IDEA) and most recently as the Individuals With Disabilities Education Improvement Act (IDEIA, 2004). As with the original legislation, the current reauthorization identifies that the purpose of early intervention and early childhood special education (ECSE) is to

- enhance the development of children with disabilities and minimize potential for developmental delay,
- reduce educational costs to our society,
- maximize potential for individuals with disabilities to live independently, and
- enhance the capacity of families to meet the special needs of their infants and toddlers with disabilities. (IDEIA, 2004)

State and local agencies have considerable flexibility in providing early intervention and ECSE. Although public school systems are typically responsible for providing ECSE for children ages 3 to 5 with disabilities, early intervention for infants and toddlers may be provided by other agencies, such as health and human services agencies. In some states, educational agencies are responsible for services to children from birth or from 2 years of age to age 21. To identify the agency responsible for early intervention (both Part C for infants and toddlers and Part B, Section 619 for preschoolers) in particular states, professionals can find the information on the Web site of the National Early Childhood Technical Assistance Center at www.nectac .org. For local information, individuals can also contact the director of exceptional child services at their local school system.

In this chapter, an overview of early intervention and ECSE is provided to help specialists in neurogenetic disorders understand the supports and services that are available to young children with disabilities and their families. In addition, summaries of the research literature on early intervention and ECSE for children with 22q11 deletion syndrome, fragile X syndrome, Turner syndrome and Klinefelter syndrome are presented. Resources for professionals and families are also described.

Early Intervention and Early Childhood Special Education

Early Intervention

In recognition of the impact of the diagnosis of a disability in very young children, Part C of IDEA requires parental involvement in early intervention. When young children have disabilities, families experience a number of stressors such as

- the need for information about the diagnosis and prognosis and the impact of the disability on the child's development,
- personal and family distress related to the diagnosis,
- the need for additional resources to meet the needs of the child with a disability, and
- threats regarding their ability to adequately parent the child with a disability (Guralnick, 2000).

Families of children with genetic disorders, particularly those with hereditary disorders, face additional unique challenges including guilt about passing the disorder to their child, reproductive decisions about whether or not to have additional children, and the potential need to inform extended family members that they, too, may be the carriers of a neurogenetic disorder. These challenges are described in detail in chapters 11 and 12 of this volume.

These stressors can impact parent–child interactions, the experiences that the family can provide to the child, and the family's ability to provide a safe, healthy, and supportive environment for the child and family (Guralnick, 2000; chapter 12, this volume). Therefore, one goal of early intervention and ECSE is to support families so that they can then facilitate the optimal development of their children with special needs.

In addition, IDEIA 2004 recognizes that infants and toddlers have specialized needs that may require the expertise of professionals from multiple disciplines (medicine, special education, speech–language pathology, occupational therapy, physical therapy, social work, psychology, etc.). Therefore, interdisciplinary collaboration is required, and the family is considered an integral member of the early intervention team.

Similar to the individualized education program (IEP) for children with disabilities between the ages of 3 and 21 years that is described in detail by Sudhalter in chapter 15 of this volume, the individualized family service plan (IFSP) is used as both a process and a document to ensure that the needs of infants and toddlers with disabilities and their families are met. Guidelines for the development of the IFSP and for the provision of early intervention are specified in Part C of IDEIA 2004. These guidelines describe time lines for assessment, development of the IFSP, the provision of services, and monitoring the IFSP. In relation to these guidelines, I will briefly describe key issues that may be of particular importance for young children with neurogenetic disorders.

Determining Eligibility for Early Intervention   Eligibility requirements for securing early intervention services may vary from state to state; however, all states are required to provide early intervention for children with established conditions that are associated with intellectual disabilities or developmental delays. Most neurogenetic disorders should meet the criteria for established risk, and a medical record with the diagnosis may be sufficient to establish eligibility. Most children with disabilities are served under the eligibility label of "developmental delay," however. Some children with neurogenetic disorders who may not be experiencing significant delays within the first year or two of life may not qualify for early intervention based on developmental delay. Therefore, professionals who support families of children with neurogenetic disorders should be alert to this possibility and should be prepared to help families advocate for services under the established condition eligibility category if needed.

Assessment for Intervention Planning and Monitoring   Even though eligibility for early intervention may be made from medical records, assessment for program planning is required in order to develop the IFSP. According to Part C of IDEIA, children must be assessed by professionals from at least two disciplines in order to describe their current levels of functioning in the areas of cognition, communication, motor development, adaptive development, socioemotional development, and physical development. In addition to using the information gathered through this assessment, families are expected to direct the assessment of their resources, priorities, and concerns in order to identify the supports and services required for them to meet the developmental needs of the infant or toddler. Families always have the right to determine their level of involvement in early intervention; however, some families are only interested in early intervention that addresses the needs of their child, rather than the needs of their entire family. Therefore, professionals must carefully balance the legal requirements of IDEIA 2004, Part C with family values and preferences. Early interventionists are also obligated to advocate for children in early intervention, and so sometimes must make recommendations that families may not want to pursue. Thus, a collaborative partnership between early interventionists and families that is respectful is important in meeting the needs of both children and their families.

The Individualized Family Service Plan   Using assessment information and information about family resources, concerns, and priorities, a written IFSP is developed by a interdisciplinary team, including the parents. The IFSP must include a written description of the appropriate transition services for infants and toddlers when they approach their third birthday, the time when they usually transition from Part C services for infants and toddlers to Part B (Section 619) services for preschoolers. The IFSP should be evaluated at least once each year and reviewed at 6-month intervals—or more often if appropriate. Because infants and toddlers grow and develop at a rapid rate, more frequent review of the IFSP may be necessary in order to provide optimal early intervention for many infants and toddlers.

Additionally, Part C of IDEIA requires that early intervention be provided, to the maximum extent, in natural environments, including the home and the community settings in which children without disabilities participate. This requirement reflects that society values inclusion of all individuals in community settings. However, Part C also requires family involvement in planning and implementing early intervention. Therefore, some families and early intervention teams may identify specialized settings for early intervention if early intervention cannot be implemented in natural environments. According to Part C of IDEIA, the IFSP must include a statement of the natural environments in which early intervention services will appropriately be provided, including a justification of the extent, if any, to which the services will not be provided in a natural environment.

The latest authorization of Part C of IDEIA (2004) includes some new features such as requiring preliteracy and language skills and the use of early intervention services that are based on peer-reviewed research. These changes appear to be related to the accountability movement spurred by the No Child Left Behind initiative. Because few early interventionists have had training in literacy and because of the lack of empirical research on effective early intervention strategies, professionals in the field of early intervention will face challenges in meeting these new requirements in the next few years.

There is considerable variability in the early intervention services provided to infants and toddlers with disabilities. Six months after entry into early intervention, most children received from two to six different services, and 80% of families received service coordination (U.S. Department of Education, 2001). About half of infants and toddlers with disabilities received speech–language therapy and about 40% received special instruction. Most (about 78% of a sample of 3,338) infants and toddlers receive early intervention in their homes (U.S. Department of Education, 2001).

Early Childhood Special Education

In most state and local education agencies, children transition from Part C to Part B services at 3 years of age. Interestingly, most states do not provide education for typically developing children between 3 and 5 years of age, and so providing ECSE in inclusive settings with nondisabled peers can be a challenge. In the past few years, schools have increasingly been encouraged to provide more inclusive services. Consequently, fewer children are being served in self-contained special education classes for preschool-age children with disabilities.

Service delivery can vary for preschoolers with disabilities, with some schools sending special educators into child care centers, preschools for typically developing children, or homes to provide specialized support. The intensity and type of services can also vary considerably for children within the same school system. Some children may attend all day self-contained classrooms, while others may receive hour-long home visits. The number and intensity of related services such as speech–language and occupational therapy may also vary considerably. IEPs for school age children are typically reviewed annually, rather than every 6 months, reflecting different rates of growth anticipated at different stages of development.

Even though preschoolers may receive services in a different manner than children in grades kindergarten and above, the guidelines used to determine eligibility, for assessment and for the development of the IEP, are the same for children ages 3 to 21 years. Families are often surprised at the change from family-centered services for infants and toddlers to the often less responsive special education system geared to older children. Rather than being oriented to both child and family, the IEP focuses on the educational needs of children.

Typically, children have to be determined eligible for special education when they transition from Part C (early intervention) to Part B, Section 619 (for 3- to 5-year-olds with disabilities) services. Many children with neurogenetic disorders will qualify for special education at age 3 years due to developmental delay. In some cases, however, children with these disorders may not qualify for services based on developmental delay. In those cases, families and neurogenetic specialists might suggest that children qualify for special education under the eligibility category of "other health impaired." The state-specific guidelines for other health impaired criteria are established by a state's department of public education, and are often provided on the Web sites of such agencies.

Transitions from infant–toddler to preschool programs and from preschool programs to kindergarten are often stressful for the families of children with disabilities. In recognition of that, Part C of IDEIA 2004 provides detailed guidelines for transition planning from infant–toddler to preschool programs. Professionals should be prepared to provide support to families of children during these transition periods.

Outcomes and Recommended and Evidence-Based Practices for Early Intervention and ECSE

Outcomes As mentioned earlier, the accountability movement spurred by the No Child Left Behind Act appears to be extending downward to early intervention and

ECSE. Because it requires promoting preliteracy skills for infants, toddlers, and pre-schoolers with disabilities and requires that intervention strategies be based on peer-reviewed research, many professionals are struggling to acquire skills, knowledge, and expertise in these areas that are not readily available. Moreover, in a recent review of federal early intervention and ECSE projects, it was noted that there was little or no evidence that early intervention and ECSE are actually effective (Early Childhood Outcomes [ECO] Center, 2004). Subsequently, the Office of Special Education Projects (OSEP) at the U.S. Department of Education funded the ECO Center to identify child and family outcomes for early intervention and ECSE, methods for assessing outcomes and for reporting outcomes to OSEP. The ECO Center began this ambitious endeavor in 2003. Its impact is now being felt in the state and local agencies responsible for reporting outcome data in 2006. Due to these demands on local service agencies and to the lack of preparation of many early intervention and ECSE personnel to address these requirements, families of children with disabilities may experience challenges as they seek to secure appropriate services for their children. Therefore, professionals who serve children and families with neurogenetic disorders should be aware of these systems changes that could potentially impact children and families in an adverse manner.

On a more positive note, the changes resulting from the accountability movement may result in better services for children and families. The child and family outcomes identified by the ECO Center for children with disabilities, ages birth to 5 years, appear to be functional and appropriate. The challenge will be to find appropriate measures and methods to assess the outcomes. As identified by stakeholders throughout the United States, young children with disabilities should achieve the following outcomes through their participation in early intervention and ECSE (ECO Center, 2005):

- Children have positive social relationships.
- Children acquire and use knowledge and skills.
- Children take appropriate action to meet their needs.

The overall goal of these child outcomes is to enable children to be active and successful participants in their early childhood years and in the future.

Family outcomes identified by the ECO Center also seem appropriate and will probably be easier to measure than the child outcomes. All five of the following family outcomes have been accepted as relevant for children being served under Part C of IDEIA; however, agencies serving 3- to 5-year-olds are only addressing the first three outcomes. Unfortunately, the proposed regulations for reporting family outcomes for 3- to 5-year-olds to the OSEP at the U.S. Department of Education are not consistent with the outcomes identified by the ECO Center.

Desired outcomes from early intervention and ECSE for families of young children with disabilities, as identified by stakeholders throughout the United States, include the following (ECO Center, 2005):

- Families understand their children's strengths, abilities, and special needs.
- Families know their rights and advocate effectively.
- Families help their children develop and learn.
- Families have support systems.
- Families access desired services, programs, and activities in their communities.

For families, the overall goal of early intervention and ECSE is to enable them to provide care for their child and to have the resources they need to participate in their own desired family and community activities. For ongoing updates about the status of child and family outcomes, their measurement, and reporting the results to OSEP, see the Web site of the ECO Center at www.the-ECO-center.org.

Recommended Practices   Even though IDEIA 2004 mandates the provision of early intervention and ECSE services that are based on peer-reviewed research, there are relatively few studies reporting successful early intervention practices. Although research has documented the efficacy of early intervention for disadvantaged children (Brooks-Gunn & Hearn, 1982; Ramey, Bryant, Sparling, & Wasik, 1985; Ramey & Campbell, 1991) and premature low-birth-weight children (Hill, Waldfogel, & Brooks-Gunn, 2003; Klebanov, Brooks-Gunn, & McCormick, 2001), there have been no large scale randomized clinical trials demonstrating the efficacy of early intervention for young children with disabilities. The heterogeneity of children with disabilities; the need for family-centered, individualized intervention; and limited resources no doubt contribute to the limited research on the efficacy of early intervention for young children with disabilities.

There is an urgent need for evidence-based practices for young children with disabilities. Unfortunately, the evidence-based practice movement is coinciding with a period of relatively low funding for research in early intervention and early childhood education. Therefore, there is currently a disconnect between the legal requirements for research and evidence-based practices and funding that supports such endeavors.

One solution to this dilemma is for early interventionists and early childhood special educators to implement recommended practices from existing sources such as the manual *DEC Recommended Practices: A Comprehensive Guide for Practical Application in Early Intervention/Early Childhood Special Education* (Sandall, Hemmeter, Smith, & McLean, 2005). DEC is the professional organization known as the Division for Early Childhood of the Council for Exceptional Children, to which many early interventionists and early childhood special educators belong. All of the practices described in *DEC Recommended Practices* were derived from published peer-reviewed research, and, therefore, are evidence-based practices. Unfortunately, the practices do not address emergent literacy, and there are no disability-specific practices such as those needed for children who are blind, who are deaf, or who have significant motor impairments. Nevertheless, this book provides important practices that serve as the foundation for effective early intervention and ECSE. This book is described on the DEC Web site, www.dec-sped.org, and can be purchased from the Sopris West Web site, www.sopriswest.com.

The DEC recommended practices book is appropriate for teachers, families, administrators, and higher education faculty and includes sections on direct services and indirect supports. Geared toward teachers and families, the direct services section includes chapters on assessment, child-focused practices, family-based practices, interdisciplinary models, and technology applications. The section on indirect services includes chapters on policies, procedures, and systems change and on personnel preparation. Next, some topics from this book that are particularly relevant for professionals who serve young children with neurogenetic disorders and their families are briefly described.

Assessment   Very often families of young children with neurogenetic disorders seek assessment from specialists in the specific disorder that has been diagnosed in their child. Under IDEIA 2004, children can be evaluated to determine their eligibility for early intervention and ECSE and assessed for program planning and monitoring progress. In some cases, children are assessed for program evaluation. Because the diagnosis of a neurogenetic disorder is documented in medical records, many local agencies will probably accept medical records as proof of eligibility. Therefore, the purpose of most assessment of young children with neurogenetic disorders will be for program planning for the IFSP or IEP and for monitoring ongoing progress. When completing such assessments, it will be helpful for specialists to consider the functional outcomes for children and families described earlier so that they provide information in a format that is consistent with that of early intervention and ECSE professionals.

In addition, specialists in neurogenetic disorders should also consider DEC recommended practices for assessment. Specifically, Neisworth and Bagnato (2005) describe the critical qualities of assessment that are developmentally appropriate for young children with disabilities, ages birth to 5 years, as

- having utility, being useful for intervention planning;
- being acceptable, being related to socially and parental valued competencies;
- being authentic, providing information about functional behaviors in natural settings and routines;

- involving collaboration, having parents and professionals work together to assess children;

- having convergence, using information from multiple sources;

- being equitable, making accommodations when needed (e.g., sensory and motor impairments);

- being sensitive, using measurement tools that document even small progress; and

- being congruent, using measures developed with a population that is similar to the children being assessed.

Most professionals will agree that these qualities are critical for appropriate assessment of young children with disabilities. Unfortunately, the assessment of all young children is somewhat controversial because assessment results for children under 5 years of age rarely predict future outcomes. For children with disabilities, few assessment tools have been developed for and standardized on this specific population, probably due to the extreme heterogeneity of young children with disabilities. When using standardized assessments, professionals may not tap into the full range of children's abilities because testing protocols do not allow for adapting the assessment to children's idiosyncratic characteristics. Therefore, appropriate assessment of young children with disabilities continues to be challenging.

For program planning, some early intervention professionals use functional assessment approaches such as routines-based assessment (RBA) to identify priorities and areas of concerns for families of children with disabilities. McWilliam (1992) developed guidelines for conducting RBA that might be useful for specialists who provide support to families of infants and toddlers. Detailed information about RBA can be found at http://www.vanderbiltchildrens.com/interior.php?mid=1173.

In addition to considering the critical qualities of assessment described earlier, Neisworth and Bagnato (2005, pp. 51–59) identify the following recommended practices for the assessment of young children with disabilities:

- Professionals and families collaborate in planning and implementing assessment.

- Assessment is individualized and appropriate for the child and family.

- Assessment provides useful information for intervention.

- Professionals share information in respectful and useful ways.

- Professionals meet legal and procedural requirements and use recommended practices.

Family-centered approach As mentioned earlier in this chapter, Part C of IDEIA (2004) acknowledges the importance of families in early intervention for infants and toddlers. Indeed, most early intervention services depend on parents and families' implementing interventions continuously throughout the week. When considering that most infants and toddlers only receive 1 to 2 hours of formal early intervention each week, it is easy to understand why a family-centered approach is so critical. Increasingly, early intervention has moved from a medical model in which a child's deficits were identified and targetted by a prescribed program of therapy to a collaborative, strengths-based approach that is the centerpiece of family-centered practices. According to Trivette and Dunst (2005), family-centered practices involve

a philosophy or way of thinking that leads to a set of practices in which families or parents are considered central and the most important decision maker in a child's life. More specifically, it recognizes that the family is the constant in the child's life and that service systems and personnel must support, respect, encourage, and enhance the strengths and competence of the family. (p. 119)

Therefore, the goal of family-centered practices is to facilitate optimal child outcomes through strengthened family functioning. This strengthened family functioning results from

• shared responsibility and collaboration between early interventionists and families,

• individualized and flexible practices, and

• strengths- and assets-based practices.

When making recommendations for young children with neurogenetic disorders, specialists should be mindful of this family-centered and strengths-based approach.

Child-focused practices   In the DEC recommended practices manual, Wolery (2005) describes several guiding principles for child-focused interventions. He notes that the purpose of intervention is to promote children's learning and development and that children's interactions with social and physical environments influence learning and development. He also emphasizes that early interventionists and early childhood special educators should maximize positive learning experiences and minimize potentially negative learning experiences. Finally, they should use research findings to organize and implement interventions.

Intervention goals and strategies for implementation should be based on authentic and appropriate child assessment and on family-directed assessment of their priorities, concerns, and resources. Increasingly, however, intervention goals for children between 3 and 5 years of age are also based on state standards and goals designed to address federal school accountability standards. Nevertheless, recommended practices for children ages birth to 5 years with disabilities require a collaborative, interdisciplinary, and family-centered approach to identify, design, implement, and monitor the progress of interventions.

Early interventionists and early childhood special educators can often benefit from the expertise of specialists in neurogenetic disorders to provide appropriate and optimal intervention. This expertise can provide information relevant to structuring children's learning opportunities, facilitating children's development and learning, and guiding when and where instructional practices are implemented (Wolery, 2005). When writing recommendations for young children with neurogenetic disorders, specialists should consider disability-specific issues that might impact children's opportunities for learning in order to promote optimal development and learning. For example, the distractibility of children with fragile X syndrome often impacts learning, and strategies for addressing it could be described.

Specialists in neurogenetic disorders, as well as early intervention professionals, should consider the different phases of learning and the implications of these phases for intervention. According to Wolery (2005), learning involves the following:

- acquisition, learning how to do something;
- fluency, learning to complete skills smoothly and naturally;
- maintenance, learning to complete skills without instruction or support; and
- generalization, learning to apply the skill to other settings when needed.

Furthermore, to promote optimal learning, families and early intervention professionals should

- design environments to promote safety, active engagement, learning, participation, and membership;
- collect ongoing data to consistently meet children's changing needs; and
- use systematic procedures within and across environments, activities, and routines to promote learning and participation (Wolery, 2005).

Increasingly, challenging and problem behaviors have been recognized as important impediments to learning for some children, as documented by the establishment of the Center for Evidence-Based Practice: Young Children with Challenging Behavior (http://challengingbehavior.fmhi.usf.edu) and the Center for Social Emotional Foundations for Early Learning (http://csefel.uiuc.edu), funded by the OSEP at the U.S. Department of Education. Challenging behavior can be of particular relevance for some types of neurogenetic disorders, such as fragile X (Hatton et al., 2002; Kau et al., 2004). For that reason, specialists in neurogenetic disorders may be particularly interested in resources related to this topic because parents and teachers may be more concerned with the impact of challenging behavior on daily life than with other features of these disorders.

To address challenging behavior, it is important to determine the antecedents, behavior, and consequences of the behavior (Wolery, 2005). Following this documentation, families, early intervention professionals, and/or neurogenetic specialists can identify and implement interventions that make the behavior

- irrelevant (environment is changed so that behavior is unnecessary);
- inefficient (a more efficient behavior is taught); and/or
- ineffective (different consequences or other reinforcements are used). (Wolery, 2005)

Interdisciplinary models   For the past 20 years, the field of early intervention/ECSE has recognized the importance of interdisciplinary models in meeting the diverse needs of young children with disabilities and their families. Over the years, practice has evolved from a deficit-based medical model in which allied health professionals saw children individually and rarely collaborated to a more integrated interdisciplinary model in which professionals with special expertise from multiple disciplines work together to help children with disabilities and their families. This approach is consistent with family-centered practices and a concern for supporting families in a positive manner rather than contributing to more stress through multiple interactions with professionals who sometimes provide conflicting information and recommendations. Transdisciplinary approaches have been recommended so that team members can collaborate and provide integrative interventions through cross-disciplinary training. McWilliam (2005) describes the following recommended practices for providing interdisciplinary intervention:

- Collective responsibility: Teamwork—different perspectives build better decisions.
- Transdisciplinary-expertise and competencies are shared among team members.
- Functionality: Interventions promote children's engagement, independence, and social relationships in natural routines.
- Practicality and parsimony for regular caregivers: Interventions must be practical for caregivers to implement.
- Teams, including family members, make decisions and work together.
- Professionals cross boundaries of their disciplines.
- Intervention is focused on function, not services.
- Regular caregivers and routines provide the most appropriate opportunities for learning and receiving intervention.

With basic knowledge of early intervention and ECSE and recognition of recommended practices in those fields, neurogenetic specialists will be better able to meet the needs of young children with specific genetic disorders and their families. In the following sections, summaries of research on early development and early intervention for specific disorders in young children ages birth to 5 years are presented, along with implications for early intervention and ECSE.

As noted in the chapters in part I of this book, children with neurogenetic disorders represent a very heterogeneous population. Many have complex medical conditions in addition to developmental delays. Therefore, early intervention and ECSE should be highly individualized to meet the needs of families and children. This individualized approach is consistent with IDEIA 2004 and with recommended practices in early intervention and ECSE.

Young Children with 22q11.2 Deletion Syndrome

As reviewed in chapter 6 (this volume), children with 22q11 deletion syndrome are diagnosed soon after birth due to obvious physical anomalies, whereas others are diagnosed later in infancy when they experience feeding problems or fail to meet developmental milestones, or even in the school age years when adults note an atypical nasal quality to their voices. Those identified within the first 3 years of life may be referred to early intervention services through Part C of IDEIA 2004. If diagnosed between 3 and 5 years of age, the children may be referred to their local education agencies for services through the exceptional children's program under Part B, Section 619 of IDEIA 2004. Some children with 22q11 deletion syndrome may not experience delays during the first few years of life; therefore, it is important to remember the established risk eligibility category for early intervention and ECSE.

Early Development

Although many reports of 22q11 syndrome in the literature include a few infants, toddlers, and preschoolers in their samples, detailed information about this age group appears relatively scarce. The only detailed peer-reviewed report exclusively examining children under 5 years of age with 22q11 deletion syndrome found in the existing literature was by Gerdes et al. (1999), who described early development in a sample of 40 children between 13 and 63 months of age. Results for the 28 infants and toddlers between 13 and 42 months were reported separately from the results of the 12 preschoolers between 42 and 63 months of age. Only 25% of the 40 children was functioning in the average range (± 1 SD of the mean of the standardized measure used). The mean score of toddlers was in the significantly delayed range (>2 SD from mean), while the mean score of preschoolers was in the borderline range. These differences, however, could be due to different assessment tools. Delays in expressive language were beyond those expected by cognitive level, and were not always related to structural anomalies of the palate. Feeding disorders were present in 67.5% of the 40 children and included decreased intake, atypical tongue movement that interfered with feeding, nasopharyngeal reflux, resistance to new foods and textured foods, and choking. Children with and without accompanying cardiac and palatal defects experienced feeding problems. Although emotional facial expressions could be elicited, many children did not spontaneously express typical facial emotions and instead displayed "minimal changes in facial expression during play and general social interaction" (p. 131).

Considerable variability in developmental outcome was evident in the toddlers with 22q11 deletion syndrome, with 21.4% functioning in the average range, 32.2% functioning in the mildly delayed range, and 46.4% functioning in the significantly delayed range (Gerdes et al., 1999). When considering motor development, 79% of the toddler group had significant delays, 13% had mild delays, and 2% had motor skills within the average range. Approximately 54% of the children had hypotonia. On language assessment, the toddler group had below average expressive and receptive language. Behavior and emotional regulation in toddlers was reported to be within the average range.

In the 12 children ages 4 to 5 years who could complete IQ assessment, the mean IQ was 78.2 ($\pm$11), with 33% functioning in the average range, 33% in the borderline range, and 33% in the mild mental retardation range (Gerdes et al., 1999). Regarding speech and language total scores, 9% of the children scored in the average range, 38% experienced mild delays, and 40% experienced significant delays. Although 53% of the children scored in the significantly delayed range on expressive language, only 26% scored in the significantly delayed range on receptive language, suggesting that receptive language may not be as severely delayed as expressive language in preschool-age children. Unlike the toddlers, 9 of the 12 preschoolers were considered highly active, impulsive, or disorganized, and 3 children were described as behaviorally inhibited. These descriptions of atypical behaviors in preschool children are consistent with Simon, Burg-Malki, and Gothelf's (this volume) synthesis of research on behavior and psychiatric disorders in older children, adolescents, and adults with 22q11 deletion syndrome.

Early Intervention for Children with 22q11 Deletion Syndrome

Preventive Approach   In discussing the implications of their findings, Gerdes et al. (1999) concluded that there was considerable variability in the developmental status of children with 22q11 deletion syndrome during the early childhood years that was not always related to cardiac defects and palate anomalies. They recommended a preventive approach to early intervention that should begin in infancy with early evaluation and interventions to support language and gross motor development. Because most of the children in their sample had no verbal communication at age 2 years and had below-average language skills overall, communication and language were of particular concern, consistent with Simon et al.'s (chapter 6, this volume) description of delayed language in young children with this disorder.

Gerdes et al. (1999) recommended early speech–language evaluation and therapy and the use of alternative communication such as sign language for children who do not speak, as well as therapy to help them acquire speech and language. Because

38 of the 40 children in their study acquired speech by entry into kindergarten, it appears that they make rapid gains in speech and language between 3 and 5 years of age. Additionally, Gerdes et al. recommend that the socioemotional behavior and health of young children with 22q11 deletion syndrome should be monitored due to decreased facial expression and potential social and attention problems. Solot et al. (2000) recommend that early intervention for children with 22q11 deletion syndrome should be provided to "stimulate development, increase communicative interactions, and decrease frustration" (p. 197).

Speech–Language Intervention   Because almost all children with 22q11 deletion syndrome experience speech and language delays and/or disorders, they should be carefully monitored even before such delays become evident, consistent with the preventive model discussed earlier (Gerdes et al., 1999; McDonald-McGinn, Emauel, & Zackai, 2003; Persson, Lohmander, Jonsson, Oskarsdottir, & Soderpalm, 2003; Ritinski-Mack, Oblser, Smooth, & Tsipis, 2005; Solot et al., 2000). As noted, some children with 22q11 deletion syndrome have decreased facial expression, making it difficult for others to respond to their communicative cues (Gerdes et al., 1999; Ritinski-Mack et al., 2005). This information is important for early interventionists, who can assist families in learning to read the more subtle cues of these young children. By taking a proactive approach to promoting communication and language through early intervention, families and clinicians may be able to lessen the impact of the disorder on development.

Most children with 22q11 deletion syndrome will experience significant speech and expressive language delays; therefore, speech–language therapy will probably be an important service for these children. Because the speech–language delays and disorders observed in children with 22q11 deletion syndrome are not always related to structural defects of the palate or to their intellectual function (Solot et al., 2000), families and professionals must be particularly alert to the need for speech–language services or for monitoring by a speech–language pathologist. For children with structural defects, surgery to correct the defects and subsequent speech–language therapy may be most effective during the preschool years (Dykens, Hodapp, & Finucane, 2000). Children's receptive language may be considerably higher than their expressive language during the toddler and preschool years (Simon et al., this volume; Solot et al., 2000); therefore, adults should be careful not to underestimate the intellectual capabilities of children due to early speech–language delays.

Feeding Problems   Feeding disorders have been described as one of the earliest clinical indicators of this syndrome. Infants might experience nasaopharyngeal reflux, as well as gagging and choking. McDonald-McGinn, Finucane, and Zackai (2003) note that feeding problems may be so severe that nasogastric or gastrostomy tube feedings may be required. They suggested specific strategies for feeding disorders including modified spoon placement, treatment for gastroesophageal reflux, postural therapy, and medication for gastrointestinal dysmotility and constipation. Therefore, early intervention or ECSE for children with this disorder may include interventions to address feeding disorders. Both speech–language pathologists and occupational therapists may have expertise in this area. In addition, an occupational or physical therapist might be involved due to hypotonia and delayed motor skills.

Motor Skills   Motor delays are probably related to the hypotonia observed in many young children with 22q11 deletion syndrome (as reviewed in chapter 6, this volume). Even though many toddlers appear to have significant impairments, considerable variability in developmental outcome is evident, reinforcing the need for individualized early intervention plans.

Multidisciplinary Assessment and Service Coordination   McDonald-McGinn et al. (2003) note the need for a multidisciplinary evaluation of individuals with this disorder, consistent with IDEIA 2004 regulations and recommended practices in early intervention and ECSE. Early interventionists may serve as service coordinators to help families efficiently access and implement help from professionals from multiple disciplines. Early interventionists and speech–language pathologists can also provide overall support to families regarding children's communicative cues and how to promote optimal development. Hearing impairment should be ruled out for children with 22q11 deletion syndrome due to its relatively high prevalence (39% in the Solot et al., 2000, sample).

Socioemotional and Behavioral Interventions   Although learning disabilities, attention deficit/hyperactivity disorder (ADHD), and intellectual disabilities may become more apparent in kindergarten and the early elementary years, children during the 3- to 5-year age range present some evidence of socioemotional and behavioral problems (Gerdes et al., 1999). Although there have been some reports of challenging behaviors and psychopathology in older children and adults with 22q11 deletion syndrome (Simon et al., this volume), relatively little is known about this topic in infants and toddlers. Dykens et al. (2000) noted six toddlers with shyness and social withdrawal who were described in a larger study of problem behavior in Dutch children with 22q11 syndrome (Swillen et al., 1997).

Because the developmental outcome of children with 22q11 deletion syndrome is so variable, it is important for families and professionals to have high expectations for them. By being alert to potential problems with communication and therefore being very responsive to communicative attempts, adults can alleviate some of the frustration that these children experience due to the structural defects that impede speech and language. By being responsive to children's interests and communication, adults can scaffold their learning within play and daily routines to promote optimal development. Consistent behavior management, responsive caregiving, and opportunities to interact and play with peers should help prepare these children for kindergarten.

Preschool Services for Children with 22q11 Deletion Syndrome

Children with 22q11 deletion syndrome between the ages of 3 and 5 might be provided a variety of services, depending on their developmental and socioemotional status. They might be enrolled in specialized classes for preschoolers with disabilities with support from related service personnel such as speech–language pathologists and occupational or physical therapists. Or perhaps, these children attend regular child care centers where the early childhood special educator makes visits to collaborate with child care staff and to work directly with the child. Some young preschool children with 22q11 deletion syndrome function in the average range of intelligence, while others experience mild to moderate delays. Therefore, services may vary considerably from child to child.

Preschoolers who attend center-based classes or child care centers may require explicit instruction for some activities such as activities to promote phonological awareness rather than a more child-centered approach (Ritinski-Mack et al., 2005). Additionally, they may benefit from small group instruction, tasks broken down into small steps, structured environments, and opportunities for participation in individual and group physical activities (Ritinski-Mack et al., 2005). Although Ritinski-Mack et al. provided additional strategies for educators of children with 22q11 deletion syndrome, many are developmentally inappropriate for preschoolers. These authors did note that there is no research to guide intervention and education of children with 22q11 deletion syndrome. Consequently, they recommended collaboration among families, teachers, and other service providers; creativity and flexibility in providing intervention and instruction; and continuous progress monitoring to promote optimal learning and development.

Young Children with Fragile X Syndrome

From 1993 through 2006, Don Bailey and his colleagues at the Frank Porter Graham (FPG) Child Development Institute at the University of North Carolina at Chapel Hill have studied young children with fragile X syndrome through the Carolina Fragile X Project. From the work of this group and others, we know that infants with fragile X syndrome as young as 9 months of age may exhibit delays on development screening tasks (Mirrett, Bailey, Roberts, & Hatton, 2004); that parents of toddler boys report delayed milestones as early as the first year of life (Roberts, Hatton, & Bailey, 2001); and that young boys with fragile X between 2 to 6 years of age develop at about half the rate of typically developing children, although there is considerable variability in the development of individual children with fragile X (Bailey, Hatton, & Skinner, 1998; see also chapter 3, this volume). In addition, this group also found that higher levels of autistic behavior were associated with poorer developmental (Bailey, Hatton, Skinner, & Mesibov, 2001) and behavioral (Hatton et al., 2002) outcomes and lower levels of adaptive behavior (Hatton et al., 2003) in their sample of young children with fragile X syndrome. These findings are consistent with those of others studying autism in young children with fragile X and its impact on development, problem behavior, and adaptive behavior (Kaufmann et al., 2004; Rogers, Wehner, & Hagerman, 2001). Higher levels of the fragile X mental retardation protein (FMRP) were associated with better developmental (Bailey et al., 2001) and adaptive behavior (Hatton et al., 2003) outcomes in children in the Carolina Fragile X Project.

We have found that challenging behavior rather than intellectual disability is of primary concern to families of young children with fragile X syndrome (Hatton & Roberts, in press) and to early interventionists, teachers (Hatton et al., 2000), and speech–language pathologists (Mirrett, Roberts, & Price, 2003). In addition to relatively high rates of autistic behavior in children with fragile X, both boys and girls with fragile X have been found to have ADHD (Cornish, Levitas, & Sudhalter, this volume; Hagerman, Farzin, & Sakimura, in press; Hatton & Roberts, in press; Hatton et al., 2002). Other behaviors that have been described in children with fragile X include anxiety, self-injurious behavior, and aggression to self and others (Cornish et al., this volume; Hatton & Roberts, in press; Hagerman et al., in press). Because of these and other challenging behaviors one important goal of early intervention and ECSE for children with fragile X should be to promote positive behavior (Hatton & Roberts, in press).

In describing the early physical and medical needs of young children with fragile X, Hagerman et al. (in press) noted that hypotonia, or low muscle tone, is often one of the first physical signs of the disorder. Hypotonia can contribute to early motor coordination problems involved in nursing or bottle feeding and/or in gastroesophageal reflux, as well as to recurrent otitis media. Otitis media can be caused by both bacteria and viruses; therefore, antibiotics are often not effective. Because of the high prevalence of otitis media in young children with fragile X and its subsequent impact on hearing and language development, Hagerman and colleagues note that the insertion of pressure equalizing tubes may be particularly helpful in cases of frequent and prolonged bouts of otitis media. Hagerman et al. acknowledge the prevalent use of medication to address challenging behaviors in children with fragile X and urge extreme caution in prescribing medication for children under 5 years of age because few if any studies have documented the safety and efficacy of medication in young children with developmental disabilities. In fact, stimulant use in children under 5 years of age may actually increase hyperactivity and irritability (Hagerman et al., in press).

Medication use for older children with fragile X syndrome is discussed in chapter 3 (Cornish et al., this volume).

As noted, one of the earliest physical symptoms of fragile X in infants may be hypotonia that likely contributes to the feeding problems, gastroesophageal reflux, and otitis media that have been documented in young children with fragile X. In addition, delayed motor milestones such as sitting up, crawling, and walking become evident in many children within the first 15 months of life (Roberts et al., 2001; Roberts, Mirrett, & Schaaf, in press). However, across all developmental domains, there is considerable variability in outcomes. In the second year of life, many parents become concerned because of language delays that become even more apparent in the third year of life (Roberts et al., in press). Indeed, spoken language may not occur until the fourth year of life in boys with fragile X (Roberts, Mirrett, Anderson, Burchinal, & Neebe, 2002; Roberts et al., in press). Expressive language appears to be more delayed than receptive, and delays in prelinguistic communication during the first 2 years of life have also been documented (Roberts et al., 2002; Roberts et al., in press). These communication and language delays often prompt parents to seek speech–language therapy for their young children with fragile X syndrome.

Hypersensitivity to sounds, visual stimuli, and touch has been described in young children with fragile X and is probably associated with descriptions of hyperarousal (increased response and anxiety to environmental stimuli) in individuals with fragile X (Cornish et al., this volume; Hatton & Roberts, in press). These sensory characteristics, combined with the hypotonia mentioned earlier, often lead to fairly early referral for occupational therapy services.

Early Intervention and Education for Children with Fragile X Syndrome

The earliest reported studies of education in school-age children with fragile X examined teacher awareness and understanding of the syndrome. Not surprisingly, special educators serving elementary-school-age children knew relatively little about fragile X (Madison, Mosher, & George, 1998; Wilson & Mazzocco, 1993; York, von Fraunhofer, Turk, & Sedgwick, 1999). Among teachers who had students with fragile X, Saunders (1999) found that the teachers of school-age children were concerned about aggression (to others, themselves, and the environment); inability to stay seated; extreme reactions to change or to things that were upsetting; distractibility; need for one-on-one assistance; and "nervous habits" (p. 78) such as hand-flapping, strange noises, and biting. Approximately 63% of the teachers said that their students with fragile X syndrome had autistic behaviors, 64% noted hyperactivity, and 56% reported attention deficit disorder. Young students with fragile X preferred practical and physical activities such as physical education, music, play, and computer time (Saunders, 1999). Teachers reported that large-group and whole-class activities that involved language-based activities were challenging for children with fragile X syndrome. "The potential for noise, bustle, lack of order and routine, and the general unpredictability of the behaviour of others make these times very difficult for the child with fragile X" (Saunders, p. 78). Children were noted to sometimes act inappropriately when asked direct questions or when faced with the need to interact with peers. Students with fragile X disliked writing and other fine motor skills.

Symons and colleagues (Symons, Clark, Roberts, & Bailey, 2001) conducted an observational study of behavior in school age boys in public school classrooms. They found that boys with fragile X had similar levels of engagement in classroom activities as did their peers in special education classes; they displayed relatively little problem behavior. The higher the quality of the classroom, the more engaged were the boys with fragile X.

There is relatively little evidence-based information to guide early intervention and early childhood education for young children with fragile X syndrome, as evident by this brief review of the existing research on this subject. To date, two such research studies have been reported on early intervention for young children with fragile X syndrome. First, Hatton et al. (2000) described early intervention services for 50 young boys with fragile X, and teacher perceptions of their students' characteristics and needs; teacher recommendations for serving young children with fragile X; parent perceptions of educational services; and the relation among service intensity, developmental status, and demographic variables. Second, Mirrett et al. (2003) interviewed 51 speech–language pathologists regarding their perceptions of their young clients with fragile X. Across these studies, the recommendations of teachers and speech–language pathologists were remarkably similar. Both groups recognized that behavior and extreme reactivity to sensory features, rather than developmental delays, might interfere with developmental outcome and achievement.

In the Hatton et al. (2000) study, the average age of entry into early intervention was 21.6 months. The first services provided were typically home visits, often followed by the addition of speech–language therapy and physical therapy. On average, boys started receiving occupational therapy at age 43 months. The amount of early intervention/ECSE increased over the age period of 12 to 71 months; however, the intensity of related services—speech–language, occupational therapy, and physical therapy—did not increase. The parents of boys with fragile X syndrome were satisfied with services and with the IFSP and IEP process. Most thought that additional occupational therapy and speech-language therapy would have been helpful (Hatton et al., 2000).

In surveys and interviews, early interventionists and early childhood special educators were more concerned about behavioral challenges than with intellectual disabilities. To address these issues, educators recommended structured routines and environmental accommodations to address both behavior and sensory reactivity.

Children with higher developmental scores received fewer services than children with more delays (Hatton et al., 2000).

According to Mirrett et al. (2003), speech–language pathologists described their clients with fragile X as visual, hands-on learners who were social, pleasant, and eager to please. They also noted that boys with fragile X need structure and accommodations to address sensory processing challenges, that they had limited nonverbal and verbal pragmatic and social skills, and that their connected speech was unintelligible. Treatment priorities included speech and articulation goals to address rapid rate of speech, poor intelligibility, and fluency; language and grammar goals to promote auditory comprehension, vocabulary, and syntactic skills; and pragmatic goals to address greetings/social responses and turn taking. Mirrett et al. recommended the use of structure and routines, as well as combined visual and auditory input, to address pragmatic and social issues, sensory defensiveness, and behavioral challenges.

Recommendations for Early Intervention and Education

Table 14.1 summarizes recommendations for early intervention and education for young children with fragile X research based on findings (Hatton et al., 2000; Mirrett et al., 2003; Saunders, 1999; Symons et al., 2001). Recommendations address promoting positive behavior, facilitating learning, and environmental adaptations.

Pharmacological Intervention

As noted in chapter 3, many children with fragile X syndrome are prescribed medication for ADHD, anxiety, or aggression. Many of these medications have not been tested in toddlers and preschoolers, however, and so families and educators should be wary regarding their use in very young children (Hagerman et al., in press). Physicians with expertise with young children with developmental disorders and with pharmacological expertise should be best able to assist families seeking medication for their young children.

Family Support

Families of children with fragile X syndrome have reported considerable stress related to the diagnosis of the syndrome in their families and related to parenting children with fragile X (Bailey, Skinner, & Sparkman, 2003; Johnston et al., 2003; Wheeler, Hatton, Reichardt, & Bailey, in press). For that reason the provision of family-centered supports described in the introduction of this chapter are particularly important for many families of children with fragile X syndrome (Bailey, in press; Hatton & Bailey, in press). In many cases, this support can be provided through early interventionists, early childhood special educators, and social workers who provide services through local early intervention agencies. Although a detailed description of family-centered practices is beyond the scope of this chapter, Bailey (in press)

Table 14.1
Research recommendations for early intervention and education for children with fragile X syndrome

Promoting Appropriate Behavior and Engagement
• Consider hypersensitivity to sensory stimuli to prevent behavior problems.
• Respect the need for medication for some children.
• Use behavior management plans tailored to individual children's needs.
• Use consistent behavior management and reinforce appropriate behavior.
• Alternate quiet and active activities.
• Ease transitions by preparing children for them.
• Motivate children with favorite toys, activities, praise, music.
• Read children's cues and be responsive.
• Use repetitive tasks to calm children.
• Be patient, persistent, and flexible.
• Collaborate with families.
• Provide high quality classrooms.

Facilitating Learning
• Focus on practical, functional tasks.
• Provide instruction in small groups or one on one.
• Avoid direct questions.
• Use visual cues, real objects, or symbols.
• Be quiet, calm, and unobtrusive and know that touch and direct eye contact may be aversive.
• Consider sensory integration needs and work with occupational therapist.
• Break tasks down into manageable steps.
• Use strategies designed for children with autism.
• Provide opportunities to practice social skills and to facilitate developmentally appropriate play.
• Build on the strengths and interests of the child.
• Recognize that writing is challenging, and provide alternatives such as worksheets and computers.

Environmental Modifications
• Have a quiet, calm, orderly environment.
• Provide a structured, consistent routine.
• Reduce distractions.
• Provide a personal work space.

provides detailed suggestions for providing such support to families of children with fragile X.

Turner Syndrome

Unlike many other neurogenetic syndromes (including several described in this book), Turner syndrome is not typically associated with mental retardation (Davenport, Hooper, & Zeger, this volume; Ross, Zinn, & McCauley, 2000; Rovet, 2004). Neuropsychological and psychosocial outcomes appear to be related to specific genotypic features, as described by Davenport et al. (chapter 1, this volume). Turner syndrome may be diagnosed incidentally through prenatal testing; during infancy through identification of physical features associated with Turner syndrome, especially slow growth; during early childhood and childhood due to physical features, particularly short stature and, in some cases, developmental delays; and during adolescence due to short stature and delayed pubertal growth spurt (Davenport et al., this volume). Thus many girls with Turner syndrome are identified at young ages when they may qualify for early intervention ECSE.

As discussed in chapter 1, Davenport et al. (this volume) note that delays in girls with Turner syndrome may occur in motor, communication, cognitive, and psychosocial functioning. Because of the variability in severity, infants, toddlers, and preschoolers with Turner syndrome may experience subtle delays that may go undetected.

Early Intervention and Education for Girls with Turner Syndrome

Because intellectual disability falling within the mental retardation range is not typically associated with Turner syndrome, young children with this disorder may not be eligible for early intervention and ECSE under the established condition eligibility category. Eligibility under the developmental delay category might be made based on state-specific criteria for this category.

Rovet (2004) noted that school-age girls with Turner syndrome are underserved by special education, even though most girls perform two grade levels below average by sixth grade. Apparently, many girls with Turner syndrome have adequate or above average language, reading, and spelling skills, even though the majority have visual–spatial and arithmetic deficits that are consistent with nonverbal learning disabilities (Ross et al., 2000; Rovet, 2004, chapter 1, this volume).

In addition to deficits in visual–spatial and math abilities, older girls with Turner syndrome have been described as lacking social competence and having low self-esteem, particularly as they enter adolescence (Davenport et al., this volume; Mazzocco, Baumgardner, Freund, & Reiss, 1998; Ross et al., 2000; Rovet, 2004). These findings are consistent with Davenport et al.'s (this volume) description of social–emotional and temperament characteristics of preschool-age girls with Turner syndrome.

Ross et al. (2000) noted that family support, high self-esteem, and access to resources are associated with more favorable outcomes for females with Turner syndrome. In particular, these authors noted that "an accepting, supportive family may override some of the major impediments of this condition" (p. 138). Therefore, specialists in neurogenetics disorder might consider the family-centered practices and family outcomes described earlier in this chapter. Providing families with information about support groups such as the Turner Syndrome Society of the United States (www.turner-syndrome-us.org) might be helpful for many families.

Even though many girls with Turner syndrome ages 5 years and younger may not be eligible for early intervention and ECSE due to relatively subtle delays, families should adopt a proactive approach to facilitating their early development and education, as well as to meeting their medical and physical needs through growth hormone replacement and other treatments described by Davenport et al. (this volume).

Neurogenetic specialists and families should also consider a preventive approach to the development of delays in very young girls with Turner syndrome as described by Ross et al. (2000). Specifically, young girls could be monitored through ongoing assessment to identify cognitive strengths and needs. Families and teachers could build upon strengths to motivate girls and to build their self-confidence and self-esteem when they are very young. In addition, families may want to consciously facilitate early friendships and play by inviting peers over to play with their daughters or by enrolling their daughters in play groups and preschools to promote access to typically developing peers.

Families and teachers might consider using daily routines and play activities to provide opportunities for girls with Turner syndrome to practice early developmentally appropriate skills. For example, because copying shapes and letters involves visual–spatial skills and because of known difficulties in early writing for many girls with Turner syndrome, families and preschool teachers should consider providing ample developmentally appropriate opportunities for scribbling, drawing, and other fine motor activities that provide the foundation for later writing.

Families and teachers should have high social expectations for girls with Turner syndrome; however, they should be alert to their potential inability to read subtle social cues. Parents and teachers can facilitate early social interactions by helping young girls with Turner syndrome read the cues of their playmates and siblings. By doing so, they may be able to compensate for deficits in visual–spatial processing that may contribute to their inability to read fast-paced nonverbal social cues. Young girls with Turner syndrome who have close friendships and successful peer relationships during early childhood and childhood may be protected from some of the social problems described during adolescence, although this notion has not been examined empirically for girls with Turner syndrome.

In addition, parents should encourage their young daughters with Turner syndrome to become responsible and independent by having them complete chores around the home and by caring for their own needs (Ross et al., 2000). By contributing to the family (helping to put away toys, clean clothes, and wash dishes; sorting flatware or laundry; taking out the garbage; helping with the yard work; etc.), young children may gain self-esteem and self-confidence.

Children with Klinefelter Syndrome

There are many reasons why individuals with Klinefelter syndrome may not come to the attention of early childhood intervention specialists. First, the hallmark physical features of Klinefelter syndrome, such as tall stature, breast enlargement, and small testes, typically emerge during puberty (as discussed in chapter 2, this volume). In fact, some males with Klinefelter syndrome are not diagnosed until adulthood when they are tested for fertility. In some cases, boys may be identified in early childhood due to poor penile growth. Second, perhaps because there are no other severe hallmark features such as intellectual disability (mental retardation), pronounced dysmorphology, and externalizing behavior problems, Klinefelter syndrome is under-diagnosed (Geschwind & Dykens, 2004; Ross, Stefanatos, & Roeltgen, this volume). As many as 75% of males with Klinefelter may be undiagnosed (Bojesen, Juul, & Gravholt, 2003). Only 25% of males with Klinefelter are diagnosed in childhood, and many of these are diagnosed prenatally in older and at-risk mothers.

Even though males with Klinefelter have normal IQs, delayed and impaired speech and language development, difficulties with word retrieval and phonologic process-ing, and internalizing behavioral problems have been documented that may not have been evident in early studies of this disorder (Geschwind & Dykens, 2004; Ross et al., this volume; Rovet, Netley, Keenan, Bailey, & Stewart, 1996).

Behaviorally, males with Klinefelter have been described as immature, shy, impul-sive, anxious, dependent, socially isolated, and with low self-esteem (Geschwind & Dykens, 2004; Ross et al., this volume). However, in a pilot study of 15 males ages 16 to 64 years, Geschwind and Dykens examined motivational preferences and found that curiosity was the primary motivating force reported by the males, with family factors and social contact also being important motivators. Prestige, independence, and vengeance-seeking were not motivating. Although only 14% had clinically signif-icant externalizing problems, 43% had internalizing problems. These authors noted that their small sample of males with Klinefelter syndrome were characterized by "empathy with others, a noncompetitive, kind-spirited orientation, a valuing of fam-ily and relationships, and a curiosity to learn new things" (p. 171).

In a review of literature describing very young boys with Klinefelter syndrome, Samango-Sprouse and Rogol (2002) note that previous studies have documented delays in walking (mean age = 18 months) and language (mean age of first word = 24 months). In their own study of 73 infants with Klinefelter who were all diagnosed prenatally, decreased motor activity was evident as early as 2 to 3 months of age, as was hypotonia. Balance problems were evident at 24 to 36 months, and problems with motor planning were also evident. Some infants had difficulties with sucking and swallowing, particularly during breast-feeding, and had delayed sound production and imitation by 12 months of age. These delays prompted Samango-Sprouse and Rogol to theorize that many infants and toddlers with Klinefelter syndrome have developmental dyspraxia, a condition characterized by difficulty in planning and integrating motor activities. They further noted that early intervention can enhance developmental outcome, as well as social and behavioral skills, while also providing the foundation for future education and independence. Though no specific recommendations were made for intervention, Samango-Sprouse and Rogol noted that interventionists could use individualized and syndrome-specific strategies to promote optimal outcomes in males with Klinefelter syndrome.

Although males with Klinefelter syndrome typically do not have intellectual disabilities, they do appear to have subtle neuropsychological impairments. Performance IQ is usually higher than Verbal IQ in children, consistent with delays and impairments in speech and language (Geschwind & Dykens, 2004; Ross et al., this volume). However, some adult males with Klinefelter syndrome do not exhibit this Verbal–Performance IQ discrepancy. Many boys with Klinefelter syndrome have moderate to severe delays in academic skills that will not be apparent until the elementary and middle school years (Ross et al., this volume; Rovet et al., 1996). Boys with Klinefelter syndrome can lag several grade levels behind peers, show academic underachievement, receive special education support at a high rate (60% to 86%), and repeat grades, and few attend college (Ross et al., this volume; Rovet et al., 1996).

Early Intervention and Education for Boys with Klinefelter Syndrome

Even though only 25% of males with Klinefelter syndrome are diagnosed during childhood, we know that many infants with Klinefelter syndrome have hypotonia and that many will experience delayed motor milestones, atypical motor patterns, impaired fine and gross motor skills, and poor balance and coordination. Delays in language are often evident by 2 to 3 years of age and are probably the first indication of lifelong impairments in language and verbal skills (Ross et al., this volume).

By recognizing these early developmental characteristics of Klinefelter syndrome, parents and neurogenetic specialists can take a proactive approach to facilitating the development of communication and language and motor skills. Even though boys with Klinefelter syndrome may not qualify for early intervention under the established condition eligibility category, parents and professionals can closely monitor the acquisition of motor and communication/language skills during infancy and toddlerhood. If it appears that boys with Klinefelter syndrome are experiencing developmental delays, the boys can be referred to early intervention under the eligibility category of developmental delay, described earlier in this chapter. Parents can request that speech–language pathologists and occupational or physical therapists be involved in the required multidisciplinary evaluation needed to determine eligibility for early intervention. Professionals from these disciplines are important members of the assessment team due to known delays in motor and communication/language development in young boys with Klinefelter. If delays are evident in these two domains and if early intervention is provided, parents and neurogenetic specialists can request that professionals from these disciplines provide services.

If children do not meet criteria for early intervention, parents may ask their sons' pediatricians to closely monitor their development and to prescribe speech–language therapy and occupational and/or physical therapy as needed to facilitate development in these areas.

According to Rovet et al. (1996), "The need for special education is clearly indicated in this population" (p. 192). Based on their research with 41 boys with Klinefelter syndrome, these researchers found that these children had lower verbal abilities with normal nonverbal abilities and difficulties with tasks that involve "auditory memory, language comprehension, and expressive abilities" (p. 192), as well as attention problems. In addition, boys with Klinefelter showed lower levels of academic achievement than their siblings and had more difficulty with word decoding, reading comprehension, spelling, written language, math, and conceptual understanding in content areas such as science. Performance on standardized tests deteriorated over time, and problems with reading and math seemed equal, while diagnoses of learning disabilities increased with age. Problems with working memory and/or auditory processing were noted as possibly contributing to the language-based learning disability. Problems in processing auditory information probably contribute to underachievement because boys with Klinefelter syndrome may not understand their teachers' instructions. As academic demands increase over time, boys with Klinefelter syndrome may have more and more difficulty in understanding instructions and information that is presented orally. Unfortunately, Rovet et al. also found that reading comprehension was poor and that it interfered with the ability to understand print. These problems with auditory and print processing probably contribute to the attention problems that have been noted in boys with Klinefelter syndrome.

Although intended for school-age boys with Klinefelter syndrome, the intervention strategies suggested by Rovet et al. (2004) may be adapted for preschool-age boys. These recommendations included early speech–language therapy stressing vocabulary development, sentence understanding, reading comprehension, and word finding; use of slower speech and short concrete sentences by teachers; reduction of ambient noise; use of strategies to enhance memory; use of advance organizers, short sessions, and continuous checks during reading instruction; and use of drills for math facts, close monitoring of math processes, and provision of extra support for word problems to facilitate understanding of math. These authors also noted that supportive families and special assistance/remediation at school were associated with better longtime outcomes in males with Klinefelter syndrome.

Geschwind and Dykens (2004) note that early intervention that addresses phonological processing may be valuable in alleviating early reading problems. Although such intervention may only be appropriate in the later preschool years, speech–language pathologists may be most knowledgeable in this area. These authors also mentioned that the impact of pharmacologic treatments used with children with ADHD or hormone replacement therapy on attention and executive function have not been investigated in children with Klinefelter syndrome.

There is limited evidence of difficulties with inhibition and working memory in school-age boys with Klinefelter syndrome (Geschwind & Dykens, 2004; Ross et al., this volume); therefore, parents of young boys with KS might consider monitoring them for signs of these impairments. They can take a proactive approach to supporting their sons by encouraging them to "slow down and wait" before responding in games and in interactions with siblings and peers to promote appropriate inhibition. Parents can play simple memory games (hide-and-seek with small toys in known locations; how many fingers did I just hold up, etc.) in a fun and playful way to promote working memory. They can also help their young children develop strategies for recalling information such as vocalizing information that has to be remembered.

By being aware of the behavioral characteristics of boys with Klinefelter syndrome, parents and neurogenetic specialists can promote higher self-esteem in these young boys by recognizing the special interests of these boys, providing a variety of opportunities for them to succeed, providing positive feedback and reinforcement for appropriate and social behavior, and providing opportunities for play dates and for these young boys to make friendships with others. By taking a proactive approach to promoting self-esteem and appropriate social behavior during early childhood, parents may be able to prevent chronic behavioral and emotional problems that have been described in older boys with KS (Ross et al., this volume).

Summary

The purpose of this chapter was to provide information about the legal basis for early intervention and ECSE and about recommended practices for these fields. To exemplify what specific information is relevant to decisions about early intervention, the literature on early intervention and ECSE was summarized for a range of neurogenetic disorders, recommendations for early intervention and education were described, and potential resources were provided. Specifically, detailed information was provided for 22q11 deletion syndrome, fragile X syndrome, Turner syndrome, and Klinefelter syndrome. These disorders range in terms of symptom severity, but also in terms of their hallmark characteristics and age at which diagnosis of the disorder typically occurs. Although it may be apparent that earlier onset of syndrome symptoms will lead to an earlier initial delivery of intervention services, a professional's awareness of these possible features and of the need to provide supportive or preventive services may facilitate prompt recognition of the symptoms. With knowledge of the phenotypic characteristics of a given syndrome, particularly a syndrome that presents early in life (such as fragile X syndrome), parents and professionals can adopt a preventive approach to promoting health and development of a young child. Recommendations for early intervention may include medical or pharmacological treatment, speech and language therapy, occupational or physical therapy, socioemotional and behavioral intervention, or preschool services to address multiple developmental needs and delays.

Just as the nature and number of intervention approaches recommended will vary across the disorders—as seen in the variety of recommendations provided for the three disorders summarized earlier in this chapter—so, too, will such recommendations vary for each individual child within a given population (e.g., children with fragile X syndrome). In fact, many of the recommended interventions discussed for one or more of these three neurogenetic disorders can be applied to other children whose developmental delay includes features similar to those described for children with fragile X syndrome, 22q11 deletion syndrome, or Klinefelter syndrome. In this regard, the recommendations may be drawn also from research carried out with children who do not have a known neurogenetic syndrome. For example, knowledge of well-established and empirically based interventions for children with reading disabilities can inform recommendations for boys with Klinefelter syndrome who have reading difficulties. However, it is necessary to empirically evaluate the efficacy of specific interventions in special populations, in view of the potential for variability in the causal mechanisms leading to phenotypic features. For this reason, understanding the mechanisms that underlie the physical, cognitive, or behavioral characteristics associated with a neurogenetic disorder will enhance decision making about appropriate treatment recommendations. This information should be helpful for both neurogenetic specialists and families. In view of the ongoing and rapid advancements in our knowledge of neurogenetic disorders, professionals working with children and their families must stay abreast of such new resources and information.

Acknowledgments

The writing of this chapter was supported, in part, by grant # 3-P30-HD003110-35S1 from the National Institute of Child Health and Human Development awarded to Deborah D. Hatton, Donald B. Bailey, and Joe Piven. Thanks go to Jennie Bollinger, Nicole Mason, and Julie Nagelson for their assistance.

Suggested Resources

22q11 Deletion Syndrome

22q and You Center: The Children's Hospital of Philadelphia
http://www.chop.edu/consumer/jsp/division/service.jsp?id=74652

The 22q11.2 Deletion Syndrome Foundation, Inc.
http://www.22q.org/index.html

The 22q11 Group
http://www.vcfs.net

Chromosome 22 Central
http://www.c22c.org

Chromosome Deletion Outreach, Inc.
http://www.chromodisorder.org

Congenital Cardiovascular Genetics
http://www.cardiogenetics.org/del22q11.asp

Velo-Cardio-Facial Syndrome Education Foundation
http://www.vcfsef.org

McDonald-McGinn, D., Finucane, B., & Zackai, E. (2000). *Faces of sunshine: The 22q11.2 deletion: A handbook for parents and professionals.* The Children's Hospital of Philadelphia.

Fragile X Syndrome

The National Fragile X Foundation
www.fragilex.org

FRAXA—Fragile X Research Foundation
http://www.fraxa.org/

Facts about Fragile X Syndrome—NIH
http://www.nichd.nih.gov/publications/pubs/fragilextoc.htm

Carolina Fragile X Project
http://www.fpg.unc.edu/~fx

Fragile X Information Center
http://www.fpg.unc.edu/~fxic

Dykens, E. M., Hodapp, R. M., & Leckman, J. F. (1994). *Behavior and development in fragile X syndrome.* Thousand Oaks, CA: Sage.

Hagerman, R. J., & Hagerman, P. J. (Eds.). (2002). *Fragile X syndrome: Diagnosis, treatment, and research* (3rd ed.). Baltimore: Johns Hopkins University Press.

Saunders, S. (2001). *Fragile X syndrome: A guide for teachers.* London: David Fulton.

Weber, J. D. (2000). *Children with fragile X syndrome: A parent's guide.* Bethesda, MD: Woodbine House.

Turner Syndrome

Turner Syndrome Society
http://www.turner-syndrome-us.org/

Turner Syndrome at NIH
http://turners.nichd.nih.gov/

Frias, J., & Davenport, M. (2003). Health supervision for children with Turner syndrome. *Pediatrics, 111*(3), 692–702.

Rovet, J. (2004). Turner syndrome: Genetics and hormonal factors contributing to a specific learning disability profile. *Learning Disabilities Research and Practice, 19,* 133–145.

Saenger, P., Albertsson Wikland, K., Conwy, G. S., Davenport, M., Graveholt, C. H., Hintz, R., et al. (2001). Recommendations for the diagnosis and management of Turner syndrome. *The Journal of Clinical Endocrinology and Metabolism, 86,* 3061–3069.

Klinefelter Syndrome

American Association for Klinefelter Syndrome Information and Support
http://www.aaksis.org/

Klinefelter syndrome—NIH
http://www.nichd.nih.gov/publications/pubs/klinefelter.htm

Klinefelter's Syndrome Association (UK)
http://www.ksa-uk.co.uk/

Klinefelter Syndrome Support Group Home Page
http://klinefeltersyndrome.org/

References

Bailey, D. B. (in press). Families and fragile X syndrome. In D. B. Bailey, S. F. Warren, D. D. Hatton, & N. Brady (Eds.), *Young children and fragile X syndrome: A primer for parents and professionals*. Baltimore: Brookes.

Bailey, D. B., Hatton, D. D., & Skinner, M. (1998). Early developmental trajectories of boys with fragile X syndrome. *American Journal of Mental Retardation, 103*, 29–39.

Bailey, D. B., Hatton, D. D., Skinner, M., & Mesibov, G. (2001). Autistic behavior, FMR1 protein, and developmental trajectories in young males with fragile X syndrome. *Journal of Autism and Developmental Disorders, 31*, 165–174.

Bailey, D. B., Skinner, D., & Sparkman, K. (2003). Discovering fragile X syndrome: Family experiences and perceptions. *Pediatrics, 111*, 407–416.

Bojesen, A., Juul, S., & Gravholt, C. H. (2003). Prenatal and postnatal prevalence of Klinefelter syndrome: A national registry study. *The Journal of Clinical Endocrinology & Metabolism, 88*, 622–626.

Brooks-Gunn, J., & Hearn, R. (1982). Early intervention and developmental dysfunction: Implications for pediatrics. *Advances in Pediatrics, 29*, 497–527.

Dykens, E., Hodapp, R. M., & Finucane, B. M. (2000). *Genetics and mental retardation syndromes: A new look at behavior and intervention*. Baltimore: Brookes.

Early Childhood Outcomes Center. (2004, May). *Uses and misuses of data on outcomes for children with disabilities*. Retrieved January 26, 2006, from The Early Childhood Outcomes Center Papers: http://www.fpg.unc.edu/~eco/pages/publications.cfm

Early Childhood Outcomes Center. (2005, April). *Family and child outcomes for early intervention and early childhood special education*. Retrieved January 26, 2006, from The Early Childhood Outcomes Center Papers: http://www.fpg.unc.edu/~eco/pages/publications.cfm

Gerdes, M., Solot, C., Wang, P., Moss, E., LaRossa, D., Randell, P., et al. (1999). Cognitive and behavior profile of preschool children with chromosome 22q11.2 deletion. *American Journal of American Genetics, 85*, 127–133.

Geschwind, D. H., & Dykens, E. (2004). Neurobehavioral and psychosocial issues in Klinefelter syndrome. *Learning Disabilities Research and Practice, 19*(3), 166–173.

Guralnick, M. J. (2000). Early childhood intervention: Evolution of a system. *Focus on Autism and Other Developmental Disabilities, 15*(2), 68–79.

Hagerman, R. J. (2000). Medical concerns and treatment for children with fragile X syndrome. In J. D. Weber (Ed.), *Children with fragile X syndrome: A parents' guide* (pp. 200–242). Bethesda, MD: Woodbine House.

Hagerman, R. J., Farzin, F., & Sakimura, J. (in press). Physical and medical needs of infants and toddlers with fragile X syndrome. In D. B. Bailey, S. F. Warren, D. D. Hatton, & N. Brady (Eds.), *Young children and fragile X syndrome: A primer for parents and professionals*. Baltimore: Brookes.

Hatton, D. D., & Bailey, D. B. (in press). Early intervention and early childhood special education for children with fragile X syndrome. In D. B. Bailey, S. F. Warren, D. D. Hatton, & N. Brady (Eds.), *Early intervention for young children with fragile X syndrome*. Baltimore: Brookes.

Hatton, D. D., & Roberts, J. E. (in press). Behavior and physiological regulation in young children with fragile X syndrome. In D. B. Bailey, S. F. Warren, D. D. Hatton, & N. Brady (Eds.), *Young children and fragile X syndrome: A primer for parents and professionals*. Baltimore: Brookes.

Hatton, D. D., Bailey, D. B., Roberts, J. P., Skinner, M., Mayhew, L., Clark, R. D., et al. (2000). Early intervention services for young boys with fragile X syndrome. *Journal of Early Intervention, 23*, 235–251.

Hatton, D. D., Hooper, S. R., Bailey, D. B., Skinner, M., Sullivan, K., & Wheeler, A. (2002). Problem behavior in boys with fragile X syndrome. *American Journal of Medical Genetics, 108*, 105–116.

Hatton, D. D., Wheeler, A. C., Skinner, M. L., Bailey, D. B., Sullivan, K. M., Roberts, J. E., et al. (2003). Adaptive behavior in children with fragile X syndrome. *American Journal of Mental Retardation, 108*, 373–390.

Hill, J., Waldfogel, J., & Brooks-Gunn, J. (2003). Sustained effects of high participation in early intervention for low-birth-weight premature infants. *Developmental Psychology, 39,* 730–744.

Individuals with Disabilities Education. Improvement Act of 2004, H.R. 1350 (2004).

Johnston, C., Hessl, D., Blasey, C., Eliez, S., Erba, H., Dyer-Friedman, J., et al. (2003). Factors associated with parenting stress in mothers of children with fragile X syndrome. *Journal of Developmental & Behavioral Pediatrics, 24,* 267–290.

Kau, A. S. M., Tierney, E., Bukelis, I., Stump, M. H., Kates, W. R., & Trescher, W. H. (2004). Social behavior profile in young males with fragile X syndrome: Characteristics and specificity. *American Journal of Medical Genetics, 126A,* 9–17.

Kaufmann, W. E., Cortell, R., Kau, A., Bukelis, I., Tierney, E., Gray, R., et al. (2004). Autism spectrum disorder in fragile X syndrome: Communication, social interaction, and specific behaviors. *American Journal of Medical Genetics, 129A,* 225–234.

Klebanov, P. K., Brooks-Gunn, J., & McCormick, M. C. (2001). Maternal coping strategies and emotional distress: Results of an early intervention program for low birth weight young children. *Developmental Psychology, 37,* 654–667.

Madison, L., Mosher, G., & George, C. (1998). Patterns of early intervention service utilization: Child, maternal, and provider factors. *Journal of Early Intervention, 21,* 217–231.

Mazzocco, M., Baumgardner, T. M., Freund, L. S., & Reiss, A. L. (1998). Social functioning among girls with fragile X or Turner syndrome and their sisters. *Journal of Autism and Developmental Disorders, 28,* 509–571.

McDonald-McGinn, D. M., Emanuel, B., & Zackai, E. (2003). *22q11.2 deletion syndrome.* Retrieved December 6th, 2005, from http://www.geneclinics.org/profiles/22q11deletion/details.html

McDonald-McGinn, D. M., Finucane, B. M., & Zackai, E. (2000). *Faces of sunshine: The 22q11.2 deletion: A handbook for parents and professionals.* Philadelphia: The Children's Hospital of Philadelphia.

McWilliam, R. A. (1992). *Family-centered intervention planning: A routines-based approach.* Tucson, AZ: Communication Skill Builders.

McWilliam, R. A. (2005). DEC recommended practices: Interdisciplinary models. In S. Sandall, M. L. Hemmeter, B. J. Smith, & M. E. McLean (Eds.), *DEC recommended practices: A comprehensive guide for practical application in early intervention/early childhood special education* (pp. 127–146). Longmont, CO: Sopris West Educational Services.

Mirrett, P. L., Bailey, D. B., Roberts, J. E., & Hatton, D. D. (2004). Developmental screening and detection of developmental delays in infants and toddlers with fragile X syndrome. *Developmental and Behavioral Pediatrics, 25*(1), 21–27.

Mirrett, P. L., Roberts, J. E., & Price, J. (2003). Early intervention practices and communication intervention strategies for young males with fragile X syndrome. *Language, Speech, and Hearing Services in Schools, 34,* 320–331.

Neisworth, J. T., & Bagnato, S. J. (2005). DEC recommended practices: Assessment. In S. Sandall, M. L. Hemmeter, B. J. Smith, & M. E. McLean (Eds.), *DEC recommended practices: A comprehensive guide for practical application in early intervention/early childhood special education* (pp. 45–69). Longmont, CO: Sopris West Educational Services.

Persson, C., Lohmander, A., Jonsson, R., Oskarsdottir, S., & Soderpalm, E. (2003). A prospective cross-sectional study of speech in patients with the 22q11 deletion syndrome. *Journal of Communication Disorders, 36,* 13–47.

Ramey, C. T., Bryant, D. M., Sparling, J. J., & Wasik, B. H. (1985). Project CARE: A comparison of two early childhood intervention strategies to prevent retarded development. *Topics in Early Childhood Special Education, 5,* 12–25.

Ramey, C. T., & Campbell, F. A. (1991). Poverty, early childhood education, and academic competence: The Abecedarian experiment. In A. Huston (Ed.), *Children reared in poverty* (pp. 190–221). New York: Cambridge University Press.

Ritinksi-Mack, L., Obler, D., Smoot, L., & Tsipis, J. (2005). *An educator's guide to understanding VCFS.* Retrieved December 6th, 2005, from http://www.cardiogenetics.org/del22q11_Guide.asp

Roberts, J. E., Hatton, D. D., & Bailey, D. B. (2001). Development and behavior of male toddlers with fragile X syndrome. *Journal of Early Intervention, 24,* 207–223.

Roberts, J. E., Mirrett, P., Anderson, K., Burchinal, M., & Neebe, E. (2002). Early communication, symbolic behavior, and social profiles of young males with fragile X syndrome. *American Journal of Speech-Language Pathology, 11,* 295–304.

Roberts, J. E., Mirrett, P. L., & Schaaf, J. (in press). Developmental skills in young children with fragile X syndrome. In D. B. Bailey, S. F. Warren, D. D. Hatton, & N. Brady (Eds.), *Young children and fragile X syndrome: A primer for parents and professionals.* Baltimore: Brookes.

Rogers, S. J., Wehner, E., & Hagerman, R. J. (2001). The behavioral phenotype in fragile X: Symptoms of autism in very young children with fragile X syndrome, idiopathic autism, and other developmental disorders. *Journal of Developmental Behavioral Pediatrics, 22,* 409–417.

Ross, J., Zinn, A., & McCauley, E. (2000). Neurodevelopmental and psychosocial aspects of Turner syndrome. *Mental Retardation and Developmental Disabilities, 6,* 135–141.

Rovet, J. (2004). Turner syndrome: Genetic and hormonal factors contributing to a specific learning disability profile. *Learning Disabilities Research and Practice, 19*(3), 133–145.

Rovet, J., Netley, C., Keenan, M., Bailey, J., & Stewart, D. (1996). The psychoeducational profile of boys with Klinefelter syndrome. *Journal of Learning Disabilities, 29,* 180–196.

Samango-Sprouse, C., & Rogol, A. (2002). XXY: The hidden disability and a prototype for an infantile presentation of developmental dyspraxia (IDD). *Infants and Young Children, 15*(1), 11–18.

Sandall, S., Hemmeter, M. L., Smith, B. J., & McLean, M. E. (2005). *DEC recommended practices: A comprehensive guide for practical application in early intervention/early childhood special education.* Longmont, CO: Sopris West Educational Company.

Saunders, S. (1999). Teaching children with fragile X syndrome. *British Journal of Special Education, 26*(2), 76–79.

Solot, C., Knightly, C., Handler, S., Gerdes, M., McDonald-McGinn, D. M., & Moss, E. (2000). Communication disorders in the 22q11.2 microdeletion syndrome. *Journal of Communication Disorders, 33,* 187–204.

Swillen, A., Devriendt, K., Legius, E., Eyskens, B., Dumoulin, M., Gewilling, M., et al. (1997). Intelligence and psychosocial adjustment in velocardiofacial syndrome: A study of 37 children and adolescents with VCFS. *Journal of Medical Genetics, 34,* 453–458.

Symons, F. J., Clark, R. D., Roberts, J. P., & Bailey, D. B. (2001). Classroom behavior and academic engagement of elementary school-aged boys with fragile X syndrome. *Journal of Special Education, 34,* 194–202.

Trivette, C. M., & Dunst, C. J. (2005). DEC recommended practices: Family-based practices. In S. Sandall, M. L. Hemmeter, B. J. Smith, & M. E. McLean (Eds.), *DEC recommended practices: A comprehensive guide for practical application in early intervention/early childhood special education* (pp. 107–126). Longmont, CO: Sopris West Educational services.

U.S. Department of Education. (2001). *Twenty-third report to Congress on the implantation of the Individuals with Disabilities Education Act.* Washington, DC: Education Publications Center.

Wheeler, A., Hatton, D., Reichardt, A., & Bailey, D. (in press). Correlates of maternal behavior in mothers of children with fragile X syndrome. *Journal of Intellectual Disability Research.*

Wilson, P. G., & Mazzocco, M. M. M. (1993). Awareness and knowledge of fragile X syndrome among special educators. *Mental Retardation, 31,* 221–227.

Wolery, M. (2005). DEC recommended practices: Child-focused practices. In S. Sandall, M. L. Hemmeter, B. J. Smith, & M. E. McLean (Eds.), *DEC recommended practices: A comprehensive guide for practical application in early intervention/early childhood special education* (pp. 71–106). Longmont, CO: Sopris West Educational Services.

York, A., von Fraunhofer, N., Turk, J., & Sedgwick, P. (1999). Fragile X syndrome, Down's syndrome and autism: Awareness and knowledge amongst special educators. *Journal of Intellectual Disability Research, 43,* 314–324.

15 The Individualized Education Program: Navigating the IEP Development Process

Vicki Sudhalter

Overview

This chapter is written for professionals who interact with parents whose children have developmental disabilities. In my experience, pediatricians are often the first professionals from whom parents seek information about developmental milestones and advice about maximizing their children's developmental gains. Additionally, these medical professionals may offer advice concerning what steps parents should follow in order to help their children gain developmental milestones. This chapter is designed to provide physicians, and other professionals who interact with parents of children with developmental disabilities, with information about the role of the individualized education program (IEP) in optimizing a child's intellectual and psychological growth. With this information, parents have the knowledge to guide their own participation in their child's education and to serve as their child's advocate. It has been my experience that many professionals who work with developmentally delayed children (and the parents of these children) have not had the opportunity to learn about the importance, function, and limitation of the IEP. This lack of information limits the effectiveness of the professional's role to serve as facilitator or to contribute to the IEP process in a way that is specifically permitted by the federal law. As such, the objective of this chapter is to help fill this existing gap in information, so as to enable parents and the professional to whom they turn to become more effective partners in the development of a child's IEP.

Introduction

The IEP is a very powerful tool that was initially created from the Education of All Handicapped Children Act (EAHCA) of 1975, and more recently reauthorized as the Individuals With Disabilities Education Act (IDEA) of 2004. The power associated with an IEP stems from the fact that it is a legal contract between the public educational system and the parents or guardians of a child with a disability. The IEP is an educational program that, ideally, is developed by the child's parents, teachers, and therapists—persons who can contribute information directly relevant to the child's education. It describes the manner in which the child will receive a free and appropriate education (FAPE) in the least restrictive environment (LRE). Most of this chapter is devoted to explaining how the IEP is created and the crucial role parents and other specialists can play in its development and implementation. However, I first provide an introduction to the IDEA, its importance, and the recent developments and changes to this law. I then discuss the process of creating, writing, and implementing the IEP for a child with a disability.

History of the IEP

The IDEA (2004) is the nation's special education law. IDEA provides federal funding to help states and local communities provide education to the approximately 6 million students (Ed Publications, 2002) with varying degrees of disability. IDEA requires the states to provide a FAPE, which means that children with disabilities are entitled to a publicly financed education that is appropriate to their age and abilities. This education is to occur in the LRE, which means that placement of students with disabilities in special classes, separate schools, or other forms of removal from the regular classroom occurs only when the nature or severity of the disability cannot be satisfactorily achieved in the regular classroom. Special education and related services will be made available to all children with disabilities; and will (a) be provided, under public supervision and direction at public expense; (b) meet the standards of the state educational agency (SEA); (c) include an appropriate preschool, elementary school, or secondary school; and (d) be provided in conformity with the IEP established for the child (Department of Education, 2006). Students have a right to a FAPE if they meet the eligibility requirements for an IEP (discussed below) and are ages 3 to 21 years (in most of the 50 states) or have not yet graduated from high school. In order to determine state-specific eligibility criteria, one should contact the appropriate local Board of Education. FAPE does *not* mean that the best possible education is offered at public expense. Courts have defined "appropriate education" as the basic minimum for a given child with a given set of behaviors, symptoms, strengths, and deficits. Thus IDEA guarantees equal opportunity, but it does not guarantee the best possible education. This is one reason why parents and the educators who have created an IEP may disagree on what is an "appropriate education." This disagreement can be resolved either around the "IEP table," or, if necessary, through "due process." At due process, the parents argue for the type of education and/or level of therapy they desire for their child. This argument is presented in front of a due process judge (in some states this is called the "impartial hearing officer"). This process is discussed at length below.

No Child Left Behind and the Updated IDEA

The No Child Left Behind law (NCLB) was created in 2001 (Public Law 107–110) and signed into law in 2002. Under NCLB, the states and local school systems are held accountable for ensuring that all children, including children with disabilities, are making advances in learning. This is accomplished by reporting yearly assessment results of all students, including those with disabilities. IDEA, as opposed to NCLB, requires that the IEP team determine how the child with a disability is to be assessed, but not whether the child is assessed. NCLB, on the other hand, holds school systems accountable for assessment and for the progress of their students regardless of disability.

Since 1997, IDEA has required that all states have alternative assessments available for children with disabilities, because children with disabilities may have atypical learning processes. In 2004, IDEA was updated to allow states to develop alternate assessments linked to alternate achievement standards. As of early 2006, not all states or municipalities had codified this concept. In view of the recent enactment of this law and the variability of its implementation across states, for up-to-date information it is advisable to consult one's local school boards to determine (a) if alternate assessments are in place, (b) what forms of alternative assessments are available, (c) how the school system decides the manner in which an individual student is assessed, and (d) how one can be involved in that decision for a given child.

The IEP

Definition

The IEP is a record of the goals established for a child and the methodologies that will be used to enable the child to meet these goals. The IEP should be considered an agreement between a child's school and parent. By law, the parents are to play a major role in the decisions made regarding their child's eligibility and educational placement. Additionally, parents *must* be given the opportunity to participate in meetings related to identification, evaluation, educational placement, and provision of an appropriate FAPE for their child.

From Identification to Education

In order to start the process of creating an IEP, the child must be identified as having a disability. Why would the parent want to initiate this rather long and arduous process? Because the IEP is the sole mechanism by which parents have a legal document detailing the therapy and education that will be provided to help their child meet developmental milestones. The initiation of the process may arise from questions asked by a pediatrician who may question the rate of motor or cognitive development, a relative or friend who may inquire about the child's progress, or a teacher who is concerned with the child's lack of academic growth. Once there is suspicion of a developmental problem, the parent can initiate the IEP process (or the Individualized Family Service Plan (IFSP) process for a younger child) at any time. The first official step toward creating an IEP is the evaluation to determine whether a child has developmental delay.

Evaluation

The Evaluation Process Can only Be Initiated with the Consent of the Parent For children of 5 years and older, the child is referred to the Child Study Team (the exact name of the evaluation team varies from state to state). This evaluation team may consist of a learning disabilities teacher or consultant, a psychologist, a social worker, a speech therapist, an occupational and/or physical therapist, and a school nurse (whose role it would be to review any pertinent medical records). An initial evaluation to determine the child's needs must include a physical examination, a psychological evaluation (if determined appropriate for school-age students, but is mandatory for preschool children), a social history, observation of the child in his or her current education setting, other tests or assessments that are appropriate for the child (such as a speech and language assessment or a functional behavioral assessment), and vocational assessments (required at age 12 years). The parents have the legal right to have input on the tests and assessments to be administered to their child. Before an evaluation is conducted, the parent should be asked for suggestions about the child's evaluation and should be given information about the kinds of tests that may be used. The results of the evaluation will not only determine eligibility for the child to receive a FAPE, but will inform the creation of the IEP.

Every Area of Suspected Disability Must Be Evaluated The testing must be individualized and validated for the purposes used. The tests should be administered by trained, knowledgeable professionals using the native language of the child. The operative word is knowledgeable. For instance, if the child is presenting with a diagnosis such as fragile X syndrome, it is important that the professional administering the assessments understand the hyperarousal issues and eye contact difficulties that many children with fragile X syndrome experience (please see chapter 3, this volume) and modify the administration of the assessments accordingly. It is inappropriate to demand that a child with fragile X syndrome maintain eye contact with the examiner, as this may compromise the child's performance; or with a teacher, as this may affect the IEP goals. All of the principles of sound psychological testing (e.g., Sattler, 2001) are of essential importance.

How is it possible to determine the strengths and weaknesses of a child with severe disabilities? Formerly, students with severe disabilities were exempted from assessments. However, the IDEA amendments and NCLB now require the states to have implemented an alternate assessment system. Alternate assessment formats are necessary because, through these mechanisms, the students are able to demonstrate their abilities, learning, and skill attainment.

Along with standardized or alternative assessments, the child also undergoes functional assessments such as a structured observation in a classroom or on the schoolyard. Parents, teachers, and others who are knowledgeable about the child are interviewed. There is a review of the child's developmental and educational history, and in cases of a reevaluation of an IEP, there is a review of the interventions already in place in the classroom.

A functional behavioral assessment (FBA) is used when the child's behavior interferes with the child's learning or the learning of others in the classroom. The FBA investigates possible explanations for the child's behavior on the basis of the nature of the child and the classroom environment. For instance, a child may become aggressive toward a peer or a teacher or may engage in a tantrum before going to lunch or out to play. The child may also have a very short attention span, roam around the room, or have difficulty remaining seated. These behaviors interfere not only with the child's learning but also with the ability of the other classroom children to learn. A behavioral specialist should create a behavioral plan that will help eliminate or diminish the maladaptive behaviors as part of the IEP. In my experience, many parents do not know that they can ask for an FBA. For many children, however, an FBA is the key component of their IEP and must be in place in order for the child to learn.

If the parents feel either that an evaluation or its results are inappropriate, they have a right to obtain, and request that the school district pay for, an independent educational evaluation (IEE). The request must be made in writing, and the parent should explicitly state the evaluations they are requesting (e.g., occupational therapy for fine motor deficits). There may be no one who specializes in these deficits or who understands the child's disabling condition (e.g., fragile X, Williams, or Down Syndrome) on the child study team. In order to obtain a thorough evaluation that will help procure the services needed, the parent would have to take the child to a knowledgeable, private (i.e., not part of the Board of Education) occupational therapist who understands the implications of the disabling condition on the fine motor system. All of these evaluations must be considered to determine eligibility and establish the IEP.

Once a child has an IEP, the child must be reevaluated every 3 years, or sooner if the teacher, parent, or therapist makes the request. This is not to say that the IEP is written every 3 years; the IEP is written at least every year; however, the child undergoes a formal reevaluation process every 3 years (known as the "triennial review"). The special education team reviews evaluation data and results and information provided by parent(s), current classroom-based assessments, and observations by teachers and related service providers. The reevaluations determine whether additions or modifications are needed to the child's program to enable the child to meet IEP goals and to participate, as appropriate, in the general curriculum. The reevaluation may result in a change of diagnosis or a determination that the child no longer needs an IEP, at which point the child is placed in a mainstream setting (i.e., a regular classroom).

Eligibility

Once the evaluation is completed, a meeting is held to review the results and determine eligibility for services. Parents must receive the evaluation reports 10 days in advance of the meeting to provide sufficient time to review the results, and prepare any questions related to the testing. The parent may also bring additional evaluation information to the eligibility meeting, such as that obtained by the IEE, which the committee must consider.

Each State Has Its Own Eligibility Criteria   For this reason, it is important that professionals in the field be familiar with their local policies. A "student with a disability" means a child with a disability as defined in education law; who does not turn 21 years old before September 1; who is entitled to attend public school; who because of mental, physical, or emotional reasons has been identified as having a disability; and who requires special services or programs. In general, eligibility is defined as students ages 5–21 years, who are identified as having a disability and who may have autism, deafness, deaf-blindness, emotional disturbance, hearing impairment, learning disability, mental retardation, multiple disabilities, orthopedic impairment, other health impairment, speech and language impairment, traumatic brain injury, or visual impairment (including blindness).

If the parent, with the committee, decides that the child does not require special education services or programs, the child based support team will provide the parent with information indicating why the child is ineligible. The parent will receive a written notice that explains the decision and the information on which the decision was made. If there is disagreement, then the parent can request mediation and or an impartial hearing to resolve the disagreement (see the Due Process section, below). The parent may also decide that the child may be served through a 504 classification (see the 504 Plan section later in this chapter).

The Writing of the IEP

Federal guidelines dictate that the IEP must be written within 30 calendar days from the time the child was determined to meet the eligibility requirements. Who creates the IEP? By law, certain individuals must be involved in writing the child's IEP. The case manager, parent, general education teacher, special education teacher, and other specialists (as the child's deficits dictate) create the IEP. If the child is in a general education classroom, the general education teacher has input into the writing of the IEP and must be present whenever issues affecting general education are discussed. The general education teacher need not participate in all decisions nor be present throughout the entire meeting but should participate in those meetings that directly influence general education. Each of the student's teachers, including general educator(s), must be informed of their responsibilities related to IEP implementation and specific accommodations, modifications, and supports that must be provided in order for the child to meet the IEP goals.

Current Performance

The first part of the IEP, the current performance section, must state the child's present levels of educational performance. This information is usually drawn from classroom tests and assignments, individual tests given either to determine eligibility or during reevaluation, and observations made by parents, teachers, related service providers, and other school staff. It is important that this section is comprehensive, because it provides the creators or modifiers of the IEP the necessary information on which to establish new IEP goals and the related teaching strategies. The statement of current performance should also include the ways in which the child's disability affects involvement and progress in the general curriculum, the student's strengths, parental concerns, and all areas of weakness each of which is linked to annual goals and objectives.

This section of the IEP may address inconsistencies between the child's performance at home and at school. If the child is performing better in school than at home, then the parent should be so informed and should further be taught how to encourage desirable performance levels in the home. If the child is performing better in the home than in the school (e.g., as a result of a home program or as a result of the child's becoming distracted by the school environment), then a change to the existing classroom environment based on the techniques used in the home should be considered.

Parents must be encouraged to voice their own concerns about the deficits their child is exhibiting and should also be shown how these concerns can be addressed by the IEP. For instance, many parents do not understand that such deficits as the child's lack of toileting ability, feeding skills, social play or playing with toys are target areas of current performance. If these deficits are interfering with the acquisition of the curriculum, they are legitimate areas to be addressed by the IEP. Additionally, maladaptive behaviors should also become part of current performance and can then be addressed in the annual goals of the IEP.

Annual Goals

Annual goals pertain to the child's deficits and, whenever possible and practical, to the curriculum. These goals must be assessed (regardless of how that assessment is designed) so that all responsible educators can be held accountable. Annual goals should be carefully crafted. As required, the IEP team must agree that the goals are attainable within an academic school year, on the basis of the child's current abilities, assessment performance, and his or her learning speed and style. To monitor the child's progress the goal itself is broken down into short-term measurable objectives, or *benchmarks*. Target dates are specified as the times at which the child is expected to have acquired the benchmarks. When the short-term objective is not met by the agreed upon date, a reassessment of the methodologies used to teach the goal should take place to determine what further modification may need to be implemented. Benchmarks should be viewed as a type of report card. If the child fails to meet these objectives, a reevaluation should take place because the child will be at risk for not meeting the annual goal.

The annual goals are written for all areas of development, including academic goals, but also social, behavioral, physical, daily living, and emotional goals. The parent will be asked to provide goals either before the initial IEP meeting, or at the initial writing of the IEP goals.

How to Write an Annual Goal   A well-written goal is a positive statement that describes an observable event. It is based upon present levels of performance with appropriate short-term benchmarks, and must include the five following elements: a) it should be clear *what* skill or behavior is being taught (e.g., the child will initiate going to the bathroom; the child will produce three word utterances); b) *where* the skill will be evaluated (e.g., in the classroom, at home and in school, with the speech and language teacher); *how* the skill will be taught (e.g., through Applied Behavior Analytic [ABA] methodology, through the use of augmentative devices, through teacher and peer interactions; through one-on-one teaching); *when* the desired behaviors will be accomplished (e.g., "By March 31, 2007"); and with what level of *frequency* (e.g., "The child will demonstrate this skill 100% of the time"; "The child will do this 4/5 times").

Case 15.1: Preparing an IEP for Tyrone   Tyrone is a 6-year-old enrolled in a kindergarten-first grade inclusion class. He has been evaluated for speech and language delay at the request of his classroom teacher. Tyrone's speech and language teacher determined that he had difficulty producing phrases longer than two words. This is his *current performance.* It was determined at the IEP meeting that an appropriate *annual goal* for Tyrone would be to increase his spontaneous and elicited phrases from two words to five- or six-word phrases. In order to accomplish this increase in the mean length of utterance, Tyrone must learn how to incorporate adjectives, adverbs, prepositional phrases, and verb phrases into his productions. Thus, one annual goal is that "Tyrone will increase the average length of his phrases to between five and six words, including adjectives, adverbs, prepositional phrases, and verb phrases." In order to meet his annual goal, Tyrone will be given speech and language therapy and oral motor therapy during the year—this is an explicit statement of how this specific IEP goal is to be achieved. To specify when and where Tyrone will produce these lengthy utterances, the IEP includes a statement that the utterances will be produced in all environments by the end of the academic year. Tyrone will produce these utterances 100% of the time an utterance is being elicited or spontaneously produced—an explicit statement of the expected frequency of the desired behavior. Intermediate *benchmarks* toward meeting this annual goal are also specified. For instance, by 3 months into the school year, Tyrone will be able to use adjectives and adverbs in elicited and spontaneously produced utterances; by 6 months, he will be able to use prepositional phrases along with adjectives and adverbs in his elicited and spontaneously produced utterances; and by the end of the school year, Tyrone will be able to use verb phrases along with adjectives, adverbs, and prepositional phrases in his elicited and spontaneously produced utterances.

Role of the Parent   It is also important that the goals of the IEP be explained to the child's parents so that the skills can be encouraged and reinforced at home. If parents require specialized training in order to reinforce targeted behaviors at home, then this should be added to the IEP. In this regard, it is also important that there be regular and frequent communication between parents and teachers. Parents should inform their children's teachers of any factors that may influence their children's behavior at school (e.g., the family is moving, a child had a bad night, a child was discovered to have a seizure disorder), and teachers should inform children's parents about their academic progress as well as any significant events that occurred at school (e.g., a child initiated an interaction with a peer, a child used adjectives for the first time, a child aggressed on a classmate). This communication is usually accomplished with a notebook passed between the home and the school. The method and frequency of this information exchange are legitimate areas to include in the IEP. If a parent does not speak English, and the teacher does not speak the parent's native language, then this communication should occur through a translator who can be a parent representative, a paraprofessional who has been assigned to the assist the child, or some other professional who speaks the parent's language. A parent's reliance on a foreign language should not be the cause of a breakdown in communication between school and home. In such cases, it is incumbent on the school staff to find a translator so that parents always have the opportunity to be involved with their child's education. Such details should be addressed in the IEP.

Related Services   Once the annual goals have been agreed upon and written as specifically as possible, the next step involves establishing what additional supports are needed to ensure that the child will meet the annual goals. Related services may include transportation services or other supportive services that are considered necessary for a child with a disability to benefit from special education (Statement of the Special Education and Related Services, Supplementary Aids and Services, Program Modifications, and Supports For School Personnel—34 CFR §300.347(a)(3)). This term includes such services as the following:

Speech–language pathology and audiology

Psychological services (counseling, play therapy, etc.)

Physical and occupational therapy

Recreation including therapeutic recreation

Counseling including rehabilitative counseling

Orientation and mobility services

Medical services for diagnostic or evaluation purposes

School health services

Social work services

Parent counseling and training.

The IEP should specify how many times per week the child is to receive these special services (e.g., two–three times per week), for how long (e.g., 30 minutes per session), in what location (e.g., in the classroom or in a separate therapy room), and in what size group (e.g., one on one or in a group of two or three). Exactly when such services are to begin should also be specified. It is usually assumed that such services will be in place when an IEP is implemented, but this is often not the case. If a child does not or cannot receive the mandated services for any reason (e.g., because there are too few hours in the school day to meet all the therapy needs or because there is no therapist who can provide the mandated therapy), then the parents may procure those services privately (i.e., from a source other than the Board of Education), and the Board of Education is responsible for paying the private provider. Frequently Boards of Education have lists of approved private providers they make available to parents. Additionally, if for some reason a child cannot receive the mandated number of sessions per week within the classroom, the parent is allowed to make up the difference from private providers. For example, it is often recommended that children with autistic disorder receive between 25 and 40 hours per week of one-on-one discrete trial ABA therapy. However, with other demands (gym, art, lunch, circle time, speech and language, occupational therapy, physical therapy, and counseling) a child may not be able to receive the mandated number of hours of ABA therapy within the school day. These hours can be made up during afterschool hours.

I next turn to services and personnel training, which, in addition to those services discussed above, may be necessary to allow certain children to meet their annual goals.

Other Services to Help the Child Meet the Annual Goals

Specialized training for staff There are many additional issues, such as professional training, assistive technology, language needs, and curriculum modifications, that should be addressed when describing how best to assist a child in achieving the annual goals. What follows is a description of some of those components that should be added to the IEP. For example, it is important that the professional who will interact with a particular child has knowledge of that child's disabling condition. Basic information is needed in order to understand how to interact with and teach a child with a known disorder. If the staff person has never worked with a child with Asperger's syndrome, Cri du Chat, fragile X, or Williams syndrome, parents should request that the child's IEP specify that the designated staff must receive specialized training. The parents may request that specialists provide an in-service training at their child's school, as occurred in the case of Uriele, a child with pervasive developmental disorder.

Case 15.2: Uriele Uriele is a 7-year-old with pervasive developmental disorder (PDD). He attends public school, where he is in a classroom with other children with a similar disorder. His mother became concerned that Uriele was not meeting his benchmarks and would not meet his annual goals. She arranged to have a meeting with his classroom teacher and quickly discerned that the teacher really did not understand how to teach the children or how to maintain discipline. Uriele's mother also sought input from an educational specialist, who documented that Uriele was not likely to meet his IEP goals in his current educational placement in view of the little progress noted from 1 year before. The educational specialist advised Uriele's mother to reopen the IEP. However, the school had only one class appropriate for Uriele, and only one teacher was assigned to teach that class. The educational specialist, who attended the IEP meeting, recommended that the teacher be supported by receiving training in working with students who have PDD. It was agreed that this was necessary to ensure that Uriele would meet his annual goals and that the school would cover the cost for the classroom teacher to attend several professional development seminars. The teacher welcomed the opportunity to receive this supportive training.

Limited English speakers The IEP team should also consider the language needs of students with limited English ability. A child who does not speak English would have significant challenges to meeting the daily benchmarks and annual goals if English were the language of instruction. Thus, these children are eligible to receive instruction in their native language if such a classroom opportunity exists. Alternatively, the child may attend English as a Second Language classes in addition to regular classes. When such opportunities are not available, the child is eligible to have an assigned paraprofessional aide whose role would be to translate that child's work until such time as the child is able to function in English and benefit from instruction in English.

There are several additional advantages of having a one-on-one paraprofessional aide who knows and can respond to a child's specific needs. For example, if a child is being toilet trained, then his or her paraprofessional could be vigilant and responsive to that task; if the child has behavior management issues, then the paraprofessional could provide necessary control; if the child elopes or engages in pica, then the paraprofessional could focus on those issues in order to ensure the child's safety.

Specific sensory or language impairments   For the visually impaired child, the instructional material should be translated into Braille. For the hard of hearing child, instructions should be administered through sign language. Many parents, especially of children with severe speech apraxia or dyspraxia, may request that their child be taught sign language in addition to other communication systems (e.g., Picture Exchange Communication System). If sign language is considered for the child, then the various professionals who work with the child will have to be able to converse with the child in sign language. This may be another opportunity for teacher training.

Assistive technology should also be considered for children who are having difficulty learning language, who have speech apraxia or dyspraxia or other disabilities that interfere with motor planning. "Assistive technology" is defined as any item, piece of equipment, or product system that is used to increase, maintain, or improve the functional capabilities of a child. In order to obtain an assistive device, a child must undergo an evaluation to determine whether the child is capable of using the device and to ensure that it does what it is intended to do. The teachers, parents, and therapists of any child who receives an assistive device must become familiar with that device's operation, so that use of the device is integrated into the child's curriculum. It is my experience that this is often a forgotten part of the solution. Many times a child is trained in how to use an assistive device, but because neither the child's parents nor the teacher are similarly trained, the device goes virtually unused.

Extended school year   The need for an extended school year (ESY) is also a valid IEP consideration. For those cases where a child would regress without continuing education, or if it is deemed necessary that a child receive more time in school than the traditional 9 months in order to meet his or her IEP goals, then ESY may be mandated. This is provided free of charge to the parents.

The examples provided above illustrate that IEPs are designed to help individual children, with particular disabling conditions and learning styles, achieve specific agreed upon annual goals. All needed services, training, personnel, and machinery deemed necessary to help a child achieve those goals must be carefully specified in the IEP.

Transition from Secondary to Postsecondary Education

"Transition" refers to activities meant to prepare students with disabilities for adult life. This can include developing postsecondary education and career goals, obtaining work experience while still in school, and establishing relationships with adult service providers such as a vocational rehabilitation agency. Beginning at age 14 years, the IEP will include a statement of the state and local graduation requirements that the student must meet. If exemptions to these graduation requirements are considered necessary, then the IEP must include a rationale for these exemptions and a description of alternate proficiencies that the child should meet in order to qualify for a state endorsed diploma. There should also be a statement of the services needed to take the student from school life to adult life and a statement of the school courses the child must take in order to reach the postschool goals. Such statements of transition services must appear in each of the child's subsequent IEPs. By at least 16 years of age, a statement of transition services that includes interagency responsibilities and necessary relationships with appropriate service providers should become part of the IEP. Transition services may include, but are not be limited to, instruction, related services, community experiences, development of employment and postschooling adult living objectives, and, if appropriate, acquisition of daily living skills and functional vocational evaluation. These services are designed to help disabled children prepare to separate from the school environment. Beginning at least 1 year before a child reaches the age of majority (21 years in most states), the child's IEP must include a statement that he or she has been told of any rights that will transfer to him or her at the age of majority. However, this statement would be needed only in states that transfer rights at the age of majority.

Classroom Placement

After a child's IEP has been agreed upon, the child's classroom placement is considered. According to the law, the first consideration for placement should always be the general education classroom in the child's neighborhood school, with appropriate supports and services. This is often referred to as supported inclusive education or an inclusionary classroom. If such a setting is acceptable to the parents and the creators of the IEP, then it is necessary to discuss what accommodations and modifications will be needed to make the classroom a viable and productive learning

Table 15.1
Modifications to be considered in a supported inclusive educational environment

Modification category	Examples
Classroom modifications	Modify physical setting of the classroom to make the child comfortable. Use study carrels or proximity seating. Use small group instruction.
Classwork modifications	Use assistive technology. Use alternatives for written assignments, such as drawing or cutting out pictures or making a tape recording. Provide extra time for assignments or tests. Provide assistance and support in advance. Provide a set of classroom books to the parents to enable preteaching.
Instructional modifications	Provide ongoing coaching and feedback. Provide organization devices and support. Break up test administration to short sessions. Test orally. Implement peer tutoring. Modify classroom management procedures. For example, use behavioral charts with rewards so child has a graphic way of understanding behavior and consequences.
Teacher–parent relationship	Report to parents daily or weekly via checklists or notebooks, or e-mail; use a child-customized template to maximize efficiency.

environment for the child. These modifiable aspects of a classroom may include the teaching style, the materials presented to the child, the ways of assessing the child, and the allowable response types of the child. Table 15.1 provides a summary of the accommodations or modifications that may be considered when describing how to teach and maintain a child in a supported inclusive environment.

Preparing Classroom Peers

Parents may choose not to place their child in a supported inclusive environment for a variety of reasons: Parents may be concerned about the reactions that the typically developing children may have toward their child, or they may fear possible danger to their child (i.e., the atypically developing children are usually eager to please their typically developing peers and so are easy prey to their less scrupulous typically developing peer); parents may also believe that the regular classroom is not the most appropriate environment in which their child should receive an education.

When parents do wish to place their child in a supportive inclusive environment, parents may request sensitivity training for the children in the classroom and peer-buddy training for the nondisabled peers so that they can better understand how to interact with a child with disabilities. In addition, the child with a disability may need training in how to interact with his nondisabled peers and not be unduly influenced by their words and behavior.

Self-contained Classroom Placements

The only time that an inclusive type of setting is not considered is when a child's IEP could not be implemented within a supported inclusive environment. If exclusion from general education is desired, such as when placement is to be in a self-contained special education classroom, this request must be made in writing as part of the IEP. In such cases, however, it is important that the child also receive some opportunity to interact with nondisabled children in order to gain socialization skills. This limited mainstream experience is most often arranged within nonacademic classes such as music, art, or physical education.

Parents' Considerations

Prior to signing an IEP and agreeing to placement, parents should be allowed to visit the school to consider whether it is an appropriate environment for their child. The physical layout of the school and the layout of the child's classroom are important factors in determining the educational success of children with various disabilities. For example, if a child requires toileting (and the FBA is in place), then the location of the bathroom relative to the classroom becomes an important factor. If a child has mobility issues, then the distance to the classroom and the need to climb stairs may determine whether (and how much) assistance will be required by the child to move around the school. Similarly, if a child is sensitive to noise and if noise interferes with the learning process, then the proximity of the child's classroom to common areas such as the school's cafeteria or gymnasium is important. These physical details are usually not discussed at IEP meetings, and the members of the IEP committee may not be familiar with the physical layout of the recommended school or classroom. Consequently, an on-site inspection will be important so that issues such as these may be considered before committing to a particular placement.

In addition to providing important information about the school itself, an on-site visit will also allow parents to become familiar with the other children in the classroom. These are some of the appropriate questions to ask: "What is the cognitive level of the other children?" "Will my child have peers with whom to interact?" "Do any of the other children exhibit behaviors that could interfere with my child's learning?" These and many other questions about the physical and social issues to be addressed can be answered only by visiting the prospective classroom before any placement is accepted.

Lack of Available Resources

In some cases, placement options that satisfy a child's IEP will not be available. For example, there may be no classrooms, no therapists, and no teachers within a school system who are trained to teach a child with a certain disability. When this occurs, the IEP committee must consider a non-public-school placement that satisfies the mandates of the IEP. Thus, the IEP should always determine the type of classroom and school that a child will attend, rather than this being determined by the availability of services offered by any given school system.

The 504 Plan

There are students who do not meet the eligibility requirements for the establishment of an IEP but whose disability nevertheless interferes with their classroom performance. The Rehabilitation Act of 1973, contains a paragraph that addresses the failure of public schools to adequately educate students with such disabilities:

No otherwise qualified individual with a disability in the United States, as defined in section 706(8) of this title, shall, solely by reason of her or his handicap, be excluded from participation in, be denied the benefits of, or be subjected to discrimination under any program or activity receiving Federal financial assistance or under any program or activity conducted by any Executive agency or by the United States Postal Service. (29 U.S.C. § 794(a) (1973) section 504).

"504-only students" are those who are entitled to the protections of § 504 but who are not eligible for special services under IDEA. Some students with disabilities in elementary, middle, or high school do not receive special education services because their disabilities do not impair their ability to learn to such a degree that such services are warranted, and parents are often unaware that they nevertheless are entitled to reasonable accommodations to support the specific needs of their less impaired children.

The general process of identifying, evaluating, and creating a "504" plan of modifications and accommodations is similar to that which we have described for those students who have more severe disabilities and therefore qualify for IEPs. These two factors play into eligibility for 504 plans: Whether there is a physical or mental impairment, and whether the physical or mental impairment substantially limits one or more major life activities. An example of such a student who would meet eligibility requirements for "504" is one who has dyslexia but has no other physical or mental disabilities. Because this student's disability would interfere with his or her classroom performance, this student is entitled to a "504 plan" that may include reading classes and/or modifications to work assignments, the administration of tests, and the student's placement within the classroom. For students with such disabilities, basic modifications to the curriculum often enable them to perform well within the regular classroom.

Due Process

What happens when a family does not agree with the recommendations made by their school system? Whenever a child's parent disagrees with the child's evaluation, eligibility status, class placement, or services, there are several options available. First, the parent may agree to a trial period under which the child's program is carefully monitored and reviewed. If, after a predetermined period of time, it is mutually recognized that the IEP is unsatisfactory, then all members can revisit the process and create a new IEP. A concern may develop over time and elicit review of an existing IEP. A review need not involve third-party contributors, but in some cases expert opinions are sought, as in the case of Victor.

Case 15.3: Victor   Victor is a 14-year-old diagnosed with fragile X syndrome and autism. When his mother noticed that Victor was becoming more agitated than is usual for him, she contacted the teachers at his school. In doing so, she learned that her son's teacher had resigned and that his bus aide had been eliminated. Believing that these classroom changes in Victor's routines would interfere with his learning, and fearing for his safety on the school bus, Victor's mother wrote a letter to his school based support team requesting that the IEP be reopened so that appropriate modifications could be made.

At the reopening of the IEP, Victor's mother was accompanied by two specialists in fragile X syndrome from whom she had sought guidance. The specialists explained to the committee why it was important to inform the mother and child of impending changes before those changes were implemented. The teachers and other IEP team members recognized the importance of these issues. Thus, one outcome of this meeting was the addition to the IEP stating that Victor and his mother would be informed, whenever possible, of any changes in Victor's teachers or routine and that Victor be introduced to new personnel before permanent staff changes were made. It was further indicated in the IEP that the purpose of this plan was to avoid possible behavioral changes as a result of staff changes. Additionally, Victor was assigned a bus aide to ensure safety.

In cases where agreements are not so readily reached, a second option is to go to mediation. "Mediation" is defined as an attempt to bring about a peaceful settlement or compromise between parties to a dispute through the objective intervention of a neutral party. Mediation is legally binding. To discourage unnecessary and costly litigation, IDEA requires states to establish and implement procedures to allow parties to resolve disputes through the mediation process. Whenever parents or the local educational agency file a complaint related to the provision of special education and related services to a child with a disability, the party filing the complaint has the right to call for a mediation hearing. These hearings are conducted by the SEA or local educational agency (LEA) and are meant to provide both parties a fair impartial venue for resolving the issues contained in the complaint.

The third option is called due process. A due process notice is an official complaint from the parent about their child's IEP or services provided under IDEA. The notice must include the name and home address of the child, the name of the school the child attends, a description of the nature of the problem, and a proposed resolution. The parties presenting the complaint must file this notice before a due process hearing can occur. The LEA must respond to the parents within 10 days of receiving the due process notice. An impartial hearing officer presides over the due process hearing. The hearing officer must not be an employee of the SEA or LEA involved and must not have a professional or personal interest that conflicts with his or her ability to be objective in the hearing. Due process rulings may be appealed, and any party who disputes the final decision of the hearing officer may bring a civil action in any state court of competent jurisdiction or in a U.S. district court. The party bringing the civil action has 90 days from the date of the hearing officer's final decision to file such a claim. If state law provides for a different timeline, the state law prevails.

Case 15.4: Wendy Wendy is a 15-year-old with severe learning disabilities, who has particular difficulty with mathematics and writing. She is mainstreamed for part of the school day and attends a self-contained classroom for the remainder of the day. At the initial writing of the IEP, Wendy's teachers and therapists recommended that she no longer receive occupational therapy. All the school professionals felt that Wendy wrote "well enough" and should not be pulled out of the class any more times than was absolutely necessary. Her father disagreed with their assessment, because he felt that Wendy still needed help with writing and with self-help skills such as buttoning, zippering, and snapping. He arranged for Wendy to receive an independent evaluation, and through that process these deficits were documented.

At first, there was no compromise when the IEP was being written. Wendy's father requested two weekly occupational therapy classes, but the school therapists did not agree that any occupational therapy was necessary. Instead of going to arbitration, the matter was taken up at due process. Both sides presented their opinions: While Wendy's father presented his concerns and elicited testimony from experts regarding Wendy's deficits, the school's therapists demonstrated that Wendy had acquired skills and argued that continued therapy was detrimental to Wendy's long-term welfare because of the class time she would miss when pulled out of class. The due process judge proposed a compromise: Instead of two classes per week, Wendy would receive one occupational therapy class per week. Moreover, the occupational therapist would provide Wendy with materials to bring home to use to practice her skills. This was agreed upon by all parties and the IEP went forward.

What happens while the new IEP is under dispute? The child remains in the "old" setting with the "old" IEP until a new one is written. This is sometimes called "stay put" or "pendency." The initial IEP is the agreed upon contract that remains in effect until a modified plan is agreed to and signed.

Timeline

Table 15.2 is a summary of the timeline for the generation of the IEP. All communication with the LEAs should be sent via certified return receipt post so that the

Table 15.2
Timeline for individualized education program (IEP)

Elapsed Time	Action	Time Counted From
	Written referral for special education by parent, teacher, or service provider	
15 days	Proposed assessment plan	Date of written referral
15 days	Parent considers proposed assessment plan Assessment of child begins	Receipt of proposed assessment plan
Early enough to ensure an opportunity to attend	IEP notification	
50 days	IEP development (team meeting)	Receipt of parents' written consent for assessment
As soon as possible	IEP implementation	IEP team meeting
30 days	Meeting to re-open IEP	Receipt of written request from parents to reexamine the IEP
At least annually	Review of IEP	Date of last IEP team meeting
3 years	Triennial reassessment	Date of last 3-year assessment

parent can maintain a dated record of communication. The parent's signature is necessary to begin the assessment and to implement the IEP. If the parent does not sign the appropriate forms, the assessments will not be completed and/or the IEP will not be implemented.

Summary

Despite reports of group characteristics associated with known disorders, individual differences prevail within special population groups. The chapters in this volume have demonstrated the breadth of variation evident across common and uncommon disorders and the need to recognize that extremes may exist at both ends of the phenotype continuum. The IEP is designed to reflect and accommodate the unique learning styles and needs of each individual child with disabilities and to help that child learn and attain the skills necessary to live a fulfilled adult life. As such, the importance of the IEP should not be underestimated, for it is the underlying mechanism that drives the education of a child with disabilities.

Acknowledgments

The writing of this chapter was supported by funds from the New York State Office of Mental Retardation and Developmental Disabilities.

The author wishes to thank Dr. Richard Belser, without whose help this chapter could not have been completed, and Laurie Yankowitz for her valuable insights and conversation.

Resources

The Council for Exceptional Children
1110 N. Glebe Road
Arlington VA 22201-5704
1-888-232-7733
TTY: 866-915-5000
Fax: 703-264-9494
E-mail: service@cec.sped.org
http://cec.sped.org

U.S. Department of Education Publication Department
P.O. Box 1398
Jessup, MD 20794-1398
877-4-ED-PUBS
877-576-7734 (TTY)
301-470-1244 (Fax)
http://www.ed.gov/pubs/edpubs.org

Office of Special Education Programs
Office of Special Education and Rehabilitative Services
U.S. Department of Education
400 Maryland Avenue, SW
Washington, DC 20202-7100
202-245-7459 (Voice/TTY)
http://www.ed.gov/about/offices/list/osers/osep/

National Information Center for Children and Youth with Disabilities (NICHCY)
P.O. Box 1492
Washington, DC 20013
800-695-0285 (Voice/TTY); 202-884-8200 (V/TTY)
E-mail: nichcy@aed.org
http://www.nichcy.org

The IDEA Partnership Projects

National Technical Assistance Center
Pacer Center
8161 Normandale Blvd
Minneapolis, MN 55437-1044
952 838 9000 – Voice
952 838 0190 – TTY/711 Relay
952 838 0199 Fax
1-888-248-0822 toll free number nationwide
E-mail: alliance@taalliance.org
http://www.taalliance.org

The Policy Maker Partnership (PMP) for Implementing IDEA 97
National Association of State Directors of Special Education
1800 Diagonal Road, Suite 320
Alexandria, VA 22314
703-519-3800; 703-519-7008 (TTY)
E-mail: nasdse@nasdse.org
http://www.nasdse.org

Regional Resource Centers

Northeast Regional Resource Center (NERRC)
Learning Innovations
At Wested
Williston, VT 05495
802-951-8226; 802-951-8213 (TTY)
E-mail: nerrc@aol.com
http://www.wested.org/nerrc/
Serving: Connecticut, Maine, Massachusetts, New Hampshire, New Jersey, New York, Rhode Island, and Vermont.

Mid-South Regional Resource Center (MSRRC)
Human Development Institute
University of Kentucky
1 Quality Street
Lexington, KY 40507
859-257-4921; 859-257-2903 (TTY)
E-mail: msrrc@ihdi.uky.edu
http://www.ihdi.uky.edu/msrrc
Serving: Delaware, Kentucky, Maryland, North Carolina, South Carolina, Tennessee, Virginia, Washington, DC, and West Virginia.

Southeast Regional Resource Center (SERRC)
School of Education
Auburn University Montgomery
P.O. Box 244023
Montgomery, AL 36124
334-244-3100; 334-244-3800 (TTY)
E-mail: ebeale@mail.aum.edu
http://edla.aum.edu/serrc/serrc.html
Serving: Alabama, Arkansas, Florida, Georgia, Louisiana, Mississippi, Oklahoma, Puerto Rico, Texas, and the U.S. Virgin Islands.

North Central Regional Resource Center (NCRRC)
Institute on Community Integration
University of Minnesota
5 Pattee Hall
150 Pillsbury Drive SE
Minneapolis MN 55455
612-624-9722
E-mail: ncrrc@umn.edu
http://www.rrfcnetwork.org/ncrrc

Mountain Plains Regional Resource Center (MPRRC)
Utah State University
1780 North Research Park Way, Suite 112
Logan, UT 84341
435-752-0238; 435-753-9750 (TTY)
E-mail: cope@cc.usu.edu
http://www.usu.edu/mprrc
Serving: Arizona, Bureau of Indian Affairs, Colorado, Kansas, Montana, Nebraska, New Mexico, North Dakota, South Dakota, Utah, and Wyoming.

Western Regional Resource Center (WRRC)
1268 University of Oregon
Eugene, OR 97403-1268
541-346-5641; 541-346-0367 (TTY)
E-mail: wrrc@oregon.uoregon.edu
http://rrfc.network.org/wrrc
Serving: Alaska, American Samoa, California, Commonwealth of the Northern Mariana Islands, Federated States of Micronesia, Guam, Hawaii, Idaho, Nevada, Oregon, Republic of the Marshall Islands, Republic of Palau, and Washington.

References

Department of Education (August 14, 2006). Assistance to States for the Education of Children with Disabilities and Preschool Grants for Children with Disabilities; Final Rule. *Federal Register* § 300.320.

Education of All Handicapped Children Act, 20 U.S.C. § 1400 et seq. (1975).

Individuals with Disabilities Education Act, Pub. L., 108-446, Stat. 2647 (2004).

No Child Left Behind Act of 2001, Pub. L., 107-110 115 STAT. 1425 (2002).

Office of Special Education and Rehabilitative Services U.S. Department of Education (July, 2002) A Guide to the Individualized Education Program. Available at http://www.ed.gov/pubs/edpubs.html

Rehabilitation Act of 1973, Pub. L. 93-112.

Sattler, J. M. (2001). Assessment of Children: Cognitive Applications San Diego: Jerome M. Sattler.

U.S. Department of Education, Office of Special Education Programs, Washington, DC. (2002). *Annual report to Congress on the Implementation of the Individuals with Disabilities Education Act* (24th ed.). Ed Publications, Education Publication Center, U.S. Department of Education. Retrieved from http://www.ed.gov/about/reports/annual/osep/2002/index.html

Contributors

Kevin M. Antshel, PhD
Department of Psychiatry and Behavioral
Sciences
SUNY—Upstate Medical University
Syracuse, New York

Georgianne Arnold, MD
Pediatric Genetics
University of Rochester School of Medicine
and Dentistry
Rochester, New York

Rosalind Brown, MD
Endocrine Division
Children's Hospital, Boston
Department of Pediatrics, Harvard
University
Boston, Massachusetts

Merav Burg-Malki, MA
The Behavioral Neurogenetics Center
Schneider Children's Medical Center of Israel
Petah Tiqwa, Israel

Kimberly M. Cornish, PhD
Neuroscience Laboratory for Research and
Education in Developmental Disorders
McGill University
Montreal, Canada

Marsha L. Davenport, MD
Department of Pediatrics, Division of
Endocrinology
University of North Carolina,
Chapel Hill, North Carolina

Laraine Masters Glidden, PhD
Department of Psychology
St. Mary's College of Maryland
St. Mary's City, Maryland

Edward M. Goldstein, MD
Child Neurology Associates
Children's Healthcare of Atlanta—Scottish
Rite Children's Medical Center
Atlanta, Georgia

Doron Gothelf, MD
The Behavioral Neurogenetics Center
Schneider Children's Medical Center of
Israel
Petah Tiqwa, Israel

Deborah D. Hatton, PhD
Frank Porter Graham Child Development
Institute
University of North Carolina, Chapel Hill
Chapel Hill, North Carolina

Agnes T. Heaney, MSed
New York State Institute for Basic Research
in Developmental Disabilities
Staten Island, New York

Veronica J. Hinton, PhD
G.H. Sergievsky Center and Department of
Neurology
Columbia University
New York, New York

Stephen R. Hooper, PhD
Center for Development and Learning
University of North Carolina
Chapel Hill, North Carolina

Andrew Levitas, MD
Department of Psychiatry
University of Medicine and Dentistry of
New Jersey
Stratford, New Jersey

Theodore I. Lidsky, PhD
Center for Trace Element Studies and
Environmental Neurotoxicology
New York State Institute for Basic Research
in Developmental Disabilities
Staten Island, New York

Michèle M. M. Mazzocco, PhD
Department of Psychiatry and Behavioral
Health Sciences
Johns Hopkins School of Medicine
Kennedy Krieger Institute
Baltimore, Maryland

Allyn McConkie-Rosell, PhD CGC
Division of Medical Genetics
Department of Pediatrics
Duke University Medical Center

Carolyn B. Mervis, PhD
Department of Psychological and Brain
Sciences
University of Louisville
Louisville, Kentucky

Bartlett D. Moore, III, PhD
Division of Pediatrics
M.D. Anderson Cancer Center
University of Texas
Houston, Texas

Colleen A. Morris, MD
Department of Pediatrics, Division of
Genetics
University of Nevada School of Medicine
Las Vegas, Nevada

Julianne O'Daniel, MS, CGC
Institute for Genome Sciences and Policy
Durham, North Carolina

David Roeltgen, MD
Cooper University Hospital
Robert Wood Johnson University
Camden, New Jersey

John F. Rosen, MD
Division of Environmental Sciences
The Montefiore Medical Center
Bronx, New York

Judith L. Ross, MD
Department of Pediatrics, Division of
Endocrinology
Jefferson Medical College,
Philadelphia, Pennsylvania

Joanne F. Rovet, PhD
The Hospital for Sick Children
Departments of Pediatrics and Psychology
The University of Toronto
Toronto, Canada

Jay S. Schneider, PhD
Department of Pathology, Anatomy, and
Cell Biology
Thomas Jefferson University
Philadelphia, Pennsylvania

Sarah A. Schoolcraft
Department of Psychology
St. Mary's College of Maryland
St. Mary's City, Maryland

Tony J. Simon, PhD
University of California, Davis
Cognitive Analysis & Brain Imaging
Laboratory
M.I.N.D. Institute
Sacramento, California

John M. Slopis, MD, UT MD
Department of Neuro Oncology
Anderson Cancer Center
Houston, Texas

Gerry A. Stefanatos, D Phil
Moss Rehabilitation Research Institute
Albert Einstein Medical Center
Philadelphia, Pennsylvania

Vicki Sudhalter, PhD
New York State Institute for Basic Research
in Developmental Disabilities
1050 Forest Hill Road
Staten Island, New York

Martha Zeger, MD
Department of Pediatrics, Division of
Endocrinology
Thomas Jefferson University
Philadelphia, Pennsylvania

Index